Patient Safety Handbook

Second Edition

Edited by
Barbara J. Youngberg, JD, MSW, BSN, FASHRM
Visiting Professor of Law
Academic Director, On-Line Legal Education
Loyola University Chicago
School of Law
Beazley Institute for Health Law and Policy
Chicago, IL

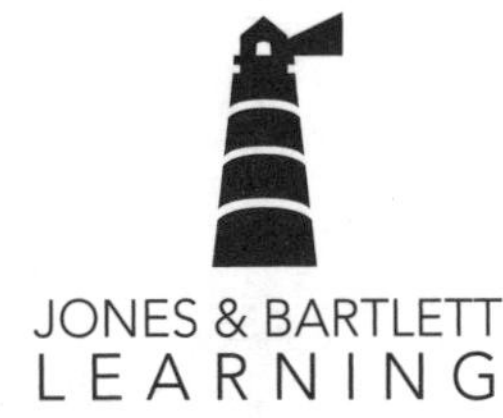

World Headquarters
Jones & Bartlett Learning
5 Wall Street
Burlington, MA 01803
978-443-5000
info@jblearning.com
www.jblearning.com

Jones & Bartlett Learning books and products are available through most bookstores and online booksellers. To contact Jones & Bartlett Learning directly, call 800-832-0034, fax 978-443-8000, or visit our website, www.jblearning.com.

Substantial discounts on bulk quantities of Jones & Bartlett Learning publications are available to corporations, professional associations, and other qualified organizations. For details and specific discount information, contact the special sales department at Jones & Bartlett Learning via the above contact information or send an email to specialsales@jblearning.com.

Production Credits
Publisher: Michael Brown
Editorial Assistant: Chloe Falivene
Editorial Assistant: Kayla Dos Santos
Production Manager: Tracey McCrea
Senior Marketing Manager: Sophie Fleck Teague
Manufacturing and Inventory Control Supervisor: Amy Bacus
Composition: Publishers' Design and Production Services, Inc.
Cover Design: Scott Moden
Cover Image: © Nagy Jozsef—Attila/ShutterStock, Inc.
Printing and Binding: Edwards Brothers Malloy
Cover Printing: Edwards Brothers Malloy

Library of Congress Cataloging-in-Publication Data
Patient safety handbook / edited by Barbara Youngberg. -- 2nd ed.
p. ; cm.
Includes bibliographical references and index.
ISBN 978-0-7637-7404-2 (pbk.)
I. Youngberg, Barbara J.
[DNLM: 1. Patient Safety. 2. Medical Errors--prevention & control. WX 185]
610--dc23

2012018525

6048

Printed in the United States of America
16 15 14 13 12 10 9 8 7 6 5 4 3 2 1

To the mothers and fathers who have lost children due to medical error, to the husbands and wives who have lost spouses, and to all of those who have lost trust in our ability to recognize the privilege of caring for you or those you love.

And to Anie, my daughter, who despite a challenging year, taught me that hard work, focus, humor, and love is really what makes for a good and meaningful life.

Contents

Preface

Tackling the second edition of *Patient Safety Handbook* initially seemed like a relatively simple proposal. The first edition, which was released in 2004, was actually conceptualized shortly after the landmark IOM report *To Err Is Human* made public what many clinicians, administrators, and patients already knew: that healthcare systems were poorly designed, preventable errors occurred frequently, and people who entrusted their lives to providers and systems that promised a great outcome were too frequently harmed or killed.

The science of safety was relatively nascent. Early leaders in the field such as Dr. Lucian Leape and James Reason helped us all to begin thinking differently about why the healthcare system was so prone to error and how the science of safety (borrowed from other high hazard industries) might be applied to health care to better understand the root causes of error and to identify potential solutions for solving specific safety problems. Early on, one of the recommendations offered by the drafters of the IOM report—to fund research to advance the science and study of safety—took root, and research into the most common types of errors and to their etiology flourished. I would guess there are very few healthcare providers who are not familiar with the common causes of medication errors, the reasons wrong-sided procedures continue to happen, and the economic and emotional impact that preventable errors have on our healthcare delivery system. Yet the ability or the willingness to translate this knowledge into strategies that yield positive change seems to lag far behind.

I have read the many articles and commentaries on safety since the release of the IOM report: some suggesting that great progress has been made and others (probably equal in number) lamenting the fact that little progress has been made. In fact, both are probably true. We know a great deal more about the complexities of the healthcare delivery system that predispose individuals to err, we know that leadership is key in setting an agenda for change and in aligning safety with the core vision and values of the organization, and we know that change (even some of the seemingly simple things) is extremely hard to bring about and sustain in a culture steeped in tradition and hierarchy.

Many providers continue to demand more and better data and fail to appreciate that they probably already have more than is necessary to begin the process of change. We have all learned that you can avoid the inevitable for a long time by simply asking for more proof. In my work with many hospitals, it is clear that it is far easier to continue to study the problem than to actually fix it and it is also easy to justify the limited effort to focus on safety by describing the current conditions and challenges faced by the healthcare industry, which often seem to compete with the safety agenda.

Clearly, many individuals and organizations have provided great leadership to stimulate the safety agenda, but far too often the impetus for change is yet another tragic event, another loved one lost, and another group of providers devastated by their role in, or proximity to, an event where significant harm to a patient is the result. We must do better, and real and lasting change will occur only when healthcare providers and organizations acknowledge that they must hold themselves and their peers accountable for safety, they must stop making excuses as to why safety is not a priority in their organizations or within their practices, and they must be willing to change practices and behaviors that we now know are counterproductive to a culture of safety.

As both a clinician and a lawyer, I have been intrigued by how often I still hear the excuse offered that "we can't be more transparent . . . we can't share information about our own errors and best practices . . . we can't hold our peers accountable" because the legal system is "so unfair," "so punitive," so "likely to deliver an unfair or unjust verdict." This excuse continues to inhibit progress in many areas. It also has the impact of allowing providers to blame someone or something else for the problems that really are under the control of the caregiver and the caregiving organization. It seems somewhat obvious that most patients enter the legal system only after harm has occurred or information has been withheld. So undoubtedly a better strategy would be to take control of the environment that is under our control and recognize that the only way to not be put at risk by the legal system is to develop strategies for keeping patients free from harm. For over 30 years, doing the opposite has not proven to be the solution.

Some looking at the table of contents of this book might be concerned that there are no specific chapters representing the patient's responsibility or the patient's role in patient safety. This was actually intentional. My position on patient safety is that once again it is first and foremost the responsibility of the provider and of healthcare organizations. It is a responsibility that we cannot pass off to a patient or a concerned family member or advocate. Of course, patients must be the reason we rededicate ourselves to changing the unsafe and overly complex systems that often give rise to error, and we must listen to them so we know what things are of greatest concern to them. But we cannot make patients and family members responsible for patient safety. I find it unnerving when campaigns are launched asking patients to "speak up" to ask their caregivers if they have washed their hands or to challenge patients to know how to escalate a concern when their loved one seems in peril. It is once again an attempt to shift responsibility away from those individuals who are responsible and in the best position to lead the change to someone who is vulnerable, frightened, and oftentimes too ill or too timid to be an advocate. My fear is we might further harm patients and their loved ones after an error by intimating that, if only they had been more assertive or more demanding of their care providers, they could have avoided or prevented the error. This shifting of our responsibility onto others adds insult to injury and often fails to allow providers to uncover the true root cause of the problem. Patients should expect that when they entrust their care to a provider or an organization that reasonable, safe, and effective care will be provided and that preventable errors will indeed be prevented, without their needing to maintain constant vigilance to protect their loved ones. The fact that so many people now state they would never leave their loved ones alone in a hospital is a testament to how little faith the public has in us, and this needs to change.

In addition, providers should know that their role in advocating for patient safety and their efforts at creating and sustaining personal and collective accountability will not only yield benefits for their patient but also for them. Errors are devastating to those experiencing them and to their loved ones, but the toll they take on the providers involved is also devastating. Working as a provider in our current healthcare delivery system is physically and emotionally exhausting, and providers deserve to be in systems that support them and that have processes in place to assure ensure both individual and collective success.

If you read the first edition of *Patient Safety Handbook*, you will recognize that a number of the chapters were retained because the authors were actually ahead of the field and the content of those chapters still provides a necessary framework detailing the science of safety, the knowledge of error, and the role of various members of the healthcare team in advancing a safety culture. More than half of the chapters, however, are completely new and reflect work that has been done over the past 10 years, along with specific strategies for making our systems, our providers, and most importantly, our patients safer. Two new and important chapters address the need to change the way we educate physicians and nurses so that they develop the competencies needed to be safety champions. This recognition of the need to create a measureable curriculum around safety is reinforced by the tools available with this second edition, which include specific learning objectives for each chapter, questions to test whether the most salient points were understood, and Microsoft PowerPoint slides to review the highlights of each chapter and to teach colleagues specific aspects of the topics presented.

It is my hope that the material provided in the second edition will enable you to see that while we are not yet where we need to be in making our systems safer, we are making progress toward achieving safer and more transparent health care for all.

Foreword

Helen Haskell

For those outside the medical profession—and to a large extent, those inside it as well—the reasons for becoming involved in patient safety are most often personal, and not in a good way. For my husband and I, this involvement was precipitated by the loss of our brilliant, vibrant 15-year-old son, Lewis, who died from a cascade of medical errors following elective surgery.

I will not go into detail, but suffice it to say that a boy we regarded as one of the outstanding young men of his generation was casually sacrificed to medication error, hierarchy, and misplaced arrogance—in short, to all the shortcomings of the teaching hospital. Lewis entered the hospital a healthy, athletic teenager wearing shorts and sandals in the last days of a late South Carolina autumn. Four days later, we emerged without him into the first bright, cold days of winter. His path in those few days can be traced in half a sentence: two hours in surgery, two and a half days in recovery, and a day and a half in calamitous decline before he died, unrescued, in his hospital bed. Through all this, our concerns and pleas for help had gone unheeded.

As we worked through Lewis's medical records to reconstruct the decisions that had been made, we were taken aback by what we found. Most chilling was the gradually dawning realization that despite their ultimately lethal mistakes, most of our son's caregivers had acted strictly by the book, even down to the language used when speaking to us. But the standards they were following came with cavernous wiggle room, enough to accommodate even the most egregious errors and then nothing was done to catch them after they had occurred. Not just the process but the structure was rife with potential for harm. In this context, James Reason's Swiss cheese metaphor—another piece of our new knowledge—seemed little more than a euphemism. The system, so implicitly trusted by so many, was simply not set up to accomplish its goal. From our perspective, there were more holes than cheese.

We saw only one way forward from this experience—to bring some good out of the disaster that had befallen us. That was the beginning of a journey of advocacy that has yet to end. In many ways, we were typical of families affected by medical harm. Like most, we sought to bring hope out of despair, and we thought that the legacy of our son and thousands of others would be the immediate reform of the system that had taken their lives. Our aspirations seem almost quaint from our current perspective. But we believed that a system so out of sync with its own mission could surely be brought back to its intended path by a small group of determined people bent on doing the right thing.

This all took place at the end of 2000, a year after the Institute of Medicine's report *To Err Is Human*. Hope was high in that moment. The problem had been delineated, and we had both the will and the outline of a plan to change it. Rereading parts of the 2004 edition of *Patient Safety Handbook*, one can still feel that hope. And yet, there and elsewhere, many people were already expressing dismay at the slow pace of reform. The fifth anniversary and then the 10th passed with much soul-searching. Few thought we had shown significant change to be proud of.

No one can say we have not made many advances. We have put to rest—in most circles, at least—the idea that patient harm is not a problem. We have meaningful support from government entities. We have dedicated champions both within and outside of the system. Thanks in large part to the path blazed by consumer advocates in many American states, we have the beginnings of a system of transparency that has the potential of giving patients a clearer idea of benefits and risks. And yet we still do not have a real-time picture of the extent of patient harm, and we do not know to what extent our efforts in the past few years may or may not have helped reduce it.

Patients overwhelmingly see patient harm as an ethical issue, and those who think about it see transparency as the essential underlying principle of reform. They are not mistaken in this. The industry of health care has been allowed to function with too little accountability to its patients, its practitioners, and its communities and in the process has often lost the virtues of openness, honesty, and altruism that the public thinks should be its hallmark. Patients will also tell you that fragmentation and high-volume medicine—lack of time with their providers—are among the most significant drivers of patient harm. The patient voice is essential to solving these problems. Left unaddressed, these difficult, overarching questions have the potential to negate all that is achieved through other patient safety programs.

The bottom line is that much remains to be done. Patients and families continue to entrust themselves to systems that are fraught with risks over which they often have no power. Technical solutions, standardization, teamwork, improved communication, culture change—these all are necessary, important, and transformative. But they are only parts of a larger solution. Above all, we need to take on patient safety as an ethical challenge, one that pays careful attention to patient concerns and aspires to broad and innovative change at a fundamental level. I urge you to read this volume with that in mind.

Contributors

Laura Ashpole, JD
Loyola University Chicago
School of Law
Beazley Institute for Health Law and Policy
Chicago, IL

Barbara Balik, RN, EdD
CEO, Common Fire
Albuquerque, NM

John Banja, PhD
Professor, Department of Rehabilitation Medicine
Medical Ethicist, Center for Ethics
Director, Ethics Section: Atlanta Clinical and Translational Science Institute
Emory University
Atlanta, GA

Raj Behal, MD, MBA
Assistant Professor
Associate Chief Medical Officer
Biostatistics and Biomedical Informatics Task Force
Rush University Medical Center
Chicago, IL

John Blum, JD, MHS
John J. Waldron Research Professor
Loyola University Chicago
School of Law
Beazley Institute for Health Law and Policy
Chicago, IL

Keshia Carswell
Loyola University Chicago
School of Law
Beazley Institute for Health Law and Policy
Chicago, IL

Carolyn Chapman, JD
Attorney
Chicago, IL

Barbara A. Connelly, RN, MJ
Director of Risk Management, MCWAH
Graduate Medical Education
Milwaukee, WI

Richard I. Cook, MD
Royal Institute of Technology
Sweden

George R. Cybulski, MD, FACS
Associate Professor of Neurological Surgery
Northwestern University
Feinberg School of Medicine
Chicago, IL

Erin Egan, MD, JD
Assistant Professor of Medicine
Division of General Internal Medicine
University of Colorado
Denver, CO

David A. Ehlert, PharmD
Vice President, Pharmacy Practice Resources
McKesson Pharmacy Optimization
Golden Valley, MN

Kathleen Ferket, RN, MSN, APN
Executive Director, Patient Care Support
Northwest Community Hospital
Chicago, IL

Shannon Flaherty
Beazley Institute for Health Law and Policy
Loyola University Chicago
School of Law
Chicago, IL

John Fromson, MD
Vice President for Professional Development
Massachusetts Medical Society
Clinical Instructor in Psychiatry
Harvard Medical School
Boston, MA

Kathy Gerwig
Vice President
Employee Safety, Health and Wellness and Environmental Stewardship Officer
Kaiser Permanente
Oakland, CA

Doni Hass, RN
Stuart, FL

David Hewett, MD
Assistant Medical Director (Litigation)
Winchester Eastleigh Healthcare
NHS Trust
England, United Kingdom

Gerald B. Hickson, MD
Assistant Vice Chancellor for Health Affairs
Associate Dean for Faculty Affairs
Joseph C. Ross Chair in Medical Education and Administration
Director, Center for Patient and Professional Advocacy
Vanderbilt University Medical Center
Nashville, TN

John Hidley, MD
Psychiatrist
Behavioral Science Technology
Ojai, CA

Marina Karp, MJ
Beazley Institute for Health Law and Policy
Loyola University Chicago
School of Law
Chicago, IL

Mark Keroack, MD, MPH
Chief Physician Executive, Baystate Health
President, Baystate Medical Practices
Springfield, MA

G. Eric Knox, MD, FACOG
Minneapolis, MN

Mahendra S. Kochar, MD, MS, MBA, JD
Associate Dean for Graduate Medical Education
University of California, Riverside School of Medicine
Riverside, CA

Thomas R. Krause, PhD
Behavioral Science Technology
Ojai, CA

Louise LaFramboise, PhD, RN
Associate Professor and Director
Baccalaureate Program
University of Nebraska College of Nursing
Omaha, NE

Laverne Largie, JD, LLM
Woodstock, MD

Richard Lauve, MD
Founder and Principal
L & A Consulting
Baton Rouge, LA

Lucian Leape, MD
Adjunct Professor of Health Policy
Department of Health Policy and Management
Harvard School of Public Health
Boston, MA

Allison Caravana Lilly, MSW, LICSW, CEAP
Employee Assistance Program
Brigham and Women's Hospital
Boston, MA

Roy Magnusson, MD, MS, FACEP
Associate Dean for Clinical Affairs
Chief Medical Officer
John A. Burns School of Medicine
University of Hawaii
Honolulu, HI

Shawn Mathis, JD, LLM
Staff Attorney
New Mexico Legislative Council Services
Santa Fe, NM

Doni M. McCoy, JD, LLM
Atlanta, GA

Wendy Tuzik Micek
Market Director, Nursing Science and Magnet
Advocate Christ Medical Center
Oak Lawn, IL

Sarah Mick, JD, LLM
Associate
Dorsey & Whitney
Des Moines, IA

Connie Miller, PhD, RN
Assistant Professor
Director, LRC Omaha Division
UNMC College of Nursing
Omaha, NE

Karla M. Miller, PharmD, BCPP
Director of Medication Usage and Safety
Hospital Corporation of America
Nashville, TN

Julianne Morath, RN, MS
Chief Quality and Patient Safety Officer
Vanderbilt University Medical Center
Nashville, TN

Laura B. Morgan, JD
Loyola University Chicago
School of Law
Beazley Institute for Health Law and Policy
Chicago, IL

John J. Nance, JD
John Nance Productions
Seattle, WA

Dennis O'Leary, MD
President Emeritus
The Joint Commission
Oak Brook Terrace, IL

James Pichert, PhD
Codirector, CPPA; Professor, Medical Education and Administration
Vanderbilt University Medical Center
Nashville, TN

Katherine A. Pischke-Winn, MBA, RN
Director, Clinical Innovation and Research
Advocate Good Shepherd Hospital
Barrington, IL

Caitlin Podbielski, JD
Beazley Institute for Health Law and Policy Fellow 2012
Loyola University Chicago
School of Law
Chicago, IL

Grena Porto, RN, MHA, ARM, CPHRM
Principal
QRS Healthcare Consulting, LLC
Hockessin, PA

Marsha Regenstein, PhD, MCP
Director
National Public Health and Hospital Institute
The Commonwealth Fund
Washington, DC

David Resnik, JD, PhD
Bioethicist and NIEHS IRB Chair
National Institutes of Health
Research Triangle Park, NC

Emily Rhinehart, RN, MPH, CIC, CPHQ
Vice President
Chartis Insurance
Atlanta, GA

Karlene H. Roberts, PhD
Professor Emeritus
Haas School of Business
University of California Berkeley
Berkeley, CA

Bethany Robertson, DNP, CNM, NM
Assistant Professor, Clinical
Academic Lead for Technology Innovation
Emory University
Atlanta, GA

Steven Rough, MS, RPh
Director of Pharmacy
University of Wisconsin Hospital and Clinics
Clinical Assistant Professor
University of Wisconsin School of Pharmacy
Madison, WI

Mary Salisbury, RN, MSN
President
The Cedar Institute, Inc.
North Kingstown, RI

Manisha Shaw, MBA, RCP
Chief Operating Officer
National Patient Safety Foundation
Boston, MA

Gwen Sherwood, PhD, RN, FAAN
Professor and Associate Dean for Academic Affairs
University of North Carolina at Chapel Hill
School of Nursing
Chapel Hill, NC

Keith Siddel, MBA, JD, PhD
Chief Marketing Officer
Health Revenue Assurance Associates
Plantation, FL

Robert Simon, EdD, CPE
Education Director
Center for Medical Simulation
Boston, MA

Kathleen Rice Simpson, PhD, RNC, FAAN
Perinatal Clinical Nurse Specialist
St. John's Mercy Medical Center Labor and Delivery
St. Louis, MO

David Van Stralen, MD
Department of Pediatrics
Loma Linda University Medical Center
Loma Linda, CA

Karen M. Stratton, PhD, RN, NE-BC
Clinical Assistant Professor and Coordinator, Graduate Administrative Studies Program Department of Health Systems Science
UIC College of Nursing
Chicago, IL

Charles Vincent, MD
Professor of Psychology
University College
London, England

David D. Woods, PhD
Professor
Ohio State University
Institute for Ergonomics
Columbus, OH

Barbara J. Youngberg, JD, MSW, BSN, FASHRM
Visiting Professor
Academic Director On-Line Legal Education
Loyola University Chicago
School of Law
Beazley Institute for Health Law and Policy
Chicago, IL

Kuo (Frank) Yu, PhD
Assistant Professor
City University of Hong Kong
Kowloon Tong
Kowloon, Hong Kong

1

Understanding the First Institute Of Medicine Report and Its Impact On Patient Safety

Marsha Regenstein, PhD, MCP

In October 1999, the Institute of Medicine (IOM) released *To Err Is Human: Building a Safer Health Care System*, a report that put the issues of patient safety and medical errors in front of the American public and on the agendas of healthcare institutions, provider associations, consumer groups, the administration, and the Congress seemingly overnight. The national news networks and other media outlets broadcast the startling finding that up to 98,000 people die in hospitals each year as a result of medical errors and countless more are seriously harmed. And, whereas other industries have worked systematically to improve error rates and adverse outcomes over the past several decades, the healthcare industry appears to have made woefully few improvements in patient safety and has essentially maintained high medical error rates over the past 15 years.

Despite its shock value and the media attention it received, the IOM report does not include new information about the prevalence of medical errors. It explains the etiology of errors in the healthcare system and describes ways that other industries have successfully tackled this problem. It also includes detailed analyses of systems failures in the delivery of care to (primarily) hospitalized patients and identifies steps that healthcare institutions can take to reduce their error rates.

The report is essentially a call to action for policymakers, providers, and the American public to create a groundswell for change. The report's real take-away message is that medical errors are infrequently the result of the lone individual. On the contrary, medical errors are the result of a complex series of system-related problems. In the report's language, the authors call for the healthcare system to "systematically design safety into processes of care."[1] Thus, error reduction and improved patient safety focus more on designing systems to reduce the likelihood of error and less on identifying the person or persons responsible for the mistake.

This chapter describes the findings in the IOM report and summarizes some of the published literature upon which the findings were based. It also describes public- and private-sector responses to the IOM report and the ways in which various groups have positioned themselves on this issue.

ERRORS, ADVERSE EVENTS, AND NEGLIGENCE: SOME COMMON TERMINOLOGY

With all of the talk about errors coming from a variety of different sources, it is important to designate a set of definitions that can be used to distinguish the types of events that take place within healthcare environments that apply to patient safety. The IOM report defines *medical error* as "the failure to complete a planned action as intended or the use of a wrong plan to achieve an aim."[2]

Despite the popular appeal of discussing "errors" in health care, most of the literature on this subject, and most of the information in the IOM report, describes *adverse events* or *potential adverse events* rather than *errors*. An adverse event is defined as an injury caused by medical management rather than by the underlying disease or condition of the patient.[3] A potential adverse event carries the potential for injury. Many, but not all, adverse events are preventable. Those that are preventable, or those that are preventable and result only in the potential for harm, are considered errors. Thus, errors may or may not result in adverse events, and adverse events may or may not be the result of errors.[4]

An example commonly used to illustrate the distinction between preventable and nonpreventable events is an adverse event related to the administration of a new antibiotic to a patient who subsequently has a severe allergic reaction. This case could be the result of medical error, or it could be an unavoidable adverse reaction. If the medical record showed a prior allergic reaction to the type of antibiotic, or the healthcare team failed to ask the patient whether he or she had any allergies to drugs, the adverse event (i.e., the allergic reaction) would have resulted from medical error. If, on the other hand, the patient was asked about allergic reactions and it was clear that there was no history of allergy to this type of medication, the result would be an adverse event that was not the result of medical error.

Medical errors can result from virtually all processes involved in healthcare delivery. Some of the most common sources are the following:

- Drug-related errors, such as those resulting from prescribing the wrong medication or dosage, misinterpreting the correct prescription or prescribing instructions, and using incorrect routes of administration
- Diagnostic error, such as misdiagnosis leading to an incorrect choice of therapy, failure to use an indicated diagnostic test, misinterpretations of test results, and failure to act on abnormal results
- Equipment failure, such as defibrillators with dead batteries or intravenous pumps whose valves are easily dislodged or bumped, causing increased doses of medication over too short a period of time
- Blood-transfusion-related injuries, such as giving a patient blood of an incorrect type
- Misinterpretation of other medical orders, such as failing to give a patient a salt-free meal as ordered by a physician

MEDICAL ERRORS AND PATIENT SAFETY: WHAT DOES THE LITERATURE SHOW?

The estimates of deaths of inpatients resulting from medical errors come from two separate studies. The first, published in two parts in 1991 in the *New England Journal of Medicine*, was conducted by Lucien Leape, Troyen Brennan, and colleagues, and is referred to as the Harvard Medical Practice Study. It estimates the number of adverse events occurring or discovered in New York hospitals in 1984 and identifies those that resulted from medical negligence. The second, by Eric Thomas and colleagues published in *Inquiry* in 1999, estimates the costs of medical injuries in Utah and Colorado and uses much the same methodology as the Harvard Medical Practice Study.[5]

This study also includes an estimate of adverse events occurring or discovered in hospitals and identifies those that are preventable adverse events.

The Harvard Medical Practice Study

Researchers reviewed more than 30,000 randomly selected records from 51 randomly selected acute care, nonpsychiatric hospitals in New York State in 1984. Using data from these records, they developed population estimates of injuries and computed rates according to the age and sex of the patients as well as the specialties of the physicians. Brennan, Leape, and associates found that adverse events occurred in 3.7% of the hospitalizations.[6] More than one quarter of these (27.6%) were due to negligence. Using weighted totals, the authors estimated that among the nearly 2.7 million patients discharged from New York hospitals in 1984, there were more than 98,000 adverse events and approximately 27,000 adverse events involving negligence.[7]

The authors found that more than half of adverse events resulted in minor impairment, with complete recovery in 1 month. About one of seven resulted in disability lasting 1 to 6 months. But about 2.6% of adverse events resulted in permanent, total disability, and 13.6% caused death. Extrapolating to the state of New York in 1984, the authors estimated that 2,550 patients suffered permanent total disability and another 13,451 died at least in part as a result of adverse events.[8]

Although the authors do not identify specifically the percentage of adverse events related to errors (they use the higher standard of negligence), they found that negligence was more frequently associated with more severe adverse events. For example, while about 22% of adverse events leading to temporary disability were caused by negligence, 51% of the deaths associated with adverse events were caused by negligence.

Additional findings from the Harvard Medical Practice Study are as follows:

- Rates of adverse events increased strongly with increasing age of the patient. This could be a result of the fact that older individuals tend to require more complex care with multiple services, drugs, and therapies. Each of these increases the risk of an adverse event.
- The authors found no significant differences in adverse events between patient sexes, although they did find significant differences across diagnosis-related groups (DRGs). For example, the rate of adverse events in vascular surgery DRGs (16%) was about 25 times higher than that for neonatal DRGs (less than 1%). Rates of negligence, however, did not vary across DRGs.
- Approximately 20% of the adverse events caused by negligence occurred during outpatient care before the index hospitalization but were discovered during the index hospitalization.[9]
- Nearly half of the adverse events (48%) resulted from operations. Wound infections were the most common surgical adverse event, accounting for 29% of surgical complications and nearly one seventh of all adverse events identified in the study.[10]
- Drug complications were the most common single type of adverse event (19%).
- There was wide variation in the type of care that resulted in negligence. For example, 17% of the adverse events related to operations were due to negligence, ranging from 13% of the wound infections to 36% of the surgical failures. Negligent care was identified as causing 75% of the adverse events resulting from problems in diagnosis and 77% of those resulting from a therapeutic mishap.
- Drug-related complications were the most common type of adverse event for patients in all age groups except those aged 16 to 44 years, among whom drug

complications ranked second to wound infections. Children had the lowest rates in all categories.

- The largest number of adverse events resulted from treatment provided in the operating room. Emergency rooms, intensive care units, and labor and delivery rooms were each the site of about 3% of the adverse events. However, 70% of the adverse events associated with the emergency room were considered to result from negligence, compared with 14% of adverse events in the operating room.
- The most common class of error for physicians, accounting for 35% of all errors, involved the performance of a procedure or operation. Errors in prevention (i.e., failure to take preventive measures) were the next most common (22%). Errors in diagnosis and prevention were the most likely to be considered negligent (75% and 60% involved negligence, respectively).

The Utah and Colorado Study

Eric Thomas and colleagues reviewed medical records of 14,732 randomly selected 1992 discharges for 28 hospitals in Utah and Colorado to estimate the costs of all types of patient injuries. Using methods very similar to those used in the Harvard Medical Practice Study, they found that adverse event rates in Utah and Colorado were similar to those in New York. In addition, they found that the total costs (in discounted 1996 dollars) were $662 million for adverse events, of which $308 million was for preventable adverse events. In the case of preventable adverse events, 46% of the costs were attributable to healthcare costs. Extrapolating these figures to the 33.6 million admissions in the United States, the authors estimated the national costs of adverse events to be $37.6 billion, of which $17 billion is for preventable adverse events.[11]

Furthermore, the results of the Utah and Colorado study imply that at least 44,000 Americans die each year as a result of medical errors. Even when using this lower estimate (in lieu of the 98,000 estimate from the New York study), deaths caused by medical errors exceed the number attributable to the eighth leading cause of death. More people die in a given year as a result of medical errors than from motor vehicle accidents (43,458), breast cancer (42,297), or AIDS (16,516).

Other Selected Studies

The health services literature is rich with studies that together portray a healthcare system that abounds with medical errors. Many of these studies address the issue of medication-related errors. For example:

- Each year, medication-related errors, occurring in or out of the hospital, are estimated to account for over 7,000 deaths. This is higher than the number of Americans who die each year from workplace-related injuries.[12]
- In a 1995 study of medication-related problems at a university hospital, an average of three clinical outcomes associated with medication-related problems were detected per patient.[13]
- A 1991 study of iatrogenic cardiac arrests in a university teaching hospital found that during a 1-year period, 28 of 203 arrests in which resuscitation was attempted followed an iatrogenic complication. Seventeen of the 28 patients (61%) died. The authors found that the most common causes of potentially preventable arrest were medication errors and toxic effects, as well as suboptimal response by physicians to clinical signs and symptoms.[14]
- In a study by Cullen and associates that looked at preventable adverse drug events in intensive care units, the authors found that the rate of preventable or potential adverse drug events was twice as high in intensive care units as in general care units. This difference was due to the quantity of drugs prescribed, and not to a high-stress environment.[15]

- David Bates and colleagues evaluated the incidence and preventability of adverse drug events in an urban tertiary care hospital over a 37-day period. The rate of drug-related incidents was 73 in 2,967 patient days, with 27 incidents judged as adverse drug events, 34 as potential adverse drugs events, and 12 as problem orders. Fifty different drugs were involved, and physicians were primarily responsible for 72% of the incidents. More than half of the events were judged to be preventable.[16]

These studies demonstrate with remarkable consistency the vulnerability of the healthcare system and the pervasiveness of medical errors. Although they tend to concentrate on hospitalized patients, most of the studies are careful to point out that errors are by no means confined to hospitals. Hospitals tend to provide more accessible records and also demonstrate a longer and more concentrated period of time caring for a patient. They have been a valuable laboratory for research on medical errors.

Hospitals, however, may carry higher error rates than other healthcare institutions, although this is not determinable in the literature. Most researchers cite the complexity of an institution or healthcare process as being a risk factor for error. Hospitals are among the most complex healthcare delivery sites and therefore are likely to carry with them significant risk for error. They also are appropriate sites to begin designing systems for error reduction.

TO ERR IS HUMAN: THE IOM REPORT AND RECOMMENDATIONS

In June 1998, the IOM formed a Quality of Health Care in America Committee[17] to develop a strategy to result in a "threshold" improvement in quality over the next 10 years.[18] The report on patient safety was the first in a series that will address issues of quality in the healthcare system.

The purpose of the committee's work on patient safety is fourfold:[19]

1. To establish a national focus to create leadership, research, tools, and protocols to enhance the knowledge base about safety.
2. To identify and learn from errors through immediate and strong mandatory reporting efforts, as well as to encourage voluntary efforts, both with the aim of making sure the system continues to be made safe for patients.
3. To raise standards and expectations for improvements in safety through the actions of oversight organizations, group purchasers, and professional groups.
4. To create safety systems inside healthcare organizations through the implementation of safe practices at the delivery level. This level is the ultimate target of all the recommendations.

The IOM recommendations fall under the four categories just listed and call for a comprehensive effort on the part of all sectors of the healthcare system and its healthcare workforce to make patient safety a priority of the industry. The report challenges the healthcare industry to reduce medical errors by half over a 5-year period. At a minimum, this requires systemwide changes in the way health care is delivered, the relationships among health professionals, and the way health professionals interact with each other and their institutions. It also requires a profound culture shift within healthcare institutions to identify and root out errors and their underlying systemic causes. It requires an explicit commitment from CEOs, boards of trustees, medical and nursing staff, and a host of other healthcare participants to view error identification not as the beginning of punitive action, but as an opportunity to learn how to redesign systems so that they are much safer for patients.

The IOM recommends that the federal government establish a new "Center for Patient Safety" that would be housed at the Agency for Healthcare Research and Quality (formerly the Agency for Health Care Policy and Research) to set national goals for patient safety, track efforts, report to the American public, develop a research agenda, and fund projects designed to improve patient safety and reduce medical errors. In what is perhaps its most controversial recommendation, the IOM calls for a mandatory reporting system for the collection of standardized information by state governments about adverse events that result in serious harm or death. (See the chapter appendix for a complete list of the IOM recommendations.) The IOM also recommends setting up voluntary reporting systems to encourage the reporting of less serious adverse events.

The IOM calls for Congressional legislation to extend peer review protections to data related to patient safety and quality improvement that are collected and analyzed for the purposes of designing safer systems. Currently, information developed outside of peer review protections is open to discovery as part of a lawsuit. Thus, calling for mandatory or even voluntary reporting of serious adverse events would require a more protected legal environment to encourage individuals who commit errors (either individually or as part of a system or group process) and those who become aware that errors have occurred to report them without fear of punishment by supervisors or retribution by peers. This appears to be an extremely challenging goal, even in the presence of legal protections, but it is certainly one that could never be achieved without some sort of protection.

It is important to note that these legal protections do not preclude use of information that is "discoverable" through other sources. In other words, the legal protections suggested previously preclude use of information developed through the patient safety reporting process. In the case of negligence or otherwise inappropriate care, information developed pursuant to a legal action outside of the patient safety reporting system would be unaffected by these protections.

THE CLINTON ADMINISTRATION'S RESPONSE TO THE IOM REPORT

Within days of the IOM report, then-President Clinton publicly underscored the administration's commitment to improving patient safety and asked a healthcare quality task force to study the report and make recommendations about how to move forward with a patient safety agenda. The task force, know as the Quality Interagency Coordination (QuIC) Task Force, which originally had been formed in 1998 to focus federal efforts on improving healthcare quality, was chaired by Department of Health and Human Services Secretary Donna Shalala and Department of Labor Secretary Alexis Herman.[20] In December 1999, it was asked to concentrate on patient safety and medical errors.

The QuIC issued a report in February 2000 that supported virtually all of the IOM's recommendations. The QuIC's report included details about ways that federal agencies could assist in the effort to improve patient safety, as well as specific proposals for the Veterans' Administration and the Department of Defense. The most important feature of this report and the president's acceptance of its recommendations was that it supported the original IOM recommendation to create a mandatory reporting system for serious adverse events. It also supported efforts to provide legal protections for reporting for patient safety purposes, while stressing that these protections would not result in the creation of safe harbors for negligent providers.

The QuIC's recommendations tended to place the monitoring components (a mandatory reporting system along with incentives to encourage voluntary reporting of lesser events) within state systems, and the research, evaluation, and advisory components within federal agencies. Some of the latter efforts would likely involve collaborative efforts between one or more federal agencies and nonprofit organizations that are experienced in the issue of patient safety.

LEGISLATIVE PROPOSALS ON PATIENT SAFETY

There appears to be a significant amount of interest in patient safety on Capitol Hill, despite the relatively few bills introduced in Congress as of late 2000 specifically on this issue. Many Hill watchers believed that with so much legislation getting bogged down in election-year politics, Congress might take a "wait and see" attitude and revisit the medical errors issue after the November 2000 elections. Since the subject has bipartisan appeal, however, it seems safe to assume that there will be some legislative action aimed at reducing medical errors in upcoming sessions of Congress.

Several of the bills that were introduced in the 106th session kept these issues in front of Congress.[21] Maryland Congresswoman Morella introduced legislation that would provide for the voluntary reporting of medication errors. Senators Grassley, Lieberman, and Kerry sponsored the "Stop All Frequent Errors (SAFE) in Medicare and Medicaid Act of 2000," proposed legislation that largely mirrored the recommendations in the IOM's and the QuIC's reports. The purpose of the legislation was to develop a nonpunitive error reduction system[22] with "pragmatic" reporting requirements and adequate legal protections to support the collection of information under such systems. Among other provisions, the legislation would have extended existing confidentiality and peer review protections to a set of "additional required reports of error" that would have had to be reported in some systematic way. These additional required reports essentially broadened the definition of what a mandatory, reportable event would be.

Senators Specter and Harkin drafted legislation that would establish a mechanism to award grants to states to implement data collection systems so that national trends could be determined and analyzed. Like the Grassley proposal, information collected through the Specter–Harkin proposal would also be confidential and protected from discovery. The legislation called for the establishment of 15 research and demonstration projects throughout the nation that would test three models for reporting medical errors: Five sites would be required to inform the Department of Health and Human Services (DHHS) (through the Agency for Healthcare Research and Quality) of any medical errors occurring at the facility; five would be required to inform the DHHS as well as the patient or the patient's family (or both) of any medical errors; and five would be asked to voluntarily inform the DHHS of any medical errors.

Both of these proposals called for larger federal investment in research that addresses the reasons behind medical errors and ways to design systems to decrease their prevalence. The two sides of the argument differed on whether to institute a mandatory or a voluntary reporting system for serious adverse events. The IOM committee, the Clinton administration, and the Grassley bill clearly favored a mandatory system. The Specter legislation would have studied and evaluated various reporting models, leaving open the possibility of a voluntary system. Specter and colleagues are not alone, however, in coming down on the side of a voluntary system, as discussed in the following sections.

CURRENT REPORTING REQUIREMENTS

State Requirements

A recent report by the National Academy for State Health Policy (NASHP) provides information on the types of reporting systems that are currently in place in the 50 states and the District of Columbia.[23] According to that report, the majority of states do not have formal mandatory or voluntary systems for reporting errors or adverse events.

Fifteen states require mandatory reporting from general and acute care hospitals of adverse events, as defined by the IOM or by the state in a way that encompasses part or all of the IOM definition.[24] These states are Colorado, Florida, Kansas, Massachusetts, Nebraska, New Jersey, New York, Ohio, Pennsylvania, Rhode Island, South Carolina, South Dakota, Tennessee, Texas, and Washington. Twelve of these states must report expected deaths; these 15 states also report one or more of the following adverse events: wrong-site surgery, major loss of function, medication error, or a defective process not resulting in harm.

Six additional states have voluntary reporting of errors or adverse events. These include the District of Columbia, Georgia, New Mexico, North Carolina, Oregon, and Wyoming. Other states have legislation pending that would require or encourage reporting of adverse events.

Most of the 15 states that require reporting indicated that they protect at least some reports from legal discovery, although they vary in the types of information and reports that are protected. They also vary in the ways that they use the data that they collect. Some make part of the information available to the public; others conduct analyses, issue reports, or develop trend data. Nine of the 15 administer sanctions as a result of reported errors.

Two thirds of the states that require reporting say they experience significant problems with underreporting. Several respondents to the survey stated that they would benefit from the development of a uniform reporting system that would include protections and incentives for reporting.

Requirements of The Joint Commission

The Joint Commission (the Commission) has for several years promulgated what is known as the "sentinel event" policy, which is a series of recommendations designed to encourage the self-reporting of medical errors. According to the Commission, its principal goal is to learn about the relative frequencies and underlying causes of sentinel events, share "lessons learned" with other healthcare organizations, and reduce the risk of future sentinel event occurrences. It disseminates the information gathered through these reports through nationwide bulletins known as *Sentinel Event Alerts*.

A sentinel event is "an unexpected occurrence involving death or serious physical or psychological injury, or the risk thereof."[25] The definition was revised in May 1998 and includes a subset of adverse events that signal the need for immediate action. Action is needed if:

1. The event has resulted in an unanticipated death or permanent loss of function, not related to the natural course of the patient's illness or underlying condition.
2. The event is one of the following, even if the outcome was not death or major permanent loss of function:
   - Suicide of a patient in a setting where the patient receives around-the-clock care (e.g., hospital, residential treatment center, crisis stabilization center)
   - Infant abduction or discharge to the wrong family
   - Rape
   - Hemolytic transfusion reaction involving administration of blood or blood products having major blood group incompatibilities
   - Surgery on the wrong patient or wrong body part

Under the policy, these events are subject to review by the Commission and may be reported to the Commission on a voluntary basis. If the Joint Commission becomes aware that a sentinel event has occurred (either through voluntary reporting or through other means), the healthcare organization is required to prepare and submit to the Commission a root-cause analysis and action plan within 45 calendar days of the event. Thus, though not required to report a sentinel event, organizations that choose to report to the Commission are required to meet various reporting deadlines and criteria once the report has been made. Furthermore, following a report, The Joint Commission may decide to conduct a "for cause" survey to determine whether there is a real or potential ongoing threat to patient safety. The Commission indicates that these surveys occur infrequently.

The Commission has elected to stay out of the debate on mandatory versus voluntary reporting systems. The Joint Commission supports the development of an "effective medical/healthcare reporting system, whether mandatory or voluntary."[26] It strongly supports the IOM's call for protection of information reported for the purpose of patient safety analyses. In testimony to Congress in 2000, the Joint Commission stated that the sentinel event program had received relatively few reports, in large part because of a lack of statutory protections from disclosure of information. The testimony stated: "We will not be successful in attaining our goals if Congress does not pass federal protections that will encourage the surfacing, evaluating, and sharing of . . . information." The Commission also responded to the IOM report.

THE RESPONSE FROM THE AMERICAN HOSPITAL ASSOCIATION

The American Hospital Association (AHA) has been very engaged in the issue of medical errors. Shortly after the release of the IOM report, the AHA sent out a Quality Advisory to its full membership, indicating that it was in the process of developing an initiative to improve patient safety. Over the next several months, the AHA contacted hundreds of its members and worked through its regional structure to approve a series of policies on patient safety.

The AHA is working with the Institute for Safe Medication Practices (ISMP) to develop tools for hospitals to improve patient safety, especially regarding the issue of medication safety. ISMP developed a Medication Safety Self-Assessment tool that the AHA sent to all of its members. Hospitals were asked to complete the self-assessment tool and send the results back to the ISMP for analysis purposes. The tool, however, has generated a fair amount of concern among risk managers, who question how the information will be used and whether there are guarantees of confidentiality.

The AHA does not support several of the key recommendations included in the IOM report. First, the AHA supports a voluntary reporting system (except in cases where the state already requires reporting of such events). AHA officials strongly believe that a voluntary system is necessary to foster open communication and error identification and reporting. Second, the AHA does not support the recommendation that the Agency for Healthcare Research and Quality (AHRQ) serve as the appropriate reporting agency. Instead, it recommends that device-related errors continue to be reported to the FDA, that medication errors go to the ISMP, and that other types of errors be reported to other currently existing expert organizations. The AHA does not consider multiple reporting entities to be a drawback.

The Institute for Safe Medication Practices agrees with the AHA in its preference for a voluntary rather than a mandatory reporting system. Its strong belief is that a voluntary system is more likely to produce the culture change necessary for encouraging individuals to come forward and report medical errors.

The AHA supports the IOM's recommendations concerning legal protections for information developed through error reporting. It also supports federal and other efforts to raise awareness about medical errors and provide additional research dollars to study appropriate mechanisms to improve patient safety.

OTHER RESPONSES

Not surprisingly, several health-related associations and professional groups have issued policy statements or have testified about medical errors. Most often, differences among these parties center on the questions of whether a reporting system should be voluntary or mandatory (or some form of both) and which entity should receive those reports.

A partial list of these organizational responses follows.

- *The American Medical Association (AMA)* supports the AHRQ's role in developing information and funding research on patient safety and medical errors. It also supports the extension of peer review liability protections to those involved in patient safety improvement initiatives and confidentiality protections for individually identifiable information reported for health system safety and quality improvement purposes. The AMA does not support a nationwide mandatory error reporting system. The AMA insists that a mandatory reporting system could have unintended consequences and elicit less information than a well-designed, well-run voluntary program. The AMA also believes that Congress should help create a "culture of safety" within healthcare organizations by allowing medical professionals to convene to discuss patient safety problems and potential solutions without having their discussions, findings, or recommendations become the basis for class action or other lawsuits.

  The AMA established the National Patient Safety Foundation as an independent, nonprofit organization of healthcare clinicians, consumer advocates, health product manufacturers, public and private employers and payers, researchers, and regulators to develop strategies for improving patient safety. The group has developed an agenda for research, convened several high-level panels to discuss reducing medication errors, and has awarded several research grants to advance patient safety.
- *The American Association of Health Plans (AAHP)* issued a "Statement of Principles" in February 2000 to promote patient safety among its member health plans. Chief among its principles was support for a mandatory, nationally uniform reporting system free from disincentives for reporting life-threatening medical errors and a voluntary system for less serious problems.[27] This essentially mirrors the recommendation included in the IOM report.
- *The American College of Physicians–American Society of Internal Medicine (ACP-ASIM)* supports the establishment of a nationwide mandatory reporting system for adverse events that result in death or serious harm, adding that reporting requirements should not be overly inclusive or excessively burdensome to institutions or physicians, and should be narrowly defined to include only major errors. The ACP-ASIM also supports a voluntary reporting system of incidents that do not result in fatalities or major injuries.
- *The American Nurses Association (ANA)* supports the creation of a mandatory reporting system but would extend it beyond so-called sentinel events to include a broader range of errors and adverse events. The ANA is particularly concerned about how staffing affects patient safety and would like to see studies that address the extent to which understaffing of nurses is a detriment to patient care.
- *The Anesthesia Patient Safety Foundation (APSF)*[28] urges the nation to move cautiously before instituting the type of mandatory reporting system called for in the IOM report. Instead it urges further study and consultation with expert groups to deliberate the benefits of a mandatory system. The APSF believes that a voluntary system can be set up immediately and, if designed appropriately, can have an enormous impact on patient safety.

REASONS FOR OPTIMISM: SUCCESSFUL STRATEGIES

Much of the rhetoric about the epidemic of medical errors is accompanied by stories of successful interventions to reduce errors, save lives, and improve patient care. Safety advances in other industries (most notably, the aviation industry) are held up as examples of successful systems redesign that have resulted in vastly improved safety outcomes. Other occupational safety measures also serve as models for health system redesign for safety.

Examples of safety improvements in healthcare organizations that have resulted in marked (albeit smaller-scale) advances in patient safety also exist. Several quality-related organizations have published *Reducing Medical Errors and Improving Patient Safety: Success Stories from the Front Lines of Medicine*, a glossy report that details eight different approaches to error reduction.[29] Among them are reports about the strides in anesthesiology safety, which has reduced death rates from anesthesiology from roughly 1 in 3,000 to 4,000 in the 1950s, to 1 in 10,000 in the 1970s, and to 1 in 200,000 to 300,000 by 1990. The Anesthesia Patient Safety Foundation attributes this dramatic improvement to the field's attention to identifying safety problems early, promoting research, disseminating information, and promoting an emphasis on patients in clinical practice. According to the APSF, the most important feature of these efforts has been the elevation of patient safety to coequal status with more traditional concerns, such as determining the molecular mechanisms of anesthesia, developing specialized drugs, or managing critically ill patients.

Also showcased in the report are efforts through the Patient Safety Improvement Initiative at the U.S. Department of Veteran Affairs (VA). The VA set up the National Center for Patient Safety, headquartered in Ann Arbor, Michigan, and run by a physician and former astronaut, James Bagian. The first accomplishment under the new initiative was field-testing a bar-coding system to reduce medication errors at two VA hospitals in Kansas. The results were dramatic, with a 70% reduction in error rates over a 5-year period. The VA planned to have the bar-coding system in place at all VA hospitals by the end of 2000. A similar bar-coding system is planned for blood products used in transfusions. Other initiatives include changes in the way medications are stored and in the use of physical restraints, and improvements in the use of data on medical errors.

Other programs highlighted in the IOM report include the following:

- Efforts at Dana-Farber Cancer Institute in Boston, Massachusetts, to make chemotherapy safer
- Encouraging physicians to use computers to write prescriptions at Brigham and Women's Hospital in Boston, Massachusetts
- Engaging the participation of a pharmaceutical company (Bristol-Myers Squibb) to redesign medication packaging and develop guidelines for naming new pharmaceuticals
- Focusing on managing a few high-risk drugs at Fairview Health Services in Minneapolis, Minnesota
- Using simulation technology at the VA/Stanford Simulation Center in Palo Alto, California, to mimic complex and realistic clinical crisis scenarios

In each of these cases, encouraging results have been shown through the interaction of technology, leadership, and a strong "corporate" commitment to error reduction and patient safety. There have also been efforts across the sites to work with teams of health professionals to stimulate a culture of change and trust—one that welcomes error detection and reporting as an opportunity for improved patient care.

According to the American Hospital Association, the Agency for Healthcare Research and Quality, and other interested organizations, hospitals and other healthcare institutions can begin a program addressing medical errors with little up-front investment other than commitment to the cause. For example, the AHA suggests that organizations review their policies and procedures for reporting and investigating errors. It also encourages hospitals to access information from organizations such as the Institute for Safe Medication Practices, the Institute for Healthcare Improvement, the Food and Drug Administration, and others who have worked for years on this issue.

The AHRQ has developed helpful lists for improving patient safety from the hospital, health professional, and patient perspective. For example, the AHRQ found through its own funded research programs that the following procedures can help reduce medical errors:

- *Computerized adverse drug event monitoring:* Although chart review has been found to be more accurate than computer tracking and voluntary reporting in identifying adverse drug events, it required five times more personnel time. Researchers concluded that the computerized method was the most efficient means of tracking drug errors.
- *Computer-generated reminders for follow-up testing:* Some diagnostic tests require repeat tests to follow up certain conditions. A computerized physician-reminder system for timing of repeat tests was suggested as a useful adjunct to these procedures to prevent patients from being subjected to unnecessary repeat tests.
- *Standardized protocols:* An AHCPR-sponsored study of ICU patients with severe respiratory disease found a fourfold increase in survival rates with computerized treatment protocols.
- *Computer-assisted decision making:* In a study of trauma cases, computerized decision algorithms were tested against physician-generated management plans and evaluated by a panel of trauma surgeons. Overall, the panel rated the computer-supported decisions as more acceptable than those based on judgment alone.

CONCLUSION

With very few exceptions, the healthcare industry has been united in its support for a comprehensive effort to reduce medical errors across all sites of care.[30] Nevertheless, as noted earlier in this chapter, there is considerable difference of opinion about the ways that systems of error detection and reporting should be designed. Some of the parties feel strongly that even in the presence of added protections of error-related information, current malpractice law places providers (most often physicians) at risk of legal action. Furthermore, this risk is increased by taking error reporting outside the bounds of the healthcare institution and placing it in an external repository of information on medical mistakes.

Despite the goodwill that exists on both sides of the debate, the success of future efforts to improve patient safety may rise or fall on issues essentially unrelated to the technical design of safer systems. A redesigned healthcare delivery system can be successful only with the buy-in from the leadership at the top of healthcare institutions and from healthcare professionals at the bedside, both of whom have their reputations on the line when it comes to patient care. Any changes to strengthen patient care by exposing medical errors—albeit for study and redesign purposes only—will have to be balanced by clear and fair protections that encourage full disclosure, regardless of the mandatory or voluntary nature of the reporting system.

APPENDIX: IOM RECOMMENDATIONS*

1. Congress should create a Center for Patient Safety within the Agency for Health Care Policy and Research. This Center should
   - set the national goals for patient safety, track progress in meeting these goals, and issue an annual report to the President and Congress on patient safety; and
   - develop knowledge and understanding of errors in health care by develop-

---

* Reprinted with permission from *To Err Is Human*, © 2000 by the National Academy of Sciences, courtesy of the National Academies Press, Washingron, DC.

ing a research agenda, funding Centers of Excellence, evaluating methods for identifying and preventing errors, and funding dissemination and communication activities to improve patient safety.

2. A nationwide mandatory reporting system should be established that provides for the collection of standardized information by state governments about the adverse events that result in death or serious harm. Reporting should initially be required of hospitals and eventually be required of other institutional and ambulatory care delivery settings. Congress should
   - designate the Forum of Health Care Quality Measurement and Reporting as the entity responsible for promulgating and maintaining a core set of reporting standards to be used by states, including a nomenclature and taxonomy for reporting;
   - require all healthcare organizations to report standardized information on a defined list of adverse events;
   - provide funds and technical expertise for state governments to establish or adapt their current error reporting systems to collect the standardized information, analyze it and conduct follow-up action as needed with healthcare organizations. Should a state choose not to implement the mandatory reporting system, the Department of Health and Human Services should be designated as the responsible entity; and
   - designate the Center for Patient Safety to:
     (1) convene states to share information and expertise, and to evaluate alternative approaches taken for implementing reporting programs, identify best practices for implementation, and assess the impact of state programs; and
     (2) receive and analyze aggregate reports from states to identify persistent safety issues that require more intensive analysis and/or broader-based response (e.g., designing prototype systems or requesting a response by agencies, manufacturers, or others).
3. The development of voluntary reporting efforts should be encouraged. The Center for Patient Safety should
   - describe and disseminate information on external voluntary reporting programs to encourage greater participation in them and track the development of new reporting systems as they form;
   - convene sponsors and users of external reporting systems to evaluate what works and what does not work well in the programs, and ways to make them more effective;
   - periodically assess whether additional efforts are needed to address gaps in information to improve patient safety and to encourage healthcare organizations to participate in voluntary reporting programs; and
   - fund and evaluate pilot projects for reporting systems, both within individual healthcare organizations and collaborative efforts among healthcare organizations.
4. Congress should pass legislation to extend peer review protections to data related to patient safety and quality improvement that are collected and analyzed by healthcare organizations for internal use or shared with others solely for purposes of improving safety and quality.
5. Performance standards and expectations for healthcare organizations should focus greater attention on patient safety.
   - Regulators and accreditors should require healthcare organizations to implement meaningful patient safety

programs with defined executive responsibility.
- Public and private purchasers should provide incentives to healthcare organizations to demonstrate continuous improvement in patient safety.

6. Performance standards and expectations for health professionals should focus greater attention on patient safety.
   - Health professional licensing bodies should
     (1) implement periodic reexaminations and relicensing of doctors, nurses, and other key providers, based on both competence and knowledge of safety practices; and
     (2) work with certifying and credentialing organizations to develop more effective methods to identify unsafe providers and take action.
   - Professional societies should make a visible commitment to patient safety by establishing a permanent committee dedicated to safety improvement. This committee should
     (1) develop a curriculum on patient safety and encourage its adoption into training and certification requirements;
     (2) disseminate information on patient safety to members through special sessions at annual conferences, journal articles and editorials, newsletters, publications and websites on a regular basis;
     (3) recognize patient safety considerations in practice guidelines and in standards related to the introduction and diffusion of new technologies, therapies, and drugs;
     (4) work with the Center for Patient Safety to develop community-based, collaborative initiatives for error reporting and analysis and implementation of patient safety improvements; and
     (5) collaborate with other professional societies and disciplines in a national summit on the professional's role in patient safety.
7. The Food and Drug Administration (FDA) should increase attention to the safe use of drugs in both pre- and postmarketing processes through the following actions:
   - develop and enforce standards for the design of drug packaging and labeling that will maximize safety in use;
   - require pharmaceutical companies to test (using FDA-approved methods) proposed drug names to identify and remedy potential sound-alike and look-alike confusion with existing drug names; and
   - work with physicians, pharmacists, consumers, and others to establish appropriate responses to problems identified through postmarketing surveillance, especially for concerns that are perceived to require immediate response to protect the safety of patients.
8. Healthcare organizations and the professionals affiliated with them should make continually improved patient safety a declared and serious aim by establishing patient safety programs with defined executive responsibility. Patient safety programs should
   - Provide strong, clear, and visible attention to safety;
   - Implement nonpunitive systems for reporting and analyzing errors within their organizations;
   - Incorporate well-understood safety principles, such as standardizing and simplifying equipment, supplies, and processes; and
   - Establish interdisciplinary team training programs, such as simulation, that incorporate proven methods of team management.
9. Healthcare organizations should implement proven medication safety practices.

References

1. Institute of Medicine (IOM) Committee on Quality of Health Care in America. *To Err Is Human: Building a Safer Health System* [Advance Copy]. Linda T. Kohn, Janet M. Corrigan, and Molla S. Donaldson, editors. Washington, DC: National Academy Press, 2000, p. vii.
2. Ibid.
3. Brennan, T. A., Leape, L. L., Laird, N. M., et al. Incidence of adverse events and negligence in hospitalized patients: Results of the Harvard Medical Practice Study I. *N Engl J Med* 1991;324:370–376.
4. The studies upon which the IOM error estimates are based discuss medical negligence, which is a term generally left out of the IOM study. *Negligence* is a legal term that relates to care that falls below the standard expected of healthcare professionals (generally physicians) in their community. Some medical errors may not rise to the level of medical negligence.
5. Thomas, E. J., Studdert, D. M., Newhouse, J. P., Zbar, B. I., Howard, K. M., Williams, E. J., Brennan, T. A. Costs of medical injuries in Utah and Colorado. *Inquiry* 1999;36(3):255–264.
6. The authors define *adverse event* as an injury caused by medical management (rather than underlying disease) and that prolonged the hospitalization, produced a disability at the time of discharge, or both.
7. These estimates, along with ones from Thomas and colleagues, were used to form the basis of the national estimates included in the IOM report. The Harvard Medical Practice Study estimates set the higher range in the estimate of 40,000 to 98,000 deaths per year.
8. Brennan et al., p. 371.
9. The Harvard Medical Practice Study identified adverse events and negligence from hospital medical records only. Some of these events occurred as a result of outpatient treatment or from hospitalization prior to the study period. All of the events occurred or were discovered during the study period hospitalization but could have resulted from prior treatments in or out of the hospital.
10. Leape, L. L., Brennan, T. A., Laird, N., et al. The nature of adverse events in hospitalized patients: Results of the Harvard Medical Practice Study II. *N Engl J Med* 1991;324:377–384.
11. The authors used 1993 data from the American Hospital Association to estimate national admission rates.
12. Phillips, D. P., Christenfeld, N., Glynn, L. M. Increase in US medication-error deaths between 1983 and 1993. *Lancet* 1998;351:643–644.
13. Schneider, P. J., Gift, M. G., Lee, Y., Rothermich, E. A., Sill, B. E. Cost of medication-related problems at a university hospital. *Am J Health-Syst Pharm* 1995;52:2415–2418.
14. Bedell, S. E., Deitz, D. C., Leeman, D., Delbanco, T. L. Incidence and characteristics of preventable iatrogenic cardiac arrest. *JAMA* 1991;265:2815–2820.
15. Cullen et al. Preventable adverse drug events in hospitalized patients: A comparative study of intensive care and general care units. *Crit Care Med* 1997;25:1289–1297.
16. Bates, D. W., Leape, L. L., Petrycki, S. Incidence and preventability of adverse drug events in hospitalized adults. *J Gen Intern Med* 1993;8:289–294.
17. The committee was chaired by William C. Richardson, president and CEO of the W.K. Kellogg Foundation. Members of the committee included representatives from health systems, academics, experts in patient safety and quality of care, major industries, consumer organizations, and medical groups. For a complete list of committee members, see page iii of the IOM report.
18. IOM, *To Err Is Human*, p. ix.
19. Ibid., p. 5.
20. The Clinton administration pointed out, in its public materials on this subject, that its efforts in patient safety and quality predated the IOM report. That may be true, but clearly the impetus for the administration's increased activity specifically on medical errors was the release of the IOM report.
21. In addition, Senators James Jeffords (R-VT), Patrick J. Kennedy (D-RI), Christopher Dodd (D-CT), and William Frist (R-TN) were drafting legislation that would begin to implement

the recommendations of the presidential QuIC.

22. See the April 3, 2000, version of the Grassley bill.
23. Rosenthal, J., Riley, T., Booth, M. *State Reporting of Medical Errors and Adverse Events: Results of a 50-State Survey.* Portland, ME: The National Academy for State Health Policy, 2000.
24. Some states require hospitals to report other types of events, such as violence and infectious outbreaks. These do not fall within the IOM's definitions of error and are not included here.
25. See The Joint Commission Web site, www.jointcommision.org for information on the sentinel event policy.
26. Reporting of Medical/Health Care Errors: A Position Statement of the Joint Commission on Accreditation of Healthcare Organizations. http://www.jcaho.org/sentinel/errors.html.
27. The AAHP's stance came as a surprise to some analysts watching this debate unfold. Some of the more skeptical in the group suggested that the AAHP position was advanced to deflect attention from the Patients' Bill of Rights.
28. The Anesthesia Patient Safety Foundation was formed in 1985 to improve the safety of anesthesia administration and reduce adverse effects. The field of anesthesia is the sole area of medicine that can point to dramatic decreases in error rates over the past two decades. These efforts are discussed in a later section of this chapter.
29. The report is the work of Accelerating Change Today (A.C.T.) for America's Health, a collaborative initiative of the National Coalition on Health Care and the Institute for Healthcare Improvement.
30. The July 5, 2000, issue of *JAMA* includes an article under the section called *Controversies* that claims that the data referenced in the IOM report concerning deaths due to medical errors are exaggerated. This claim is refuted by one of the principal authors of the Harvard Medical Practice Study. See McDonald, C. J., Weiner, M., Hui, S. L. Deaths due to medical errors are exaggerated in Institute of Medicine report. *JAMA* 2000;284:93–94; and Leape, L. L. Institute of Medicine medical error figures are not exaggerated. *JAMA* 2000;284:95–97.

2

Patient Safety Movement: The Progress and the Work That Remains

Manisha Shaw, MBA, RCP and Karla M. Miller, PharmD, BCPP

INTRODUCTION

One need only turn on the news to see that health care is still at the forefront of national consciousness. Twelve years after the release of the landmark Institute of Medicine (IOM) report,[1] *To Err is Human: Building a Safer Health System*, preventable errors continue to occur, systemic frailties in every aspect of the healthcare delivery system exist, and seemingly simple solutions gain limited traction.[2] It is difficult to determine whether media coverage has caused or increased consumer concern or whether the public's desire for information prompts the media to scrutinize events more closely. What is certain is that keeping patients safe is now an expectation in health care.

Accountability to ensure safety of all patients is expected at all levels of leadership, from individual clinicians to national legislators who oversee healthcare regulations. Recent events have ensured that patient safety is never far from the minds of caregivers, patients, payers, and regulators.[2] Although advances in patient safety have been made, countless numbers of patients continue to suffer preventable medical errors. More and more attention is being paid to system issues. Wachter graded the progress from a C+ in 2004 to a B– in 2010, noting advancement in many areas such as error reporting and involvement by leaders. However, he also noted a lack of progress in areas such as health information technology and malpractice system reform.[3] Efforts to improve patient safety are not limited to hospitals and healthcare institutions. Healthcare institutions are not the only ones coming under scrutiny; the public is growing wary of medical device manufacturers and the pharmaceutical industry. The existence of several device recall registries, the fact that often the labeling practices of drugs have been shown to be one of the root causes of many medical errors, and the fact that product recalls make the news on a regular basis attest to the fact that device malfunctions and drug safety are not isolated incidents.[4]

Much progress has been made in patient safety over the past decade. Yet, as an industry, health care has only scratched the surface. In this chapter, the authors will review the foundation of patient safety by exploring the historical events that have shaped patient safety as it is known today. We will discuss critical issues that continue to gain attention. By examining the issues health care faces and the history of patient safety in America, we will show that a more cohesive and united effort is needed to have a meaningful effect on both quality of care and patient safety.

A HISTORY OF PATIENT SAFETY

The frequency and magnitude of avoidable adverse patient events was not well known until the 1990s, when multiple countries reported staggering numbers of patients harmed or killed by medical errors. Recognizing that healthcare errors affect 1 in every 10 patients around the world, the World Health Organization called patient safety an endemic concern.[5]

The first big step toward improving patient safety was the formation of the Institute of Medicine (IOM). Established in 1970, the IOM is the health arm of the National Academy of Sciences, chartered under President Abraham Lincoln in 1863.[6] The IOM asks and answers the nation's most pressing questions about health and health care. The Institute's goal is to provide unbiased, reliable information about health care, especially as it pertains to public health and policy. Information is furnished primarily by committees in the form of formal reports. The IOM arranges forums for sharing information and conducts its own research.[5] Information and research provided by the IOM has been invaluable for advancing the cause of patient safety. As a nonprofit, nonpartisan organization, policy makers highly regard and give considerable weight to findings from the IOM. *To Err Is Human* is one of the recognized contributions from the IOM. Additionally, because the IOM has completed numerous studies and reports on issues pertaining to patient safety, it is an excellent source of information for those advocating for safer care both at the patient and the provider levels. Many of the studies that the IOM undertakes begin as specific mandates from Congress, whereas others are requested by federal agencies and independent organizations.

The IOM tackles questions about general patient safety and quality, whereas the newer FDA MedWatch (developed in 1993) focuses more on medical products, such as medications and devices.[7] MedWatch provides medical product safety alerts, recalls, withdrawals, and important labeling changes that may affect the health of all Americans via its Web site and the MedWatch E-list. MedWatch allows healthcare professionals and consumers to report serious problems that they suspect are associated with the drugs and medical devices they prescribe, dispense, or use. It also has played a pivotal role in incorporating consumers into improving patient safety.

The catalyst for addressing patient safety concerns was initiated by three major publications put out by IOM: *To Err Is Human* (1999),[1] *Crossing the Quality Chasm* (2001),[8] and *Preventing Medication Errors* (2006).[9] The first report sent shock waves through the industry and the nation by awakening everyone to the level of preventable medical errors occurring in the United States. *To Err Is Human* was the inspiration for the Institute for Healthcare Improvement's 100,000 Lives Campaign,[10] which in 2006 claimed to have prevented an estimated 124,000 deaths in a period of 18 months through patient safety initiatives in more than 3,000 hospitals. *Crossing the Quality Chasm*[7] urgently called for changes to healthcare system processes to improve patient care. It analyzed this dilemma and explored potential ways in which change could be implemented in the healthcare delivery system at all levels. These two documents were instrumental in raising patient safety awareness in health care and among policy makers. Most recent, the report *Preventing Medication Errors*[8] put forth a national agenda for reducing medication errors predicated on estimates of the incidence and cost of such errors and presented evidence on the efficacy of various prevention strategies. This report proved to be more of a call to action than were the other two, providing specific strategies for medication safety improvement rather than more general information detailing the errors in health care and specific patient safety concerns.

Efforts to improve patient safety have been made in the past, and the report built on this earlier work. In the early part of the century, two important pieces of legislation were passed: the Biologics Control Act and the Food, Drug and Cosmetics Act.[6] The former, passed in 1902, was spurred by the deaths of 13 children who had received a diphtheria vaccine. It regulated the production of biological products to ensure the safety of consumers.[8] The latter, passed in 1938, required that drugs be proven safe before advertised to the public, set quality standards for packaged products, and authorized inspections of production facilities.[6] The importance of this legislation cannot be overstated. Medications and vaccines are indispensable for consumer health but can do more harm than good if not properly regulated. The legislation of 1902 and 1938 set precedents for product regulation and demonstrated the willingness of the government to step in on behalf of consumers. The next landmark event in patient safety occurred in 1951 with the founding of The Joint Commission (TJC).[11] At its inception, the TJC provided accreditation to hospitals based on adherence to its published standards. In 1965, adherence to TJC standards became mandatory for hospitals that wished to participate in Medicare or Medicaid, ensuring compliance by even more institutions. Over time, standards became more complex, and councils were formed to oversee accreditation for mental health facilities, facilities for persons with disabilities, hospice facilities, and long-term care facilities, among others.[10] Although accreditation is an important part of its mission, the TJC also conducts research on patient safety and healthcare quality, provides tools to help hospitals measure performance, and periodically issues reports on the state of patient safety.[12]

Two decades after the founding of the IOM, another critical piece of legislation was passed. The Safe Medical Devices Act was passed in 1996 and gave the FDA power to regulate the medical device industry. The law stipulates that hospitals and other healthcare providers must report and track undesirable events related to medical devices. Additionally, manufacturers must create tracking methods for each device they produce, such as a unique serial number or bar code.[13] This legislation greatly expanded the regulatory capabilities of the FDA and officially brought medical devices into the realm of patient safety concerns. In 1994, *Error in Medicine* was published, drawing attention to the need for human factors research in the prevention of medical errors.[14] In 1997, the National Patient Safety Foundation[15] was created with a singular mission of ensuring safe care of patients.[14] Several other organizations, such as the Agency for Healthcare Research and Quality,[16] the Institute for Healthcare Improvement (IHI),[17] and the Leapfrog Group,[18] have as central to their missions the improvement of quality and patient safety.

Although much was accomplished before *To Err Is Human*[1] was published, the report spurred a wave of interest and action in the realm of patient safety and established it firmly as a movement rather than a collection of isolated efforts. In 2002, the TJC created the National Patient Safety Goals program to help organizations target areas most in need of improvement.[19] The following year, in 2003, the National Quality Forum (NQF) published a set of guidelines called Safe Practices for Better Healthcare, an evidence-based list of 30 practices to be employed by all healthcare facilities to increase safety and quality.[20] The guidelines address topics such as safety culture, transfer of information, and medication safety, and suggest ways to improve them.

Two years later, another important piece of legislation was passed, the Patient Safety and Quality Improvement Act (PSQIA) of 2005.[21] This law lead to the creation of the patient safety organizations with the goal of learning from collated event data to improve patient safety. This law laid a framework in which providers and organizations could collect patient safety data without fear of legal retribution. Malpractice suits are a serious concern for healthcare organizations and providers; for them to be forthcoming about errors, a certain level of protection needed to be ensured. The PSQIA[15] also emphasized the need for a comprehensive database of adverse safety events. It is hoped that ultimately this reporting initiative will collect information in a standardized way and will be useful to compare geographic regions and track national trends.[15]

The latest development in patient safety is the creation of the Partnership for Patients program.[22] Launched in 2011, the Partnership has two main goals: to reduce patient harm in healthcare environments and improve transitions from hospitals to less-acute care settings to lessen the rate of readmission. To accomplish these goals, the Partnership for Patients has identified nine areas of concentration: adverse drug events, catheter-associated urinary tract infections, central line-associated bloodstream infections, inpatient falls, adverse obstetrical events, pressure ulcers, surgical-site infection, venous thromboembolism, ventilator-associated pneumonia, and other unspecified hospital-acquired conditions.[23] If the goals of this program are met, the federal government estimates that $35 billion and 60,000 lives could be saved over the next three years.[16]

The above-mentioned organizations and legislation are testimony to the leadership and movement in patient safety. Despite the consistent efforts of many in health care, this industry continues to be faced with critical issues that have a profound effect on patient outcomes. We will discuss some of these critical issues and their prevalence later in this chapter in more detail. Creating a culture of safety is considered to be the foundation for all patient safety activities and perhaps, given the tradition and hierarchy in our healthcare delivery system, has proven to be one of the most challenging issues.

CREATING A CULTURE OF SAFETY

According to the Institute of Medicine,[1] changing patient safety culture is the biggest impediment to improving outcomes. Workplace culture makes a difference in clinical outcomes. All healthcare organizations must recognize that patient safety is a top priority and make decisions based on that priority. Several omnipresent elements that support a culture of safety include a blame-free work environment, transparency, and a process designed to prevent errors. A just and fair culture of transparency is essential to empowering employees to create safe processes and improve the safety of the care they deliver. In organizations committed to patient safety, leadership must recognize patient safety as its top priority and describe the factors that must be present in an organization to support a culture of safety. Among these factors are a pervasive commitment to patient safety, which is evident in all decisions made by leadership; open communication, where everyone in the organization feels free to report potential safety concerns; a blame-free environment, where such reporting is rewarded rather than ignored; and the use of tools, techniques, and processes that have been proven to prevent future errors.

Safety culture can be defined as the set of values, beliefs, and norms about what is important, and how to behave and what attitudes are appropriate when it comes to patient safety in a work group.[24] Many organizations measure patient safety culture through the use of the Safety Attitude Questionnaire, developed by the Agency for Healthcare Research and Quality (AHRQ).

The dimensions measured by the AHRQ patient safety culture tool are as follows:

- Supervisor/manager expectations and actions promoting patient safety
- Organizational learning—continuous improvement
- Openness of communication
- Feedback and communication about errors
- Hospital management support for patient safety
- Nonpunitive response to error (blame-free environment or a *just* culture)
- Staffing
- Teamwork within units
- Teamwork across hospital units
- Hospital handoffs and transitions

The University of Texas Patient Safety Attitudes Questionnaire is also frequently used to assess safety culture. Healthcare organizations can use the survey to measure caregiver attitudes about six patient safety-related domains to compare themselves to other organizations, to prompt interventions to improve safety attitudes, and to measure the effectiveness of these interventions.[25]

Assessing the culture of patient safety allows organizations to delineate the areas where improvement is needed. At present, these are the most standardized tools available for assessing culture. It must be noted that questionnaires are somewhat subjective because they collect data on the perceptions of respondents, not on their actual activities or habits.

Currently, there are few proven interventions that have been successful in completely changing the culture of a healthcare organization. However, a nonpunitive, blame-free culture is essential as a foundation for a culture of safety.

MOST COMMON PATIENT SAFETY CONCERNS

Over the past 12 years, research specific to patient safety has accelerated, and though clearly we have yet to fully operationalize the solutions, we have a much clearer understanding of the problems. Analysis of specific event types is bringing us closer to the development of specific strategies for reducing or eliminating these patient safety risks.

Medication Errors

One of the most common preventable medical errors relates to the ordering, dispensing, preparing, and administering of medication. Medication errors injure 1.5 million people per year and amass an additional $3.5 billion in additional healthcare costs.[8] According to National Coordination Council for Medication Error Reporting, a medication error is any preventable event that may cause or lead to inappropriate medication use or patient harm while the medication is in the control of the health care professional, patient, or consumer. Such events may be related to professional practice, healthcare products, procedures, and systems, including: prescribing; order communication; product labeling, packaging, and nomenclature; compounding; dispensing; distribution; administration; education; monitoring; and use.[26] An adverse medication event denotes some type of harm, from unexpected side effects to serious injury and death. Some medication errors result from patients taking their medications incorrectly, but others result from errors by healthcare providers. Examples of these errors include errors in transcription, errors in dispensing, errors in prescribing, and errors in administering drugs. Together, errors by clinicians and patients send more than 282,500 people to the emergency department each year. Of those, 98,000 are children, 177,000 are elderly, and 7,500 are middle aged.[27] Clearly, the elderly are at the most risk, but this may also be because they take the most medications and fill the most prescriptions of any age group.

Research has identified many of the reasons for medication errors, which include hard-to-read paper prescriptions, confusing labeling or packaging, unclear directions, low health literacy, and an unwillingness of patients to ask questions about their medications. Means of prevention include bar-coded medications, electronic medical records, rewriting medication directions so they are easier to understand, higher health literacy in general, and closer monitoring of at-risk groups, such as infants and the elderly. Establishing standards by which to identify and assess gaps in the medication management process is a first step to prevention of medication errors.

Hospital-Acquired Infections

Hospital-acquired infection (HAI), also referred to as a nosocomial infection, is an infection acquired during the course of treatment at a healthcare facility that was not present prior to the visit. The infection often occurs within 48 hours of admission, but infections that occur after discharge are also considered HAIs if the pathogen was acquired during the patient's stay.[28]

The World Health Organization[29] estimates that around 8.7% of hospital patients worldwide have an HAI at any given time. In the United States, one out of 20 hospitalized patients contracts an HAI and 100,000 die each year,[30] but as of 2010 only 27 states had laws requiring hospitals to report their rates of infection.[31] For patients, the cost of an HAI is high: the length of the hospital stay increases by seven to nine days and they pay $40,000 more on average. For the healthcare system as a whole, HAIs add between $4.5 and $5.7 billion each year to medical costs.[32] There are many types of HAIs, but the most common are central line-associated bloodstream infections, catheter-associated urinary tract infections, and ventilator-associated pneumonia. Although surgical-site infections and MRSAs (methicillin-resistant *Staphylococcus aureus*) are also grave concerns, the aforementioned infections account for more than two-thirds of all HAIs.[33]

Fortunately, HAIs are preventable. The World Health Organization (WHO)[27] and the Centers for Disease Control (CDC)[34] recommend several steps to reduce infection: hand washing of the proper length and frequency, proper cleaning and sterilization of the patient's environment, proper staff attire, and reduction of unnecessary injections and surgical procedures.[35] It has been demonstrated through clinical research that strict adherence to these recommendations has the potential to prevent infections or reduce infection rates to extremely low levels. Ensuring that the recommendations are followed correctly and uniformly, however, has proved difficult.

Surgical-Site Errors

Surgical-site errors result in procedures being performed on the wrong site, correct procedures performed on the wrong person, incorrect procedures being performed at a site, and procedures that are more invasive than intended or necessary. Causes vary, but some are cited by The Joint Comission (TJC) as risk factors because of their prevalence in cases where wrong-site surgeries have occurred. These include time constraints (caused by emergency surgery or a full schedule), room or staffing changes, multiple procedures being performed, and patient characteristics, such as obesity or physical deformities, that prompted a change in operating room setup.[36]

Wrong-site surgeries, though uncommon, are preventable. Between 1995 and 2010, 956 wrong-site incidents were reported to The Joint Commisssion.[37] However, these numbers are believed to represent only 10% of actual occurrences because reporting to the TJC is voluntary.[34] One study surveyed surgical procedures from 28 hospitals and found the incidence of wrong-site surgeries to be approximately one in 112,994 procedures. For the average hospital, this means one error every five to 10 years. This study also surveyed the costs of these incidents to the hospitals. The median payment to the patient was $12,000, and the cost of defense was $1,500, for a total of $13,500 per case on average.[38]

To address the problem of surgical-site errors, The Joint Commission chaired a summit that produced the "Universal Protocol for Preventing Wrong Site, Wrong Procedure, and Wrong Person Surgery." The Protocol makes three central recommendations to prevent errors: a preprocedure verification, marking the procedure site clearly, and taking a time-out before the surgery to conduct a final check.[34]

Device Malfunctions

According to the Food and Drug Administration (FDA),[39] a medical device is any object used for the diagnosis, prevention, or treatment of disease in humans or animals. The device can be internal or external but excludes substances metabolized by the body, commonly known as drugs or pharmaceuticals.[40] A device malfunction is any function of a device that causes harm or is unintended even if the patient is not injured. Adverse events of this type are required to be reported to the FDA because its Center for Devices and Radiological Health oversees the regulation of medical devices. Unfortunately, not all adverse events are reported, and of those reported, the FDA releases information only about products that could cause patients to be seriously injured or to die. In the year 2011, 27 such press releases were issued by the FDA in addition to those done by the manufacturers themselves.[41] In almost all cases, recalls are initiated by the company and completed voluntarily; the difficulty lies in getting information about recalled items out to the affected consumers.

Error in Diagnosis

Misdiagnosis is of serious concern to both patients and their doctors. Besides the cost in patient lives, misdiagnosis—defined as an incorrect diagnosis, an incomplete diagnosis, errors in testing, and mishandling of lab or diagnostic test data—places heavy financial costs on the healthcare system. In 2004 alone, $4.2 billion was paid out for malpractice lawsuits, and of these, the vast majority were brought for misdiagnosis or failure to diagnose.[42] The threat of misdiagnosis and its aftermath keeps malpractice insurance premiums and healthcare costs high. The possibility of such a suit is particularly high for primary care physicians because they are often the first healthcare providers patients present to deal with a problem. The primary care physician is often responsible for the patient's course of care.

The effects on patients are even more sobering because early detection and a proper course of treatment are crucial for fighting chronic conditions such as cancer, diabetes, asthma, and other autoimmune disorders. Meta-analyses have shown the diagnostic error rate to be between 4.1% and 49.8%, with 4% of cases displaying preventable, lethal errors. Diagnostic error is difficult to study, however, because it often goes undetected or unreported.[43] Present studies rely heavily on autopsy findings and malpractice suits for data, which is problematic because such methods preferentially select for a population that has already been seriously harmed by errors. Nonetheless, the effects of diagnostic error—poor prognoses, lost productivity, increase in costs for patients and healthcare systems—are known, but the scope and prevalence are yet to be determined.

THE IMPACT OF LITERACY ON PATIENT SAFETY

It is well acknowledged that informed patients make better decisions. The ability to obtain and analyze information pertaining to health and wellness is called health literacy. Health literacy is necessary to navigate the healthcare system and to make decisions about one's health care; unfortunately, many Americans have low health literacy. This has negative consequences for patient safety for several reasons. First, patients with low health literacy are more likely to misunderstand medical instructions or ignore advice from their doctors. This can lead to adverse medication events, a worsening of medical conditions, and repeat visits to the hospital for the same problem. Second, patients with low health literacy are less likely to speak up or ask a question when something is amiss, which removes a source of protection against clinician errors. Finally, patients with low health literacy incur more costs than those with high literacy. This places an additional strain on already strapped health systems and diverts money from improvement initiatives.[44]

Health literacy is recognized as an important facet of patient safety, and improvements are already under way. Centers for health literacy have been created as a part of existing organizations and as free-standing groups. With these centers has come the position of consumer health librarian, an individual who creates community partnerships and teaches people to access and understand health information. Another point of focus is on making healthcare materials—prescription information, device recalls, and Web pages—simpler and easier to understand. Most sources of healthcare information are written at a college level, and many Americans' reading comprehension is below this. Advocates hope that by conducting outreach and making materials more accessible, the public can make better healthcare decisions.[42]

MAKING CARE SAFER THROUGH RESEARCH

It is impossible to overstate the importance of research to patient safety. One can speculate about the causes and consequences of medical errors, but scientific research provides a more concrete basis for large-scale changes in law and policy. Research also helps solve problems because it can answer questions about the nature, scope, and prevalence of an issue, as well as determine whether a certain process or policy is effective at preventing error. From preliminary investigations to meta-analyses, research is helping to improve patient safety. There is still much to be done, however. The importance of research for patient safety is well recognized, but the resources are limited. A large amount of research has been done, but there are still questions left to be answered and future projects that will require analysis.

EMERGING TRENDS

As an industry, health care is testing new tools to help improve patient safety. Risk management has historically focused on ameliorating damage once it occurs and minimizing legal retributions. Safety officers and risk management experts are focusing more on prevention as a result of the new emphasis on patient safety, being proactive and learning from close calls and near misses. Sharing these outcomes is imperative to improving the safe care of patients.

Many industries have identified teamwork as a critical factor in developing a culture of safety. Rather than praising clinicians exclusively for their individual skills and encouraging them to solve problems on their own, healthcare systems are emphasizing teamwork skills as important for clinical outcomes and preventing medical errors. Utilizing skills from other industries, team building has become an important tool in healthcare facilities. Working in teams puts an emphasis on an interdisciplinary approach to providing care to patients. Instead of working in silos, the emphasis is on collaborative care among physicians, patients, and the entire healthcare team.

Before the patient safety movement, responsibility for medical errors was considered to be solely that of the clinician. Slowly, this mindset is changing and there is a realization that breakdowns in the system are to be blamed for most medical errors.

TECHNOLOGY

From electronic health records to palm-scanning devices, many believe that new technology can help prevent medical errors. The Obama administration passed the Health Information Technology for Economic and Clinical Health (HITECH) Act[46] as part of the recently enacted stimulus bill, demonstrating its support of health information technology (HIT) as a means of addressing quality and cost issues. $19.2 billion allocated to motivate increased use of electronic health records, which in turn shall improve the processes of healthcare delivery documentation and record keeping for safer care. However, there is skepticism too that the lack of a completely integrated health information technology system is a risk to patient safety. The infrastructure does not allow for the plethora of systems to seamlessly integrate data, hence creating a gap in the patient record. An infrastructure to enable multiple care settings and systems to integrate data is the key to safer care.

CONCLUSIONS: WHERE WE STAND TODAY

Improving patient safety is a daunting task, not least of all because the well-being of millions is at stake. Most can agree on the importance of keeping patients safe, but the agreement often ends there. There is a plethora of proposed solutions, and we continue to search for solutions that will be accepted by all stakeholders. Compounding the problem is the fact that the body of knowledge gleaned from research is not always consistent. It varies tremendously in source, scope, and reliability. This is in part due to the nature of what we are trying to study—behavior is intensely subjective both for the performer and the observer—and in part because different research groups are seeking different results. It is commonly understood that being observed changes the nature of an action and that the way in which a question is phrased determines the nature of the answer received. Therefore, the different interests of stakeholder groups create different understandings of patient safety and different ideas about what action is necessary. The problem of patient safety can be stated thus: the pursuit for an understanding of the full scope of the problem and exact solutions remains a work in progress.

Despite these hurdles, the patient safety movement has made great strides. The central issues have been identified, which means that the healthcare industry now has a direction in which to focus in terms of research and policy developments. The system level weaknesses are evident, now the industry must agree on concrete solutions for conditions to change considerably. Additionally, there is a growing realization across different sectors that everyone has a stake in and responsibility for patient safety. There is an increasing emphasis on patient safety in areas such as patient engagement, health literacy, medication management, safer devices, prevention of healthcare acquired infections, and hospital acquired conditions. This development shows that different sectors of the healthcare industry are beginning to consider their roles in improving safety and understand how critical it is at each system juncture.

Creating change is always difficult. For all striving to create sustainable culture of safety, the below provides a solid foundation. The inaugural meeting of the LLI at NPSF, cast the vision for the transformation of the healthcare delivery system by proposing five key areas: transperancy, care integration, consumer engagement, restoration of joy and meaning in work, and medical education reform.[45] Stakeholders must be honest with themselves about shortcomings and willing to compromise with one another to make the necessary changes. It won't be easy, but with acceptance of the problem, transparency, cultural evolution, and a blame-free environment, patient safety will improve drastically.

References

1. Kohn LT, Corrigan JM, Donaldson MS, eds. *To Err Is Human: Building a Safer Health System*. Committee on Quality of Health Care in America, Institute of Medicine. Washington, DC: National Academy Press; 2000.

2. Partnerships for Patients. Available at: http://www.healthcare.gov/center/programs/partnership/index.html. Accessed December 15, 2011.
3. Wachter RM. Patient safety at ten: Unmistakable progress, troubling gaps. *Health Aff (Millwood)*. 2010 Jan-Feb;29(1):165–73.
4. List of Device Recalls. The Federal Food and Drug Administration. Available at: http://www.fda.gov/MedicalDevices/Safety/RecallsCorrectionsRemovals/ListofRecalls/default.htm. Accessed December 15, 2011.
5. "World Alliance for Patient Safety." Available at: www.who.org.
6. A Short History of the National Institutes of Health: Biologics. National Institutes of Health. Available at: http://history.nih.gov/exhibits/history/docs/page_03.html. Accessed December 14, 2011.
7. Significant Dates in U.S. Food and Drug Law History. U.S. Food and Drug Administration. Available at: http://www.fda.gov/AboutFDA/WhatWeDo/History/Milestones/ucm128305.htm. Accessed December 14, 2011.
8. *Crossing the Quality Chasm: A New Health System for the 21st Century*. Committee on Quality of Health Care in America, Institute of Medicine. Washington, DC: National Academy Press; 2001.
9. Preventing Medication Errors: Quality Chasm Series. Committee on Preventing and . . . 2006
10. http://www.ihi.org/about/Pages/InnovationsContributions.aspx
11. The Joint Commission History. Available at: http://www.jointcommission.org/assets/1/18/Joint_Commission_History_20111.PDF. Accessed December 14, 2011.
12. Facts About the Joint Commission. Available at: http://www.jointcommission.org/assets/1/18/The%20Joint%20Commission%203%207%2011.PDF. Accessed December 14, 2011.
13. Alder HC. 1993. Safe Medical Devices Act: management guidance for hospital compliance with the new FDA requirements. *Hospital Technology Series*. Vol. 12, no. 11. (October 1, 1993): 1.
14. Leape LL. Error in medicine. *JAMA*. 1994 Dec 21;272(23):1851–7.
15. NPSF Mission and Vision. Available at: http://www.npsf.org/about-us/mission-and-vision. Accessed June 23, 2012.
16. AHRQ Mission. Available at: http://www.ahrq.gov/about/stratpln.htm. Accessed. June 23, 2012.
17. About IHI. Available at: http://www.ihi.org/about/pages/default.aspx. Accessed June 23, 2012.
18. About Leapfrog. Available at: http://www.leapfroggroup.org/about_leapfrog. Accessed June 23, 2012.
19. National Patient Safety Goals. Available at: http://www.jcrinc.com/National-Patient-Safety-Goals/. Accessed December 14, 2011.
20. Safe Practices for Better Health Care Fact Sheet, AHRQ Publication No. 05-P007. Rockville, MD: Agency for Healthcare Research and Quality, March 2005.
21. The Patient Safety and Quality Improvement Act of 2005. Available at: http://www.ahrq.gov/qual/psoact.htm. Accessed December 14, 2011.
22. Making Care Safer. Available at: http://www.healthcare.gov/center/programs/partnership/safer/index.html. Accessed December 15, 2011.
23. Partnerships for Patients. Available at: http://www.healthcare.gov/center/programs/partnership/index.html. Accessed December 15, 2011.
24. Nieva VF, Sorra J. Safety culture assessment: A tol for improving patient safety in healthcare organizations. *Quality & Safety I Healthcare*. 2003;12:ii17-ii23.
25. The Safety Attitudes Questionnaire: psychometric properties, benchmarking data, and emerging research, John B Sexton1*, Robert L Helmreich1, Torsten B Neilands2, Kathy Rowan3, Keryn Vella3, James Boyden4, Peter R Roberts5 and Eric J Thomas, BMC Health Services Research 2006, 6:44 doi:10.1186/1472-6963-6-44.
26. What Is a Medication Error? Available at: http://www.nccmerp.org/aboutMedErrors.html. Accessed June 23, 2012.
27. Hafner JW, Belknap SM, Squillante MD, Buchelit KA. Adverse Drug Events in Emergency Department Patients. *Anals of Emergency Medicine*. 2002;39(3):258–267.
28. Hospital-Acquired Infections. Available at: http://emedicine.medscape.com/article/967022-overview. Accessed December 15, 2011.
29. About the World Health Organization. Available at: http://www.who.int/about/en/. Accessed June 23, 2012.

30. Healthcare-associated Infections: the Burden. Available at: http://www.cdc.gov/HAI/burden.html. Accessed December 15, 2011.
31. Methicillin-Resistant Staphylococcus aureus (MRSA) and Other Healthcare-Associated Infections. Available at: http://www.ncsl.org/default.aspx?tabid = 14084. Accessed December 15, 2011.
32. de Lissovoy G, Fraeman K, Hutchins V, Murphy D, Song D, Vaughn B. Surgical site infection: incidence and impact on hospital utilization and treatment costs. *American Journal of Infection Control*. 2009;37:5:387–397. Retrieved December 15, 2011 from SciVerse Science Direct database.
33. Healthcare-associated Infections: Infection Types. Available at: http://www.cdc.gov/HAI/infectionTypes.html. Accessed December 15, 2011.
34. Healthcare Infection Control Practices Advisory Committee. Available at: http://www.cdc.gov/hicpac/pubs.html. Accessed June 23, 2012.
35. World Health Organization. Prevention of Hospital-acquired Infections: a Practical Guide (2nd ed.). [document]. Ducel, G., Fabry, J., Nicolle, L. http://www.who.int/csr/resources/publications/whocdscsreph200212.pdf. 2002.
36. Mulloy DF, Hughes RG. Wrong-site Surgery: a Preventable Medical Error. In Patient Safety and Quality: An Evidence-Based Handbook for Nurses (ch. 36). Agency for Healthcare Research and Quality Publishing. 2008.
37. Total Number of Sentinel Events. Available at: http://www.jointcommission.org/assets/1/18/Stats_with_all_fields_hidden30September2010_(2).pdf. Accessed December 15, 2011.
38. Kwaan MR, Studdert D, Zinner M, Gawande A. Incidents, patterns and prevention of wrong-site surgery. *Archives of Surgery*. 2006;141:353–358.
39. Is the Product a Medical Device? Available at: http://www.fda.gov/MedicalDevices/DeviceRegulationandGuidance/Overview/ClassifyYourDevice/ucm051512.htm?utm_campaign = Google2&utm_source. Accessed June 23, 2012.
40. Is the Product a Medical Device? Available at: http://www.fda.gov/MedicalDevices/DeviceRegulationandGuidance/Overview/ClassifyYourDevice/ucm051512.htm. Accessed December 15, 2011.
41. List of Device Recalls. Available at: http://www.fda.gov/MedicalDevices/Safety/RecallsCorrectionsRemovals/ListofRecalls/default.htm. Accessed December 15, 2011.
42. McDonald C, Hernandez MB, Gofman Y, Schreier W. The five most common misdiagnoses: a meta-analysis of autopsy and malpractice data. *The Internet Journal of Family Practice*, 7(2). Accessed December 15, 2011.
43. Diagnostic Error in Acute Care. Pennsylvania Patient Safety Advisory, 7(3), 76–86. Available at: http://www.patientsafetyauthority.org/ADVISORIES/AdvisoryLibrary/2010/Sep7(3)/Pages/76.aspx. Accessed December 15, 2011.
44. Health Literacy. Available at: http://nnlm.gov/outreach/consumer/hlthlit. Accessed December 15, 2011.
45. Leape L, Berwick D, Clancy C, Conway J, Gluck P, Guest J, Lawrence D, Morath J, O'Leary D, O'Neill P, Pinakiewicz D, Isaac T. Lucian Leape Institute at the National Patient Safety Foundation. Transforming healthcare: a safety imperative. *Qual Saf Health Care*. 2009 Dec;18(6):424–8.

3

Accelerating Patient Safety Improvement

Thomas R. Krause, PhD and John Hidley, MD

INTRODUCTION

In this chapter, we argue that despite much activity, patient safety improvement has been surprisingly sluggish, and we describe an integrated strategic policy designed to accelerate improvement. The approach has three concurrent components: (1) establish a mandatory standard of patient safety performance that is valid, reliable, and universal in its application; (2) initiate specific interventions to improve the healthcare workplace and the safety of workers and patients; and (3) upgrade the knowledge and skills of healthcare leaders and workers to build organizational cultures of safety.

To pick up the pace of patient safety progress, execution of all three components is essential. To execute just one or two leaves gaps in reporting, gaps in safe and productive work environments, or gaps in cultural imperatives.

SLOW PROGRESS

At a recent conference for healthcare board members and CEOs, one of the conference organizers—a physician and CEO of one of the largest healthcare organizations in the United States—said the following: "My father is having surgery in the next month. I will be at the hospital and in his room because I fear that he will not receive the optimal care he deserves. I do not fear for his medical condition or the ability of his doctors to treat it, but I do fear for his safety in the hospital."

This is not an exceptional point of view among healthcare workers. The year 2009 marked the 10-year anniversary of the groundbreaking *To Err Is Human* report, published by the U.S. Academy of Sciences' Institute of Medicine (IOM).[1] The milestone report triggered assessments of how the healthcare industry has responded to the 1999 report's call for a national effort to reduce medical errors. Frustration, disappointment, and concern are the major findings:

- Lucian Leape et al.[2] laments that "the slow progress is not for want of trying."
- The Consumers Union[3] summarizes the situation this way: "Ten years later, we don't know if we've made any real

progress, and efforts to reduce the harm caused by our medical care system are few and fragmented."

- Stevens[4] says that healthcare is running out of excuses and notes that "the prescription from . . . patient safety leaders . . . seems to collide with inertia that defies explanation."

The picture is not entirely bleak. Perhaps Wachter's[5] is the most positive of the progress reports. He writes that patient safety at the 10-year mark has made "unmistakable progress," and he gives "safety efforts a grade of B–, a modest improvement since 2004 (the five-year anniversary)." He specifically praises The Joint Commission for developing its National Patient Safety Goals, the National Quality Forum for developing its *never events* list as the scaffolding for more robust and insightful reporting systems, and the 27 states that now require hospitals to report never events.

Wachter mentions other significant milestones as well:

- In 2004 the World Health Organization formed the World Alliance for Patient Safety (later renamed WHO Patient Safety).
- The Institute for Healthcare Improvement launched two massive nationwide campaigns to promote the use of patient safety interventions.
- The U.S. Congress authorized the creation of patient safety organizations to promote voluntary error reporting.
- The *New England Journal of Medicine* published the Michigan ICU study, which demonstrated significant reductions in catheter-related bloodstream infections through the use of an observation checklist and other interventions.
- In 2008 Medicare initiated its *no pay for errors* policy, the first use of the payment system to promote patient safety.

But note that most of these accomplishments are at the governmental level and have yet to drive universal patient safety improvement at the level of the individual healthcare institution, be it the system, hospital, or private practice.

Perhaps the intervention that has produced the most widespread benefit at the level of individual hospital practice is The Joint Commission's ongoing endeavor to institute and improve performance measures. In The Joint Commission's 2010 annual report on quality and safety,[6] substantial improvement is apparent among The Joint Commission accredited hospitals in their performance of their 24 accountability measures. Although these process measures represent only a narrow slice of patient safety exposure—they cover only five issues—the improvement they demonstrate is real. Nevertheless, the report also indicates that improvement is uneven and concludes that more improvement is needed.

One issue may be that hospital CEOs are not always comfortable in their role as patient safety leaders. A 2008 survey of hospital CEOs found few "feel strongly confident about practices in place to prevent or manage" patient safety incidents.[7] Seventy percent of the CEOs agreed that consumer concerns about safety in hospitals are justified and that very few patient safety interventions have focused on educating CEOs.

To summarize, although effort is being expended to improve patient safety, progress is slow. Too many healthcare institutions are deficient in the cultural values needed for patient safety improvement: mutual respect, teamwork, and transparency.[2] Healthcare leaders are far too timid about organizational cultural transparency. Workforce and training issues have been "surprisingly inert in recent years," and progress in nursing safety has been "surprisingly sparse."[8] These problems have resulted in calls to accelerate what Leape et al. describe as "sputtering progress."[2]

GETTING IN GEAR

Leaders understand the need for patient safety improvement. What is hard to understand is why change is so slow in coming. One way to understand this sluggish response is that broad societal norms implicitly condone the status quo, norms such as those manifested in comments like these:[9]

- The so-called patient safety crisis is exaggerated; we don't have a problem here.
- Health care is not like other industries; what works there won't necessarily work here.
- Medicine is an art; you can't just impose cookbook solutions.
- There may be a problem, but fixing it is not my job.
- The problem is complex and needs more study.
- We are already doing everything we can.
- Some adverse events are unavoidable.

To get beyond the status quo requires both healthcare and policy leadership committed to improvement. Leaders in other industries know that leaders create culture and what gets measured, gets done. These truisms lead to three practical recommendations for shifting patient safety improvement into high gear: (1) establish a mandatory standard of patient safety performance that is valid, reliable, and universal in its application; (2) initiate specific interventions to improve the safety of workers and patients and the healthcare workplace; and (3) upgrade the knowledge and skills of healthcare leaders and workers to build organizational cultures of safety.

All three components of this approach are essential and should be implemented concurrently. As previously noted, utilizing only one or two would leave gaps in reporting, safe and productive work environments, or cultural imperatives. Nevertheless, urgency is such that no one component should wait on the others.

The rationale for this strategy rests on three principles:

1. A mandatory, universal, and publicly accessible patient safety performance reporting metric, parallel in concept to the U.S. Bureau of Labor Statistics' annual report on workplace injuries and illnesses, will set the bar for driving improvement in both patient safety and worker safety.
2. Emphasizing the well-being of healthcare workers and their work conditions will engage workers in the effort and create needed consistency in safety climate and culture, at the same time improving quality of care and patient safety.[10]
3. Although the first two prongs of this strategy underwrite the development of a culture that fosters patient safety, building culture requires skills, knowledge, and abilities that local leaders may not have.

The use and ultimate success of this approach depends on the willingness of healthcare and policy leaders to confront and correct these issues:

- The lack of a nationally mandated, universal metric for patient safety performance[3] forfeits the meaningful context within which to drive patient safety performance.
- Health care is plagued by high rates of work injuries and illnesses, particularly back injuries and falls. These produce absences from work or restricted duty and affect operations, organizational culture, quality of care, and patient safety.[11]
- Barriers exist to institutional and physician commitment to patient safety, such as the absence of strong market incentives, lack of a budget line item for patient safety, lack of reimbursement to physicians for time spent on patient safety, vague guidelines about what constitutes a patient safety activity, insufficient physician and/or administrator buy in regarding the magnitude of the problem, and malpractice liability concerns and the litigious culture of blame that has a chilling effect on error reporting.[12]

A UNIVERSAL METRIC FOR PATIENT SAFETY

The 1999 Institute of Medicine's (IOM) report, *To Err Is Human*, propelled medical errors into the spotlight of public and policy-maker awareness. Among the report's strong recommendations was the proposal to create a mandatory reporting system for medical adverse events.[1] Today, variability remains rampant in the quality and utility of the healthcare safety measures used across geographic locations and delivery institutions.[13,14] There is no mandatory reporting system. We believe the lack of adequate metrics is a major impediment to patient safety progress and will remain so, absent a mandatory, standardized performance statistic.

Contrast this circumstance to the same need for standardization and benchmarking in almost any manufacturing, agricultural, maritime, construction, or service industry. Companies are required under the 1970 Occupational Safety and Health Act[15] to maintain a standard log and are periodically surveyed for their employee illness and injury statistics. These data encompass work-related deaths, injuries, and illnesses.

When the Department of Labor's Bureau of Labor Statistics (BLS) was delegated responsibility for developing this employee safety measurement system, it was not obvious how different types of injuries should be categorized and summarized. How should the severity of different types of injuries be handled? How should the variance in exposure between and within industries be dealt with? Many factors can influence counts and rates of injuries and illnesses in a given year.[15] Variability includes not only the year's injury and illness experience but also employer understanding of record-keeping guidelines. The number of injuries and illnesses reported in a given year can also be affected by changes in the level of economic activity, working conditions and practices, and worker demographics, experience, and training.

Despite such obstacles—which are notably similar to those faced today in patient safety—a system was developed and successfully implemented. Neither the inherent difficulty of this task nor difficulties due to variability of the data have impeded private industry's acceptance and use of the data. Today, information collected under this system is valued by industry, policy makers, the safety community, and employees.

The effect of the employee health and safety record-keeping and reporting mandate can be viewed in historical terms. From 1940 to 1970, work-related injury rates improved 45%, but after the creation of the Occupational Safety and Health Administration and its record-keeping requirements, rates improved by 75% from 1970 to 2000.[16] The earlier period saw a 42% improvement in work-related fatalities, but the subsequent OSHA-led period bested that with 78% improvement.[17]

Incidence rates permit comparison and fair competition in safety performance. Rates express various injury and illness events in terms of a constant: hours of exposure to the work environment (for example, 200,000 employee hours or the equivalent of 100 full-time employees working for one year). This creates a common statistical base across industries regardless of size or level of activity.[15] Rates are also useful for trending safety performance over time and comparing geographic variations in an industry's safety record.

National and state policy makers use the survey as an indicator of the magnitude of occupational safety and health problems. OSHA uses the statistics to help determine which industries clearly need to improve safety programs. The agency annually sends approximately 15,000 letters to workplaces with the highest rates of severe injuries and illnesses, namely those resulting in days away from work, restricted work activities, or job transfers. This metric is known as the DART rate. Employers receiving the letters are provided copies of their injury and illness data, along with a list of the most frequently cited OSHA standards for their specific industry. The letter offers assistance in reducing workplace injuries and illnesses by suggesting, among other things, the use of OSHA's free safety and health consultation services for small businesses provided through the states.[18]

OSHA also uses the data for targeted industry- or hazard-specific inspection programs, called national emphasis programs (NEP) and regional/local emphasis programs (REPs/LEPs). In July 2009, OSHA was operating seven NEPs focusing on amputations, lead, crystalline silica, shipbreaking, trenching/excavations, petroleum refinery process safety management, and combustible dust. OSHA also conducted approximately 140 REPs/LEPs.[19]

Within organizations, both labor and management use the estimates in evaluating safety programs. The log serves as an important source of information for employees regarding the safety and/or healthfulness of their workplace. OSHA requires that employees have direct access to the log and that companies post the summary of injuries and illnesses by February 1 of each year.[20] Other users include insurance carriers involved in workers' compensation, industrial hygienists, manufacturers of safety equipment, researchers, and others concerned with job safety and health.[15]

Within the industrial safety world these measures are viewed as essential. They provide support for or directly enable the following: [21,22]

- Distinguishing safety approaches that work from those that do not
- Tracking progress over time
- Pinpointing the effect on safety performance of organizational and process changes
- Analyzing cost–benefit performance
- Making judicious use of scarce resources
- Gaining and maintaining employee, management, and leadership support
- Pinpointing incidents that require further investigation and prioritizing issues that require attention
- Benchmarking with others with similar exposures and issues
- Supporting safety accountability processes

Health care likewise needs a mandatory metric to drive patient safety improvement and enable benchmarking.[1] We believe a widely shared patient safety metric will facilitate fair patient safety accountability and vigorous comparison and competition across organizations, just as the BLS data have generated for employee safety and health. We need the metric so we can set patient safety targets and create plans and budgets to achieve them, just like we do in occupational safety and health. We need it to measure progress, both within healthcare institutions and between them. And the metric needs to be mandatory. The IOM recognized that practitioners might be reluctant to voluntarily report medical mistakes. At the time of the IOM report, underutilization was a recognized, serious problem for error-reporting programs,[23] and in many institutions underreporting remains a serious problem today.

In the face of the missing mandatory metric, delivery organizations that are serious about improving patient safety improvise, but improvisation generates a hodgepodge of indicators that defy performance comparison across and within organizations, and fails to provide the many benefits of a standard metric described above. These measures range from simple incident counts to complex dashboards which allow for the aggregation and trending of data over time.

The mandatory metric for patient safety should be a simple set of standard outcome measures. An outcome metric is one that quantifies performance against the desired end result. Profit is an example of a financial outcome measure. One could not successfully operate a business without a measure of profit. Patient outcome measures are what the public needs to judge performance and what institutions need to drive performance and to develop and maintain a clear picture of their standing among peer organizations.[24]

The rate of sentinel events is an example of a patient safety outcome metric. The sentinel event rate and several other measures like it should be standardized and mandated. Doing this properly requires refining a taxonomy for adverse events with operational definitions and classification decision rules. Considerable work in this direction has already been accomplished. For example, excellent work has been done to develop chart-auditing protocols (trigger tools) that result in reliable incident counts for specific types of adverse events. Although time consuming and resource intensive when performed manually, this method can be automated in systems that use electronic health records, and it provides the raw incident data from which standard event rates can be computed.[25]

HEALTHCARE WORKER SAFETY

Employee safety metrics already exist and are well-tested in industry to quantify how well the organization performs on dimensions of worker safety outcomes. Health care, like all industry, tracks these measures. But, unlike other industries, health care does not use them effectively to drive organizational improvement.[10]

Access to health care is a recognized problem in the industry. There is increasing recognition that patient safety performance and access to health care are linked through healthcare worker well-being. Both the access problem and patient safety difficulties are compounded by staff shortages due to morale problems and time lost to injuries, illness, and long-term disability, as well as by the increased demands on staff of quarantines for hospital-acquired infections.[10]

Joseline Sikorski, president and CEO of the Ontario Safety Association for Community and Healthcare (OSACH), states:[26]

> The health care sector must make a fundamental shift to equate worker safety with patient safety. It must also make this shift a strategic priority if it is to deliver exemplary patient care and ensure the health and safety of workers, patients and the public. Failure to do so puts the sector at risk and makes it vulnerable to crises.

In the United States, more than three-quarters of respondents in a 2001 survey conducted by the American Nurses Association indicated that unsafe conditions interfere with nurses' ability to deliver high-quality care.[27] Bureau of Labor Statistics data on healthcare worker safety underline the extent of the problem and highlight the need to focus time and resources on employee health and safety. In 2008, the most recent year for which data are available, hospitals had a total recordable incidence rate of 7.6 cases per 100 equivalent full-time workers. That is double the national average for all of private industry (which is only 3.9 cases).[19] The total recordable case rate for nursing and residential care facilities is even higher: 8.4 cases per 100 full-time workers.

Moreover, injuries and illnesses in health care are more serious than in other industries. The DART rate (injuries requiring days away from work or job restriction or transfer) for hospital employees is 3.0 per 100 workers compared to only 2.0 for workers in other industries. For nursing and residential care facilities, the DART rate is 5.0. Nursing aides, orderlies, and attendants suffered more DART cases (44,610) in 2008 than construction workers (31,310) and required a median of five days to recuperate. This clearly represents a substantial unnecessary drain on staffing.

Of particular concern in health care are injuries involving musculoskeletal disorders (MSD). Healthcare support occupations were one of seven occupational categories with an MSD-related DART case rate three times greater than the all-worker rate. Among healthcare workers, MSD cases relating to the back caused on average five lost workdays; the shoulder, eight; the arm, eight; the wrist, six; and the knee, 11. Lifts and transfers of patients using awkward postures, adverse psychosocial aspects of work such as high job demands with low decision authority and job control, and low social support and low job satisfaction at work are all deemed to contribute.[10]

For many years, other industry sectors have recognized a connection between a safe, engaged workforce and excellent customer care.[22] These sectors have pursued systems and processes to ensure employee safety and well-being, often implementing the *hierarchy of controls*. This model, which is enforced by OSHA, calls for first engineering out the hazard. If that is not feasible, administrative controls such as rotating employees in and out of jobs with hazardous exposures should be used. If administrative controls are not feasible, the last line of defense is the use of personal protective equipment.

These methods are often not standard practice in health care. Reasons for this include:[26]

- Workplace health and safety is infrequently understood or addressed as a strategic priority by healthcare boards of directors, leadership, and management.
- Often there is limited sustained leadership commitment and allocation of adequate health and safety resources.
- Health and safety resources often are not aligned with corporate planning and the budgeting cycle.
- Health care has a well-entrenched, hierarchical, and tradition-bound professional and organizational culture that does not view safety as an important value.
- There is often fragmented accountability and inadequate communication of health and safety matters in healthcare settings.
- Often there is an absence of comprehensive corporate analysis to identify, monitor, mitigate, and manage health and safety risks.
- The healthcare workplace has complex, trained groups of professionals who have experienced different training and who are used to working independently and in silos.
- There is limited cross-enterprise communication on solution management.

More research on the linkages between employee and patient safety are needed, and some studies are indeed under way. Projects include investigating the effect of working conditions in ICUs on elderly patient outcomes and the safety and health of healthcare workers, and assessing how staffing levels and other organizational parameters act as risk factors for injury for both patients and workers in acute- and long-term care facilities.[28]

In terms of intervention, performance improvement requires systematic feedback, whether the performance area is patient or employee safety.[9,24] Methods from industrial engineering can be adapted to health care to improve both quality of care and employee safety.[29] By viewing patient and employee safety as different manifestations of the same issue, health care would benefit from increased employee engagement in patient safety, higher employee morale, intervention synergies, a more cohesive culture, more coherent vision of safety, and greater bang for the intervention buck.

A HEALTHCARE CULTURE OF SAFETY

Measurement, as we have stressed, plays a central role in driving performance. But it is not the sole driver.[2] Culture is pivotal to both a high level of performance and its sustainability. Creating a culture of safety is a difficult leadership challenge,[8] and part of the challenge consists of leadership understanding culture and how leadership practices shape organizational culture.[9] The first step in culture change is not to give another survey on the climate for safety but to understand what unspoken assumptions are being made that create the culture leaders want to change.

What unspoken assumptions underlie the lack of attention to patient and worker safety? Such assumptions involve what healthcare institutions expect from their people and from leadership. "Medical practitioners have their own view of the world," writes Dr. Robert Wachter and Dr. Kaveh G. Shojania in *Internal Bleeding*. "We speak of the art of medicine . . . teamwork, checklists, standard operating procedures, systems thinking—none of that comes naturally to us."[30] Many physicians are dead set against giving up their autonomy and authority for what some call *cookbook medicine*, although this is emphatically not what patient and employee safety actually requires of them.

Interestingly, the first author found a similar cultural dynamic at NASA after the Columbia tragedy. At NASA we found brilliant scientists who were genuinely motivated to accomplish nearly impossible tasks, who took on challenges with enthusiasm, and who inadvertently compromised safety in the process.[22] Wachter calls these same traits in medical personnel, "hubris, elitism, and wishful thinking."[30] In health care, as at NASA, these sentiments are understandable, and they have served a purpose in fostering individual rigor and dedication among healthcare providers. They explain why many healthcare providers take personal responsibility for medical errors, why they are personally demanding, prone to blame, and inclined to fire employees who make mistakes. These traits produce individual excellence but are maladaptive for optimal health care as a system, and they set up a culture that supports heroes but impedes safety.[9,30,31] The good news in all this is that worker safety and patient safety are inextricably linked and can be used to motivate culture change.

The leading attributes of organizational culture that influence operational performance—the credibility of management, procedural justice, and receptiveness to upward communication—also drive outcomes in both patient and worker safety.[32,33,34] Improvement tools needed to address patient safety are the same tools and strategies needed to address worker safety, and both can be used by leaders with cultural know-how to foster and sustain an organizational culture that supports safety: root cause analysis, behavioral observation and feedback, assessment of safety leadership capability, cultural diagnostics, and powerful intervention design.

CONCLUSION

The opportunity exists to shift patient safety into drive with the three-pronged strategic policy described here. A universal and mandatory patient safety outcome metric is required, and health institutions should transparently post worker and patient incident frequencies. Reinvigorated initiatives to improve worker safety and combine or coordinate them with patient safety will engage patient well-being and improve quality of care and employee well-being. The third and crucial element of the strategy is supporting leadership's systematic analysis of the organization's culture and upgrading the culture-shaping skills of leaders.

References

1. Kohn L. T., Corrigan, J. M., Donaldson, M. S. (Eds.), for Committee on Quality of Health Care in America and Institute of Medicine (1999). *To err is human*. Washington, DC: National Academies Press.
2. Leape, L., Berwick, D., Clancy, C., Conway, J., Gluck, P., Guest, J., . . . Isaac, T. (2009). Transforming healthcare: A safety imperative. *Quality & Safety in Health Care, 10*, 424–428.
3. Consumers Union Safe Patient Project. *To err is human—To delay is deadly*. Retrieved from http://cu.convio.net/site/PageNavigator/spp_To_Delay_Is_Deadly_Executive_Summary.
4. Stevens, D. P. (2010). Safe healthcare: We're running out of excuses. *Postgraduate Medicine Journal, 86*, 129–130.
5. Wachter, R. M. (2010). Patient safety at ten: Unmistakable progress, troubling gaps. *Health Affairs, 29*(1), 1–9.

6. The Joint Commission. (2010). *Improving America's hospitals—The Joint Commission's annual report on quality and safety*. Retrieved from http://www.jointcommission.org/annualreport.aspx.
7. VHA Foundation. (2008, May 6). *New survey finds that hospital CEOs recognize patients' safety concerns, but lack confidence about best ways to create safer environment*. Retrieved from https://www.vhafoundation.org/PressReleases/Pages/NewSurveyFindsthatHospitalCEOs.aspx.
8. Wachter, R. M. (2008). *Understanding patient safety*. New York: McGraw-Hill.
9. Krause, T. R., & Hidley, J. H. (2009). *Taking the lead in patient safety: How healthcare leaders influence behavior and create culture*. Hoboken, NJ: Wiley.
10. Yassi, A., & Hancock, T. (2005). Patient safety-worker safety: Building a culture of safety to improve healthcare worker and patient well-being. *Healthcare Quarterly, 8*, 32–38.
11. U.S. Department of Labor, Bureau of Labor Statistics. (2009). *Workplace injury and illness summary*. Retrieved from http://www.bls.gov/news.release/osh.nr0.htm.
12. Devers, K. J., Pham, H. H., & Liu, G. (2004). What is driving hospitals' patient-safety efforts? *Health Affairs, 23*(2), 103–115.
13. U.S. Department of Health and Human Services, Agency for Healthcare Research and Quality. (2008). *2007 national healthcare quality report*. Retrieved from http://archive.ahrq.gov/qual/nhqr07/nhqr07.pdf.
14. U.S. Department of Health and Human Services, Agency for Healthcare Research and Quality. (2008). *2007 national healthcare disparities report*. Retrieved from http://archive.ahrq.gov/qual/nhdr07/nhdr07.pdf.
15. U.S. Department of Labor, Bureau of Labor Statistics. (1997). *BLS Handbook of Methods* Chapter 9: Occupational Safety and Health Statistics. Retrieved from http://www.bls.gov/opub/hom/homch9.htm.
16. National Safety Council. *Injury facts: 2005–2006*, pp. 36–37. Itasca, IL: National Safety Council. Retrieved from https://www.usw12775.org/uploads/InjuryFacts08Ed.pdf.
17. National Safety Council. *Accident facts: 1997*, p. 49. Itasca, IL: National Safety Council. Retrieved from https://www.usw12775.org/uploads/InjuryFacts08Ed.pdf.
18. U.S. Department of Labor, Occupational Safety and Health Administration. (2010). *US Labor Department's OSHA notifies 15,000 workplaces nationwide of high injury and illness rates*. Retrieved from http://ehssafetynews.com/2010/03/10/.
19. U.S. Department of Labor, Occupational Safety and Health Administration. (2009). *Site-specific targeting 2009* (SST-09). Retrieved from http://www.osha.gov/pls/oshaweb/owadisp.show_document?p_table = DIRECTIVES&p_id = 4002.
20. Seligman, P. J., Sieber, W. K., Pedersen, D. H., Sundin, D. S., & Frazier, T. M. (1988). Compliance with OSHA record-keeping requirements. *American Journal of Public Health, 78*(9), 1219.
21. Petersen, D. (2006). The problem with macro measures. *Industrial Safety & Hygiene News, 40*(10), 110.
22. Krause, T. R. (2005). *Leading with safety*. Hoboken, NJ: Wiley.
23. Yale Journal of Health Policy, Law, and Ethics Editorial Staff. (2008). A national survey of medical error reporting laws. *Yale Journal of Health Policy, Law, and Ethics, IX*(1), 202–286.
24. Pronovost, P., Nolan, T., Zeger, S., Miller, M., & Rubin, H. (2004). How can clinicians measure safety and quality in acute care? *Lancet, 363*, 1064.
25. For example, see Eckstrand, J. A., Habib, A. S., Williamson, A., Horvath, M. M., Gattis, K. G., Cozart, H., & Ferranti, J. (2009). Computerized surveillance of opioid-related adverse drug events in perioperative care: A cross-sectional study. *Patient Safety in Surgery, 3*,18.
26. Sikorski, J. (2009). Connecting worker safety to patient safety: A new imperative for health-care leaders. *Ivey Business Journal*. Retrieved from http://wwwold.iveybusinessjournal.com/article.asp?intArticle_ID = 808.
27. American Nurses Association. (2002). *Analysis of American Nurses Association staffing survey*. Warwick, RI: Cornerstone Communications Group. Retrieved from http://ana.nursingworld.org/MainMenuCategories/OccupationalandEnvironmental/occupationalhealth/HealthSafetySurvey.aspx.

28. U.S. Department of Health and Human Services, Agency for Healthcare Research and Quality. (2002). *Impact of working conditions on patient safety*. Retrieved from http://www.ahrq.gov/news/workfact.htm.
29. Brennan, T. A., & Berwick, D. M. (1996). *New rules: Regulation markets and the quality of American health care*. San Francisco: Jossey-Bass.
30. Wachter, R. M., & Shojania, K. G. (2004). *Internal bleeding: The truth behind America's terrifying epidemic of medical mistakes*. New York, NY: Rugged Land.
31. Bohmer, R. M. J. (2009). *Designing care: Aligning the nature and management of health care*. Cambridge, MA: Harvard Business Press.
32. Coyle-Shapiro, J., Kessler, I., & Purcell, J. (1985). Reciprocity or "it's my job": Exploring organizationally directed citizenship behavior in a national health service setting. *Journal of Applied Psychology, 70*, 777–781.
33. Mark, B., & Hoffman, D. A. (2006). An investigation of the relationship between safety climate and medication errors as well as other nurse and patient outcomes. *Personnel Psychology, 9*, 847–869.
34. Katz-Navon, T., Naveh, E., & Stern, Z. (2005). Safety climate in healthcare organizations: A multidimensional approach. *Academy of Management Journal, 48*, 1075–1089.

4

The Importance of Leadership to Advance Patient Safety

Barbara Balik, RN, EdD

The signature of mediocrity is not the unwillingness to change. It is chronic inconsistency.

Jim Collins[1]

The consistent behaviors of senior leaders create organizational results. Safer outcomes for patients stem from the consistent behaviors of senior leaders and all who work with them in the unrelenting pursuit of safer, more reliable care. Studies inside and outside health care identify the powerful role of leaders in creating environments where others thrive.[2–6] Ultimately, senior leaders and the boards of directors of healthcare organizations are accountable for the safety of those who entrust us with their care. The behaviors of senior leaders and boards prevent harm and save lives.

National quality organizations and regulatory bodies such as the National Quality Forum and The Joint Commission are growing in their emphasis on leadership accountabilities for safe, reliable care as well as excellence in the experience of care. Healthcare reform adds intensity to changes in how care is provided, its outcomes, and its value for which leaders are held accountable.

Healthcare leaders often distinguish between organizational accountability for business outcomes (market share, financial performance, bond rating, and capital projects) and accountability for clinical quality and safety outcomes. The more traditional business aspects are clearly viewed as senior leader accountability whereas clinical quality and safety are frequently seen as the responsibility of clinical team members and clinical executives. The result is delegation of these essential aspects of healthcare delivery solely to clinical leaders. In short, many healthcare leaders display a mindset that says they take care of the business end and clinicians take care of the clinical end.

This mindset does not stem from lack of concern about safe patient care. Leaders frequently voice concerns about the safety of care in their organizations but acknowledge they lack the skills to know where to begin, to know where this work fits with the myriad of other demands on them, and to know how to sustain the difficult, complex work of safer care. The distinction between leadership for business aspects of care and accountability for quality and safety creates gaps in leadership behavior and resulting gaps in safety outcomes.

In this chapter, specific behaviors drawn from relevant literature are provided to aid leaders, senior executives, midlevel leaders, and governing boards in developing their skills to achieve safer care. This chapter will describe both what to do—the tactics—and how to do it—the personal and specific behaviors used as a reflective leader—to achieve different outcomes.

DEFINITION: LEADERS

The content focuses on the senior executive team and board of directors. Senior leaders include the chief executive officer, chief nurse officer, chief medical officer, chief finance officer, chief patient safety officer/quality officer, administrator, and the board of directors of the organization. Ultimately, the behaviors exhibited by leaders that advance safety in an organization must be present in all leaders throughout the organization. Frontline clinical leaders—nurses, pharmacists, physicians, imaging, and others—are crucial in translating organizational vision into daily action. It requires committed senior leaders, informed and challenging boards, and talented frontline leaders to achieve safer care.

DEFINITION: HEALTHCARE ORGANIZATION

All healthcare organizations—hospitals, clinics, outpatient and ambulatory centers, and other community-based care settings including home care, hospice, and skilled nursing facilities—are included in the scope of this chapter. Leadership behavior transcends settings and pertains to the complexity of healthcare services. The growing emphasis on safe, effective cross-continuum care demands that competency within an individual setting is not enough. Cross-continuum competency is a new leadership requirement for excellence in care.

HOW TO USE THE CONTENT

Options for use of the content include:

- Content for board retreats and ongoing board development.
- Leadership development in structured formats—organized groups of leaders using a facilitated process for self-assessment and action planning. This is followed by ongoing assessment through individual and group reflection, practice developing clear behavior changes, progress on action steps, and ultimately improved safety results.
- Lighting the path for others to follow: individual use for self-assessment, identifying key areas for change, and coaching for positive behaviors.
- Development of dramatically revamped leadership recruitment, hiring, evaluation, promotion, and recognition systems. Hiring and promoting for demonstrated patient safety values is a powerful means of changing organizational safety culture. This requires extensive revision of most existing human resources practices and policies.

ANOTHER WAY

> Here is Edward Bear, coming downstairs now, bump, bump, bump, on the back of his head, behind Christopher Robin. It is, as far as he knows, the only way of coming downstairs, but sometimes he feels that there really is another way, if

> only he could stop bumping for a moment and think of it.
>
> **—Winnie-the-Pooh**

There is no magic place to start the journey of performance excellence in healthcare safety leadership. The key is to recognize that the current state is intolerable and there is another way to lead for safe care. Optimally, this would be led by the board of directors.

BOARD OF DIRECTORS LEADERSHIP OF QUALITY AND SAFETY

The Institute for Healthcare Improvement (IHI) developed content called Boards on Board with the launch of the 100,000 Lives Campaign in December 2006. In addition to several demonstrated clinical interventions to save lives, IHI recognized that without commitment to the safety and well-being of patients by the highest level of healthcare leadership, the ambitious aims would not be achieved or sustained. Since then hundreds of governing board members have participated in development that clearly outlines their accountabilities and the actions required to fulfill them.

The reframing of governing accountability for all quality and safety outcomes—not solely financial, capital, and market growth—has been a revolutionary discovery for many board members. At times it has even been frightening, when as one board member put it, "We don't know what we don't know! I'm not a clinician. How am I supposed to evaluate our clinical care and safety?" Board member development focuses on four key areas. See Figure 4.1.

The key areas are reviewed in detail.

Governance Role and Accountability for Safety

> Governance is ultimately accountable for safe patient care.
>
> Governance is responsible for identifying patient safety as an organizational imperative and ensuring that resources necessary for the delivery of safe care are available.
>
> Executive and clinical leaders are accountable for developing and implementing systems that assure safe care is provided, for modeling commitment and engagement in achieving patient safety within their organizations.
>
> From the bedside to the board room, patient safety goals, measurement, and improvement processes must be aligned throughout the organization.[7]

The National Patient Safety Foundation (NPSF) principles, endorsed by the NPSF Board in 2007, succinctly assign governance and executive leadership accountability for safe care. A variety of materials are available to aid governing boards in taking the next steps to put the principles into action. In addition to the NPSF Stand Up for Patient Safety materials, the IHI developed a how-to guide widely used to aid boards in fulfilling their commitment to achieving safe, effective care in their communities.

The following content from the IHI's *Governance Leadership How-To Guide* provides steps for boards to take to achieve their accountabilities.[8]

> I think that we should declare 2007 "The Year of Governance" and start to put back on the table of the boards not just a request, but an absolute sense of obligation, thatw learning who does better and then doing at least that well is central to proper stewardship of health care. Until leaders own that problem, I don't think spread is going to happen. The buck stops in the board room.
>
> **—Donald Berwick[9]**

> Leaders are responsible for everything in the organization, especially everything that goes wrong.
>
> —**Paul O'Neill, Former Secretary of the Treasury and Chairman and CEO of Alcoa**

Assessment of Specific Behaviors to Govern for Safety

Boards can begin or continue their development through self-assessment as part of the evaluation of their board effectiveness. The board self-assessment tool, based on the Six Things All Boards Should Do (see Figure 4.2), is one effective means to assess current status and progress of the board in leading quality and safety. The intent of the tool is to provide specific behaviors to discuss and to reflect on their actions as a board. After completing the tool, the focus is not on the score but on why members scored the assessment tool the way they did and the questions the tool raises. Questions may include "How do we know we have set specific aims to reduce harm?" "How often have we heard a patient story?" "Why haven't we heard a story directly from a patient rather than stories relayed to us by a staff member?"

Board Self-Assessment Tool

For each of the items in Figure 4.3, discuss and then rate your board's performance on a scale of 0 to 5 where 0 indicates the board has not begun an effort with this item and 5 indicates that the board is performing routinely at a high level.

FIGURE 4.1 Board Development Focuses on Four Key Areas

Their overall governance role and accountability for safety and quality
Assessment of specific behaviors to govern for safety and quality
Questions designed to understand the safety strategy and policy implementation
Safety science and just culture skills

Questions Designed for Board Members to Understand the Safety Strategy and Policy Implementation Within the Organization

An additional tool to assist boards is a list of sample questions to use during review of quality/safety reports and program proposals. The questions are especially helpful for boards that may be early in the journey of leading for quality and safety.

Community board members are often intimidated by a lack of clinical background, asking "How can I evaluate the reports provided and the outcomes of care when I am not a clinician?" Community board members may also overly defer to clinicians since they are not clinical experts, thus missing the opportunity to challenge and understand the strategies and policies at work.

Board members may need reassurance of the expertise they bring—expertise of an informed, concerned community member who has the capacity to ask pertinent questions on behalf of the larger community he or she represents. It is the obligation of senior leaders and those sharing information with the board to translate terms so that everyone can understand. Clinicians do this type of translation with patients and families they work with to be successful in communicating healthcare information to lay people. They can apply these same translation skills with board members. If they are unable to provide clear, unambiguous information, it signals a problem with those sharing the information, not with board members' grasp of it.

The sample questions in Figure 4.4 provide a starting point for developing board confidence in asking challenging questions on the path to safety. Executive and midlevel

FIGURE 4.2 Six Things All Boards Should Do[10]

Goal

Boards of trustees in all hospitals will undertake the six key governance leadership activities to improve quality and reduce harm in their hospitals recommended in this Guide. At a minimum, boards should start by spending more than 25% of their meeting time on quality and safety issues and by conducting, as a full board, a conversation with at least one patient, or family member of a patient, who sustained serious harm at their institution within the past year.

Six Things All Boards Should Do

1. **Setting Aims:** Set a specific aim to reduce harm this year. Make an explicit, public commitment to measurable quality improvement (e.g., reduction in unnecessary mortality and harm), establishing a clear aim for the facility or system.
2. **Getting Data and Hearing Stories:** Select and review progress toward safer care as the first agenda item at every board meeting, grounded in transparency, and putting a "human face" on harm data.
3. **Establishing and Monitoring System-Level Measures:** Identify a small group of organization-wide "roll-up" measures of patient safety (e.g., facility-wide harm, risk-adjusted mortality) that are continually updated and are made transparent to the entire organization and all of its customers.
4. **Changing the Environment, Policies, and Culture:** Commit to establish and maintain an environment that is respectful, fair, and just for all who experience the pain and loss as a result of avoidable harm and adverse outcomes: the patients, their families, and the staff at the sharp end of error.
5. **Learning . . . Starting with the Board:** Develop your capability as a board. Learn how "best in the world" boards work with executive and physician leaders to reduce harm. Set an expectation for similar levels of education and training for all staff.
6. **Establishing Executive Accountability:** Oversee the effective execution of a plan to achieve your aims to reduce harm, including executive team accountability for clear quality improvement targets.

leadership should spend time answering the questions before the board conversation. The questions add to the common understanding of the current safety culture.

Safety Science and Just Culture Skills

Beginning with the quality committee of the board, develop basic skills in safety science and just culture taught by executive leaders. Teach safety science and just culture skills based on a hypothetical or real case and teaching tools used within the organization. Board members do not need to be experts in these skills, but as they receive quality/safety reports, especially of sentinel events, claims reports, and other critical events, their skills in safety science and just culture will reinforce the behaviors in senior leaders.

Quality committee members then need to teach the skills to all board members. Each quality/safety report is an opportunity to reinforce and deepen skills in all board members.

FIGURE 4.3 Board Self-Assessment Tool[10]

Element	Assessment					
	0	1	2	3	4	5
Setting Aims: Set a specific aim to reduce harm this year. Make an explicit, public commitment to measurable quality improvement (e.g., reduction in unnecessary mortality and harm), establishing a clear aim for the facility or system.						
Getting Data and Hearing Stories: Select and review progress toward safer care as the first agenda item at every board meeting, grounded in transparency, and putting a "human face" on harm data.						
Establishing and Monitoring System-Level Measures: Identify a small group of organization-wide "roll-up" measures of patient safety (e.g., facility-wide harm, risk-adjusted mortality) that are continually updated and are made transparent to the entire organization and all of its customers.						
Changing the Environment, Policies, and Culture: Commit to establish and maintain an environment that is respectful, fair, and just for all who experience the pain and loss as a result of avoidable harm and adverse outcomes: the patients, their families, and the staff at the sharp end of error.						
Learning . . . Starting with the Board: Develop your capability as a board. Learn how "best in the world" boards work with executive and physician leaders to reduce harm. Set an expectation for similar levels of education and training for all staff.						
Establishing Executive Accountability: Oversee the effective execution of a plan to achieve your aims to reduce harm, including executive team accountability for clear quality improvement targets.						

LEADERSHIP BEHAVIORS FOR SAFETY

> We are all faced with a series of great opportunities—brilliantly disguised as insoluble problems.
>
> —**John Gardner**

The question of leadership behaviors for safety arises when current progress toward safety is examined. More than a decade ago, *To Err Is Human*,[10] with its call to reduce deaths from preventable medical errors, ignited a renewed focus on and vigor for safety and quality improvement, accompanied by a wide range of proven processes and evidence-based practices with the potential to reach that goal. What has happened since that landmark Institute of Medicine report? Nationally, the number of people who die annually from medical errors is estimated to be as high or higher than previously thought,[11] and the gap between identifying a life-saving, evidence-based practice and its full implementation is a staggering 17 years.[12] How can so little have changed when the tools, processes, and knowledge to improve safety and quality of care are far more widely known than a decade ago? And why do some healthcare organizations stand out positively in safety, quality performance, engagement, and financial health?

Executive leaders rarely ignore the imperative of safe care in their organizations but struggle with the immensity of the problems, the lack of skills to design safe systems, where this work fits with the myriad of other demands, and how to sustain the difficult, complex work of safer care. Given these struggles, it is easy to understand why other activities, all of pressing concern, can crowd out time and attention to safety.

This question of why some succeed when others struggle with competing demands and requirements for new skills stimulated a study intended to understand healthcare leaders with transformational results in quality, safety, and other domains of organizational outcomes. The authors[6] predicted that it was not about the tools, processes, and knowledge that are available, but rather it is about the focus and implementation shaped by a certain kind of leadership that produces and sustains dramatic improvement in safety, quality, financial condition, and organizational vitality. The work sought to understand and describe what is distinct in this leadership by interviewing 10 transformational leaders and those who work with them, then presenting in their own words their background, experience, and what is at the heart of their leadership. None of the leaders interviewed or those who work with them will say they are perfect—far from it. They continue to challenge themselves as leaders. Transformational leaders have a compelling story to tell about leadership for safety.

The study echoes findings by Collins, Keroack, Kouzes and Posner in describing what effective leaders do.[2,5,13] For example, Keroack and colleagues describe behaviors associated with better quality and safety outcomes in academic health centers. This research reinforces findings from leadership literature that link behaviors and outcomes. Leadership studies offer a *both/and* option for leaders. Leaders can ensure both safer care *and* better operational functioning. In short, these studies uncovered key characteristics that illustrate leadership behaviors for results—not solely safety results but overall organizational performance. They noted that not only did leadership make a *difference* in patient outcomes; leadership is *essential* for the outcomes to which we aspire. This study is highly consistent with other well-researched assessments of leadership and high performance (see Resources). This is an imperative in the demanding, chaotic healthcare world undergoing dramatic reform.

MODEL FOR LEADING AND SUSTAINING TRANSFORMATIONAL CHANGE

In the study, strong common themes were found among those interviewed. They are represented in Figure 4.5. Of the themes identified, a dominant thread weaves together the personal passion for patient care (their own and others in the organization) *and* the organization's vision and goals. Not every one of these leaders is a great speaker. But they all speak from the heart and communicate what is important to the organization in words that listeners can hear and connect with. In so doing, they touch the hearts and minds of others at all levels in every role. This attribute is pervasive and resonates beyond any single theme.

At the heart of the model are four shared personal characteristics—what makes them tick as they perform their role as leaders. The next circle shows the organizational characteristics they foster—how their personal characteristics express in organizational action. At the head of the model are the major outcomes in performance their organizations produce. From the authors' view, it all adds up to what is expressed as a "single brain" organization whose aim is that every person, every process, every system, and every action is focused on the vision and mission and is reflective of the values of the organization.[6]

Personal Characteristics

The most important point the authors make about the personal characteristics is that

FIGURE 4.4 Board and Board Quality Committee Questions: Fostering a High Bar in Innovation in Clinical and Leadership Processes

- Who is the best in the world at this service, program, or intervention?
  - How close are we to that performance?
- What would the theoretical limit of performance look like (e.g., zero surgical site infections, 100% completion of the WHO surgical checklist)?
- What plans do we have to close the gap between our current performance and the best in the world or theoretical limit?
- Is this a transformational change to achieve safe care?
  - What measures would help us to know that it is?
- How do we demonstrate evidence-based practice in clinical and leadership processes to enable safe outcomes?
- How do we know something expected happened? What happens when something unexpected occurs? Who knows about it when it happens?
- How do we know leaders, staff, and providers have adequate skills to solve safety problems in daily work?
- How do we know we have enough resources devoted to achieving safe care? How are resources aligned to achieve best safe practices?
- What is a recent example of spread of safety learning across the organization (or healthcare system) from other healthcare settings (e.g., What adverse event at another setting have we learned from in the past three months?)?
- Define what we mean by a safety culture.
  - How do we measure our safety culture?
  - Do we demonstrate principles of justice and fairness in our culture?
  - What do our employee and provider engagement surveys tell us about their view of our safety culture?
- What is our definition of respectful behavior?
  - What standards for respectful behavior do we have for all providers and staff?
  - What examples do we have of addressing disrespectful behavior?
  - Is it a fair and consistent process?
- The National Quality Forum's 30 Safe Practices for Better Healthcare expects team behavior at all levels.
  - How are we doing in team development?
  - How do we know if we are getting better or worse?
  - What are the biggest challenges?
- How do we actively involve patients and families in all aspects of our work to achieve safety (e.g., program design, improvement teams, listen to them and stop 100% of the time if they raise a safety concern)?
- How are safe practices incorporated into the credentialing and recredentialing process for medical staff?
  - How do we know if the safe practice metrics which are measured as part of the credentialing and recredentialing process are reliable in ensuring safe care?

FIGURE 4.4 Board and Board Quality Committee Questions: Fostering a High Bar in Innovation in Clinical and Leadership Processes (*Continued*)

  - What about respectful communication and team skills?
  - Do we require simulation proficiency with high-risk procedures?
- Where are our biggest gaps in safe practices?
  - What is under way to achieve best safe practices?
- How are the human resources systems aligned to support safe care (e.g., hiring for values, safety training, just culture)?
- Why were results flat in the last quarter?
  - What are we doing to improve our results in safe care?
- How are we linking quality, safety, regulatory, and risk activities?

For Program and Capital Design Projects:

- What patients/family members sat at the table in the design of this program or capital project?
- Are patient/family needs met in this program?
  - How do we know?
- What is the ROI for quality/safety on this project?

When Things Go Wrong:

- What actions do we take when something goes wrong in care?
  - Do we apologize every time?
  - How do we train people to apologize to patients/families?
  - Who speaks to the patient/family?
  - How quickly do we talk to them?
- How do we learn from the causal analysis?
  - How do we communicate this information so everyone can learn?
- Could an incident in another healthcare organization happen here?
  - What have we done to learn from their safety event?
- What are we doing differently as a result of that lawsuit?
- Is the frequency of claims declining?
- What are our financial settlement principles when harm has occurred that we caused? How do we avoid conflict between our settlement principles (as it was correct) and physicians?

they are not what these leaders *do* (a role they play); it is *who they are*. These characteristics pervade their lives and their leadership in every context, every conversation, whomever they are speaking to—the board, a housekeeping aide, a physician, the community—and are as natural to them as breathing.

A description of the personal characteristics and examples are listed in Figure 4.6. Each example begins with a quote from a colleague inside the organization.

The organizational chart these leaders work with may look similar to other charts, but the areas the organizations emphasize and the action of the CEOs to create this emphasis are distinct and fuel their effectiveness and success. The organizational characteristics they foster—how their personal characteristics express themselves in organizational action—are

FIGURE 4.5 Board and Board Quality Committee Questions

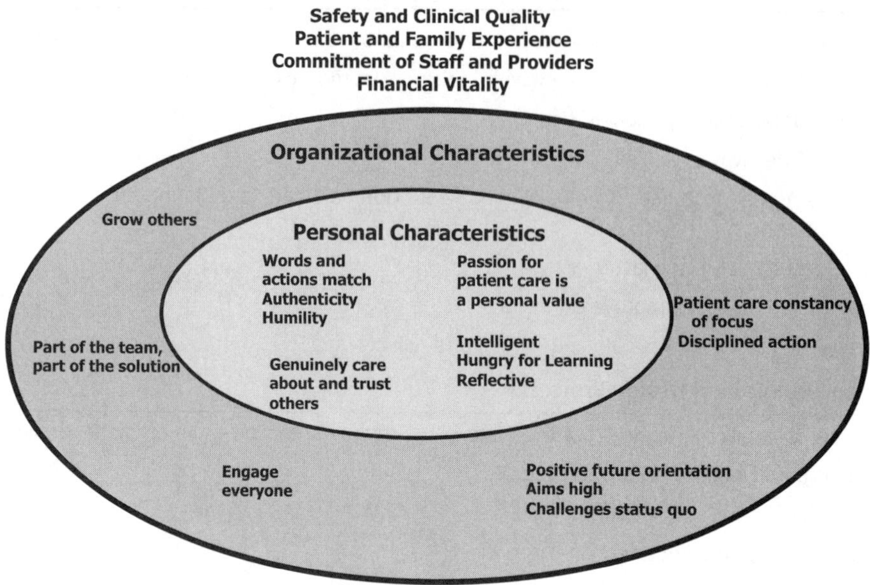

Courtesy of Barbara Balik and Jack Gilbert.

described in Figure 4.7. Each example begins with a quote from a colleague inside the organization.

A Single-Brain Organization

Taking these organizational characteristics as a whole, they add up to what the authors call a single-brain organization, one in which:

- Every person's contribution is needed for optimal performance.
- Different parts work together for a common goal.
- Every part needs to be nurtured for the health of the whole.
- Diminishment of the value of one function, one level, or one person diminishes performance of the whole.
- The wisdom of every person combined far outweighs the wisdom of one person or group, including the executive and the leadership team.

These elements, combined with the organizational characteristics, which are fueled by the personal characteristics of the leaders interviewed, paint a picture of possible paths to transformational results.

Knowledge to Lead Complex Organizations Plus Skills in the Science of Safety, Just Culture, and Team Development

Leadership for safety requires knowledge of the science of safety, just culture, and team development applied to leaders' work. It is a skill that cannot be delegated to others in the organization to master or reserved for a select group.

Additional emerging content that enhances healthcare leadership comes from studies of successful complex organizations. Health care is the most complex of any organizations, and this work has great relevance. Steven Spear offers extensive insight into

FIGURE 4.6 Examples of Personal Characteristics of Leaders

Personal Characteristics	Examples
Their words and actions match, they are authentic, and they demonstrate humility.	"She is impeccably true to her words—she is a servant leader." • Their employees talk about them as being "real," "genuine," "not arrogant," "easy to talk to." • They are consistent in their actions, are transparent, have no hidden agendas, and easily give credit to others for success and assume responsibility themselves for failure. • Their behaviors include spending time on activities they say are important for the mission, being humble learners, being comfortable with not knowing the answers, developing new skills to improve outcomes, saying they made a mistake and what they learned from it, respectfully listening to all.
Their passion for patient care is a personal value.	"He is unwavering about the mission; he has a constancy of purpose." • A focus on patient safety, quality of care, and community health is not a strategy or an important organizational emphasis—it is why they are in health care and it is what drives them every day—it is their North Star and the context by which they organize their thinking. Patient safety and patient care are so important to them that they do not delegate accountability for it. • They avoid the cost–quality trade-offs. • Their confidence in the focus on safety and quality is clear—always. • Behaviors may include time spent reviewing all serious patient harm events, overseeing performance improvement, storytelling to illustrate the link between the mission and an individual's role—making meaning for others—asking others why they are in health care and thereby nurturing the passion that brought them to it, learning anything they can to improve care.
They are intelligent, hungry for learning, and reflective.	"She continues to expand her personal management tool kit and inspires me to do the same." • Innate intelligence is complemented by a hunger for learning (e.g., joining book clubs, reading articles and books). They go outside the organization, and they listen to their leadership team, their employees, and other stakeholders and engage them in dialogue in order to learn. • They match their intelligence and desire for learning with their ability to be reflective—to take the learning and to consider how what they have learned can improve themselves, their colleagues, the life of patients, and the welfare of the communities they serve. Reflection on learning is a major source of organizational improvement.

(continues)

FIGURE 4.6 Examples of Personal Characteristics of Leaders (*Continued*)

Personal Characteristics	Examples
	• They understand the organization as a compilation of complex processes and have the improvement knowledge required to achieve organizational results. Frequently, senior leaders miss process knowledge, safety science, and improvement expertise in their executive leadership portfolios. • Effective leaders are curious at their core; they demonstrate passionate interest through honest questions that prompt different thinking. Their process knowledge helps them recognize that safe systems, which result in safer care, stem from a million small things in service to the purpose. They know that there is no small problem and that absence of news of unsafe events is a warning sign, not a cause for celebration. Part of their curiosity stems from being very close to, not removed from, daily work. They rely on what they see and hear and the experiences of others, in addition to standard management reports, to understand what is going on within the organization. Executive leaders who *go see, listen, and learn* have a greater depth of understanding, which fuels their curiosity. • Curiosity is also demonstrated through transparency of data, stories, and adverse events—any information that contributes to organizational learning. Transparency in service to the purpose trumps all other concerns about legal issues, looking bad to others, or fears of repercussions.
They genuinely care about and trust others.	"He has a desire to be with and around people to hear what is important to them, what they need." • They show a genuine spirit of engagement because they deeply care about others and what they have to say. They trust others, believing that they want to do the right thing and make a positive impact during their workday. • Their behaviors include behaving consistently and respectfully with everyone, exhibiting no difference in behavior depending on role; asking others for their advice and tapping into what they know from their role; and listening with singular, full attention.

Courtesy of Barbara Balik and Jack Gilbert.

leading complexity, or what he calls high velocity organizations:

> A common problem these organizations face is that they . . . provide complex services, requiring many varied forms of skill and expertise. . . . Eventually, so much is connected to so much else that the system becomes "unknowable." . . . It is in designing and operating their complex work . . . [which is] how they deal with the problem of unknowable, unpredictable systems . . . and set themselves apart.[14]

It is the recognition of the complexity within the organization that allows leaders in these types of settings to excel. They follow principles recognized by safety experts—they treat each problem of something not working as expected as a signal, as insight into the reliability of the system. Lessons learned from understanding these problems improve the function in small ways every day—a steady, relentless pace of ongoing improvement, not reliance on large projects or big breakthroughs. Leaders make sure the lessons learned are shared and used throughout the organization. They also assure managers know a disciplined way to recognize and problem solve in this type of environment of constant attention to the voice of the operations and teach others to work this way.

Spear[14] and Kenagy[15] identify capabilities of high velocity organizations. Detailed review is beyond the scope of this chapter; however, the descriptions resonate with other safety literature and studies of effective leaders. Use of this content as an ongoing source of leadership and staff development in seeking safe systems is a productive path to greater safety.

The capabilities of learning to see and learning to problem solve include:

- Observation of current work to fully understand the current state; no assumptions about how the care processes actually work; with assumptions we do not see the gaps and workarounds present.
- Based on the observations, specify the design of all work to capture existing knowledge and build in tests to immediately reveal problems.
- Building on previous best-known knowledge, observing closely how current work occurs, and specifying what, who, how, and when of each step leads to the ability to detect defects quickly.
- Standardization is not the means to safety; it provides an opportunity to know when something happened that was not anticipated, thus offering a surprise view of the system we did not know before. We can develop more reliable systems based on this surprise rather than simply working around it.
- Disciplined swarming and solving problems as they are seen to build new knowledge.
- Assumptions and workarounds are banned in this type of environment. Staff, rather than patching together any solution to meet immediate patient needs, signal the problem to leaders who can assist in both addressing the immediate needs and find the root cause of the problem.
- This unrelenting focus on small problems leads to more reliable systems.
- New learnings are shared across the organization.
- Learnings are shared in a disciplined way. Sharing information is aided through problem solving based on a consistent disciplined improvement approach. The lessons learned include what, how, why and in what context the problem solving occurred. Frequently, lessons learned include what and how but omit crucial information on why the solution worked and the context in which it happened. Why and context offer a fuller description for others to assess this solution's applicability to their setting.
    - For example, What: "We experienced a failure in a new smart pump we did not see in our trials or training." How: "We tested how the pump failed and attached is our new procedure." Missing Why: "We discovered that if the nurse attempts to change the syringe without a key step, a potential overdose can result. This was identified in direct observation of loading the pump when it was both attached to the patient and in preparation to connect to a patient." Context: "We discovered this on a busy surgical unit when a variety of patients required syringe changes in a short time period."
- Multiple methods are used to share learning but all methods are based on a similar discipline.

The capabilities of learning to lead include:

- Leaders focus on developing the capabilities that are often lacking.
- Leaders reflect the success factors listed in Figure 4.7 and strive to continually make the organization more capable in

FIGURE 4.7 How Leadership Characteristics are Expressed in Organizational Attributes

Organizational Characteristics	Examples
Patient care constancy of focus; disciplined action	"She is not distracted by the crisis of the day; she doesn't jump around or vacillate." • Their eyes on the prize commitment to patient care is communicated by the way they approach decisions and what they talk about with others, leaving not a shred of doubt that patient care trumps everything else. • While responsible for the financial health of the organization—that is evident from the results they have produced—finances, processes, management systems, strategies, goals, personnel decisions, and day-to-day actions are viewed through the screen of patient safety, patient care, and community health. • They combine their sensitivity to the needs of patients and staff with well-ordered and disciplined accountability-driven approaches to decision making, leaving their leadership team and employees in no doubt about the leader's expectations of them. There is a disciplined approach to achieving the mission. • Alignment stems from a shared purpose, not from a goal cascade management system. While carefully developed systems of goal connections are important, they become enablers of the shared purpose, not the reason for alignment. • One essential step in a leader's disciplined approach is selecting and developing leaders who embody the commitment. A leadership system, not a solo charismatic leader, is essential to make the purpose a reality. The entire process of interviewing, selecting, developing, promoting, and recognizing leaders in a range of positions throughout the organization is consistently identified as core to achieving the culture and results required for safe care. • Improvement skills are widely developed; no one expert team is relied on for improvement knowledge. While expert teachers are constantly used, the intent is to disseminate skills to everyone for improvement in daily work.
Positive future orientation; aim high; challenge the status quo	"We can always be better. She's always asking, 'What's the next best?'" • Happy to celebrate success, but are always conscious that there is more to do; are never satisfied. This dissatisfaction energizes rather than distresses them. • Dissatisfaction with the current state, regardless of the level of performance, is combined with a disciplined approach to achieving greater results. The dissatisfaction conveys aspirational belief in the ability of the organizational members to reach further in service to others. • They convey a positive spirit to the organization and look to the future with appreciation for present challenges and those to come with an underlying optimism and commitment. They are undaunted.

FIGURE 4.7 How Leadership Characteristics are Expressed in Organizational Attributes (*Continued*)

Organizational Characteristics	Examples
Engage everyone	"She has the ability to make people belong and matter and want to work hard for themselves and the institution." • They engage through clarity about organizational priorities and especially the primacy of patient care (as opposed to other cases where primacy of the bottom line dampens the passion for care in the organization). They engage by being transparent about the organization's condition, goals, successes, and failures and by expecting everyone to step up and embrace their own accountability by doing their part in realizing the vision and meeting goals. In these organizations, the sense is that people are accountable, not *held* accountable. • They understand that if everyone in the organization is successful, whatever his or her role, then the organization will prosper; they recognize that the effectiveness of every individual and the effectiveness of the organization are inextricably linked.
Part of the team; part of the solution	"He seeks advice from others, and you can see your thoughts reflected in the outcome. . . . He believes you get the best thinking when you get the positives and negatives of a decision." • They do not see themselves as *the* decision maker, nor will they make a decision alone for the sake of appearing decisive or because they think it is their job as CEO. They see their job in decision making as enabling the best possible decision or solution. • Use of teams is not situational but part of their philosophy of leadership. They look to teamwork throughout the organization as a fundamental vehicle to get work done well, and they see themselves as team members. This collaboration also engages others in the work of safety and quality. They know they have a unique role but not as the brains of the operation. The whole organization is the brain, and they are part of it. • Respectful interactions are pervasive; collaboration and teamwork are role-modeled by leaders with everyone they encounter, regardless of position, role in the hierarchy, or organizational power. Contributions of all are respected and celebrated.
Grow others	"She finds out what is good in people, exposes it, grows it, and helps you master it in pursuit of the group goal." • These leaders make others better. They show this in many ways: by having a strong presence in every employee orientation; by creating training and development structures that provide for employees to grow in ways personally and professionally beyond their job requirements; and by unpredictable personnel choices that reflect the leader's identification of a potential hidden to all, including the candidate. They get deep satisfaction when their people succeed; they are mindful that personal success will usually translate into greater organizational success.

Courtesy of Barbara Balik and Jack Gilbert.

seeing, diagnosing, and solving problems every day.

- They understand that safety problems reflect aspects of a system we do not understand and have not adequately protected against. The reliance on vigilance, memory, and individual effort is seen as totally inadequate in operating complex systems.
- Skills in immediately reflecting on actions that resulted in problems require the best of just culture, teamwork, and respectful relationships.

Leadership for safety requires extensive development of personal and organization skills—many not currently identified as leadership competencies. Understanding the personal and organizational characteristics described, reflecting on if and how they show up in your leadership practice, developing the skills of safety science, and expertise in leading, innovating, and improving in complex organizations are all part of the path to greater success for healthcare leaders.

ASSESSMENT TOOL—INDIVIDUAL LEADERS OR TEAMS

The sample questions in Figure 4.8 are a beginning for an assessment. Add questions to meet your unique needs.

References

1. Collins, J. (2008). Paper presented at New Mexico Quality Forum, Albuquerque, NM.
2. Collins, J. (2001). *Good to great: Why some companies make the leap . . . and others don't.* New York, NY: Harper Business.
3. Collins, J. (2005). *Good to great and the social sectors: A monograph to accompany good to great.* New York, NY: HarperCollins.
4. Collins, J. (2009). *How the mighty fall.* New York, NY: HarperCollins.
5. Keroack, M., Youngberg, B., Cerese, J., Krsek, C., Prellwitz, L., & Trevelyan, E. (2007). Organizational factors associated with high performance in quality and safety in academic medical centers. *Academic Medicine*, 82(12), 1178–1186.

FIGURE 4.8 Personal Characteristics

Personal Characteristics

Primacy of Patient Care as a personal value	I don't know if others know of my commitment 1	Others fully know of my commitment 10
Integrity, Authentic, Humility	Most would say "I guess s/he is" 1	I get positive feedback on this in my 360 evaluations 10
Intelligence, hunger for learning, reflective	I rarely read leadership books/articles 1	Our team & I read something daily & identify how it might apply 10
Genuinely cares about and trusts others	I am not confident I demonstrate this 1	I demonstrate this daily 10

Courtesy of Barbara Balik and Jack Gilbert.

6. Balik, M. B., & Gilbert, J. A. (2010). *The heart of leadership: Inspiration and practical guidance for transforming your health care organization*. Chicago, IL: Health Forum.
7. National Patient Safety Foundation. *Stand up for patient safety program*. Retrieved from http://www.npsf.org/membership-programs/members/.
8. 5 Million Lives Campaign. Getting Started Kit: Governance Leadership "Boards on Board" How-to Guide. Cambridge, MA: Institute for Healthcare Improvement; 2008. (Available at www.ihi.org) you will need to register to get this resource but it is free upon registration, which is also free.
9. An Interview with Donald Berwick. (2006). *Joint Commission Journal on Quality and Patient Safety*, 32(12), 666.
10. Institute of Medicine. (1999). *To err is human: Building a safer health system* Washington, DC: National Academies Press.
11. Hearst Newspapers. (1999). Dead by mistake. Retrieved from http://www.hearst.com/press-room/pr-20090809b.php.
12. Melnyk, M. B., & Fineout-Overhold, E. (2004). *Evidence-based practice in nursing and healthcare: A guide to best practice*. Philadelphia, PA: Lippincott Williams & Wilkins.
13. Kouzes, J., & Posner, B. (2003). *Encouraging the heart: A leader's guide to rewarding and recognizing others*. San Francisco, CA: Jossey-Bass.
14. Spear, S. (2010). *High velocity edge*. New York, NY: McGraw-Hill.
15. Kenagy, J. (2009). *Designed to adapt: Leading healthcare in challenging times*. Bozeman, MT: Second River Healthcare Press.

Additional Resources

16. Bridges, W. (1991). *Managing transitions: making the most of change*. Cambridge, MA: Perseus Books.
17. Brookfield, S. (2000). The concept of critically reflective practice. In A. Wilson and E. Hayes (Eds.), *Handbook 2000 of adult and continuing education*. San Francisco, CA: Jossey-Bass.
18. Heifetz, R. (1994). *Leadership without easy answers*. Cambridge, MA: Belknap Press.
19. Heifetz, R., Grashow, A., & Linsky, M. (2009). *The practice of adaptive leadership*. Boston, MA: Harvard Business Press.
20. Kouzes, J., & Posner, B. (2002). *The leadership challenge*. San Francisco, CA: Jossey-Bass.
21. Moss Kanter, R. (2004). *Confidence: How winning streaks and losing streaks begin and end*. New York, NY: Crown Business.
22. Patterson, K., Grenny, J., Maxfield, D., McMillan, R., & Switzler, A. (2008). *Influencer: The power to change anything*. New York, NY: McGraw-Hill.
23. Rother, M. (2010). *Toyota Kata: Managing people for improvement, adaptiveness, and superior results*. New York, NY: McGraw-Hill.
24. Schein, E. (1999). *The corporate culture survival guide: Sense and nonsense about cultural change*. San Francisco, CA: Jossey-Bass.
25. Schein, E. (2004). *Organizational culture and leadership*. 3rd ed. San Francisco, CA: Jossey-Bass.
26. Senge, P., Kleiner, A., Roberts, C., Ross, R., Roth, G., & Smith, B. (1999). *The dance of change: The challenges of sustaining momentum in learning organizations*. New York, NY: Doubleday.
27. Seven Leadership Leverage Point for Organization-Level Improvement in Health Care. (2007). IHI Innovation Series White Paper. Cambridge, Massachusetts. Retrieved from http://www.ihi.org/NR/rdonlyres/C84E1503-C05E-4D1B-B8D5-C74CEFE68F7F/0/LeadershipWhitePaper2007.pdf.
28. Weick, K., & Sutcliffe, K. (2001). *Managing the unexpected: Assuring high performance in an age of complexity*. San Francisco, CA: Jossey-Bass.

5

An Organization Development Framework for Transformational Change in Patient Safety: A Guide for Hospital Senior Leaders

Raj Behal, MD, MBA

Patient safety has emerged as a study of paradoxes in health care: Highly educated and rigorously trained professionals dedicated to patient care are training the future generation of health care professionals, counseling patients and the public in behavior modification, and continually learning—all in a day's work—while at the same time shifting responsibility for patient safety to others, dismissing sobering statistics on harm to patients, resisting reporting of adverse events, and showing reluctance to change their own behaviors or to participate in fixing systems of care. It is like walking into a brightly lit room and flicking off all the lights—suddenly the room that was coherent and reasoned is filled with amorphous shapes and chaos. One must painstakingly find all of the light switches and flick them back on, one at a time.

Senior leaders at hospitals face the enormous challenge of improving patient safety at their respective organizations. The Institute of Medicine (IOM) report *To Err Is Human* suggested that a large number of deaths in the nations' hospitals are attributable to medical errors.[1] The National Quality Forum and other safety experts have recommended creation of a "culture of safety" and a "blame-free culture." A culture of blame, reports suggest, prevails at many health care institutions and acts as a barrier to accurate measurement of adverse events. Health care workers fear blame and reprisal if they report an error occurring on their watch. Some organizations that have historically performed well in traditional quality improvement initiatives may find themselves struggling to get everyone to willfully support the patient safety agenda. According to a Kaiser/Harvard survey, although a third of the responding physicians acknowledged personal experiences with errors in the past year, only a small minority of the physicians surveyed rated medical errors as a top concern.[2] A phenomenon known as "normalization of deviance"—an incremental process by which a system gradually adjusts to safety problems—is considered a barrier to achieving safety goals.[3] A dysfunctional level of collaboration between physicians and nurses is cited as a barrier, and researchers have proposed a model for improving this relationship.[4] The importance of teamwork in organizational learning is well recognized.[5] A shift from the traditional functions of risk management programs to a more proactive role in hospitals is recommended to assure a culture of safety.[6] Reports of early successes in implementation of a model focusing on practitioner frailties and latent system failures[7] and of an approach to using selfassessment tools and formation of oversight committees[8] are encouraging. A framework that collates the aforementioned interventions into a unified approach to improving patient safety is not available.

Little guidance is available to senior leaders at large medical centers regarding a comprehensive and integrated approach to nurturing an organization that supports the agenda of patient safety. How does one go from a culture of blame to a culture of safety? Is a culture of safety both necessary and sufficient to promote patient safety? What are some of the other key components that must be in place to support the safety agenda? In the absence of empirical data on the effect of management strategies on culture and performance in health care, it is suggested that safety practitioners look to a rich literature on this topic from other industries.[9] This chapter presents an organization development framework shown to be successful in other industries for understanding organizational performance and for implementing lasting change. In addition, it provides guidance on how to adapt this framework for improving the state of patient safety within complex health care organizations.

SCENARIO

Let us begin with a scenario. The CEO of the University Hospital announces a new policy that calls for mandatory reporting of all errors. If errors are reported within 48 hours of occurrence, there will be no punitive action against the reporter. There will be disciplinary consequences for nonreporting once an error is recognized by other means. Reaction of physicians and nurses to this policy is one of the following:

1. Distrust and questioning of the "real reason" the policy is announced
2. Shrugging it off as just another administrative hassle—"safety is someone else's responsibility"
3. Meeting it with enthusiasm as "the right thing to do so we can learn from these adverse events and improve patient care"

What are the organizational conditions that lead to such varied responses? Is the answer to this question "organizational culture"?

WHAT IS CULTURE?

First, why does one care about the organization's culture? Isn't it organizational performance that leaders should be concerned about? During the following discussion, it should become apparent that culture drives individual and collective behavior, and collective behavior drives organizational performance. It also should become evident that culture is a necessary, but not sufficient, lever for sustainable change. A strong safety culture eventually wilts in the absence of systems support.

An organization's prevailing culture is a set of beliefs and expectations about life within that organization. Culture is deeply rooted in *assumptions*, which are "truths" taken for granted by individuals in the organization. These assumptions are interwoven into the fabric of organizational life to such an extent that they are rarely even thought about or questioned. From assumptions arise *values* and *norms*: what members of the organization consider worthwhile and what is considered to be acceptable behavior in specific situations, respectively. Any change that threatens existing values and assumptions is met with resistance. *Behavior* and tangible products of such behaviors (*artifacts* such as physical buildings, office space layout, policies, etc.) are readily observed and provide an entrée into an organization's culture. Whereas culture describes what the expectations are, *organizational climate* tells us to what extent the expectations are being met. Climate refers to a psychological state that is strongly affected by policies, supervisor behavior, and systems. It is typically perceived at the local work unit level. Organizational climate is amenable to change over a short period of time, whereas culture is more enduring and requires multifaceted interventions over a longer duration in order to change.

REVISITING THE SCENARIO

Let's assume that the intent of the aforementioned policy is to change staff behavior: a shift from nonreporting of adverse events to prompt reporting. Clearly, different cultures will assign very different meanings to the same policy. The concept of "cultural censorship" may be useful to consider here, as applied by Hart and Hazelgrove.[10] They describe the silence produced by cultural censorship—a socially shared silence that is not forced upon others or conspired and only implicitly agreed upon—that can drive adverse events and malpractice even deeper into the "underside of the organization" when mandatory reporting is introduced. As apparent in the first two responses in the scenario, the local effect of the policy may be to create a psychological state of fear or frustration within the work units. Reporting of errors may increase, but it occurs without the staff "buying in." Under these circumstances, nurses may begin to report pharmacist errors, and physicians may start reporting nursing errors. *Self-reporting*, one of the hallmarks of a safe, nonpunitive culture, may never occur. Learning from errors thus never occurs, and a culture of blame persists.

FIRST-ORDER VERSUS SECOND-ORDER CHANGE

Policies alone do little to promote a culture of safety. They can only effect a first-order, or *transactional*, change without changing the fundamental nature of the organization. If the primary goal is to increase reporting of errors, a first-order intervention may suffice. A change in the organizational structure, new policies and procedures, and a new electronic event-reporting system may be all that is needed. Each new policy must, however, go through the "lens" of culture first. If the new policy does not pose a threat to the values and underlying assumptions held by the staff, it is more likely to be accepted, though not necessarily with any enthusiasm.

If the goal is to improve patient safety and reduce the likelihood of inadvertent harm to patients, a first-order intervention will not be successful. In this case, a second-order, or *transformational*, change is required. Second-order change comes from a combination of multilevel, multidimensional interventions that focus on organizational mission and strategy, leadership style, and the culture of the organization. In a large organization, this type of effort is expended over several years before results are seen.

A conceptual model for understanding the role of reporting errors in the design of a safer health care system is presented in Figure 5.1. Reason has asserted that errors arise from a combination of active human failures and latent system conditions.[11] When holes in various layers of the Swiss-cheese defense system line up just right, errors reach and sometimes harm patients. If an error is intercepted before it reaches the patient, it is referred to as a *near miss*. Once these errors are recognized and reported, they can be further studied so that the staff can learn from what happened and why. More important, this learning can be applied to fix those *latent system conditions* that allowed the error to occur or to propagate. Environmental conditions, such as distractions, and staff fatigue may be the contributory root causes of some of the errors. These conditions can be addressed to reduce the occurrence of *active failures*. Reducing the occurrence of active failures and redesigning systems lead to a safer patient care environment. Learning is incrementally and sometimes exponentially

FIGURE 5.1 A Conceptual Model of the Role of Event Reporting in Improving Patient Safety

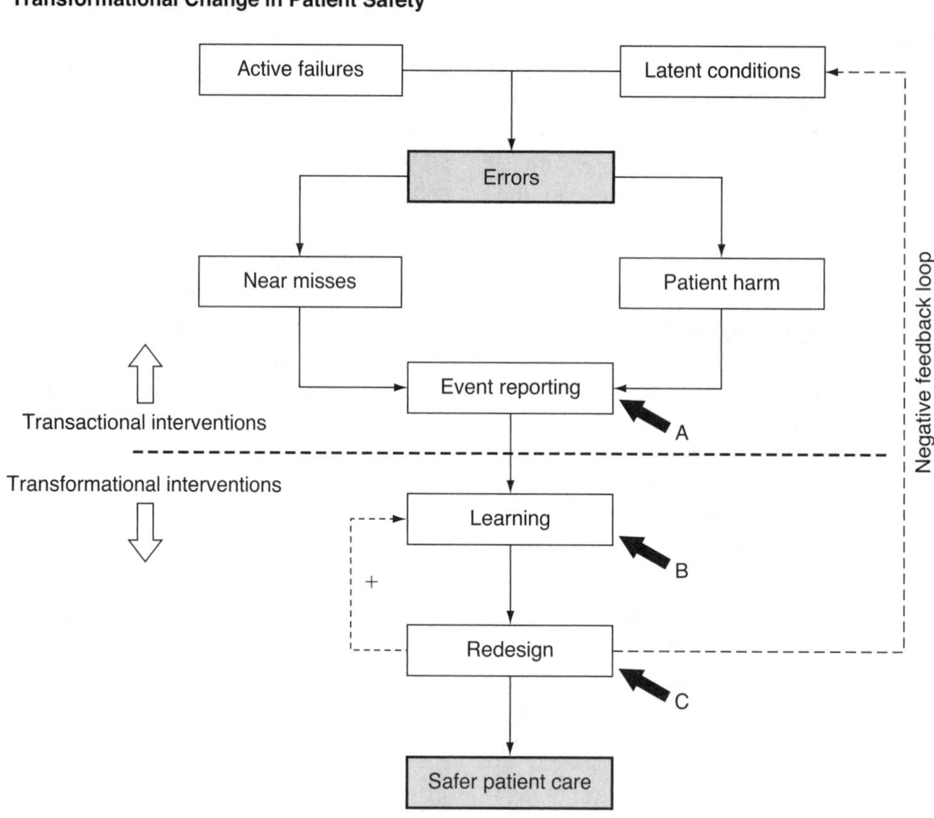

reinforced when staff members observe the outcomes of reporting and making changes.[12] Over time, common latent system conditions are identified and eliminated, incrementally building a safer system for care.

Policies for mandatory reporting and structural changes can increase event reporting (solid arrow A in Figure 5.1). In order to get to the next steps (solid arrows B and C), however, transformational interventions are needed. Without organizational values and norms that motivate learning behaviors, broad participation in development and incorporation of redesign is unlikely to occur.

CREATING AN URGENCY FOR CHANGE WHILE PROVIDING AN INFRASTRUCTURE FOR CHANGE TO TAKE HOLD

Organization development (OD) is the planned approach to improving organizational capabilities to be more effective in achieving an organization's goals. One of the basic tenets of OD is that organizational effectiveness is contingent upon developing the appropriate systems, structures, and processes. It emphasizes the need to integrate individual needs with organizational goals and to engage individuals in decisions that directly affect their work activities. This approach appears to have validity in the health care setting in the context of improving patient safety.

Health care organizations are examples of complex sociotechnical systems. This perspective emphasizes that technical and human dimensions of work are interrelated.[13] New strategies, structures, policies, performance measurement systems, and training programs are technical solutions adopted to solve specific operational problems. These technical solutions perturb the social system in place, often challenging existing notions of power, autonomy, self-esteem, status, relationships, and security. Failure to consider the social system inevitably leads to resistance and cynicism about "management fads" and eventually erodes organizational trust.[14] Consider what might happen in a tertiary care medical center if a computerized physician order entry system were installed one morning with the expectation that all physicians would use the system and follow the decision rules embedded within.

The Burke–Litwin Model of Organizational Performance and Change

Top-down efforts that are planned and driven by the senior leadership can quickly put in place appropriate structures and policies, whereas bottom-up interventions gradually prepare the front-line staff for effective participation. The latter approach to change relies on OD interventions focusing on culture and brings about "emergent" change.[14,15] A coordinated application of top-down and bottom-up interventions allows the managers and the staff to see results quickly while a "cultural infrastructure" is being erected to sustain long-term performance.

The Burke–Litwin model[16] combines transactional interventions with transformational interventions to bring about sustained improvement in organizational performance (Figure 5.2). Leadership, mission and strategy, and organizational culture are the three key targets for transformational interventions. Transactional interventions are applied to structures, systems, and management practices. The net effect of these interventions is to modify the work unit climate, which in turn contributes to alignment of essential tasks with individual needs and skills. Individuals thus motivated and given appropriate resources improve the organizational performance. Each of the components of the Burke–Litwin framework is described next in the context of patient safety.

External Environment

One of the strongest drivers of organizational change is the external environment. In health care, the external environment is rife with reports on medical errors and the national agenda on patient safety and quality. Several regulatory groups and national organizations, such as The Joint Commission, National Quality Forum, and Agency for Healthcare Research and Quality, have promulgated patient safety goals. A few third-party payers have introduced incentives for demonstrable improvements in quality and safety. Television and print media frequently highlight news of medical mishaps as human-interest stories. The environment is sending strong signals to health care professionals and leaders that attending to patient safety issues must be made a higher priority.

Leadership

Leaders need to continually scan the external environment for important trends and signals, and realign their strategy when necessary. The IOM report on medical errors heralded the era of patient safety in the year 2000. Since then the momentum for change has built, albeit slowly. Federal and public agencies as well as the media have embraced this issue and urged action. In the post-Enron era, the call for executive accountability is loud and clear. Although a crisis can be a very effective motivator for change, harm done to organizational

FIGURE 5.2 Translating External Demands and Internal Needs for Improving Patient Safety into Organizational Performance (Adapted from Reference 16)

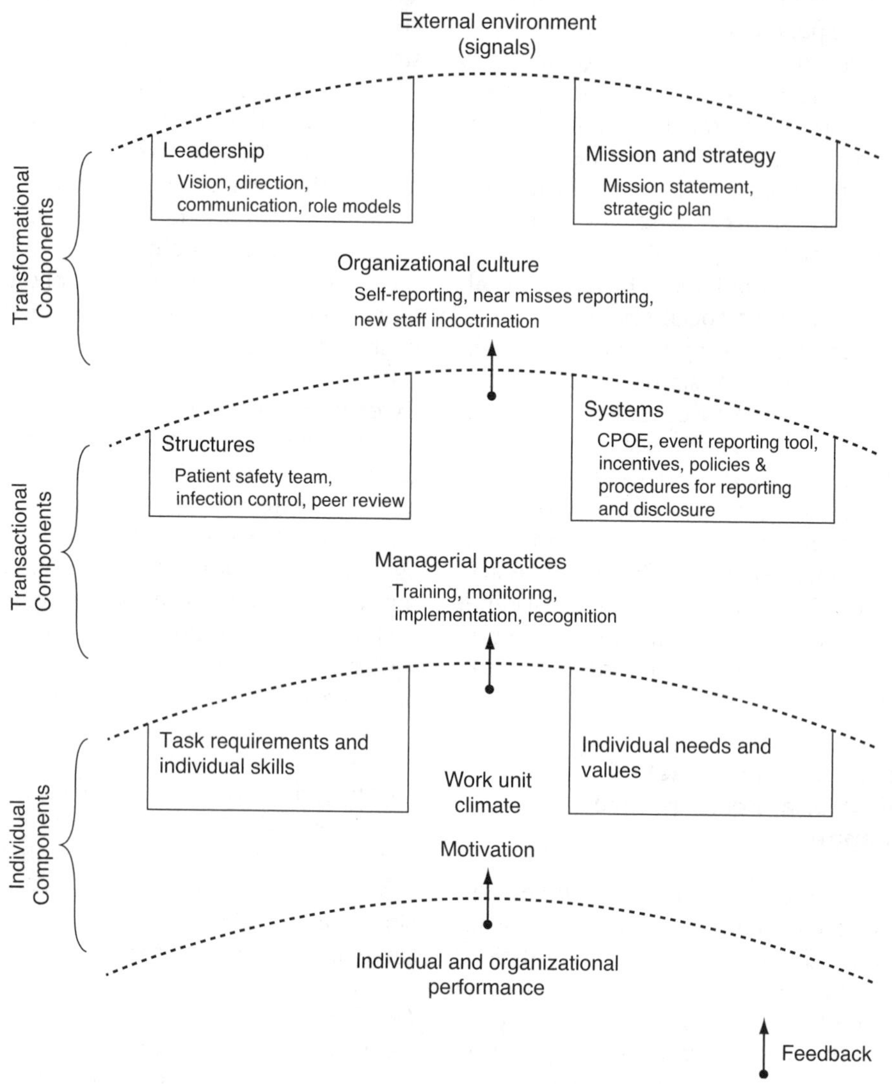

morale and reputation may take a very long time to repair.

Senior hospital leaders may find themselves being urged to address two related tasks: creating a culture of safety and learning, and implementing an error reporting system. Without an integrating vision and a structured approach, the outcome may be a few policies that are inconsistently followed and a reporting system that is seldom used. In this undesirable scenario, physicians continue to see safety as someone else's problem, nurses remain silent when unsafe practices are in plain view, and leaders keep pressing for change, while the chief medical officer expresses frustration at being caught in the middle. To break through this impasse, senior leaders have to set direction, align people, and provide motivation.[14,17] They need to consider the following guidelines:

- Develop a vision of safety: what the desired future state of patient safety in the organization looks like.
- Communicate this vision to all staff: what it means to them, and what must change and why.
- Make patient safety an explicit component of the mission.
- Serve as behavioral role models: Adopt transparency in decision making, and hold yourselves accountable to the board of trustees.

In aligning staff around patient safety, the work of the senior leadership begins with a clear and succinct definition of the current problem: what's wrong with the current state of affairs, what is the estimated magnitude of the problem (present or future), what may happen if the problem is not addressed, and what are some of the internal and external drivers for change. This is especially important when the staff does not perceive an imminent problem. If the leadership team cannot answer these questions or communicate their vision with clarity, a call to action to the staff is unlikely to be heard. Storytelling—putting a human face to the safety issue—may prove much more effective in moving staff than precise data on the magnitude of the problem. Statistics on patient falls carefully trended over time are very useful for continuous quality improvement but not for motivating staff. Compare the emotional appeal of a control chart to conversational storytelling such as the following:

> Last month we cared for a 69-year-old grandmother who was admitted for elective hip replacement. She was sedated and anticoagulated. When she got out of bed at 2 AM confused, she tripped over her IV line and landed head first and developed a massive subdural hematoma, which went unrecognized until the morning shift. She required emergency craniotomy followed by repair of a 4-cm tear in her urethra (her Foley catheter bag with balloon inflated was secured to the bedside when she fell). Despite our efforts to resuscitate her, she died the next day. How could this happen here?

The issue and the change must be explained in terms that are meaningful to staff and relevant to their daily work. Outlining what is *not* going to change can be instrumental in alleviating some anxiety. Instead of simply announcing a new policy, the leaders should outline the vision, present an open and transparent leadership style, and ask for commitment. Finally, leaders should accept the ultimate accountability for patient safety and engage the board of trustees' interest and support. Two critical effectors of the leaders' vision that cannot be delegated are mission and strategy, and organizational culture, which are described next.

Mission and Strategy

With the vision of a highly reliable, safe, and effective organization in mind, leaders need to reexamine the organization's stated mission, modify it if necessary, and then communicate it to staff with clarity and resolve. It is important to involve the staff in designing specific tactics that will help create a safer organization. Instead of resigning themselves to the mantra that "culture eats strategy for lunch around here," leaders have to be cognizant of the local culture and anticipate resistance when crafting strategy. Deadlock with the staff is as much a reflection of weakness of the strategy as it is evidence of a stagnant culture. The strategic plan should delineate how the mission is to be carried out. Important elements of the organization's strategy for ensuring patient safety include effective communication of the vision, proactive evaluation and redesign of high-hazard processes, development of appropriate structures and systems, and focus on shifting the organization's culture.

Organizational Culture

Culture is a set of beliefs and values that allows organizational members to interpret the events they experience and assign meanings to those events.[16] It is "the way we do things here." Changing culture takes sustained effort over time and should not be the sole initial intervention. Cultural change is best pursued in parallel with results-oriented interventions. Capitalizing on small wins over time, leaders can raise awareness among staff and demonstrate that change is possible. More important, improved performance may begin to resonate with individual values of patient care and thereby facilitate incorporation of new behaviors. Senior leaders with a recent tenure may aid their understanding of the organizational culture by examining the practices and values of the founders.

Cultural change is sometimes brought about at the fringes of the organization, often by newcomers. Hiring of new staff members that bring with them a desired set of values in visible positions is an important step. Indoctrination of new staff with a desired set of values and norms relating to a culture of safety may be a useful tactic, with an important caveat: If the newly hired staff members encounter behaviors in the "old culture" that seem to contradict what was just presented to them, they may find it difficult to adhere to the espoused values. Therefore, it is important to work at the same time on changing the old guard. If specific staff members remain irresponsible and unprofessional in their conduct after counseling and confrontation, removal may be the only option. Although difficult, this can be a powerful signal to the remaining staff members that the organization is serious about patient safety. Between the two extremes of hiring and firing lies a middle ground where behavioral change can be attempted.[18] A practical three-stage model for behavioral change is presented later in this discussion.

The role of cultural communications is often underestimated in changing and sustaining cultures: Although explicit modes of communications such as newsletters, announcements, and all-staff meetings are commonly used, implicit cultural messages such as stories, metaphors, and creation of cultural heroes (for example, a surgeon who reported his own error, explained the error, and apologized to the patient, and then helped change the latent conditions so it wouldn't happen again) can be much more powerful in sustaining the new culture.

Management Practices

Management involves planning and budgeting, organizing and staffing, providing control, and solving problems. These activities are distinct from but complementary to what leaders do.[17] Managers reduce complexity and increase predictability in day-to-day activities. Chairs of clinical departments, the chief medical officer, the chief nursing officer, nursing unit managers, the director of quality improvement, and the director of the pharmacy are some of the important stakeholders who manage clinical activities within and across work units. A shared purpose of safe and effective care of patients *within* work units is just as important as it is across the organization, if not more so. After all, it is here, in work units, where patient care, harm, reporting, or blame occurs. Because work units are necessarily multidisciplinary, coordination of functional department-based interventions is crucial for success. Physicians (including house staff in training), nurses, pharmacists, and other front-line workers must hear the leadership and the management team speak in one voice about patient safety. Various management practices such as those related to nurse staffing, house staff training, attending physician accountability, and implementation of computerized physician order entry are effective in improving patient safety when they are woven into the organizational strategy toward this goal.

Whether the management should use incentives to encourage behavior change remains an open question. Use of incentives assumes that individual behavior is the main constraint that limits performance. Faced with financial incentives, individuals attempting to work harder soon reach a performance plateau. To break through this plateau, support from systems and structures must be present. Incentives may be more effective if directed at the organization or at least at the department level. Incentives may be more effective in reinforcing desired behaviors than in creating new behaviors.

Structures and Systems

Structure refers to an arrangement of human resources required for execution of a strategy. Organizing staff into specific functions and roles, bestowing decision-making authority, and facilitating relationships are examples of structural interventions. Creation of a Patient Safety Team or appointment of a Patient Safety Officer is a structural change for the specific purpose of advancing patient safety. This entity or individual should report to the senior leadership and have decision-making authority. Members of this team should be carefully selected, keeping in mind that personal relationships can often accomplish more than a policy directive. The infection control and epidemiology staff should work closely with this team. The existing physician peer-review and recredentialing arrangements may not be effective in inculcating physician accountability for patient safety; some organizations will need to re-examine these relationships in this new context.

Systems interventions involve policies and procedures for facilitating the daily work; examples include policies for reporting adverse events, for full disclosure to patients who are harmed, and for disciplining malicious practitioners. Computerized physician order entry systems with decision support, electronic event-reporting tools, ICU alarms, incentive mechanisms, and the use of various forcing functions are examples of systems. There is a well-established role for process and systems redesign in eliminating latent conditions that allow errors to propagate. Making it difficult to use hazardous equipment incorrectly is a simple yet powerful example of system constraints. As a reminder, structural and systems interventions can only bring about first-order change. Used in isolation, they do nothing to change the fundamental nature of the organization. They do nothing to change a "blame culture" into a "safety culture" when other aspects of organizational life are left unattended.

Task Requirements and Individual Skills

Some staff members may resist change because they lack the skills required for participation. What is required of individuals and the skills they possess must match. Training in communication, use of electronic reporting systems, analysis of data, and use of specific tools such as failure mode analysis and root cause analysis can provide essential skills for the required tasks.

Work Unit Climate, Individual Needs, and Motivation

When individuals possess the right skills for the required tasks, are working under a resourceful work unit climate in a supportive and open culture, have their professional needs and values fulfilled, are hearing a clear and consistent message from the senior leaders, and know without a doubt what is required of them, they are motivated to achieve organizational goals of improving patient safety. Incentives, which may be monetary or in the form of professional recognition, can help sustain new behaviors that are consistent with a safety culture.

CHANGING BEHAVIOR

Three-Stage Change Model

Staff behavior is an overt manifestation of the organizational culture. A model for approaching behavior change includes the following three stages:[19,20]

1. Unfreeze old behavior.
2. Introduce new behavior.
3. Refreeze new behavior.

Each stage requires a specific intervention. In the first stage, motivation and readiness for change are introduced by (1) creation of discomfort with the current situation, (2) introduction of anxiety or guilt, and (3) provision of psychological safety. Old behaviors can be unfrozen by providing reasons why the status quo is undesirable; this may include presentation of data, trends, and stories to make the case for change. Availability of data in itself does not guarantee that the information will be assimilated or even perceived by the staff. Organizational behavior experts have long established that disconfirming information must connect to what individuals deeply care about before they will take any action.[20] Not meeting important professional goals creates anxiety, whereas violation of personal ideals generates guilt. This type of communication does not have to be negative as long as the triad of disconfirming information, important goals, and personal ideals is recognized in planning change. Finally, recipients of disconfirming information must feel safe in accepting it. If acceptance means losing face or credibility or feeling worthless, defense mechanisms will rise and information will be discarded. One way to provide psychological safety is by reassuring staff that the problem is not unique: Others have faced it and succeeded in implementing change.

Once individuals are motivated to discard old behaviors, the next step is to identify role models, peers, or other respected members of the professional network who already have incorporated new behaviors in their work. When this is not sufficient or role models are not available, a scan of the external environment may reveal individuals or organizations in other industries that are operating under the values espoused. A frequently used example of an external entity exemplifying a culture of safety is the airline industry.

In the third stage, new behaviors are reinforced to ensure that change is not transient. The work environment and significant relationships with peers, superiors, and other team members should provide positive feedback. The positive impact on patient outcomes should resonate with professional values.

SUMMING UP

Culture is an important lever for introducing and sustaining change in an organization. Nurturing a culture of safety is necessary but not sufficient for improving the state of patient safety within organizations. Transactional interventions that focus on organizational structure, systems, and policies are unlikely to produce lasting new behaviors. Measurement of near misses and patient harm is an important component of a patient safety program. In order to bridge the chasm in safety, however, these changes must be reinforced by a fundamental shift in the organizational life. Leaders must set a new direction, align people, and provide motivation. Organization development interventions that have long been used in other industries can now be used to diagnose an ailing patient safety program or, better yet, to design a highly reliable and safe health care organization.

References

1. Institute of Medicine. *To Err Is Human: Building a Safer Health System*. Washington, DC: National Academy Press, 2000.
2. Blendon, R., DesRoches, C., Brodie, M., et al. Views of practicing physicians and the public on medical errors. *N Engl J Med* 347:1933–1967, 2002.
3. Gaba, D. Structural and organizational issues in patient safety: A comparison of health care to other high-hazard industries. *California Management Review* 43:83–102, 2000.
4. Zwarenstein, M., Reeves, S. Working together but apart: Barriers and routes to nurse-physician collaboration. *Jt Comm Qual Improv* 28:242–247, 2002.
5. Firth-Cozens, J. Cultures for improving patient safety through learning: The role of teamwork. *Quality in Health Care* 10(Suppl II):26–31, 2001.
6. Kuhn, A., Youngberg, B. The need for risk management to evolve to assure a culture of safety. *Qual Saf Health Care* 11:158–162, 2002.
7. Ketring, S., White, J. Developing a systemwide approach to patient safety: The first year. *Jt Comm Qual Improv* 28:287–295, 2002.
8. Wong, P., Helsinger, D., Petry, J. Providing the right infrastructure to lead the culture change for patient safety. *Jt Comm Qual Improv* 28:363–372, 2002.
9. Davies, H., Nutley, S., Mannion, R. Organizational culture and quality of health care. *Qual Saf Health Care* 9:111–119, 2000.
10. Hart, E., Hazelgrove, J. Understanding the organizational context for adverse events in the health services: The role of cultural censorship. *Qual Saf Health Care* 10:257–262, 2001.
11. Reason, J. Human error: Models and management. *BMJ* 320:768–770, 2000.
12. Carroll, J., Edmondson, A. Leading organizational learning in health care. *Qual Saf Health Care* 11:51–56, 2002.
13. "Organization Development and Change," in Bowditch, J., Buono, A., *A Primer on Organizational Behavior* (New York: John Wiley & Sons, 2001), 312–338.
14. Beer, M. How to develop an organization capable of sustained high performance: Embrace the drive for results-capability development paradox. *Org Dynamics* 29:233–247, 2001.
15. Beer, M., Nohria, N. Cracking the code of change. *Harvard Business Review* 133–141, May–June 2000.
16. Burke, W., Litwin, G. A causal model of organizational performance and change. *Journal of Management* 18:523–545, 1992.
17. Kotter, J. What leaders really do. *Harvard Business Review* 103–111, May–June 1990.
18. "Organization Culture and Effectiveness," in Bowditch, J., Buono, A., *A Primer on Organizational Behavior* (New York: John Wiley & Sons, 2001), 285–311.
19. Lewin, K. *Field Theory in Social Science* (New York: Harper & Row, 1951), 228–229.
20. Schein, E. *Process Consultation, Volume 2: Lessons for Managers and Consultants* (New York: Addison-Wesley, 1987).

6

The Role of the Board of Directors in Advancing Patient Safety

Sarah Mick, JD, LLM and Shawn Mathis, JD, LLM

"Quality and safety will never be assured if the Board [of Directors] doesn't take a leading role in demanding accountability and measurement in those areas," said David Classen, MD, vice president of First Consulting Group, based in Long Beach, California, and a patient safety expert.[1] "It should be as important to the board as the financial metrics reported to them."[1] As Dr. Classen stated, hospital boards play a critical role in patient safety and overall quality improvement. Leadership is an essential element in an effective patient safety program, and it cannot be delegated.[2] Without the board's dedication and support, the process of establishing a culture of honesty and transparency necessary to enhance patient safety cannot fully take root.

In the past, the board viewed its sole or primary responsibility as concerning the organization's financial health and reputation. It merely examined the monthly financial documents and assumed that clinicians and healthcare executives were more adept in matters pertaining to health care.[3] The board then acted by deferring judgment on medical issues and signing off on the healthcare-related items without much thought.[3] However, this lack of direct oversight negatively affected accountability, often resulted in diminished focus on quality and safety, and failed to establish quality and safety as an essential business strategy. Boards have to recognize that their duties do not end with financial stewardship.[4] Everyone, from Standards and Poor's to the IRS, holds boards accountable for the quality of care and services. Boards bear a direct responsibility for upholding the organization's mission to provide the best possible care and to avoid harm to patients.[4] They exist to represent the owners, and in the case of hospitals, which are mostly not for profit, the *owners* are the communities, including the patients and families for whom they care. It is not possible to represent these people without protecting them from harm. Finally, even from a financial perspective, when it comes to patient safety and quality, there is nothing worse for the bottom line than repetitive and/or persistent quality problems.

Over time there has been a growing awareness that hospital boards must place patient safety among their top priorities because the success of the organization is dependent on its ability to provide safe and high-quality care to each patient it sees.[5] The authors of one study interviewed 23 board chairs and correlated their knowledge and practices with clinical quality in their respective institutions. The authors found a modest relationship between board practices and quality.[6] Authors of another study surveyed hospital leaders, primarily CEOs, and found that when boards were engaged in quality-of-care issues, hospitals were more likely to have effective quality-improvement programs;[7] however, the authors of that study did not directly examine the relationship of board practices to quality of care. The author of another study focused on board practices and their effect on quality through individual case studies.[8] In related research, H. Joanna Jiang and colleagues surveyed CEOs and found that among the 12% who responded to the survey, those whose hospital boards were more engaged with quality generally had lower mortality rates and better performance on process measures for common medical conditions.[9,10] Finally, Thomas Vaughn and colleagues used a Web-based survey of CEOs in eight states and found that hospitals with boards that were more engaged in quality management performed better on a quality index related to hospital outcomes.[11]

THE IMPACT OF SARBANES-OXLEY REFORMS ON HOSPITAL GOVERNANCE AND PATIENT SAFETY

A 2010 report from the Office of the Inspector General (OIG) for the Department of Health and Human Services (OIG adverse events report) indicated that one of every seven Medicare beneficiaries who are hospitalized is harmed as a result of poor hospital care.[12] The OIG reports that unexpected and preventable adverse events in hospitals have cost U.S. taxpayers at least $4.4 billion annually and contributed to the deaths of approximately 180,000 patients per year.[13] More disconcerting, it appears that not much has changed since the high incidence of substandard hospital care in the United States gained widespread attention following a 1999 report by the Institute of Medicine, titled *To Err Is Human: Building a Safer Health System*. That report, released more than a decade ago, estimated that 44,000 to 98,000 Americans die each year as a result of preventable medical errors in hospitals.[13]

In the United States, a board of directors governs every private hospital regardless of whether the hospital is for profit or not for profit. Unfortunately, the statistics in the OIG adverse events report do not give the impression that the boards of U.S. hospitals are doing enough to ensure quality care despite recent reforms to increase their accountability for patient safety. In this chapter, we review the traditional duties of corporate directors, discuss the genesis of reforms that have increased the accountability of for-profit and not-for-profit boards of directors generally, and make the business case for focusing hospital governance on patient safety to ensure compliance with federal healthcare regulations.

A hospital corporation, like any other corporation, is a creature of state law. Whether the hospital is for profit or not for profit, it is organized and exists according to the laws of the state in which it is incorporated.[14] Corporate law principles, as interpreted by the courts of the state of formation, define the duties of a corporation's board of directors. Under traditional corporate doctrine, both for-profit and not-for-profit board members owe the corporation the fiduciary duties of care and loyalty.[15]

The duty of loyalty is fairly straightforward: it prohibits board members from placing their own financial interests before those of the organization.[15] The duty of care is a more amorphous concept. It requires board members to make decisions in good faith and to use the same level of care and skill as would a reasonably prudent person under similar circumstances.[15] The duty of care focuses on the process by which the board members inform themselves about the transaction at issue.[15]

Embedded within the duty of care is the concept of reasonable inquiry; directors are expected to make inquiries to management to obtain the information necessary to satisfy their duty of care.[16]

The seminal case on the duty of care owed by board members of a healthcare provider is *In re Caremark International, Inc. Derivative Litigation*.[17] There, a shareholder derivative suit was filed against Caremark's board of directors after the corporation was fined for violating federal and state health program laws and regulations. Specifically, Caremark's board was accused of violating its duty to actively monitor corporate performance by permitting circumstances to develop, and continue, which exposed the corporation to enormous legal liability.

In *Caremark*, the court focused on two ways the duty of care can arise: from a board decision that results in a loss because the decision was ill-advised or *negligent*, and from an *unconsidered failure of the board to act* in circumstances in which due attention would arguably have prevented the loss.[18] In the former, the board's decision itself (whether *wrong, stupid, egregious,* or *irrational*) does not result in director liability as long as the *process* that resulted in the decision was either rational or employed in a good-faith manner to advance the organization's interests.[18] This is the so-called business judgment rule, which insulates board members from liability for erroneous, harmful, or negligent decisions, absent bad faith.[15] So the business judgment rule is process oriented and informed by deep respect for all board decisions made in *good faith*.[19]

In the latter case of a board's failure to monitor, *Caremark* holds that a director has a duty to attempt in good faith to ensure that proper corporate information and reporting systems exist; if not, a director may be held liable for losses caused by the corporation's noncompliance with applicable legal standards.[20] Further, the level of detail that is appropriate for such information systems is also a question of *business judgment*. No system can guarantee that a corporation will not violate laws or regulations, or that senior officers or directors will not be misled or fail to detect acts material to the corporation's compliance with the law. Nevertheless, the board must in good faith determine that systems are adequate to ensure that appropriate information will come to its attention "in a timely manner as a matter of ordinary operations."[20]

An additional duty is required of nonprofit board members: obedience. The duty of obedience requires board members to act in accordance with the organization's mission and to refrain from engaging in transactions at odds with the stated mission.[15] In 2008, three out of four private hospitals in the United States were not for profit.[21] One need look no further than a hospital's Web site to find a statement of mission that refers to patient care, with an implied (if not express) commitment to patient safety.[22,23] An argument can be made that a not-for-profit hospital's patients, while not shareholders, are the ultimate stakeholders of the organization. In many states, attorneys general oversee not-for-profit hospitals, protecting interests of patient–stakeholders and the public at large.[24]

Within the healthcare industry, hospital board oversight of quality has emerged as a core fiduciary responsibility.[16] One could argue that ensuring quality of care properly falls under both the duty of care and the duty of obedience to the hospital's mission. Some states have enacted laws that place responsibility for quality of care on the hospital board but are generally silent as to specific measures that must be taken to fulfill this duty.[15] New Jersey law holds board members responsible for maintaining quality of care. Under New York law, hospital board members are responsible for "maintaining quality of patient services," and the board is required to establish a coordinated plan to oversee hospital activities to ensure quality of care.[25] Irrespective of the presence or absence of state laws that hold the board responsible for quality of care, board members should be mindful when discharging their fiduciary duties that quality has been—and after the 2010 OIG adverse events report will continue to be—an enforcement priority for federal healthcare regulators.[16]

Sarbanes-Oxley and Its Legacy

Although day-to-day hospital operations have long been subject to federal regulation by virtue of participation in federal healthcare programs, federal laws enacted to address the corporate and accounting scandals of Enron and its ilk have spilled over into the area of not-for-profit governance. The Sarbanes-Oxley Act of 2002 (Sarbanes-Oxley or the Act) changed corporate governance, including the responsibilities and accountabilities of officers and directors. With two notable exceptions,[26] the Act applies primarily to U.S. and non-U.S. companies that have registered debt or equity securities with the Securities and Exchange Commission under the Securities and Exchange Act of 1934.[27]

Although Sarbanes-Oxley did not target nonprofits, several state legislatures have already passed or are considering legislation containing elements of the Act to be applied to nonprofit organizations.[28] In many instances, nonprofit organizations have chosen to adopt policies and alter governance practices in response to the Act.[29] Nonprofit leaders are advised to review provisions of Sarbanes-Oxley and the law of the state of their organization's formation. Even if not required by law, nonprofit boards should consider using the Act as a best practices template for governance.[29] An analysis of the major provisions of the Act will identify some aspects that might serve to create greater board-level accountability for healthcare organizations.

Sarbanes-Oxley mandates enhanced disclosure of a company's finances. Under the Act, management and auditors must annually assess the company's internal controls and related disclosures. Additional disclosure of off-balance sheet financing and financial contingencies is required. Pro forma information is now required. The timing for disclosure of insider stock transactions has been accelerated; disclosure of certain information must be made in real time.[30] Under the Act, the integrity of financial information is ensured through regulations requiring an audit committee composed of independent directors. Sarbanes-Oxley addresses the role and composition of only the audit committee; standards for board directors serving on other committees are found in NYSE and NASDAQ listing requirements.[31]

A majority of board members must be independent under NYSE listing requirements.[32] An *independent director* is defined as not having a *material relationship* with a listed company either directly or as a partner, shareholder, or officer of an organization that has a relationship with the company.[33] If a director or any member of his or her immediate family receives direct compensation from the listed company of more than $120,000 per year, excluding director compensation or deferred compensation for prior service, the director is presumptively disqualified.[34] A current employee of the company can never serve as an independent director.[35] If a director or a member of his or her immediate family is affiliated with the company's external auditors, or with a customer accounting for the greater of 2% or $1 million of the listed company's gross revenues, the director is not independent.[36] If a director or a family member is an executive for another company whose compensation committee includes an executive of the listed company, the director is not considered independent.[37] Furthermore, a director is not independent if any of these disqualifying relationships took place within the three previous years.[38] Additionally, any contributions made by the listed company to any tax-exempt organization in which any independent director serves as an executive officer must be disclosed if the contribution in any single year exceeded $1 million or 2% of such tax-exempt organization's consolidated gross revenues.[39]

NYSE rules require independent directors to meet in regularly scheduled executive sessions without management.[40] The name of the director presiding at the executive sessions must be disclosed in the company's proxy statement for its annual meeting or in its annual report, and describe how interested parties can communicate with either the presiding director or the independent directors as a group.[41] Listed companies must have an audit committee, a compensation committee, and a nominating and corporate governance committee, each composed entirely of independent directors.[42]

NYSE requires that a nominating and corporate governance committee have a written charter stating the committee's purpose.[43] The charter must include identifying individuals qualified to become board members consistent with the criteria approved by the board. The charter must address selecting or recommending that the board select the director nominees for election at the annual shareholders meeting, and developing and recommending to the board a set of corporate governance principles for the corporation.[43] Importantly, the charter should give the committee the sole authority to hire and fire any search firm used to identify director candidates.[44]

NYSE listing rules, and not Sarbanes-Oxley, address the compensation committee. As with the nominating and corporate governance committee, the compensation committee must be composed of independent directors and have a written charter addressing the committee's purpose.[45] Its purpose must include discharging the board's responsibilities for compensating the company's executives and producing an annual report on executive compensation for inclusion in the proxy statement or the annual report.[46] The committee's duties and responsibilities must include reviewing and approving corporate goals and objectives relevant to compensating the chief executive officer, evaluating his or her performance in light of these goals and objectives, having sole authority to determine his or her compensation based on this evaluation, and making recommendations to the board for non-CEO compensation, incentive compensation plans, and equity-based plans.[47] The committee must also evaluate its own performance annually.[48] The charter must give the committee the sole authority to hire and fire any consulting firm to assist in evaluating the compensation of directors or senior executives, including sole authority to approve the firm's compensation and other retention terms.[49]

The newly revised Internal Revenue Service Form 990, the tax return for tax-exempt organizations (including not-for-profit hospitals) reflects increased interest in governance and management. It seeks information about governance from tax-exempt organizations that publicly traded companies are required to disclose under Sarbanes-Oxley and under exchange listing rules, including:

- the number of voting members of the governing body who are independent;
- whether any officer, director, trustee, or key employee has a family or business relationship with any other officer, director trustee, or key employee;
- whether the organization delegated control over management duties customarily performed by or under the direct supervision of officers, directors, or trustees or key employees to a management company or other person;
- whether the organization became aware in the past year of any material diversion of the organization's assets;
- whether the organization has any members, stockholders, or other persons who may elect one or more members of the governing body;
- whether any of the decisions of the governing body are subject to approval of other members, stockholders, or other persons;
- whether the organization contemporaneously documents meetings held, or written actions undertaken, during the year by the governing body and by each committee with authority to act on behalf of the governing body;

- whether the organization has a written conflict of interest policy;
- whether the organization regularly and consistently monitors and enforces compliance with the conflict of interest policy;
- whether the organization has a written whistleblower policy;
- whether the organization has a written document retention and destruction policy;
- whether the process for determining compensation of the CEO, executive director, top management official, other officers, and key employees of the organization includes a review and approval by independent persons, comparability data, and contemporaneous substantiation of the deliberation and decision; and
- the way in which the organization makes its governing documents, conflict of interest policy, and financial statements available to the public.[50]

Tax-exempt bonds, which are considered securities and are the primary method for not-for-profit hospitals to raise capital, have also come under scrutiny of the Senate Finance Subcommittee. The Committee's recommendations included requiring both the CEO and CFO to certify the organization's Form 990.[51]

How Governance Impacts Financial Performance and Ratings

A charitable board is essentially a caretaker of the not-for-profit corporation and its assets.[52] Accordingly, the board must concern itself with quality of care as one of many metrics affecting the hospital's access to capital. Moody's Investors Service is the bond-rating agency for healthcare nonprofits seeking tax-exempt financing. According to Moody's, governance is more challenging for nonprofit hospitals than it is for for-profit institutions. This is due to the complexity of such organizations, rapid changes in technology, shifting governmental policy, intense market competition, burdensome liability exposure, difficult labor relations, and frequent local media attention.[51] Recruiting unpaid board members with relevant expertise, usually from the local community, is extremely difficult.[51] This has resulted in the delegation of more key decisions to management by hospital boards than is typical in other sectors.[51]

According to Moody's, not-for-profit healthcare governance has become a more important credit variable as corporate governance and accounting issues have been scrutinized in the for-profit sector.[51] Although much of the Sarbanes-Oxley legislation is not applicable to not-for-profit institutions, Moody's notes that many nonprofits are voluntarily adopting various aspects of its reforms. This trend is driven in part by board members of not-for-profit organizations who are also corporate executives or board members of publicly traded corporations that have been required to comply with Sarbanes-Oxley.

Moody's assessment of governance is an important component of the credit profile of the nonprofit hospital. Noting that governance is one of the most difficult factors to assess due to lack of quantifiable measures, Moody's looks at the following core dimensions of governance:

- Development of the organization's mission
- Selection and evaluation of senior management
- Board composition and preference
- Understanding and interpretation of financial reporting
- Use of performance metrics based on external benchmarks to regularly review the organization's performance
- Maintaining and building the organization's financial resources
- Avoidance of conflicts of interest[51]

Governance can significantly affect a hospital's bond rating, particularly if it is on the borderline between two ratings. Although the credit effect of governance may not be apparent in the short run, it frequently emerges during times of crisis. Poor governance is often a contributing reason for financial troubles or other problems of a hospital that may be difficult to identify and correct.[51]

Moody's believes that board composition is another critical dimension of effective governance.[51] Moody's examines a number of key factors when assessing board composition, including:

- the background of board members
- the selection process for new board members
- committee structure and processes
- the size of the board
- tenure of board members
- development of board members[51]

Particularly critical to Moody's rating is the background of the board members. A board member who does not understand the hospital's operations or industry dynamics will be unable to effectively evaluate the management or know when it might be necessary to step in to address problems.[51] A hospital's board tends to be composed primarily of individuals from the local community. Members of an effective board should have a diverse set of skills, including sector-specific knowledge. Desirable skill sets include clinical experience; an understanding of quality and safety issues; familiarity with third-party reimbursement methodologies; accounting, legal, and business management; and investment management.[51] The board's commitment to self-education is critical in helping members gain familiarity with issues or facets of the hospital's operations that will make for effective governance.[51]

The board's selection and evaluation of senior management are of utmost importance to the not-for-profit hospital. Unlike a for-profit hospital, a nonprofit hospital has no owners or shareholders who demand a return on their investment. In addition to patient stakeholders, hospitals have constituencies such as the physicians who have privileges at the hospital, third-party payers (including Medicare and Medicaid), regulators, and bondholders.[51]

The board has primary responsibility for creating written performance objectives and appropriate measures of performance for the CEO. These performance goals provide transparency and serve as an objective basis for compensation decisions. Moody's suggests that, along with achieving financial or industry benchmarks, it is appropriate to tie compensation to reductions in clinical errors and increases in patient and employee satisfaction—criteria that directly affect patient safety.[51]

Board Oversight of Quality and Patient Safety

The relationship between healthcare quality and cost efficiency is also becoming more widely understood. Efficiency, by definition, means avoidance of unnecessary and often unsafe care.[16] Contemporary healthcare quality, patient safety, and cost efficiency initiatives provide an opportunity for healthcare organizations to promote their missions while enhancing financial success.[16] Increasing emphasis on quality measurement techniques is now generating process and outcomes data that hospital boards of directors can use to monitor and assess the quality, and thus safety, of patient care consistent with the hospital's mission and their own fiduciary obligations.[15]

Healthcare providers operate under an extensive federal and state regulatory scheme increasingly designed to tie the healthcare provider's reimbursement to quality of care. Medicare and Medicaid conditions of participation require hospitals to monitor quality through credentialing of medical staff and through effective quality assessment and performance improvement programs. These conditions of participation specify that the medical staff be accountable to a hospital's governing body for the quality of care provided to patients.[16]

Corresponding to the regulatory trend of payment for quality, government enforcement authorities have become increasingly focused on the quality of care provided to federal health program beneficiaries. The submission of a claim for reimbursement to the government is the predicate act that establishes jurisdiction over the provider. The Office of the Inspector General, the U.S. Department of Justice, and state attorneys general are collaborating to prosecute providers who seek payment for substandard care.[16] Healthcare providers can be subject to civil and criminal monetary fines, exclusion from state and federal health programs, and even incarceration for providing unnecessary or substandard care. Even individuals who are not directly involved in the provision of health care can be subject to exclusion if they cause or permit others to provide substandard care. Consequently, all levels of a healthcare organization, from the direct caregiver to the governing body of an institutional provider, face liability for failing to meet the quality of care obligations of government program providers.[16]

The government relies on civil and criminal fraud theories to prosecute providers of substandard care. Consider the following examples of enforcement resulting from conditions that compromised patient safety:

- A Colorado rehabilitation center entered into a $1.9 million civil False Claims Act settlement to resolve allegations that it provided worthless services to patients, resulting from systemic understaffing at the facility where deficient services and abuse caused the deaths of six patients.[16]
- In Missouri, a long-term care management company, its CEO, and three nursing homes were charged with imposing budgetary constraints that they knew or should have known would prevent facilities from providing adequate care to residents. The CEO was sentenced to pay $29,000 in criminal fines and to 18 months in jail. The management company and nursing homes were each sentenced to pay nearly $200,000 in criminal fines. In a related civil case, the defendants paid $1.25 million to resolve False Claims Act allegations and agreed to exclusion from federal health programs.[16]
- A Pennsylvania hospital entered into a $200,000 civil False Claims Act settlement to resolve substandard care allegations related to the improper use of restraints.[16]

The foregoing examples make clear that systemic conditions that adversely affect the quality of care threaten to materially affect the financial condition, if not the very existence, of a healthcare organization. Unlike medical malpractice liability, there is no insurance coverage for fines and penalties imposed for violating government healthcare laws and regulations. Charitable endowments are typically restricted in use and cannot be used to pay for a hospital's fines. In addition to fines and penalties that will affect the hospital's operating income, settlements with the government routinely require ongoing oversight of the organization and may force the hospital to hire and pay for an independent monitor for a period of years. The sanction of exclusion from federal health programs may put a hospital out of business. As a result, directors need to elevate quality and patient safety to the same level of focus that financial and regulatory compliance currently command.[16]

Well before the 2010 OIG adverse events report, the Office of the Inspector General viewed the board's role as *critical* in advancing clinical improvement initiatives in healthcare organizations. To develop an understanding of the relevant quality and patient safety issues, the OIG has suggested that boards ask the following series of questions:

1. What are the goals of the organization's quality improvement program? What metrics and benchmarks are used to measure progress toward each of these performance goals? How is each goal specifically linked to management accountability?
2. How does the organization measure and improve the quality of patient/resident care? Who are the key management and clinical leaders responsible for these quality and safety programs?

3. How are the organization's quality assessment and improvement processes integrated into overall corporate policies and operations? Are clinical quality standards supported by operational policies? How does management implement and enforce these policies? What internal controls exist to monitor and report on quality metrics?
4. Does the board have a formal orientation and continuing education process that helps members appreciate external quality and patient safety requirements? Does the board include members with expertise in patient safety and quality issues?
5. What information is essential to the board's ability to understand and evaluate the organization's quality assessment and performance improvement programs? Once these performance metrics and benchmarks are established, how frequently does the board receive reports about the quality improvement efforts?
6. How are the organization's quality assessment and improvement processes coordinated with its corporate compliance program? How are quality of care and patient safety issues addressed in the organization's risk assessment and corrective action plans?
7. What processes are in place to promote the reporting of quality concerns and medical errors and to protect those who ask questions and report problems? What guidelines exist for reporting quality and patient safety concerns to the board?
8. Are human and other resources adequate to support patient safety and clinical quality? How are proposed changes in resource allocation evaluated from the perspective of clinical quality and patient care? Are systems in place to provide adequate resources to account for differences in patient acuity and care needs?
9. Do the organization's competency assessment and training, credentialing, and peer review processes adequately recognize the necessary focus on clinical quality and patient safety issues?
10. How are adverse patient events and other medical errors identified, analyzed, reported, and incorporated into an organization's performance improvement activities? How do management and the board address quality deficiencies without unnecessarily increasing the organization's liability exposure?[16]

THE MCNULTY MEMORANDUM

The submission of a claim for reimbursement to a federal healthcare program for substandard care is considered a violation of the False Claims Act and can be prosecuted as healthcare fraud. The Department of Justice has had "unprecedented success" in prosecuting corporate fraud following the scandals that led to the passage of Sarbanes-Oxley.[53] Even before the passage of the Patient Protection and Affordable Care Act in 2010, healthcare quality had become an area of keen interest to enforcement authorities. Armed with data that are publicly reported or mined from the Medicare and Medicaid databases, state adverse events reporting systems data, and sentinel events reported to The Joint Commission, federal and state prosecutors have recovered False Claims Act settlements and judgments in the billions of dollars since 2006 from healthcare defendants.[3]

The Department of Justice (DOJ) has announced that indicting corporations (or any other type of business organization) for wrongdoing enables the government to address and be a force for positive change of corporate culture, alter corporate behavior, and prevent, discover, and punish white collar crime.[53] When determining whether to bring charges against a corporation and when negotiating plea agreements, DOJ policy requires prosecutors to consider the existence and adequacy of the corporation's preexisting compliance program.[53] Prosecutors are also instructed to consider the corporation's remedial actions, including any efforts to implement an effective corporate compliance program or to improve an existing one, to replace responsible management, and to discipline or terminate wrongdoers.[53]

Federal sentencing guidelines provide for the possibility of a reduced sentence if the hospital had an effective compliance and ethics program in place at the time of the offense for which it is being sentenced. However, the guidelines are optional and not binding on judges. To qualify for sentencing credit, the compliance program must meet certain criteria that serve as the foundation of the hospital's compliance program.[54] Clearly, as part of their duties of care and obedience, hospital board members must ensure themselves that a proper compliance program, which addresses quality and patient safety, is in place to mitigate the severity of penalties should any violation of federal healthcare laws and regulations ever arise.

Corporate governance reforms rooted in Sarbanes-Oxley, combined with federal health program regulations that condition payment and participation on quality of patient care, have substantially increased the hospital board's accountability over the past decade. Fortunately, there are a number of state, federal, and industry resources to which the nonprofit hospital board can turn to fashion policies and systems to ensure that it continues to meet its evolving fiduciary duties of care, loyalty, and obedience. Furthermore, heightened government enforcement action for poor-quality health care provided to beneficiaries of federal healthcare programs creates a powerful incentive for boards to focus on patient safety.[3]

CREATING VIGILANCE FOR SAFETY AT THE BOARD LEVEL

When researchers looked at the common characteristics among high-performing organizations, they found that they include the following:[55]

- The board spends more than 25% of its time on quality issues.
- The board receives a formal quality performance measurement report.
- The CEO is held accountable for quality and safety goals and retains ultimate responsibility.
- Senior executive compensation is based in part on quality initiative performance.
- The board participates in the development of explicit criteria to guide medical staff credentialing and privileging.
- The board quality committee performs an in-depth annual review of patient satisfaction scores, at a minimum.
- The board sets the board agenda for quality.
- There is a high level of interaction between the board and the medical staff on quality strategy.

Unfortunately, there is still a long way to go in translating the undeniable connection linking board activity to quality in the boardroom into action in clinical units of the organization. A recent study demonstrated there are still questions about whether hospital boards are sufficiently educated about and engaged in oversight of quality.[56] The authors of the study surveyed a nationally representative sample of board chairs from 1,000 U.S. hospitals and found that fewer than half of the boards rated quality of care as one of their top two priorities. Further, only a minority of the boards reported receiving training in quality. In accordance with previous studies, the authors found a large difference in related board activities between high-performing and low-performing hospitals. They concluded that governing boards are likely an important target for intervention to improve care in U.S. hospitals.

In the remainder of this text, we will explore ways in which boards of directors should work to become knowledgeable about the science of quality and safety and to advance patient safety and quality in their organizations.

IHI GOVERNANCE INTERVENTION: GETTING BOARDS ON BOARD

In February 2007, the Institute for Healthcare Improvement (IHI) launched its "Boards on Board" program as part of its 5 Million Lives Campaign. The IHI's intervention focuses on what it describes as "deeply engaged leadership starting with the Board of Trustees," which it states is "one of the most crucial attributes of organizations that have demonstrated the greatest sustained progress in patient safety."[4] The program aims to offer insight into the behavior of effective boards, to apply what is learned about governance to the IHI Framework for Leadership for Improvement, and to suggest several straightforward steps for developing effective governance activity in organizations.[4] With this program, the IHI provides powerful tools to increase board involvement in patient safety.

The program begins by applying the IHI Framework for Leadership for Improvement to governance and recommends specific actions for governing boards to take within each of the framework's following five categories:[4]

1. Establish the mission, vision, and strategy.
   a. Set direction and monitor performance.
      i. Integrate strategy and quality.
      ii. Monitor the culture of quality and safety.
      iii. Establish aims for safety and quality improvement.
2. Build the foundation for an effective leadership system.
   a. Establish an interdisciplinary board quality committee.
   b. Bring knowledgeable quality leaders onto the board.
   c. Set and achieve educational standards for the board members.
   d. Build a culture of real (not pro forma) conversations about improving care at board and committee meetings, with physician and nursing leaders and with administration.
   e. Allocate adequate resources to ongoing training of employees and medical staff about quality improvement.
3. Build will.
   a. Establish a policy of full transparency about data on quality and safety.
   b. Insist on the review of both data and stories from patients and families.
   c. Help patients and families tell their stories directly to staff, senior leaders, and the board.
   d. Establish policies and practices with respect to errors and injuries that emphasize, through communication, respectful practice, disclosure, apology, support, and resolution.
   e. Understand both the current performance of your organization and the performance levels of the best organizations in the world.
   f. Show that you own the problem and are driving the agenda by placing quality first on the board agenda and devoting 25% or more of the board's agenda to it.
   g. Show courage: don't flinch.
4. Ensure access to ideas.
   a. Boards should ask management for idea-generating questions when reviewing progress against quality and safety aims:
      i. Who is the best in the world at this?
      ii. Have you talked to them to find out how they do it?
      iii. How many ideas have you tried out?
      iv. What ideas did our patients and families and front-line staff have for improvement?
5. Attend relentlessly to execution.
   a. Establish executive accountability for achievement of aims.
   b. Establish an effective oversight process, including:

   i. Devoting 25% of board meeting time to quality and safety.
   ii. Monitoring your own system-level measures for improvement (rather than being comforted by benchmarks).
   iii. Reviewing data generated weekly or, at a minimum, monthly.

c. Ask hard questions, including:
   i. Are we on track to achieve the aim?
   ii. If not, why not? What is the improvement strategy? What are key steps planned toward full-scale execution?

Next, IHI asks governance leadership to implement the program by beginning, at a minimum, to focus on the following six activities:

1. **Setting Aims:** Set a specific aim to reduce harm this year. Make an explicit, public commitment to measurable quality improvement (e.g., reduction in unnecessary mortality and harm), establishing a clear aim for the facility or system.
2. **Getting Data and Hearing Stories:** Select and review progress toward safer care as the first agenda item at every board meeting, grounded in transparency, and putting a human face on harm data.
3. **Establishing and Monitoring System-Level Measures:** Identify a small group of organization-wide roll-up measures of patient safety (e.g., facility-wide harm, risk-adjusted mortality) that are continually updated and are made transparent to the entire organization and all of its customers.
4. **Changing the Environment, Policies, and Culture:** Commit to establish and maintain an environment that is respectful, fair, and just for all who experience the pain and loss as a result of avoidable harm and adverse outcomes: the patients, their families, and the staff at the sharp end of error.
5. **Learning . . . Starting with the Board:** Develop your capability as a board. Learn about how *best in the world* boards work with executive and physician leaders to reduce harm. Set an expectation for similar levels of education and training for all staff.
6. **Establishing Executive Accountability:** Oversee the effective execution of a plan to achieve your aims to reduce harm, including executive team accountability for clear quality improvement targets.

ADDITIONAL ORGANIZATIONS THAT AFFIRM THE BOARD'S ROLE IN PATIENT SAFETY

Other organizations have worked to further engage boards in the areas of quality and safety. The National Quality Foundation (NQF) issued its Safe Practice Revisions and its first chapter, titled Culture of Safety, which addresses governance, executive leadership, and quality.[57] The Joint Commission revised its governance and leadership standards in 2008 to reflect board activity and began scoring the governance and leadership standards in 2009 to give hospitals adequate time to change their practices.[58] The Office of Inspector General (OIG) with the American Health Lawyers Association (AHLA) issued a report on corporate responsibility and healthcare quality that was designed to help boards ask knowledgeable and appropriate questions related to healthcare quality requirements, measurement tools, and reporting requirements.[59] Business coalitions, including the National Business Group on Health Toolkit, have acknowledged that the executives of companies who are members of their organizations are often the people who are sitting on hospital boards. As a result, the National Business Group have implemented training programs for hospital board members.[60] Additionally, organizations such as the Leapfrog Group have also forced Boards to consider their role in advancing organizational quality and safety.[61]

CHALLENGES BOARDS MAY FACE

Boards can face numerous challenges when working to advance patient safety, including, but not limited to, the following:[62]

- apathy by board members, perhaps due to lack of knowledge or competing priorities;
- a CEO who doesn't provide sufficient information to the board to enable them to fully understand the quality and safety challenges to support the program;
- complexity of restructuring the reporting mechanism to channel patient safety data to the safety officer and ultimately to individual board members;
- a reluctance to readily share information due to concerns about public opinion and suspicion fueled by a lay press exposition of medical errors;
- chronic history of denial by hospital administration, the board, and physicians that errors occur;
- lack of awareness by the board and or administration that a problem exists (e.g., poor information reporting);
- a traditional medical culture of individual responsibility and blame and inadequate allocation of resources for quality improvement and error prevention;
- inadequate knowledge by the board and administration about the frequency, cause, and impact of errors, as well as about methods for error prevention;
- belief that the current error rate is acceptable given the complexity of patients served, current budgetary challenges, and competing priorities; and
- the notion that problems can be fixed as they happen (i.e., no proactive approach).

IHI MENTOR HOSPITALS

Although there are substantial challenges to "getting boards on board," the IHI, along with other organizations, provides numerous tools to enable success. Specifically, the IHI has compiled a list of mentor hospitals that have volunteered to provide support, advice, clinical expertise, and tips to hospitals seeking help with their implementation efforts.[63] Currently, the list consists of 10 hospitals. The list of mentor hospitals sets forth demographic information so hospitals can identify a mentor that is similar in composition to them. The Web site also provides a wealth of information and insight into how each of these mentor hospitals is currently addressing the six activities that the IHI advocates all boards should implement.

BOARD EDUCATION: PROVIDING BOARDS WITH THE TOOLS THEY NEED TO SUCCEED

It is essential that board members are positioned to be effective in the areas of patient safety and quality oversight. With every meeting, boards should work to improve quality and safety literacy. They need to understand the data they are receiving and put names and faces to the vast sea of numbers. This requires providing them with the information in a way that is comprehensible to them and that allows them to answer the difficult questions, including how many people were harmed or died in their hospital and how the organization compares to similar organizations relative to quality and safety. I have shown that boards often perceive quality as being significantly better than do the administrators, doctors, and nurses.[64] When asked in a survey whether patient safety trumped productivity in the respondents' work organizations, on a scale of one to five, with one being every day and five being not at all, only 27% of middle management scored it positively, whereas 72% of board and c-suite members (chief executive officer, chief operating officer, chief financial officer, etc.) did.

Content for Effective Board Meetings

Safety and quality must be discussed at every board meeting to effectuate improvement in patient safety. Safety and quality issues should be the first items on the agenda, and the conversation should not be cut short due to lack of time. Data must be presented to provide an accurate view of not only the frequency and severity of preventable events but also the root causes giving rise to them.

Ideally, a board member should lead the discussion with management support. He or she should use language that allows other board members to apply their personal learning and highlight key issues with which the quality committee is dealing (assuming there is a quality committee). This should be an actual discussion that opens up the floor for feedback and questions and results in recommendations for policy changes. If possible, pertinent senior management and clinical staff should attend this portion of the meeting, and board members should have the opportunity to ask questions of them.[65]

As boards review cases, they should make every attempt to personalize the stories and be provided with background information on each patient. All patient stories should bring the data to life by putting a face on the data. The stories should explain how the incidents affected both the lives of patients and their families. The board should understand why the story was told and how it relates to the big picture of patient safety. In hearing these stories, boards must also understand that their role is to set priorities, foster culture and values, and hold management accountable for system improvement.

Use of Patient Safety Dashboards

To optimize results, boards must set clear expectations and goals for reducing harm to patients and monitor the progress toward those goals. They must demand to see reports on quality and safety performance as often as they do financial reports. Boards should receive dashboard-type key performance indicator reports at each meeting, one quadrant of which covers patient safety. A dashboard is a powerful tool that allows the board to focus on the organization's key issues and strategies. It displays key indicators in a highly visual and easily readable format that helps identify areas that are doing well and those that need improvement.

Board members' obligations don't end with just glancing at the dashboards and reports, though. Instead, they must actively analyze the reports and constantly question how many medical errors occurred, how many near misses were identified, what is being done about them, and probably most important, the impact of the actions taken. Regularly reported quality and safety metrics provide a useful and user-friendly source of information to assess whether care is getting better and whether the hospital is on track to achieve its key quality and safety objectives. If regularly reported user-friendly reports are not provided to the Board they should be provided with sufficient information to investigate why care is not getting better and to determine whether they need to amend their strategies for improvement or to amend the execution of those strategies.

Dashboard

The aims should be clearly displayed and understood. A few system-level measures should be graphically displayed over time, perhaps as a rolling 12-month report. The measures should be displayed monthly and should be close to real time. Measures do not necessarily need to be risk adjusted. Measures of critical initiatives (projects that must be executed to achieve the aim) should be available if needed to answer the board's questions. The full board should review the system-level measures. The board quality committee should review both the system-level measures and the key drivers of those measures. Occasionally, but not often, the board will need to see measures of key projects, but these key projects are generally the responsibility of management to oversee and execute.

CONCLUSION

In conclusion, boards bear the ultimate responsibility for quality and patient safety. They must always put patients first and make patient safety central to their strategic plan because their actions are required to reduce harm and save lives.

References

1. Appleby, C. (2003). Industrial strength: Patient safety means leading preindustrial health care into a postindustrial world. In K. Gardner (Ed.), *The excellent board: practical solutions for health care trustees and CEOs* (pp. 326–336). Chicago, IL: AHA Press.
2. Botwinick, L., Bisognano, M., & Haraden, C. (2006). Institute for Healthcare Improvement. *Leadership Guide to Patient Safety*. IHI Innovation Series white paper. Cambridge, MA: Institute for Healthcare Improvement. Retrieved from http://www.ihi.org/knowledge/pages/ihiwhitepapers/leadershipguidetopatientsafetywhitepaper.aspx
3. Miller, T. E., & Gutmann, V. L. (2009). Changing expectations for board oversight of healthcare quality: The emerging paradigm. *Journal of Health & Life Sciences Law, 2*(4) 31, 33–77.
4. 5 Million Lives Campaign (2008). *Getting Started Kit: Governance Leadership "Boards on Board" How-to Guide*. Cambridge, MA: Institute for Healthcare Improvement. Retrieved from http://www.ihi.org/knowledge/Pages/Tools/HowtoGuideGovernanceLeadership.aspx.
5. Keroack, M. A., Youngberg, B. J., Cerese, J. L., Krsek, C., Prellwitz, L.W., & Trevelyan, E.W. (2007). Organizational factors associated with high performance in quality and safety in academic medical centers. *Academic Medicine, 82*(12), 1178–1186.
6. Joshi, M. S., & Hines, S. C. (2006). Getting the board on board: Engaging hospital boards in quality and patient safety. *Joint Commission Journal on Quality and Patient Safety, 32*(4), 179–187.
7. Weiner, B. J., Shortell, S. M., & Alexander, J. (1997). Promoting clinical involvement in hospital quality improvement efforts: The effects of top management, board and physician leadership. *Health Services Research, 32*(4), 491–510.
8. Dulworth, S. (2003). Hospitals and the competitive edge: How educated boards make a difference. *Journal for Healthcare Quality, 25*(6), 28–30, 41.
9. Jiang, H. J., Lockee, C., Bass, K., & Fraser, I. (2008). Board engagement in quality: Findings of a survey of hospital and system leaders. *Journal of Healthcare Management, 53*(2), 121–134.
10. Jiang, H. J., Lockee, C., Bass, K., & Fraser I. (2009). Board oversight of quality: Any differences in process of care and mortality? *Journal of Healthcare Management, 54*(1), 15–29.
11. Vaughn, T., Koepke, M., Kroch, E., Lehrman, W., Sinha, S., & Levey, S. (2006). Engagement of leadership in quality improvement initiatives: Executive quality improvement survey results. *Journal of Patient Safety, 2*(1), 2–9.
12. Department of Health and Human Services, Office of Inspector General. (2010). Adverse Events in Hospitals: National Incidence Among Medicare Beneficiaries. Retrieved from http://oig.hhs.gov/oei/reports/oei-06-09-00090.pdf.
13. Wilson, D. (2010, November 15). Mistakes chronicled on Medicare patients. *The New York Times*. Retrieved from http://www.nytimes.com/2010/11/16/business/16medicare.html.
14. See, for example, the Illinois Business Corporation Act of 1983, 805 ILCS 5/1 et seq. (Thomson West 2004); and the Illinois General Not For Profit Corporation Act of 1986, 805 ILCS 105/101.01 et seq. (Thomson West 2004).
15. Jacobson, P. D., & Mathur, S. K. (2010). Health law 2010: It's not all about the money. *American Journal of Law & Medicine, 36*(2–3), 389–404.
16. Callender, A. N., Hastings, D. A., Hemsley, M. C., Morris, L., & Peregrine, M. W. (2007).

Corporate Responsibility and Health Care Quality: A Resource for Health Care Boards of Directors, United States Department of Health and Human Services, Office of the Inspector General, American Health Lawyers Association, p. 2. Retrieved from http://oig.hhs.gov/fraud/docs/complianceguidance/CorporateResponsibilityFinal%209-4-07.pdf.

17. In re Caremark International, Inc. Derivative Litigation, 698 A. 2d 959 (Del. Ch.1996).
18. 698 A. 2d at 967.
19. 698 A. 2d at 967-68.
20. 698 A. 2d at 970.
21. American Hospital Association. (2010). Fast Facts on U.S. Hospitals. Retrieved from http://www.aha.org/aha/resource-center/Statistics-and-Studies/fast-facts.html.
22. Northwestern Memorial Hospital. Mission & Core Values. Retrieved from http://www.nmh.org/nm/about+us+mission+core+values.
23. The University of Chicago Medicine. Website states its mission is "to provide superior healthcare in a compassionate manner." Retrieved from http://www.uchospitals.edu/pdf/uch_005118.pdf.
24. Nixon Peabody. (2006). New York's Not-for-Profit Law Empowers Attorney General Spitzer to Pursue Former NYSE Chairman Richard Grasso for Excessive Compensation. http://www.nixonpeabody.com/services_pubdetail.asp?ID=1293&SID=62.
25. N.Y. Comp. Codes R. & Regs. tit. 10 §405.2 (a).
26. Whistleblower and obstruction provisions of the Act apply to all companies, whether publicly traded or not. It is a criminal offense to punish whistleblowers who report truthful information about the possible commission of a criminal offense to law enforcement officials under 18 U.S.C. §1514A (a) (2). Under Sections 802(a) and 1102 of the Act, it is a criminal offense to alter, destroy, or conceal a document, record, or other object with the intent to impair its integrity or availability for use in an official proceeding, or otherwise to obstruct, influence, or impede an official proceeding. 18 U.S.C. 1519 and 1512(c).
27. 15 U.S.C. § 7201, et seq. (2010).
28. For example, see N.Y. Not-for-Profit Corp. Law, Article 7, §717.
29. BoardSource (formerly the National Center for Nonprofit Boards) and Independent Sector. (2006). The Sarbanes-Oxley Act and Implications for Nonprofit Organizations. Retrieved from http://www.boardsource.org/dl.asp?document_id=558.
30. Lander, G. P. (2004). *What is Sarbanes-Oxley?* (p. 3). New York, NY: McGraw-Hill.
31. Lander, G. P. (2004). *What is Sarbanes-Oxley?* (p. 46). New York, NY: McGraw-Hill. Because NASDAQ listing requirements are similar in most respects to those of the NYSE, we focus only on the NYSE for purposes of this discussion.
32. NYSE Listed Company Manual, § 303A.01 (NYSE-2009-89), November 25, 2009.
33. NYSE Listed Company Manual, § 303A.02 (a).
34. NYSE Listed Company Manual, § 303A.02 (b) (ii).
35. NYSE Listed Company Manual, § 303A.02 (b) (i).
36. NYSE Listed Company Manual, § 303A.02 (b) (iii) and (v).
37. NYSE Listed Company Manual, § 303A.02 (b) (iv).
38. NYSE Listed Company Manual, § 303A.02 (b) (i), (ii), (iii), (iv), (v).
39. NYSE Listed Company Manual, § 303A.02(b) (v), Disclosure Requirement.
40. NYSE Listed Company Manual, § 303A.03.
41. NYSE Listed Company Manual, § 303A.03, Disclosure Requirement.
42. NYSE Listed Company Manual, §§ 303A.04, 303A.05 and 303A.06.
43. NYSE Listed Company Manual, § 303A.04 (b).
44. NYSE Listed Company Manual, § 303A.04 (b), Commentary.
45. NYSE Listed Company Manual, § 303A.05.
46. NYSE Listed Company Manual, § 303A.05, Disclosure Requirements.
47. NYSE Listed Company Manual, § 303A.05 (b) (i)(A).
48. NYSE Listed Company Manual, § 303A.05 (b) (ii).
49. NYSE Listed Company Manual, § 303A.05, Commentary.
50. IRS Form 990 (2009), Part IV.
51. Moody's Investors Service. (2005). Governance of Not-for-Profit Healthcare Organizations, pp. 1–2, 4. Retrieved from http://www.healthlawyers.org/Members/PracticeGroups/blg/ExecSumms/Documents/Moody_Report.pdf.

52. Manhattan Eye, Ear & Throat Hospital v. Spitzer, 186 Misc. 2d 126, 151; 715 N.Y.S. 2d 575, 593 (N.Y. Sup. Ct. 1999).
53. U.S. Department of Justice, Office of the Deputy Attorney General, Paul McNulty. (2010). Principles of Federal Prosecution of Business Organizations. Retrieved from http://www.justice.gov/dag/speeches/2006/mcnulty_memo.pdf.
54. Gouraige, H., & Scielzo, A. (2010, June). *The intersection of compliance and governance: Overcoming challenges*. Paper presented at the annual meeting of the American Health Lawyers Association, Seattle, WA.
55. Lockee, C., Kroom, K., Zablocki, E., & Bader, B. (2006). *Quality*. San Diego, CA: The Governance Institute. Retrieved from http://www.google.com/search?client = safari&rls = en&q = Lockee + C, + Kroom + K, + Zablocki + E, + Bader + B.&ie = UTF-8&oe = UTF-8.
56. Jha, A., & Epstein, A. (2010). Hospital governance and the quality of care. *Health Affairs, 29*(1), 182–187.
57. National Quality Forum, Safe Practices for Better Health Care, Washington DC, April 2010.
58. http://www.jointcommission.org/assets/1/18/WP_Leadership_Standards.pdf accessed May 4, 2012.
59. http://www.healthlawyers.org/hlresources/PI/InfoSeries/Documents/OIG_CorpResp HealthcareQuality.pdf accessed May 4, 2012
60. http://www.businessgrouphealth.org/pdfs/National%20Business%20Group%20on%20Health%20Position%20Statement%20on%20Health%20Care%20Quality%20and%20Patient%20Safety.pdf accessed may 5, 2012
61. http://www.leapfroggroup.org/home acessed May 5, 2012
62. Mycek, S. (2003). Patient safety: It starts with the board. In K. Gardner (Ed.), *The excellent board: Practical solutions for health care trustees and CEOs* (pp. 350–362). Chicago, IL: AHA Press.
63. Institute for Healthcare Improvement. Mentor Hospital Registry. Retrieved from http://www.ihi.org/offerings/Memberships Networks/MentorHospitalRegistry/Pages/default.aspx.
64. Nursing Leadership from Bedside to Boardroom: Opinion Leaders' Perceptions Diane Pinakiewicz et al., Leadership from Boardroom to Bedside, CMS Summit (Fall 2006).

7

Toward a Philosophy of Patient Safety: Expanding the Systems Approach to Medical Error

David Resnick, JD, PhD

THE PROBLEM OF MEDICAL ERROR

The publication in 1999 of the report from the Institute of Medicine (IOM) entitled *To Err Is Human* has sparked considerable discussion about the incidence and etiology of errors in medicine, as well as policies and procedures for minimizing errors.[1] The IOM report estimated the annual deaths from medical errors to be between 44,000 and 98,000, or more than the annual deaths from motor vehicle accidents (43,458) or breast cancer (42,297).[2] The IOM arrived at this number by extrapolating from error rates from three different studies of medical error. Studies of hospital errors conducted in Colorado and in Utah in 1992 placed the death rate from errors at 44,000 annually.[3] The third study, which was conducted in hospitals in New York, placed the death rate at 98,000 annually.[4] The IOM estimated that the total national costs resulting from medical errors, which included healthcare costs, lost income and productivity, and disability costs, was between $37.6 billion and $50 billion per year.[5]

The IOM report also analyzed some of the probable causes of medical errors. It drew a distinction between two types of causes of error in medicine: *individuals* and *systems*.[6] For example, if a patient in a hospital receives the wrong dose of medication, one might look for an individual to blame for this mistake, such as the doctor who wrote the prescription, the pharmacist who filled it, or the nurse who administered it. Medical malpractice lawsuits encourage this type of thinking because plaintiffs often name individuals as defendants. For example, a hospital patient who is harmed as a result of receiving the wrong dose of a medication might sue the doctor, the nurse, and the pharmacist, as well as the hospital. Healthcare institutions have also accepted this individualistic framework because a hospital, nursing home, or managed care organization may discipline or fire a member of its staff who makes errors. Medical licensing boards reinforce this approach to error because they frequently discipline practitioners who make mistakes. For example, a pharmacist who makes too many errors could have his or her license suspended.

The IOM report redirects the analysis of medical error from individuals to systems: "the emphasis . . . is about how to make systems safer; its primary focus is not on 'getting rid of bad apples,' or individuals with poor records of performance. The underlying assumption is that lasting and broad-based safety improvements in industry can be brought about through a systems approach."[7] The IOM reports draws on the work of Charles Perrow and James Reason, who studied the role of systems and individuals in causing accidents, such as the space shuttle *Challenger* disaster.[8]

The IOM report defines a system as a "set of interdependent elements interacting to achieve a common aim."[9] For example, a system relating to the administration of medications in a hospital would include the media used to communicate prescription orders, such as paper, phone, or email; methods for verifying communications; computer programs to record medication orders and to check for drug interactions; protocols for checking prescriptions; terminology for referring to different medications, dosages, and means of administration; and procedures for identifying patients and storing and marking medications on the ward.[10] There are many different ways that the system for administering a medication may break down. For example, there might be a miscommunication between the doctor and the nurse or pharmacist; the hospital might use similar names to refer to different medications, which may result in confusion at times; the patient may receive the wrong medication because of unclear labeling, and so on.

The important point to glean from the IOM report is that when errors happen, it may be more useful to focus on systems rather than on individuals as sources of error. Indeed, since human beings are far from perfect, we should expect that they will make mistakes. The best way to improve safety in an industry is to design systems that eliminate or minimize errors.

The IOM report is a key milestone in the development of patient safety, and it has helped to stimulate other agencies to focus on patient safety, such as the Department of Health and Human Services, the American Hospital Association, and The Joint Commission. This chapter will go one step beyond the general tenor of the IOM report and argue that those who are concerned with patient safety should rethink and critique some of the foundational ideas and assumptions that play a key role in reducing error and improving safety. Although it is important to address healthcare systems, it is also important to address the basic ideas and assumptions—the philosophies (or worldviews)—that people use to implement and design systems. The IOM report addresses some philosophical issues related to patient safety without referring to them as philosophical issues. For example, the IOM report recommends that "health care organizations and the professionals affiliated with them should make continually improved patient safety a declared and serious aim by establishing patient safety programs."[11] The report also recommends that "performance standards and expectations for health professionals should focus greater attention on patient safety."[12]

This chapter identifies and describes several different ideas and assumptions that play an important role in medical error and explains why the healthcare industry should address the foundational issues related to medical error. The key components of a patient safety philosophy that this chapter examines include the definition of "medical error," the degree of commitment to error reduction, and the acceptance of error.

FROM SYSTEMS TO PHILOSOPHIES

To get a better understanding of the difference between a system and a philosophy or worldview, it is useful to refine the distinction between an individual and a system. For the purpose of this chapter, an individual could be any individual thing that can be uniquely identified. For example, cars, marbles, trees, and planets are "individuals" in this sense of the word. Human beings can also be individuals, of course. If we have a group of individuals, then this group could be called a collection or assortment, if it is not organized in any particular way. For example, a pile of books on the floor might be a collection. The difference between a collection of individuals and a system of individuals is that a system involves some method for organizing the individuals and assigning them different roles (or places) within the system.[13] All of the individuals are organized (or controlled or regulated) for the sake of some common aim or goal. For example, the Dewey Decimal System is a method for arranging books in a library according to a particular organization based on numbers and letters assigned to different types of books. Our solar system organizes the planets, asteroids, moons, and comets around a common focal point, the sun.

If we think of systems as types of organizations, it follows that there can be systems of different sizes, depending on the level of the organization. Nowhere is this more evident than in the biological world, where there are levels of organization ranging from molecules, organelles, and membranes at the lowest level; to cells, tissues, and organs at the intermediate level; to organisms, populations, and ecosystems at the highest level. The IOM report recognizes this point: "Systems can be very large and far-reaching, or they can be more localized."[14] However, the report does not expand on this idea and focuses on particular, localized systems in health care.

What would be a "large and far-reaching" system relating to medical error? How would this system differ from more localized systems? If we think of systems relating to human beings, lower-level systems might include families, businesses, professional associations, community associations, and volunteer organizations. Intermediate-level systems might include social institutions, such as marriage, sports, or medicine, as well as governments. At the very highest level of organization, we would find those systems that we can regard as philosophies in society. These might include political ideologies, such as democracy, communism, and fascism; economic systems, such as capitalism and socialism; religious traditions, such as Christianity, Islam, and Buddhism; and even scientific ideas and assumptions, such as determinism, the uniformity of nature, and Darwinism.

A philosophy (or worldview) consists of a set of basic ideas and assumptions that address fundamental questions in a discipline or human activity. The academic discipline known as "philosophy" studies these basic ideas and assumptions. Philosophies are much more abstract than intermediate- or lower-level systems. A dollar bill is a concrete thing that is part of the United States' monetary system. But capitalism is an abstract idea (or theory) that consists of a set of beliefs and assumptions about the organization of production, the generation of wealth, and the distribution of goods and services in society. As we shall soon see, abstract ideas also define the healthcare industry's approach to medical error.

It follows from this analysis that it is very important to understand these philosophies if one wants to understand human behavior, since higher-level principles and goals may explain and justify behavior at lower levels. For example, no explanation of marriage in the United States would be complete without some reference to the particular marital arrangements and rituals adopted by various religious practices as well as their religious beliefs. No explanation of voting behavior in the United States would be complete without some reference to particular political races as well as the idea of democracy. Also, a justification of a particular policy or procedure may refer to some higher-level goal or principle. For example, one might justify the rules of the patent system by arguing that they promote the advancement of science and the practical arts by giving incentives to inventors and entrepreneurs.

While it is important to understand philosophical ideas and assumptions in order to explain events that occur at lower organizational levels, it may be more difficult to change these ideas than it is to change lower-level systems. For example, it is much easier to change a particular regulation designed to promote good working conditions for employees than it is to change capitalism. It is much easier to change the time that a church offers its worship services than it is to change Christianity or Hinduism. This does not mean that it is impossible to change philosophies or worldviews. However, attempts to change a worldview may meet with a great deal of resistance for the simple reason that a worldview affects so many different lower-level systems. A change in a worldview is like a political or scientific revolution because it results in a new way of thinking about the world—new ideas, new beliefs, and new values.[15] We will return to this point when we examine the healthcare industry.

PHILOSOPHICAL IDEAS AND ASSUMPTIONS AND MEDICAL ERROR

Having laid some groundwork for the significance of philosophical ideas and assumptions in understanding human behavior, we can now apply this framework to the analysis and etiology of medical error. As noted earlier, the IOM report has provided an excellent discussion of the systems approach to medical error. To develop a philosophical approach, we should try to understand the basic ideas and assumptions that can reduce medical error and enhance patient safety. These ideas could be held by different individuals in the healthcare industry, including practitioners, managers, and patients. To identify some of these different ideas, it will be useful to ask the following key questions: What ideas are likely to improve patient safety and minimize error? and, conversely, What ideas are likely to worsen patient safety and increase error? This chapter identifies some fundamental ideas that play a key role in patient safety.

Idea 1: The Definition of Medical Error

The definition of error itself plays a very important role in reducing errors, since one cannot reduce something if one does not know what it is. Ever since the time of Socrates, philosophers have attempted to answer definitional ("what is it?") questions. What is a medical error? Let's start with the prior question, What is an error? This question seems easy to answer, but it is not. A great deal hinges on the type of system we are analyzing. For example, if our system is a mechanical measuring device, such as a thermometer, we could say that the thermometer makes an error when the temperature it indicates is not the same as the actual temperature.[16] Thus, an *incorrect* measurement is one type of error. The measurement is incorrect because it does not accurately represent the state of the world.

In scientific research, errors occur when we unintentionally hold beliefs that are incorrect (i.e., not true). A false belief (or epistemological error) is a belief that does not correspond to the facts. For instance, if we accept the hypothesis that a particular drug is safe and effective, when in fact it is not, then we have committed what is known as a type I error (false positive). If we accept the hypothesis that the drug is not safe and effective, when in fact it is, then we have committed a type II error (false negative).[17] Scientists confront errors constantly in research and have developed methods and procedures for reducing and eliminating them. Hence, the scientific method is often said to be "self-correcting." Some scholars have argued that the only way that science can move toward the truth is by eliminating errors.[18]

If we move away from science and consider the practical arts, then we may view errors as mistaken (or incorrect) actions (i.e., practical errors) rather than as mistaken beliefs. Since actions are not true or false, we must measure actions against some type of standard other than correspondence with the facts. We could say that an action is correct if it corresponds to the rules and norms that govern that action, and an action is incorrect if it does not correspond to the rules and norms that govern it. For example, various rules and norms govern the game of baseball. An error could occur when someone performs an action that fails to conform to those rules and norms, such as dropping a ball or making a poor throw.

We might consider some incorrect actions to be unethical or illegal rather than erroneous. For example, if a person accidentally takes someone else's umbrella, we would consider this to be a mistake. If a person *intentionally* takes someone else's umbrella, we would consider that to be theft. The same point also applies to erroneous beliefs: A person who intentionally publishes erroneous data might be guilty of fraud or misconduct, but a person who unintentionally publishes erroneous data might be guilty only of error or negligence.[19]

Thus, whether we are considering epistemological or practical errors, some elements of the definition of error are the same: (1) Errors are *deviations* from the correct belief or conduct, and (2) Errors are *unintentional*. The major difference between erroneous beliefs and erroneous actions is that the former are beliefs that do not agree with the facts, whereas the latter are actions that do not conform to the appropriate norms. If there is a situation in which there are no facts or norms (i.e., a "gray" area), it follows that there can be no errors but only disagreements or differences of opinion.

How should one define "error" in medicine? If we construe medicine as a science, then its errors should be understood as epistemological errors. If, on the other hand, we view medicine as a practical art, then its errors should be practical errors. So is the aim of medicine to obtain correct beliefs or to perform correct actions? Is it a science or a practical art? This is a complex question that will not be addressed in detail here. For the purposes of this chapter, we will assume that medicine is both an art and a science: It is concerned with forming correct beliefs as well performing correct actions.[20] Thus, errors in medicine could be epistemological or practical.

Moreover, in medicine, incorrect beliefs may lead to incorrect actions. For example, suppose that an emergency room doctor examines a 32-year-old patient with chest pain and determines that he has not had a heart attack, when, in fact, he has had a heart attack. The doctor diagnoses the chest pain incorrectly and sends the man home with a prescription for a tranquilizer. The man subsequently has a heart attack and dies. In this case, the doctor formed an erroneous belief as a result of poor clinical judgment. She acted on that erroneous belief by performing an incorrect action: She sent the man home when she should have kept him in the hospital for more medical tests and supervision. The belief was erroneous because it did not agree with facts, and the action was erroneous because it did not conform to the rules and norms of medicine, that is, the standard of care.

The IOM report adopts a definition of error that encompasses incorrect actions and beliefs: "An error is defined as a failure of a planned action to be completed as intended (i.e., error of execution) or the use of the wrong plan to achieve an aim (i.e., error of planning)."[21] In this definition, a "failure of a planned action" could be viewed as an incorrect action, and a "use of the wrong plan" could be viewed as an incorrect belief.

Although this definition of error seems clear enough, it requires some interpretation to apply it to actual cases. What is a "failure of a planned action"? If a nurse gives a patient a dose of a drug 1 hour too late, would this be a failure of a planned action? What if the dose is given only 5 minutes late? Perhaps the only planned action is that the patient should receive the dose of the medication at an appropriate time, left to the discretion of the nurse. Thus, it might not be an error if the dose is given 5 minutes or even 1 hour too late. Also, what is the "use of the wrong plan"? If a doctor writes a prescription for the wrong drug, would this be "the wrong plan"? Suppose that the drug is not the "wrong drug" but is simply a drug that is not as effective as a different drug; would this be the "wrong plan"? If one thinks long and hard about medical error, it would appear that each practitioner may make dozens of minor mistakes on a daily basis, because each practitioner will deviate from the proper beliefs or actions. Should we count all of these deviations as errors?

Thus, while the IOM's definition offers some useful guidance, one must interpret the definition in order to apply it to particular cases. In interpreting and applying the definition of error, one confronts problems relating to the scope of the definition: Should it have a broad scope or a narrow scope? If one adopts a very narrow and limited interpretation of the definition of error, then one is less likely to report errors or make serious attempts to improve safety. If one adopts a broader and more comprehensive interpretation, then one is more likely to report errors and make serious attempts to improve safety. On the other hand, an interpretation of a definition could be too broad to be useful. If one sees errors everywhere, it is practically impossible to report all of them or do anything about them.

So what is the proper way to interpret the scope of the definition of error? One useful way of restricting the scope of the definition is to distinguish between *harmful* and *harmless* errors. A harmful error is one that *has caused or could cause* harm; a harmless error is an error that has not caused harm and is not likely to cause harm. For example, giving a dose of a drug 5 minutes late would probably be a harmless error; failing to give the dose at all would probably be a harmful error.

Suppose that a nurse is about to give a patient the wrong drug, due to a labeling problem, but another member of the healthcare team catches him before he makes this error. Although many people might be tempted to not report this error because it did not result in harm to the patient—"no harm, no foul"—healthcare professionals should avoid this temptation. They should report these near misses because these are events that could have caused harm and might cause harm the next time they occur. To promote patient safety, healthcare professionals should learn from their near misses and make changes to prevent "direct hits."

Another way of restricting the scope of the definition would be to distinguish between *preventable* and *unpreventable* errors. It would seem to be pointless to spend time and effort trying to identify or analyze errors that are not preventable. An error is preventable if there is something that someone could have realistically done to stop the error from occurring. For example, if a doctor has a heart attack while operating on a patient, this is an error that is probably not preventable. Amputating the wrong foot is an error that is probably preventable.

The IOM report recognizes the relationship between errors and preventable adverse events. The IOM report defines an adverse event as an "injury caused by medical management rather than the underlying condition of the patient. An adverse event attributable to error is a preventable adverse event."[22] Thus, it appears that the IOM report would recommend that the healthcare industry focus its efforts on errors that led to or could lead to preventable adverse events.

To summarize this section, the definition of error is a basic idea that plays a key role in the prevention of error. Because healthcare providers and industry leaders must know how to recognize errors in order to report them, a comprehensive and useful definition of error is essential. Because medical errors may involve incorrect beliefs as well as incorrect actions, the definition should encompass a wide range of activities in health care, ranging from diagnosis and decision making to the administration of medications and the preparation of patients for surgery. Furthermore, the scope of the definition should not be too narrow or too broad. It should focus on errors that are harmful (or potentially harmful) and preventable, that is, errors that have caused or could cause preventable adverse events.[23]

Idea 2: The Priority of Patient Safety

The second idea is self-explanatory: The healthcare industry will not make significant progress toward reducing errors unless healthcare industry leaders, practitioners, and even patients have a strong commitment to error reduction. As noted earlier, the IOM report recognizes the importance of a strong commitment to error reduction and patient safety. The report makes several recommendations that speak to a national commitment to patient safety, including the creation of a national center for patient safety, mandatory reporting of adverse events,[24] peer review protections for patient safety inquiries,[25] and performance standards for patient safety.[26] The IOM report also recommends that healthcare institutions take several steps to demonstrate their commitment to patient safety, including developing patient safety programs, implementing systems for reporting and analyzing errors, and implementing well-understood safety principles, such as standardization of equipment and processes.[27] Many organizations have already begun to implement these recommendations.

Although these recommendations make a great deal of sense and suggest a strong commitment to patient safety, they still do not answer some of the fundamental questions about the priority of patient safety, such as, How important is error reduction? Does it have a high priority or a low priority? and Is it viewed as valuable for its own sake or only as valuable for the sake of some other goal, such as patient satisfaction? These questions are important to answer, because a patient safety program is doomed to failure if people in the healthcare industry have only a superficial commitment to patient safety. To succeed in reducing medical errors, industry leaders, practitioners, and patients must have a sincere commitment to safety and error avoidance. They must back up their public endorsements of patient safety with time, money, and resources.

One simple way to determine how much a person (or organization) values something is to determine whether he or she values it for its own sake (i.e., intrinsically) or only for the sake of something else (i.e., extrinsically). A person who values something intrinsically will continue to value that thing even when his or her circumstances change, whereas a person who values something only extrinsically will value that thing only as long as it is necessary to achieve some other goal. For example, a person who values exercise for its own sake will continue to exercise when he does not need to exercise to lose weight, control his diabetes, attract a mate, or achieve some other goal. A person who does not value exercising intrinsically will stop exercising regularly whenever the occasion permits. Likewise, an organization that values patient safety intrinsically will continue to value patient safety even when the organization does not need to emphasize patient safety to achieve some other goal, such as patient satisfaction or profitability. On the other hand, an organization that does not value patient safety for its own sake will cut corners on patient safety whenever the occasion permits.

One way of restating this point is to say that patient safety should be one of the core values of the healthcare industry. It should receive equal billing with other core values, such as quality improvement, patient satisfaction, health promotion, medical education, and medical research and development. Healthcare organizations can demonstrate their commitment to patient safety by touting the importance of patient safety in their brochures, policies, Web pages, and public communications; by developing patient safety programs; by hiring patient safety officers; and by collecting, analyzing, and interpreting patient safety data. Healthcare practitioners can demonstrate their commitment to patient safety by talking to other professionals about safety issues, by following patient safety guidelines, by reporting errors, and by helping to develop systems that are designed to improve safety. Last but not least, patients can play a key role in the patient safety movement by helping to prevent errors. Patients should be more than mere passive recipients of health care; they should be active participants. For example, a patient could ask a nurse if he or she has double-checked a medication order, and could ask a pharmacist about dangerous drug interactions and precautions for use. A patient should also discuss issues related to her own safety with her doctor, such as potential risks and steps that she can take to minimize those risks.

In other words, everyone in the healthcare industry—from doctor to patient to CEO—needs to think "safety first." This may sound like an obvious or even trivial point, but if it is, then why is error such a big problem in health care? Somehow, somewhere, many people have forgotten this simple point. There is nothing wrong with reemphasizing this point time and again, if this is what it takes to improve patient safety.

Although it is important to emphasize the intrinsic value of patient safety, it may be strategically wise to argue for the importance of patient safety by providing evidence that it tends to promote other worthwhile goals, such as quality improvement, customer satisfaction, and even profitability. Healthcare industry leaders will be hesitant to invest in patient safety programs unless they can see how these programs are likely to affect the bottom line. Although it seems rather obvious that reducing and preventing medical errors would increase patient satisfaction, quality improvement, and profitability, it would still be useful to study the relationship between patient safety and these other values in order to build the case for patient safety and to understand how it affects different aspects of health care. Is a hospital with a good safety program less likely to be sued than one without a good safety program? This would be a question worth investigating. Thus, it may be useful to invest some time, money, and effort in conducting research on the relationship between patient safety and other goals.

Idea 3: The Acceptance of Error

Another idea that can play an important role in patient safety is the acceptance of errors (or lack thereof). It sounds a bit paradoxical that one should accept errors in order to prevent them, but it is true. Although errors should be avoided, people and systems are not perfect. Healthcare practitioners who do not acknowledge and accept this important fact may deny, rationalize, and refuse to report errors. The most effective way of dealing with errors is to acknowledge that they happen and are likely to happen, again and again. Indeed, one might argue that errors are necessary in order to improve human conduct and to design better systems, since one can learn from one's mistakes. Experience is the best teacher. It is unfortunate that patients and healthcare professionals must suffer the consequences of error, but this is unavoidable. The only way to completely avoid errors in medicine would be to never practice medicine.

There is considerable evidence that doctors have a hard time dealing with their own mistakes.[28,29] Doctors tend to not talk about their mistakes, or, when they do, they may try to rationalize or deny them.[30] Evidence also indicates that doctors suffer from stress, anxiety, guilt, and depression when they make mistakes.[31] Albert Wu relates his personal experience of a medical error he encountered:

> When I was a house officer another resident failed to identify the electrocardiographic signs of the pericardial tamponade that would rush the patient to the operating room that night. The news spread rapidly, the case was tried repeatedly before an incredulous jury of peers, who returned a summary judgment of incompetence. I was dismayed by the lack of sympathy and wondered secretly if I could have made the same mistake—and, like the hapless resident, become the second victim of medical error.[32]

Wu then diagnoses the problem that is affecting the profession of medicine:

> Strangely, there is no place for mistakes in modern medicine. Society has entrusted physicians with the burden of understanding and dealing with illness. Although it is often said that "doctors are only human," technological wonders, the appar-

> ent precision of laboratory tests, and innovations that present tangible images of illness have in fact created an expectation of perfection. Patients, who have an understandable need to consider their doctors infallible, have colluded with doctors to deny the existence of error. Hospitals react to every error as an anomaly, for which the solution is to ferret out and blame the individual.[33]

According to Wu, doctors have a difficult time dealing with medical error because they and their patients have come to expect perfection, and because hospitals also expect perfection and blame individuals instead of examining systems. Other doctors have expressed similar sentiments. Some argue that medical culture and the myth of infallibility prevent doctors from facing their mistakes.[34]

Atul Gawande, a surgical resident, argues that the threat of medical malpractice liability plays an important role in the problems that doctors have in responding to error:

> The deeper problem with medical malpractice suits is that by demonizing errors they prevent doctors from acknowledging them and discussing them publicly. The tort system makes adversaries of patient and physician, and pushes each to offer a heavily slanted version of events. When things go wrong, it's almost impossible for a physician to talk to a patient honestly about mistakes.[35]

Risk managers and hospital attorneys have had a change of heart in recent years about disclosing errors to patients. At one time, hospital risk managers and attorneys would strongly discourage healthcare professionals from disclosing errors to patients. This policy was based on the idea that the patient would be likely to sue the practitioner or the hospital if he or she discovered the error. However, a growing body of evidence indicates that the consequences of nondisclosure are worse than the consequences of disclosure, since a patient who discovers an undisclosed error may become angry and vindictive. He may think that the hospital has tried to cover up the error, and he may sue the hospital out of spite or just to acquire information.[36] Today, most risk managers recommend that physicians communicate honestly and openly with patients and their families about medical errors that result in adverse events.[37]

However, there is a legal and ethical dilemma in communicating to patients honestly about medical errors, because what practitioners say to patients may be admitted into evidence in court as an admission of guilt.[38] But how can one communicate "honestly" with a patient without admitting that one has made a mistake or is at fault? This is a difficult ethical and legal issue, which this chapter will not attempt to solve.[39] On the other hand, it is important to develop an appropriate response to this issue in order to promote the acceptance of medical errors and effective communication about medical errors.

How can the healthcare industry increase the acceptance of medical errors? The first place to begin would be to implement programs that offer psychological counseling and support to practitioners who make mistakes. This program should go beyond the peer review activities that occur in health care, which usually focus only on particular episodes and tend to involve finger pointing. A support program should address the long-term consequences of medical errors for practitioners and should not be an exercise in finger pointing. Such a program should offer doctors, pharmacists, and nurses sympathy and empathy. An ideal model would be a support group similar to the groups that offer support to cancer patients, grieving families, and alcoholics and drug addicts. As Wu notes, "the kind of unconditional sympathy and support that are really needed are rarely forthcoming."[40] He also observes that there can be some very drastic consequences for doctors when they have trouble dealing with mistakes: "some physicians are deeply wounded, lose their nerve, burn out, or seek solace in alcohol and drugs."[41]

However, the inability of healthcare professionals to deal effectively with medical error has roots that extend deep into the heart of medicine. Thus, to increase acceptance of error, one must do more than just offer counseling and support, one must also change medical education and training, since it is likely that healthcare professionals learn how to respond to error while they are students and interns. Pilpel, Schor, and Benbasset argue that the medical curriculum should include discussions of medical error so that students may learn how to cope with error and come to understand that it is inevitable but also preventable.[42]

Speaking from his own experience as a surgical intern, Gawande claims that doctors need to acknowledge their fallibility but that medical education and practice teach the opposite lesson.[43] *Fallibilism* is simply the idea that one could be mistaken. In the 19th century, the prominent American philosopher Charles Peirce argued that science is fallible because today's scientific theories and hypotheses may be refuted some day. Nevertheless, science can make progress toward a more complete understanding of nature, even though it will make many mistakes along the way.[44] Almost 30 years ago, two other philosophers argued that medicine is fallible.[45] If doctors adopted this philosophy, they would be more scientific because they would strive to recognize and correct their mistakes, and they would also be, ironically, more humanistic because they would accept their mistakes as an inevitable part of the advancement of medical knowledge and practice.

It is also important to develop programs that help patients come to understand and accept errors in medicine. Patient educational materials in hospitals should include information on medical errors. Hospitals and healthcare organizations should also provide counseling and support for patients and families who are the victims of medical error. Finally, there should also be programs for healthcare administrators.

CONCLUSION

This chapter has expanded on the systems approach to medical error and considered how philosophies (or worldviews) can play a role in patient safety and error prevention. It has identified, described, and discussed three foundational ideas that play a key role in patient safety.

The first idea is the definition of "medical error." The definition should include errors related to incorrect actions as well as errors related to incorrect beliefs, and it should focus on errors that are preventable and cause harm or are likely to cause harm.

The second idea is the commitment to patient safety. Healthcare professionals, healthcare administrators, and patients should make patient safety one of the core values in health care. They should value safety for its own sake, not just for the sake of its effect on other values, such as quality improvement, patient satisfaction, or profitability.

The third idea is the acceptance of medical error. Healthcare professionals, healthcare administrators, and patients should learn to accept medical error so they may deal with it effectively. Healthcare organizations should provide support and counseling for practitioners who make mistakes, and medical, pharmacy, nursing, and other healthcare schools should include a discussion of medical error in their curricula. Risk managers and hospital attorneys should also develop policies for dealing with the dilemmas involved in honest and open communication about medical errors with patients.

References

1. Institute of Medicine, *To Err Is Human: Building a Safer Health System* (Washington, DC: National Academy Press, 1999).
2. Ibid., 22.
3. Ibid.
4. Troy Brennan et al., "Incidence of Adverse Events and Negligence in Hospitalized Patients: Results of the Harvard Medical Practice Study," *New England Journal of Medicine* 1991;324:370–376.
5. IOM, *To Err Is Human*, 22.
6. Ibid., 44–45.
7. Ibid., 42.
8. Charles Perrow, *Normal Accidents* (New York: Basic Books, 1984); James Reason, *Human Error* (New York: Cambridge University Press, 1990).
9. IOM, *To Err Is Human*, 44.
10. Ibid., 31–33.
11. Ibid., 12.
12. Ibid., 10.
13. These distinctions between "individuals," "groups," and "systems" are part of the standard vocabulary of the branch of philosophy known as ontology, which studies the basic constituents of the universe. For further discussion, see W. V. Quine, *Word and Object* (Cambridge, MA: MIT Press, 1964); and Nelson Goodman, *The Structure of Appearance* (Indianapolis: Bobbs-Merrill, 1966).
14. IOM, *To Err Is Human*, 44.
15. This observation is based on the work of Thomas Kuhn, who argued that scientific revolutions involve changes in worldviews. Kuhn also held that scientists tend to resist changes of belief that threaten their worldviews. See his *The Structure of Scientific Revolutions*, 2nd ed. (Chicago: University of Chicago Press, 1970).
16. Alvin Goldman, *Epistemology and Cognition* (Cambridge, MA: Harvard University Press, 1988).
17. Donald Brown, Kenneth Michels, and Benjamin Winer, *Statistical Principles and Experimental Design* (New York: McGraw-Hill, 1991).
18. Karl Popper, *Conjectures and Refutations* (New York: Basic Books, 1962).
19. The definition of "misconduct" in research does not include error. "Misconduct" is intentionally fabricating or falsifying data, or intentionally plagiarizing research. See Panel on Scientific Responsibility and the Conduct of Research, *Responsible Science*, Vol. 1 (Washington, DC: National Academy Press, 1992).
20. Daniel Albert, Ronald Munson, and Michael Resnik, *Reasoning in Medicine*, 2nd ed. (Baltimore: Johns Hopkins University Press, 1999).
21. IOM, *To Err Is Human*, 28.
22. Ibid., 24.
23. The risk management department at University Health Systems of Eastern Carolina has developed a comprehensive event reporting form that distinguishes among nine different categories of reportable events, ranging from "Category I: An event occurred that may have contributed to or resulted in the patient's death" to "Category A: Circumstances or events that have the capacity to cause error, harm, loss." The form also has a category for reporting errors that occur but do not reach the patient. University Health Systems of Eastern Carolina, Event Reporting form, 0289-RM/Rev.12-01/Event Report, 2001.
24. IOM, *To Err Is Human*, 7.
25. Ibid., 9.
26. Ibid.,10–11.
27. Ibid., 12.
28. David Hilfiker, "Facing Our Mistakes," *New England Journal of Medicine* 1984;310:118–122.
29. John Christensen, William Levinson, and Paul Dunn, "The Heart of Darkness: The Impact of Perceived Mistakes on Physicians," *Journal of General Internal Medicine* 1992;7:424–431.
30. Theo Mizrahi, "Managing Medical Mistakes: Ideology, Insularity, and Accountability Among Internists in Training," *Social Science and Medicine* 1984;19:135–146.
31. Albert Wu, "Medical Error: The Second Victim: The Doctor Who Makes the Mistake Needs Help Too," *British Medical Journal* 2000;320:726–727.
32. Ibid., 726.
33. Ibid.
34. Paul McNeill and Merrilyn Walton, "Medical Harm and the Consequences of Error for Doctors," *Medical Journal of Australia* 2000;176:222–225.

35. Atul Gawande, *Complications: A Surgeon's Notes on an Imperfect Science* (New York: Metropolitan Books, 2002).
36. Gerald Hickson et al., "Patient Complaints and Malpractice Risk," *Journal of the American Medical Association* 2000;287:2951–2957.
37. See, for example, Vanderbilt University Medical Center, Guide to Risk Management. <http://www.vanderbilt.edu/RiskMgmt/quality.htm#report>. Accessed December 4, 2002.
38. John Strong et al., *McCormick on Evidence*, 5th ed. (St. Paul, MN: West Publishing, 1999), 372–393.
39. McNeill and Walton, "Medical Harm."
40. Wu, "Medical Error," 727.
41. Ibid.
42. David Pilpel, Robert Schor, and John Benbasset, "Barriers to Acceptance of Medical Error: The Case for a Teaching Program," *Medical Education* 1998;32:3–7.
43. Gawande, *Complications*, 187–201.
44. Charles Peirce, "The Scientific Attitude and Fallibilism." In: J. Buchler (ed.), *Philosophical Writings of Peirce* (New York: Dover Publications, 1955), 42–60.
45. Samuel Gorovitz and Alisdare MacIntyre, "Toward a Theory of Medical Fallibility," *Journal of Medicine and Philosophy* 1976;1:51–71.

8

MISTAKING ERROR

David D. Woods, PhD and Richard I. Cook, MD

INTRODUCTION

Throughout the brief history of the patient safety movement (Hatlie, 1996), stakeholder groups have asked the authors for definitions and taxonomies of human error grounded in science. The questions are of the same form: Each group feels that their progress on safety depends on having a firm definition of human error. Each group seems to believe that this definition will enable the creation of a scorecard that will allow them to gauge where organizations stand in terms of being "safe."

Each group's search for the definition, first in the medical literature and then in the general scientific literature, becomes mired in complexity and terms of reference. As definitions appear in the medical literature about patient safety, they seem too specific to particular areas of health care or too vague if broad enough to cover health care in general. The definitions offered are often the product of committee consensus processes and thus too ad hoc to have scientific standing. The definitions offered involve arbitrary and subjective methods of assigning events to categories (e.g., "definitions" that propose to include as errors those events that "could have led to harm"). The resulting counts and extrapolations seem open to endless reassessment and debate (Leape et al., 1991; Kohn et al., 1999; Brennan, 2000; McDonald et al., 2000; Leape, 2000; Woods and Cook, 2001; Leape and Berwick, 2005). As the search intensifies, the definition of error becomes more elusive.

Some within the stakeholder groups turn to social and behavioral science researchers who have grappled with the "human error problem" that has dogged progress on safety in other high-risk industries. Nuclear power, aviation, manufacturing, and the military have invested heavily in basic and applied research on human error over the past 30 years. Although some of this research—and some outspoken researchers—rely on human error being a discrete, well circumscribed, static entity, progress on safety in these industries has come, in large part, from abandoning efforts to attack error directly and as weakness of people, specific ones or in general.

Driven partly by spectacular failures—the reactor failure at Three Mile Island in 1979 is the archetype, but the series continues with the Columbia Space Shuttle in 2003—researchers have developed new means for looking into how systems fail and how people in their various roles contributed to *both* success and failure. The research, collectively known as the "New Look" (Rasmussen, 1997; Reason, 1997; Woods et al., 1994; Hollnagel et al., 2006), drew on many different disciplines including cognitive science, organizational theory, cognitive engineering, and most recently, resilience engineering, but it has consistently focused on empirical studies of people at work. The results of these efforts challenge the conventional "folk" assumptions about the relationship between "error" and failure.

To researchers, beginning with the question "What is error?" misleads stakeholders into a thicket of difficulties where answers seem always just around the corner but never actually come into view. The efforts to answer this seemingly simple question—efforts that inevitably become entangled with social factors and lose sight of the research base—actually block progress on safety (Cook, Woods, Miller, 1998). The New Look offers an alternative to "error" as the target of efforts to improve safety (Hollnagel, 2004; Dekker, 2005; Hollnagel, 2009; Woods et al., 2010).

The need to redirect effort away from error seems counterintuitive when health care is so obviously confronted by a "human error problem." But this is precisely the situation that confronted researchers at the beginning of the development of the New Look. At that time, the folk model of accident causation was firmly in place amongst researchers and error seemed a plausible target for work on safety. It was only after a long period of empirical research on human performance and accidents that it became apparent that answering the question of what is error was not the first step, was not a useful step, but only a dead end.

How are we to respond to those who seek definitions and taxonomies in their efforts to improve safety? Faced with an equally difficult problem in 1897, Frank Church replied to a letter from an 8-year-old girl named Virginia who asked if there really was a Santa Claus. As a way of summarizing what the New Look has revealed about error and safety, we propose our own version of both Virginia's letter and Church's response.

> Dear David and Richard,
>
> Our professional group just sponsored a consensus meeting on patient safety and medical error. We were all shocked by the Institute of Medicine reports. As highly motivated professionals committed to serving our patients, we decided to take proactive steps to improve patient safety in our area of medicine.
>
> In our consensus meeting we developed an agenda for progress and strategic action. At the top of our list, we put the need for agreement on definitions of medical errors. Until we reach agreement on this we will be unable to create the error-tracking programs we need to measure the size of the problem and to evaluate the effectiveness of new interventions. However, despite much struggle, we have been unable to achieve consensus on a set of acceptable and workable definitions.
>
> We are soliciting input from different experts on human error outside health care to help us develop these definitions. *What is human error?*
>
> Thank you for your help.
>
> Virginia

Here is our reply:

> Dear Virginia,
>
> You are not the first to ask us about "human error." When researchers began studying the role of human performance in system failure, they asked the same ques-

tions, thinking that they would find the answers if only they worked hard enough and long enough.[1]

There were good reasons for them to look for the answer. Accidents, sometimes very big ones, seemed to involve human error, and the costs of these accidents were such that getting a clear idea of what human error is seemed essential for progress on safety. The researchers did not have much success however. Instead, they found a different sort of way of looking at accidents and failures, a way we now call the New Look. This is a way of understanding how systems fail and how people in their various roles contribute to both success and failure.[2]

To answer the question as you have posed it would require us to accept a set of conventional assumptions about error. We now understand that these assumptions are incorrect. The focus on defining and counting error has distracted other industries from productive work on safety. The research results can help you find more useful questions to ask.

First off, we want you to understand that the term "error" is used inconsistently in our everyday conversations about safety and accidents.[3] There are at least three ways that the term is used:

- Sense #1. Error as the *cause* of failure: "This event was due to human error." The assumption is that error is some basic category or type of human behavior that precedes and generates a failure. It leads to variations on the myth that safety is protecting the system and stakeholders from erratic, unreliable people.
- Sense #2. Error as the *failure itself*, i.e., the consequences that flow from an event: "The transplant mixup was an error." In this sense the term "error" simply asserts that the outcome was bad and produced negative consequences (e.g., injury to a patient).
- Sense #3. Error as a *process*, or more precisely, *departure from the "good" process*. Here, the sense of error is of deviation from a standard, that is a model of what is good practice, but the difficulty is there are different models of what is the process that should be followed: e.g., what standard is applicable, how standards should be described, and what it means when deviations from the standards do not result in bad outcomes. Depending on the model adopted, very different views of error result.

While you might think that it would always be clear from the context which of these senses

[1]Cook (1999) traces how individuals and organizations recapitulate the learning steps that gave rise to the current understanding of the relationship between safety, systems, and human performance (cf., Part V of Woods et al., 2010).

[2]The core of the New Look results can be seen in the work of Jens Rasmussen (1990a; 1990b; 1997; 1999); Erik Hollnagel (2004; 2009); Hollnagel and Amalberti, 2001); Jim Reason (1997); and Woods et al. (1994; 2010). Dekker (2005) provides a good entry point. Overviews of parallel work on high reliability organizations can be found in Rochlin (1999) and Weick and Sutcliffe (2007).

[3]The work of Jens Rasmussen and Erik Hollnagel have led the way. The description of the first 3 senses is drawn from Hollnagel's work.

people mean when they talk about error, in practice the senses are often confused with each other. Even worse, people sometimes slip from one sense to another without being aware that they are doing so.

Of course, what people are interested in is "error" in the second sense of bad outcomes and how to prevent them. You can see this yourself by this simple thought experiment. Imagine that we have managed to eliminate all accidents from health care but that many errors remain (third sense). Would anyone be interested in error? Probably not. Now suppose instead that we somehow eliminated all the *errors* from health care but that accidents continued to occur. Would anyone be interested in error? Again, probably not.

The motivation to explore error comes from accidents. The research that forms the New Look has two main sources: (1) the base of behavioral science about how individuals and groups cope with complexity and conflict in real-world settings and (2) a growing set of empirical studies on accidents, near-accidents, and real-world work, sometimes called "technical work" studies. The research view of "error" derived from the New Look has produced five conclusions pertaining to "error":

Conclusion #1: *Defining error-as-cause (Sense #1) blocks learning by hiding the lawful factors that affect human and system performance.*

The critical observation that gave rise to the New Look was that errors were *heterogeneous* and not directly comparable events that could be counted and tabulated. The standard way we say this today is that the label error should be the starting point of study and investigation, not the ending point.

It is tempting to stop the analysis of an adverse event when we encounter a person in the chain of events. Continuing the analysis *through* individuals requires workable model cognition of individuals and of coordinated activity between individuals. It turns out to be quite hard to decide where to halt the causal analysis of a surprising event. Although there are theoretical issues involved in this *stopping rule problem*,[4] the decision about when to stop most often reflects our roles as stakeholders and as participants in the system. We stop when we think we have a good enough understanding, and this understanding is, not surprisingly, when we have identified human error as the source of the failure.

The idea of error-as-cause also fails because it trivializes expert human performance. Error-as-cause leaves us with human performance divided in two: acts that are errors and acts that are non-errors. But this distinction evaporates in the face of any serious look at human performance.[5] What we find is that the sources of successful operation of systems under one set of conditions can be what we label

[4]See Rasmussen (1990b) is the standard statement of the difficulty and see Hollnagel and Amalberti, 2001), Amalberti (2001). For examples of the difficulty in health care, see Cook et al., *A Tale of Two Stories* (1999) and follow ups such as Wears and Nemeth (2007), Wears (2008), Patterson and Wears (2009), and Cook and Nemeth (2010).

[5]The best introduction to the complexity of expert performance is found in Gary Klein's book, *Sources of Power: How People Make Decisions* (MIT Press, Cambridge MA, 1998).

errors after failure occurs. Jens Rasmussen likes to quote Mach (1905) on this point:

"Knowledge and error flow from the same mental sources, only success can tell one from the other."

Instead of finding error and non-error, when we look deeply into human work we find that the behaviors there closely match the incentives, opportunities, and demands that are present in the workplace. Rather than being a distinct class of behavior, we find the natural laws that influence human cognition and performance are *always at work*, sometimes producing good outcomes and sometimes producing bad ones. Trying to separate error from non-error makes it to harder to see these factors.

Conclusion #2: *Defining error-as-consequences (Sense #2) is redundant and confusing.*

Much of the time in health care, the word "error" is used to refer to harm—generally *preventable* harm—to patients. This sort of definition is almost a tautology: it simply involves renaming preventable harm as error. But there are a host of assumptions that are packed into "preventable" and these are almost never made explicit. We are not interested in harm itself but, rather, *how harm comes to be*. The idea that something is preventable incorporates a complete (albeit fuzzy) model of how accidents happen, what factors contribute to them, and what sorts of countermeasures would be productive. But closer examination of "preventable" events shows that their preventability is largely a matter of wishing that things were other than they were.

To use "error" as a synonym for harm gives the appearance of progress where there is none. It would be better if we simply were clear in our use of language and referred to these cases in terms of the kind of harm or patient injuries. Confounding the label error with harm simply adds a huge amount of noise to the communication and learning process.

Conclusion #3: *Defining error-as-deviation from a model of "good" process (Sense #3) collides with the problem of multiple standards.*

The critical aspect of error-as-process-deviation is deciding how to determine what constitutes a deviation. Some have proposed normative models, e.g., Bayes Theorem, but these are rarely applicable to complex settings like healthcare domains, and efforts to use this approach to assess human performance are misleading.[6]

Some have argued that strict compliance with standard operating practices and procedures can be used to define deviation. In other fields, however, it was quickly discovered that standard operating practices capture only a few elements of work and often prescribe practices that cannot actually be sustained in work worlds. In transportation systems, for example, where striking may be illegal, labor strife has sometimes led workers to adopt a "work-to-rule" strategy. By working exactly to rule, workers can readily make complex

[6]Humans are not Bayesian machines and their success in the world is not the result of Bayesian statistics so comparing their performance to Bayesian models necessarily misrepresents the nature of work, cf. Gigerenzer F., *Simple Heuristics: Things that make us smart* (Oxford University Press, 1999) and Klein's *Sources of Power*.

systems stop working. Attempts to make complete, exhaustive policies that apply to all cases creates or exacerbates double binds or to make it easy to attribute adverse events to "human error" and stop.[7]

Choosing among the many candidates for a standard changes what is seen as an error in fundamental ways. Using finer or coarser grain standards can give you a very wide range of error rates. In other words, by varying the standard seen as relevant, one can estimate hugely divergent "error" rates. Some of the "standards" used in specific applications have been changed because too many errors were occurring or to prove that a new program was working. To describe something as a "standard" when it is capable of being changed in this way suggests that there is little that is standard about "standards."

This slipperiness in what counts as a deviation can lead to a complete inversion of standardizing on good process: rather than describing what it is that people need to do to accomplish work successfully, we find ourselves relying on bad outcomes to specify what it is that we want workers not to do. Although often couched in positive language, policies and procedures are often written and revised in just this way after accidents. Unfortunately, hindsight bias plays a major role in such activities.[8]

Working toward meaningful standards as a means for assessing performance and defining error as deviations might be a long-term goal but it is fraught with hazard. To make standards work requires not only clear statements about how to accomplish work but clear guidance about how conflicts are to be handled. Specifying standards for performance for only *part of the work* to be done creates double binds that undermine expert performance creating conditions for failure. To use standards as a basis for evaluating performance deviations requires the continuous evaluation of performance against the standard rather than (as is often the case) simply after bad outcomes become apparent. One practical test of this is whether or not deviations from standards are actually detected and treated in the same way independent of the actual outcome.

To limit the damage from the multiple standards problem, all must carry forward in any tabulation the standard used to define deviations. *This is absolutely essential!* Saying some behavior was an error-as-process-deviation has no meaning without also specifying the standard used to define the deviation.

There are three things to remember about the multiple standards problem. First, the standard chosen is a kind of *model* of what it means to practice before the outcome is known. A scientific analysis of human performance makes those models explicit and debatable. Without that background, any count is arbitrary.

Second, a judgment of error is not a piece of data which then can be tabulated with other like data; instead it is the end result of an *analysis*. Its interpretation rests on others

[7]Lucy Suchman's (1987) book illustrates how expert practice is more than just following standard policies and procedures; *Behind Human Error* captures the double binds that can arise.

[8]Woods et al. (2010), Part V, covers factors such as hindsight bias that block learning after (and before) adverse events occur.

being able to deconstruct and critique that analysis. The base data is the *story* of the particular episode—how multiple factors came together to produce that outcome. Effective systems of inquiry about safety begin with and continually refer back to these base stories of failure and of success in the learning process.

Third, being explicit about the standard used is also essential to be able to critique, contrast, and combine results across events, studies, or settings. When these standards are dropped or hidden in the belief that error is an objective thing in the world, communication and learning collapse.

In the final analysis, the science has shown that "error" is an example of an *essentially contestable* concept. In fact, any benefit to the search for error only comes from the chronic struggle to define how different standards capture and fail to capture our current sense of what is expertise and our current model of the factors that make the difference between success and failure.

Gradually, the research activities that comprise the New Look have led to recognition of a fourth sense of "error."[9]

Conclusion #4: *Labeling an act as "error" marks the end of the social and psychological process of causal attribution.*

If you really want a definition of error, Virginia, we suggest you use this one.

Taken together, the research on how people actually apply the term "error" shows that "error" is a piece of data about reactions to failure, that is, it serves as a placeholder for a set of *socially derived beliefs* about how things happen. As stakeholders, our judgments after the fact about causality are used to explain surprising events. *Thus, in practice, the study of error is nothing more or less than the study of the psychology and sociology of causal attribution.* There are many regularities and biases—e.g., the hindsight bias—that determine how people judge causality. The heterogeneity and complexity of real-world work make these regularities and biases especially important: because the field of possible contributors includes so many items, biases may play an especially important role in determining which factors are deemed relevant.

These results are deeply unsettling for stakeholders because it means the use of the term "error" is less revealing about the performance of workers than it is about ourselves as evaluators. As researchers, advocates, managers, and regulators, we are at least as vulnerable to failure, susceptible to biases and oversimplifications, and prone to err as *those other people*. Fallibility has no bounds in a universe of multiple pressures, uncertainty, and finite resources.

Error is not a fixed category of scientific analysis. It is not an objective, stable state of the world. Instead, it arises from the interaction between the world and the people who create, run, and benefit (or suffer) from human systems for human purposes—a relationship between hazards in the world and our knowledge, our perceptions, and even our dread of the *potential* paths toward and forms of failure.

What is the consequence of error being the result of processes of attribution?

[9]This sense of error was first articulated in Woods et al. (1994) and Cook and Woods (1996).

Although you did not say so explicitly, the question of what is error was predicated on the notion that we can and should treat error as an objective property of the world and that we can search for errors, tabulate them, count them. This searching and counting is futile.

The relationship between error and safety is mirage-like. We find ourselves in a desert, seeing safety glimmering somewhere in the far distance. To begin the journey, we feel we must gauge the distance to our goal in units of "error." This presumption about the location of safety is illusory. Efforts to measure the distance to it are little more than measuring our distance from a mirage. The belief that estimates of this number are a necessary or even useful method of beginning an effort to improve safety are predicated on the apparent location of the mirage.

The psychology of causal attribution, however, tells us that it is our beliefs and misconceptions about failure and error that have combined to make the mirage appear where it does. The New Look research tells us that progress toward safety has more to do with the metaphorical earth underneath our feet than it does with the tantalizing image off in the distance. When we look down, we see how healthcare workers are struggling to anticipate forms of/paths toward failure, actively adapting to create and sustain failure-sensitive strategies, and working to maintain margins in the face of pressures to do more and do it quickly. Looking closely under our feet we see:

1. How workers and organizations are continually revising their approach to work in an effort to remain sensitive to the possibility for failure;
2. How we and the workers are necessarily only partially aware of the current potential for failure;
3. How change is creating new paths to failure and new demands on workers and how revising their understanding of these paths is an important aspect of work on safety;
4. How the strategies for coping with these potential paths can be either strong and resilient or weak and mistaken;
5. How the culture of safety depends on remaining dynamically engaged in new assessments and avoiding stale, narrow, or static representations of risk and hazard;
6. How overconfident nearly everyone is that they have already anticipated the types and mechanisms of failure, and how overconfident nearly everyone is that the strategies they have devised are effective and will remain so;
7. How missing side effects of change is the most common form of failure for organizations and individuals; and
8. How continual effort after success in a world of changing pressures and hazards is fundamental to create safety.

In the final analysis, safety is not a commodity to be tabulated, it is a chronic value "under our feet" that infuses all aspects of practice. *People create safety under resource and performance pressure* at all levels of the sociotechnical system. They continually learn and adapt their activities in response to information about failure. Progress on safety ultimately comes from helping workers and managers create safety.

The folk models about human error are pervasive and seem self-evident. Challenging those folk models calls into question not only closely held beliefs, but also policy and investment decisions. The dissonance between belief and results is uncomfortable at best. Yet, Virginia, the need to make real progress on safety leaves us no choice but to point out how easy it is for all of us to fall back into fallacies and myths about human error. We must make the contrast very stark:

> The misconceptions and controversies about error and safety are rooted in the collision of two mutually exclusive paradigms or world views. One view is that erratic people degrade an otherwise safe system. Thus, work on safety is protecting the system (us as managers, regulators, and consumers) from unreliable people. This is a Ptolemaeic world view (the sun goes around the earth). To defend this world view in the face of the data on human performance and how complex systems fail takes ever greater effort (more and more epicycles by analogy).
>
> The other paradigm or world view is that *people create safety under resource and performance pressure* at all levels of the sociotechnical system by learning and adapting to information about how we all can contribute to failure (this is the basic lesson from New Look research about human performance, success and failure). This is a Copernican world view (the earth goes around the sun). Progress comes from helping people create safety. This is what the science says, despite how odd it sounds: *help people cope with complexity under pressure to achieve success.*
>
> We can blame and punish under whatever labels are in fashion but that will not change the natural laws that govern human performance, nor will it make the sun go round the earth. The paradigm shift demanded if real progress is to be made on safety is, not surprisingly, extraordinarily difficult. We have windows of opportunity for improving safety, but only if all of us are up to the sacrifices involved in building, extending, and deepening the ways we can help people create safety.
>
> So are people sinners or are they saints? An old debate, but neither view leads anywhere near to improving safety. Making safety begins with recognizing the paradox that, simultaneously, we are both the source of success and of failure. How could it be otherwise?—as we create, operate, and modify human systems for human purposes.[10]

Virginia, you wanted a simple, pragmatic answer and did not expect to walk into this onslaught

[10]Many resources are available now on the new paradigm and how it can lead to a new set of methods and means to improve safety. A sampler includes Hollnagel et al. (2006), Nemeth et al., 2008, and Hollnagel (2009) on resilience and safety; studies of resilience in health care systems such as Brown (2005), Patterson et al., 2007, Miller and Xiao (2007), Wears et al. (2008); methods to see patterns of systemic breakdown in analyses of accidents such as Dekker (200x), Nemeth et al. (2004), Nemeth et al. (2006) and Patterson et al. (2004); and Weick and Sutcliffe (2007) summarizes the work on how high reliability organizations show high resilience.

of complexities. But accidents arise from the complexities of the domain, not from its apparent simplicity. The attraction of error as a target for work on safety is illusory. No progress or success is possible if we remain trapped in a Ptolemaeic search for erratic other people or if we try to straddle the two paradigms. Either you are working in the Ptolemaeic paradigm, or you throw it off *completely* and move onto the fascinating and productive challenges of deepening the Copernican paradigm of observing, modeling, and enhancing how we cope with complexity and create safety under pressure.

Virginia, adopt the new paradigm and begin by looking for ways to understand the changing vulnerabilities and pathways that expose patients to risks of injury as a result of care. Investigate how people cope with complexity—usually successfully. Search out the sources of resilience that allow them to produce success when failure threatens.[11] In combination, these efforts will allow you to *create foresight*, to recognize, anticipate, and defend against paths to failure that arise as healthcare organizations and technology change, and to do so *before any patient is injured.*

David Woods and Richard Cook

SUMMARY OF THE NEW LOOK RESEARCH FINDINGS

Doing things safely, in the course of meeting other goals, is and has always been part of operational practice. As people in their different roles are aware of potential paths to failure, they develop failure-sensitive strategies to forestall these possibilities. Failures occurred against this background when multiple contributors—each necessary but only jointly sufficient—combine. Work processes do not choose failure but *move toward it* as production pressures and change erode the defenses that normally keep failure at a distance. This process is the result of systematic, predictable organizational factors at work, not simply erratic individuals (Cook and Rasmussen, 2005). To understand how failure sometimes happens one must first understand how success is obtained—how people learn and adapt to create safety in a world fraught with hazards, tradeoffs, and multiple goals (Cook et al., 2000; Woods and Cook, 2002).

It is clear that high levels of performance are achievable. For example, researchers have studied organizations that have been remarkably successful in managing potentially hazardous technical operations, and the empirical results match the New Look (Rochlin, 1999). Achieving such high levels of performance does not flow from rooting out error, but rather through anticipating and planning for unexpected events and future surprises. Past success is not a reason for confidence; instead, continued investment in anticipating the changing potential for failure is energized by the deeply held understanding that our knowledge base is fragile in the face of the hazards inherent in work and the changes omnipresent in the environment.

The theme that leaps out from the New Look results is that failure represents *breakdowns in adaptations* directed at coping with complexity (Woods et al., 2010; Cook, 2010. Success relates to organizations, groups, and individuals who produce resilient systems that recognize and adapt to change and surprise (Hollnagel et al., 2006; Woods and Branlat, 2011). The measure of success for groups and organizations is the ability to "create foresight—anticipate the changing shape of iatrogenic risk, *before* patients are injured" (Woods, 2005; 2009).

References

1. Amalberti, R. (2001). The paradoxes of almost totally safe transportation systems. *Safety Science*, 37, 109–126.
2. Brennan, T. A. The Institute of Medicine Report on Medical Error—Could It Do Harm? *N Engl J Med* 2000;342:1123–1125.
3. Brown, J. P. (2005). Key themes in healthcare safety dilemmas. In M. S. Patankar, J. P. Brown, & M. D. Treadwell (Eds.), *Safety Ethics: Cases from Aviation, Healthcare, and Occupational and Environmental Health* (pp. 103–148). Aldershot, UK: Ashgate.
4. Cook, R. I. (1999). Two Years Before the Mast: Learning How to Learn About Patient Safety. In Hendee, W. (ed.), Proceedings of *Enhancing Patient Safety and Reducing Errors in Health Care*. National Patient Safety Foundation, Chicago IL (held at Annenberg Center for Health Sciences, Rancho Mirage, CA, Nov. 8–10, 1998).
5. Cook, R. I. (2010). How Complex Systems Fail. In J. Allspaw and J. Robbins (eds.), *Web Operations: Keeping the Data On Time*. O'Reilly Media.
6. Cook R. I. and Nemeth, C. P. (2010). "Those found responsible have been sacked": some observations on the usefulness of error. *Cognition, Technology, and Work*, 12: 87–93.
7. Cook R. I. and Woods, D. D. (1996). Adapting to new technology in the operating room. *Human Factors*, 38(4), 593–613.
8. Cook, R. I., Woods, D. D., and Miller, C. (1998). *A Tale of Two Stories: Contrasting Views on Patient Safety*. National Patient Safety Foundation, Chicago IL, April 1998. (http://www.npsf.org/wp-content/uploads/2011/11/A-Tale-of-Two-Stories.pdf).
9. Cook, R. I., Render, M. L., and Woods, D. D. (2000). Gaps in the continuity of care and progress on patient safety. *British Medical Journal*, 320, 791–794, March 18, 2000.
10. Cook, R. and Rasmussen, J. (2005). "Going Solid": A model of system dynamics and consequences for patient safety. *Quality and Safety in Health Care*, 14, 130–134.
11. Dekker, S. W. A. (2005). *Ten questions about human error: A new view of human factors and system safety*. New Jersey: Lawrence Erlbaum Publishers.
12. Hatlie, M. (1996). *Examining Errors in Health Care: Developing a Prevention, Education and Research Agenda, October 13–15, 1996* (Rancho Mirage, CA: Annenberg Center for Health Sciences at Eisenhower).
13. Hollnagel, E. (2004). *Barriers and Accident Prevention*. Aldershot, UK: Ashgate.
14. Hollnagel, E. (2009). *The ETTO Principle: Efficiency-Thoroughness Trade-Off: Why Things That Go Right Sometimes Go Wrong*. Aldershot, UK: Ashgate.
15. Hollnagel, E., and Amalberti, R. (2001). The Emperor's New Clothes or Whatever Happened to "Human Error"? Proceedings of the Fourth International Workshop on Human Error, Safety, and Systems Development (HESSD-01), Linköping, Sweden, June 11–12, 2001.
16. Hollnagel, E., Woods, D. D., & Leveson N. G. (2006). *Resilience Engineering: Concepts and Precepts*. Aldershot, UK: Ashgate Publishing.
17. Klein, G. A. (1998). *Sources of Power: How People Make Decisions*. Cambridge, MA: MIT Press.
18. Kohn, L. T., Corrigan, J. M., and Donaldson, M., eds. (1999). *To Err is Human: Building a Safer Health System*. Washington D.C.: Institute of Medicine.
19. Leape, L. L. (2000). Institute of Medicine medical error figures are not exaggerated. *JAMA*, 284, 95–97.
20. Leape, L. L., Brennan, T. A., and Laird, N. M. (1991). Incidence of adverse events and negligence in hospitalized patients: Results of the Harvard Medical Practice Study II. *N Engl J Med*, 324, 377–384.
21. Leape L. L. and Berwick D. M. (2005). Five years after to err is human: what have we learned? *JAMA*, 293, 2384–2390.
22. Mach, E. (1905). *Knowledge and Error*. Dordrecht: Reidel Publishing Company.
23. McDonald, C. J., Weiner, M., and Hui, S. L. (2000). Deaths due to medical errors are exaggerated in Institute of Medicine report. *JAMA*, 284, 93–95.
24. Miller, A. and Xiao, Y. (2007). Multi-level strategies to achieve resilience for an organisation operating at capacity: a case study at a trauma centre. *Cognition, Technology & Work*, 9, 51–66.

25. Nemeth, C. P., Cook, R. I., Patterson, E. S., Donchin, Y., Rogers, M. L. and Ebright, P. R. (2004). Afterwords: The Quality of Medical Accident Invstigations and Analyses. Proceedings of the Human Factors and Ergonomics Society 48th Annual Meeting. 20-24 September, New Orleans LA.
26. Nemeth, C., Dierks, M., Patterson, E., Donchin, Y., Crowley, J., McNee, S., Powell, T., and Cook, R. I. (2006). Learning from Investigation. 2006, October. *Proceedings of the Human Factors and Ergonomics Society Annual Meeting*. San Francisco.
27. Nemeth, C., Wears, R. L., Woods, D. D., Hollnagel, E., and Cook, R. I. (2008). Minding the Gaps: Creating Resilience in Health Care. In K. Henriksen, J. B. Battles, M. A. Keyes and M. L. Grady (Eds.), *Advances in Patient Safety: New Directions and Alternative Approaches, Vol. 3. Performance and Tools*. AHRQ Publication No. 08-0034-3. Rockville, MD: Agency for Healthcare Research and Quality; August 2008. http://www.ahrq.gov/qual/advances2/
28. Patterson, E. S., Cook, R. I., Woods, D. D., and Render, M. L. (2004). Examining the Complexity Behind a Medication Error: Generic Patterns in Communication. *IEEE SMC Part A*, 34(6), 749–756.
29. Patterson, E. S., Woods, D. D., Cook, R. I., and Render, M. L. (2007). Collaborative Cross-Checking to Enhance Resilience. *Cognitive Technology and Work*, 9(3), 155–162.
30. Patterson, E. S., and Wears, R. L. (2009). Beyond "communication failure". *Annals of Emergency Medicine*, 53(6), 711–712.
31. Rasmussen, J. (1990a). The role of error in organizing behavior. *Ergonomics*, 33, 1185–1199.
32. Rasmussen, J. (1990b). Human Error and the Problem of Causality in Analysis of Accidents. *Phil Trans R Soc Lond*. B 327, 449–462.
33. Rasmussen, J. (1997). Risk management in a dynamic society: A modeling problem. *Safety Science*, 27(2–3), 183–213.
34. Rasmussen, J. (1999). The concept of human error: Is it useful for the design of safe systems in health care? In C. Vincent and B. deMoll (Eds.), *Risk and Safety in Medicine*. London: Elsevier.
35. Reason, J. (1997). *Managing the Risks of Organizational Accidents*. Brookfield, VT: Ashgate Publishing.
36. Rochlin, G. I. (1999). Safe operation as a social construct. *Ergonomics*, 42(11):1549–1560.
37. Suchman, L. (1987). *Plans and situated actions. The problem of human machine communication*. Cambridge: Cambridge University Press.
38. Wears, R. L. (2008). The error of counting "errors". *Annals of Emergency Medicine*, 52(5), 502--503.
39. Wears, R. L. and Nemeth, C. P. (2007). Replacing hindsight with insight: toward better understanding of diagnostic failures. *Annals of Emergency Medicine*, 49(2), 206–209.
40. Wears, R. L., Perry, S. J., Anders, S., and Woods, D. D. (2008). Resilience in the Emergency Department. In E. Hollnagel, C. Nemeth and S. W. A. Dekker, eds., *Resilience Engineering Perspectives 1: Remaining sensitive to the possibility of failure*. Ashgate, Aldershot, UK, pp. 193-209.
41. Weick, K. E., Sutcliffe, K. M., and Obstfeld, D. (2007). *Managing the Unexpected: Resilient Performance in an Age of Uncertainty* (second edition). Jossey-Bass.
42. Woods, D. D. (2005). Creating Foresight: Lessons for Resilience from Columbia. In W. H. Starbuck and M. Farjoun (eds.), *Organization at the Limit: NASA and the Columbia Disaster*. pp. 289–308. Malden, MA: Blackwell.
43. Woods, D. D. (2009). Escaping Failures of Foresight. *Safety Science*, 47(4), 498–501.
44. Woods, D. D. and Branlat, M. (2011). How Adaptive Systems Fail. In E. Hollnagel, Paries, J., Woods, D.D., and Wreathall, J., Eds., *Resilience Engineering in Practice*. Ashgate, Aldershot, UK, pp. 127–143.
45. Woods, D. D. and Cook, R. I. (2001). From Counting Failures to Anticipating Risks: Possible Futures for Patient Safety. In *Lessons on Patient Safety*. L. Zipperer and S. Cushman, Editors, National Patient Safety Foundation.
46. Woods, D. D. and Cook, R. I. (2002). Nine Steps to Move Forward from Error. *Cognition, Technology, and Work*, 4(2), 137–144.
47. Woods, D. D., Dekker, S. W. A., Cook, R. I., Johannesen, L. L., and Sarter, N. B. (2010). *Behind Human Error (2nd Edition)*. Ashgate, Aldershot, UK.
48. Woods D. D., Johannesen, L., Cook, R. I., and Sarter, N. B. (1994). *Behind Human Error: Cognitive Systems, Computers and Hindsight*. Human Systems Ergonomic Information and Analysis Center, Wright Patterson Air Force Base, Dayton OH.

9

The Investigation and Analysis of Clinical Incidents

Charles Vincent, MD and David Hewett, MD

Why do things go wrong? Human error is routinely blamed for disasters in the air, on the railways, in complex surgery, and in health care generally. However, quick judgments and routine assignment of blame obscure a more complex truth. The identification of an obvious departure from good practice is usually only the very first step of an investigation. Although a particular action or omission may be the immediate cause of an incident, closer analysis usually reveals a series of events and departures from safe practice, each influenced by the working environment and the wider organizational context. Presently, this more complex picture is gaining acceptance in health care,[1–3] but still is seldom put into practice in the investigation of actual incidents.

In a series of papers, the Clinical Risk Unit, University College London, has developed a process of investigation and analysis of adverse events for use by researchers.[4–8] Two years ago a collaborative research group was formed between the Clinical Risk Unit and members of the United Kingdom Association of Litigation and Risk Management (ALARM). This group has adapted the research methods to produce a protocol for the investigation and analysis of serious incidents for use by risk managers and others trained in incident analysis. The full protocol gives a detailed account of the theoretical background, process of investigation, and analysis, with detailed case examples and standard forms for use in the investigation process.[9]

We are, of course, well aware of the pioneering work carried out by The Joint Commission (the Commission) on sentinel event analysis in the United States,[10] and we share a similar perspective. Other formal approaches have also been developed.[11] There are a number of other types of investigation both within medicine and in other high-risk environments, which we are currently reviewing. Our aim is not to compete directly with The Joint Commission approach, but rather to suggest that incident analysis and investigation in health care is at a very early stage of development, and that a substantial research program is needed. Moreover, it is not clear what concepts in the investigation of error are appropriate in health care, what methods are most appropriate for different settings, or what the ultimate value of each approach may be. Very probably, several different approaches could be of value, as other settings have demonstrated.[12]

Our own approach diverges from that of The Joint Commission in a number of significant respects. First, we draw directly on Reason's organizational accident model.[13,14] Although The Joint Commission refers to it, and their approach has clearly been influenced by "systems" thinking, it does not seem to be based on a specific model. Second, our approach is very much investigator-led, in comparison with The Joint Commission's team-based, reflective, and brainstorming approach. It seems likely to us that, on this score at least, different approaches will be preferred in different contexts. Third, our approach is deliberately formal and may lend itself to greater precision. This feature might be useful in a research context, or indeed any setting where a more rigorous method is required. Equally, one might imagine The Joint Commission's approach to be more appropriate when an open process is required to maximize team involvement. Fourth, The Joint Commission's method relies on a wide variety of techniques and offers a number of ways to conceptualize the causes of an incident. This suggests to us that neither we nor The Joint Commission are yet confident of how best to conceptualize accidents or represent the findings. We believe that this remains a matter for further research and investigation. It cannot, in the long run, be acceptable to rely on the personal preferences of the investigator, whoever that may be.

In summary, therefore, we believe that the investigation and analysis of clinical incidents is still at a very early stage, both in terms of practical experience and especially in terms of research. There is much to be gained by exploring and researching different approaches, with the long-term aim of a greater common understanding of this important topic. In this chapter we introduce the main ideas and methods of our own approach and present sections of a case analysis to illustrate the methods in practice.

RESEARCH FOUNDATIONS

The basic theory underlying our protocol and its application derives mainly from research previously undertaken in settings outside health care. In the aviation, oil, and nuclear industries, for instance, the formal investigation of incidents is well-established procedure.[13,14] Studies in these areas have led to a much broader understanding of accident causation, with less focus on the individual who makes the error and more on preexisting organizational factors. Such studies have also illustrated the complexity of the chain of events that may lead to an adverse outcome.[1,2,5,6] The root causes of adverse clinical events may lie in factors such as the use of locum doctors and agency nurses, communication and supervision problems, excessive workload, and educational and training deficiencies as well as resource allocation decisions made in isolation from their practical consequences.

In health care, the development of preventive strategies from such analyses has not yet been fully exploited. However, the potential for these approaches is apparent in other domains. For instance, the inquiry into the Piper Alpha oil disaster led to a host of recommendations and the implementation of a number of risk reduction strategies, which covered the whole industry and addressed a wide range of issues. These included the setting up of a single regulatory body for offshore safety, relocation of pipeline emergency shutdown valves, the provision of temporary safe refuges for oil workers, new evacuation procedures, and requirements for emergency safety training. Most interestingly, oil companies had henceforth to actively demonstrate that hazards had been minimized and had been reduced to levels that are as low as could reasonably be expected.[15–17]

Incidents are opportunities to learn about the gaps and shortcomings in the way organizations manage processes or technologies within which accidents occur. This "organizational learning" paradigm is very different from the more traditional approaches, which are often more judicial in character,[18] a fact also emphasized by The Joint Commission.

Reason's Organizational Accident Model

The protocol and the methods described in this chapter are firmly rooted in Reason's organizational accident model.[13,14] Reason's model was originally developed for use in complex industrial systems as a means of understanding the relationships among the various factors involved in the genesis of accidents and, by extension, of identifying methods of accident prevention. The method of investigation implied by the model is first to recognize the institutional context within which an accident has occurred, and then to examine the chain of events that led to an adverse outcome and consider the actions of those involved. Finally, the investigator, crucially, looks further back through the organizational hierarchy at the conditions in which staff were working and the general context in which the incident occurred.[7,8]

The first step in any analysis is to identify active failures—unsafe acts or omissions committed by those at the "sharp end" of the system (pilots, air traffic controllers, anesthetists, surgeons, nurses, etc.) whose actions can have immediate adverse consequences. These may be slips (such as picking up the wrong syringe), lapses of judgment, forgetting to carry out a procedure, or, rarely, deliberate departures from safe operating practices, procedures, or standards. In our work we have substituted the term *care management problems* (CMPs) for *active failures*. In practice, care management problems may encompass a series of active failures, such as failure to monitor over a period of time. Having identified the CMPs, however, the investigator then considers the conditions in which errors occur and the wider organizational context. These are the significant factors that influence staff performance and that may precipitate errors and affect patient outcomes.

A Framework for the Analysis of Risk and Safety in Medicine

We have extended Reason's model and adapted it for use in a healthcare setting, classifying the error-producing conditions and organizational factors in a single broad framework of factors affecting clinical practice.[7]

At the bottom of the framework are patient factors. In any clinical situation, the patient's condition will have the most direct influence on practice and outcome. Other patient factors, such as personality, language, and any disability, may also be important because they can influence communication with staff, and hence the probability of an incident.

Higher up in the framework are individual (staff) and team factors. Individual factors include the knowledge, skills, and experience of each member of staff, which will obviously affect their clinical practice. Each staff member is part of a team within the inpatient or community unit, and part of the wider organization of the health service. The way an individual practices, and his or her individual impact on the patient, is both constrained and influenced by other members of the team in the way they communicate, support, and supervise each other. In turn the team is influenced by line management actions and by more distant decisions made at a higher level in the organization. These decisions are likely to include policies regarding the use of agency staff, continuing education, training, and supervision, as well as the availability of equipment and supplies. Management decisions also affect the conditions in which the team works, including staffing levels, workload, and the physical conditions of the building together with the environment at large. The organization itself is affected by the institutional context, including politically imposed financial constraints, external regulatory bodies, and the broader economic and social climate. Each level of analysis can be expanded to provide a more detailed specification of the components that make up each major factor. For example, "team factors" includes items of verbal communication between junior and senior staff as well as between different healthcare professions; the quality of written communication, such as the completeness and legibility of notes; and also the availability of supervision and support.

DEFINITIONS AND ESSENTIAL CONCEPTS

Reason's model and our framework provide the conceptual foundations for the investigation process. Before describing the procedural steps contained within the investigation process, we will define some basic terms. These are explained in greater detail in what follows, and examples are given in the case analyses.

The Incident

Essentially, an incident is something that happened to a patient, a clinical outcome with harmful or potentially harmful effects. The criteria for selecting an incident for investigation are discussed further later in the chapter.

Care Management Problems

Care management problems are actions or omissions by staff in the process of care. They have two essential features, both of which are required to be present if a particular CMP is to be selected for detailed investigation and analysis:

1. Care deviated beyond safe limits of practice.
2. The deviation had a direct or indirect effect on the eventual adverse outcome for the patient. (In cases in which the impact on the patient is not immediately apparent, it is sufficient that the CMP had a potentially adverse effect.)

Note that each CMP is to be identified individually and each will be analyzed separately to determine the reasons for its occurrence.

Clinical Context and Patient Factors

For each CMP identified, the investigator records salient clinical events relating to the condition of the patient at the relevant time (for example, bleeding heavily, blood pressure falling). Other patient-related factors affecting the process of care (for example, patient very distressed, patient unable to understand instructions) are also recorded.

Specific Contributory Factors

For each CMP, the investigator uses a process, both during interviews and afterward, to identify the factors that led to that particular CMP. For example:

- Individual factors may include a lack of knowledge or experience in either a member of staff or a group.
- Task factors might include the nonavailability of test results or specific treatment protocols.
- Team factors might include poor communication between staff.
- Work environment factors might include high workload or inadequate staffing.

All or any of these might contribute to the occurrence of a single CMP.

General Contributory Factors

A further distinction needs to be drawn between specific contributory factors and general conditions in the unit. The investigator will differentiate between those contributory factors that are only relevant on that particular occasion and those that are long-standing or permanent features of the unit or, perhaps, of a member of staff. For instance, a failure of communication between two midwives may have contributed to a care management problem. If this is unusual and seldom occurs, then it is a specific contributory factor and not a general factor with wider implications. If, on the other hand, this problem is quite frequent, then the investigator would note a general contributory factor of "poor communication," something that would have clear implications for the safe and effective running of that unit.

Similarly, the investigator might ask:

- Does the lack of knowledge shown on this occasion imply that this member of staff requires additional training?
- Does this particular problem with this guideline mean that the whole guideline needs to be revised?
- Is the high workload due to a temporary and unusual set of circumstances, or is it a more general problem affecting patient safety?

THE INVESTIGATION PROCESS

Reviewing the Case Records

Accounts may be taken from written reports of staff members, case notes, or interviews with staff. Analysis may be limited if only written reports are considered, because it may not be possible to explore the full range of conditions that allowed the event to occur, as can be done in an interview.

The first task, from the necessarily incomplete and sometimes incorrect information immediately available when an incident is first reported, is to make an initial summary of the event and record it. Next, identify the most obvious CMPs. In some instances there may only be one, but nearly always with a serious incident several problems conspire to create the event. At this point we recommend assigning a preliminary grading to the incident. This will be based on factors such as the seriousness of the outcome for the patient, the likelihood of recurrence, the threats to the organization that are posed by it, and the costs that may be incurred in both compensation and system recovery. The grading will indicate the depth and completeness of investigation and analysis that may be required. Before starting the interviews, the key staff involved are listed and decisions are made about who should be interviewed and in what order they should be seen.

Framing the Problem

The next task is to decide which section of the process of care to examine. This is not always a straightforward task. It depends less on the condition of the patient at any particular time and more on when and where problems first arose, something that may only become apparent during the investigation. For instance, a hemorrhage may have been badly managed, leading ultimately to the patient's death 2 weeks later. The chronology may summarize 3 weeks of care, most of which may be of high standard. However, the analysis must concentrate on those aspects where problems were apparent, for example, in the preparation for surgery, conduct of the surgery, and postoperative monitoring, in order that appropriate lessons may be learned.

Undertaking the Interviews

Interviews should be undertaken in private and, if at all possible, away from the immediate place of work in a relaxed setting. The purpose of the interview is simply to find out what happened, a fact that must be clearly explained at the outset. The style adopted should be supportive and understanding, not judgmental or confrontational. Where it becomes clear that a professional shortcoming has occurred, it is best that this should be allowed to emerge naturally from the conversation, and should definitely not be extracted by cross-examination. Most staff members are genuinely disturbed when it becomes clear that something they have done has contributed to an incident. Normally, additional support is essential at this point, and the staff member should be allowed, through supportive discussion, to start to come to terms with what has happened.

There are several distinct phases to the interview, and it will generally be more effective to move through these in order. Each interview should take between 20 and 30 minutes, depending on the degree of involvement. Ideally two interviewers are used, one leading the interview and the other taking notes and asking more detailed supplementary questions. The phases are detailed in the following subsections.

What Happened? Establishing the Chronology and Outcome

The investigator should first establish the role of the member of staff in relation to the incident as a whole, and record the limits of his or her involvement. Next the chronology of events is established as the staff member recalls them.

How Did It Happen? Identifying the Care Management Problems

In the second phase, the investigator should first explain the concept of a care management problem. Next, the member of staff is asked to identify the main CMPs as he or she sees them, without worrying about whether or not anyone is or is not to blame for any of them. The task is to identify all important acts or omissions, or other breakdowns in the clinical process, that were (with hindsight) important points in the chain of events leading to the adverse outcome. Subsequent questions may elicit the reasons behind specific actions (for example, Why did you not call for help at that stage?) and explore references to strong emotions, such as anxiety or anger, which sometimes highlight crucial points.

Why Did It Happen? Identifying the Contributory Factors

In the third phase, the investigator goes back and asks separately about each of the care management problems that the staff member may have information about or direct experience of. Questions should cover contributory factors at all levels of the framework. Each care management problem may be associated with several factors at different levels of the framework that were implicated in its occurrence. These might include, for example, poor motivation (Individual), lack of supervision (Team) and inadequate training policy (Organization and Management). Although the framework has higher-level, organizational factors at the top, it may be more natural in clinical terms to begin by inquiring about patient factors, then moving up the table through task factors, individual factors, and so on. The full protocol contains a much more detailed framework of factors that may be helpful when formulating questions.

Distinguishing Specific and General Contributory Factors

When a member of staff identifies a clearly important contributory factor, the investigator should be sure to ask a follow-up question. Was this factor specific to this occasion or would you regard this as a more general problem on the unit? The prevention of future incidents relies on identifying general, systemic problems, rather than isolated difficulties that are unlikely to recur.

Finally, the investigator should ask the staff member if he or she has any other comments to make or questions to ask. The approach is quite structured, and, although encouraging staff contributions, it is still important to allow time for more open reflection and comment.

Analysis of the Case

The core of the process is to ask: What happened? How did it happen? Why did it happen? What can we learn from this and what changes should we make, if any? In the analysis the same basic format is followed, this time drawing together the material from the case records, interviews, and the investigator's own observations.

The first step in the analysis is to produce an agreed-upon chronology of events, identifying any important areas of disagreement between accounts or between the case notes and the memories of the staff. The starting point for the chronology will generally be the point at which the patient entered the hospital, though relevant events before the patient's arrival (for example, previous treatment, a misleading referral letter) may also need to be recorded. However, it is important to identify and focus on the most important part of the chronology (see "Framing the Problem").

The next stage is to identify the key care management problems. These will normally have been provided by the staff themselves during the interviews, as well as from the investigator's own clinical knowledge and expertise. The investigator should look back over the list and ensure that all the care management problems are specific actions or omissions rather than more general observations on the quality of care, which should be recorded elsewhere. It is easy to note down "poor teamwork" as a care management problem, which may be a correct description of the team, but it should properly be recorded as a contributory factor within specific CMPs.

The next step is to attempt to specify the conditions associated with each of the care management problems, using the framework as a guide and as a way of reflecting on the many factors that may affect the clinical process. Interviews with staff will already have provided lists of both specific and general contributory factors. Where these conflict, it may be necessary to make a judgment as to the most important causes of the events.

A separate analysis should be carried out for each care management problem, though the depth and detail of the contributory factors identified may vary for each one. It is particularly important to distinguish *specific contributory factors*, which describe the reasons for the care management problem on that particular occasion, from *general contributory factors* that the investigator judges to be more long-standing features of the individual, team, or working conditions. Factors that are specific to the occasion and that do not reflect more general problems will usually have no long-term implications for the quality and safety of practice. They do not normally require action or changes of any kind. The final list of general contributory factors for each care management problem is examined, and those that have implications for action are identified. The protocol contains blank forms with appropriate headings to facilitate both the interview and analysis.

Preparation of the Report

Once the interviews and analysis are completed, make a composite of all of them, detailing the whole incident from start to finish. If the protocol is followed systematically and the interviews and analysis conducted thoroughly, the report and implications of the incident should emerge from the analysis in a relatively straightforward fashion. When the composite is complete, there should be a clear view of the problem and the circumstances that led up to it. The flaws in the care process will be readily apparent. The final report can be drawn up using the documentation, which by now will include the following:

- A summary of the chronology
- A list of the care management problems with their contributory causes, giving most emphasis to general contributory factors and emphasizing any positive features of the care given
- Recommended action and time scales for each one of the general factors requiring attention

CASE EXAMPLES

Attempted Suicide in an Inpatient Psychiatric Unit

This case example is based on real clinical events but has been altered in various respects to preserve the anonymity of those involved.

Eight members of staff were interviewed, six nurses and two junior doctors. Three of these people were closely involved in the incident reported. The other five staff members had been peripherally involved but had also been disturbed by the incident and approached the interviewer directly because they wanted to discuss it.

- There was no formal risk assessment in the ward round, confirmed by the medical notes, which are very sketchy in this respect. The junior doctor (MR) stated that B (the patient) was not specifically asked about urges to self-harm or suicidal ideation.
- When the junior doctor saw B the day before the incident, he recorded that B was not depressed and not suicidal.
- B subsequently attempted to harm or kill herself by cutting her wrists. When found by the nurses, attempts to care for this patients' needs were chaotic and unsupervised, contributing to greater patient harm.
- To avoid the risk of fainting, B should have been taken to the clinical room in a wheelchair. In addition, she should have been put on oxygen and had her pulse and BP taken before the duty doctor reached the ward. B's wrist had not been bandaged properly.
- When B was first taken to the clinical room, the nurses did not lie her down as a precaution against fainting. When the doctor arrived, B was sitting with her arms hanging down. The nurses should have had her hold her arms up above her head to prevent further bleeding.
- The second junior doctor could not insert a cannula for an IV infusion.
- Staff had to look for supplies to clean B's neck and wrist. Although this did not take long, any delay could have severe consequences with more serious cases.
- There was no formal, structured, and supportive discussion of the incident focusing on how staff felt and whether the incident could have been dealt with better or even prevented. Some staff talked about it briefly with one or two colleagues when they had time, while others went home still disturbed and discussed it with friends.

Whether or not this incident is regarded as preventable, lessons can certainly be learned from it. B was seen by several doctors at different times, many of whom were inexperienced or unsupervised, or coming to grips with a new job. Actions of some of the staff could have been questioned, but when the broader picture is considered and the contributory causes are examined, more general, and perhaps more worrying, problems can be identified. The junior doctors, through no fault of their own, were acting beyond their competence on several occasions. Clear training needs are apparent in regard to the induction of new staff and the medical abilities of psychiatric nurses. Equipment and supplies were poorly maintained, and no one appeared to have had overall responsibility for this important task. The poor design of the ward also appears to have been a contributing factor in that B was able to harm herself without fear of being observed and without much chance of being discovered quickly.

The lack of support and supervision involved in the incident is perhaps the most glaring problem, at least in the view of the junior doctors. On his first day, another patient had a medical problem that MR had never encountered before. He had not been told how to contact the consultant for help, and the consultant's secretary did not know how to contact him either. MR eventually managed to get help from another junior doctor. He tried subsequently to discuss the issue with the consultant, who was very dismissive. MR was quite disturbed by his unhelpful and unsupportive attitude. MR felt very strongly that he did not have enough experience to deal with a patient like B, and was keen to discuss the difficulties he had encountered because he considered them to have had profound implications for the safe functioning of the unit.

It is sometimes too easy to concentrate only on what went wrong or what could have been done better in relation to a case. This analysis also revealed several positive features in the management of the incident. Pointing these out explicitly is important for staff morale and helps present a more balanced picture of the functioning of the team and the system in general. For instance, staff had correctly advised B to stay in the hospital when she had wanted to return home; there were no delays or difficulties in summoning and getting help, either from other nurses on the ward, the junior doctor, or the emergency services; once B had been discovered, the staff worked efficiently, calmly, and effectively as a team; and staff recognized the seriousness of the incident and subsequently put B on total observation.

Implementation of the Protocol in a British Hospital

The implementation of clinical risk management throughout the hospital has been an evolutionary process that spanned four years, starting in 1995. There was already in place a reasonable infrastructure for dealing with nonclinical risks, but it was not capable of processing clinical incidents. (It is important to note that in Britain, clinical risk management encompasses active patient safety programs and is not restricted to medico-legal and insurance matters.)[19]

From the outset it was obvious that the maternity department posed the greatest risks to the organization as a whole. This could be inferred from data about complaints and litigation (85% of the costs of claims). Although there was no evidence that the quality of care was of a particularly low standard, the consequences of clinical problems were potentially very severe. Thus it made sense to start in that department. The approach adopted was to build on the existing well-established arrangements for perinatal death reviews.

First of all a small group designed an incident reporting form with help from a large firm of defendant lawyers who had experience designing these. The notion that the form had to collect all possible incidents no matter how trivial was rapidly rejected in favor of a targeted approach concentrating on a list of indications for reporting. These included stillbirth, suspected birth asphyxia, postpartum hemorrhage, third-degree tears, delayed caesarean section, and so forth. At the same time, one of the senior midwives was given protected time to investigate incidents and to prepare reports for the senior obstetrician and gynecologist to review. The latter individual then proposed service changes to the managers and his clinical colleagues when this was indicated. The lawyers also made a presentation to the medical and midwifery staff to explain why the system should be introduced.

This system started well, largely because of the enthusiasm of the senior obstetrician. It became clear, however, that the senior midwife needed support and further training, which was not readily available. Fortunately, the protocol research had just been proposed, and she joined with the authors and others to participate in the work of the research team. This experience helped to fill the gap in formal training as the methodology evolved.

As experience with collecting information about incidents grew, it became clear that the role of the midwife was crucial. Not only did she investigate incidents, but staff started to tell her a great deal more about matters that concerned them. As a well-known staff member who had worked in the department for many years, she was able to tactfully identify incidents that might otherwise not have been reported. Slowly the culture began to change. After the senior obstetrician retired, impetus faltered for a while, but with the arrival of a new head of midwifery, it was reestablished. The process became formalized, with a monthly risk management meeting being established. Also, the need to formally grade incidents for severity was recognized. The monthly meeting was set up to ensure that recommendations were followed through into practice. The protocol for investigation, described previously, became an important tool for collecting information about the most serious incidents that were being reported.

At around this time the entire National Health Service in the United Kingdom was required to implement a new process of clinical quality management referred to as "clinical governance."[20] In order to implement this, a central clinical governance committee was set up supported by committees based on the clinical directorates in the hospital. Risk management became one of the four main areas of activity for these committees. The structure and processes that had evolved in the maternity department now became applicable to the rest of the hospital. By this stage, the scale of the risk management undertaking meant that structures had to become even more formalized. A risk management strategy for the whole hospital was in place, with a clinical risk policy subordinate to it. The policy statement made specific reference to the relationship between investigation and discipline:

> We consider that a clear statement which indicates that a blame culture will not be encouraged is a crucial requirement before sufficient trust can be established to create an open climate in which reporting and investigation will flourish.

The severity grading system relies on assessments relating to the severity of outcome for the patient, the probability of recurrence, the magnitude of any public relations problems, and the potential for litigation. These, applied to a matrix, produce one of four colored grades: green, yellow, amber, or red. The color then indicates the correct administrative pathway for investigating and reporting the incident.

- Green incidents are simply counted and noted. The counts are then regularly reported to the directorate managers. Examples of green-coded incidents would include mislabeled specimens, simple drug administration errors, and lost documents. Action follows not on the basis of a single event, but on the identification of a rising trend.
- Yellow incidents require a straightforward commonsense investigation with a minimum of documentation. Recommendations are usually clear and need to be monitored by local managers to ensure implementation. Some of these incidents will require reporting to external agencies for follow-up. Examples might include prescription errors identified by the ward pharmacist, equipment malfunctions (with minimal harm to patients), imaging the wrong body part, patients falling out of bed and sustaining fractures, and detained patients leaving without proper authorization. These incidents are reported to the directorate-based governance committees.
- Amber incidents require a less detailed investigation using the protocol, usually at the level of the main headings and principal factors. Often there are only one or two CMPs, but the impact is such that the most senior levels of management need to be aware of the problem. Examples might include issuing erroneous pathology test results that caused an incorrect line of treatment to be followed, serious drug administration errors, incorrect minor operations, missed fractures, and inappropriate discharges followed by immediate readmission.
- Red incidents are very serious and require a full and detailed report, followed by recommendations. These incidents are reported at the central clinical governance committee and may also be reported to the main hospital board. Such incidents might include inappropriate interpretation of a cardiotocograph tracing leading to birth asphyxia and death or brain damage, inappropriate discharge from the Accident and Emergency Department followed by death due to a cause present but not recognized when seen in the ER, and a major diagnostic equipment failure leading to inaccurate reports in a screening program.

DISCUSSION

The protocol has been found to be of considerable assistance in investigating and writing up reports on serious events. It is time consuming, but so is any other form of detailed investigation. An important advantage is that it encourages investigators to be systematic and to review the incident as a whole rather than becoming fixated on one aspect. Clinicians faced with reviewing an incident often concentrate exclusively on the medical process and will overlook obvious systemic failures and totally ignore environmental factors. Similarly, those who are trained to interpret health and safety legislation will often fail to see clear-cut clinical failures. The protocol, both by its structure and content, avoids bias and forces a comprehensive review.

A structured and systematic approach means that the ground to be covered in any investigation is, to a significant extent, already mapped out. The protocol helps to ensure a comprehensive investigation and facilitate the production of formal reports. Although the procedure may initially appear complicated and time consuming, our experience is that using the protocol actually speeds up complex investigations by focusing the investigators on the key issues and bringing out the systemic factors that must ultimately be the target of the investigation. These systemic features are addressed when long-term risk reduction strategies are implemented. Once the general contributory factors are identified, these lead automatically to the implications and action points. The final report almost writes itself.

We have noted that even very experienced clinicians find that following a systematic protocol brings additional benefits in terms of comprehensiveness and investigation expertise. Clinicians are accustomed to identifying the problematic features in the management of a case, and so can easily identify the care management problems. However, the identification of contributory factors and the realization that each care management problem may have a different constellation of contributory factors are less familiar tasks. A systematic approach pays dividends when exploring these. The protocol does not attempt to supplant clinical expertise. Rather, the aim is to utilize clinical experience and expertise to the fullest extent.

A formal, systematic approach also brings benefit to the staff involved. The methods used are designed to promote a greater climate of openness and to move away from finger pointing and the routine assignment of blame. This is quite different from the quasi-judicial approach that can be brought to bear in formal inquiries. If a consistent approach to investigation is used, members of staff who are interviewed tend to find the process less threatening than traditional unstructured approaches, especially when the same procedure is being followed with everyone involved.

We have found that formal training and practice with the protocol is needed before it can be used to its full effectiveness. Presentations and training sessions have suggested that the basic ideas can be grasped relatively quickly, but that the full method must be absorbed relatively slowly. Guided practice on the investigation of incidents, preferably in a local context, is essential to become familiar with the methods. Investigators who can carry out an investigation with agreed-upon guidelines can then be designated in each clinical area. Each of these investigators requires specific training, time, and support to carry out detailed investigations using this protocol. The provision of these resources is a test of management resolve in dealing effectively with major incidents and learning from them.

Although we believe that the protocol is an effective and valuable tool, we consider that it is still at a relatively early stage of development, both conceptually and practically. Formal evaluation is needed, and a great deal more practical testing is required. We plan to revise and develop the protocol in the light of experience and formal evaluation. We also believe that the protocol has potential as a research instrument, in that analyses of case series of incidents will be considerably more powerful if a common method is applied to all. In the meantime, however, it is already proving a powerful means of investigating and analyzing clinical incidents and drawing out the lessons these incidents have for enhancing patient safety.

ACKNOWLEDGMENTS AND FURTHER INFORMATION

Members of the ALARM research group, who developed the protocol with the two authors, are Jane Chapman, Sue Prior, Pam Strange, and Ann Tizzard.

Copies of the full protocol are available from the Association of Litigation and Risk Management, Royal Society of Medicine, 1 Wimpole Street, London W1, United Kingdom.

References

1. Eagle, C. J. et al., "Accident Analysis of Large-Scale Technological Disasters: Applied to Anaesthetic Complications," *Canadian Journal of Anaesthesia* 39 (1992):118–122.
2. Cook, R. I., and Woods, D. D. "Operating at the Sharp End: The Complexity of Human Error," *Human Error in Medicine*, ed. M. S. Bogner (Hillsdale, NJ: Lawrence Erlbaum Associates, 1994).
3. Reason, J. T. "Human Error: Models and Management" *British Medical Journal* 320 (2000):768–770.
4. Vincent, C. A., and Bark, P. "Accident Analysis," in *Clinical Risk Management*, ed. C. A. Vincent (London: BMJ Publications, 1995).
5. Stanhope, N. et al., "Applying Human Factors Methods to Clinical Risk Management in Obstetrics," *British Journal of Obstetrics and Gynaecology* 104 (1997):1225–1232.
6. Taylor-Adams, S. E. et al., "Applying Human Factors Methods to the Investigation and Analysis of Clinical Adverse Events," *Safety Science* 31 (1999):143–159.
7. Vincent, C. A., Adams, S., and Stanhope, N. "A Framework for the Analysis of Risk and Safety in Medicine." *British Medical Journal* 316 (1998):1154–1157.
8. Vincent, C. A., Taylor-Adams, S., Chapman, E. J. et al., "How to Investigate and Analyse Clinical Incidents: Clinical Risk Unit and Association of Litigation and Risk Management Protocol." *British Medical Journal* 320 (2000):777–781.
9. Vincent, C. A. et al., *The Investigation and Analysis of Clinical Incidents: A Protocol* (London: Royal Society of Medicine Press, 1999).
10. Joint Commission on Accreditation in Healthcare Organizations, *Root cause analysis in healthcare* (Oakbrook Terrace, CA: JCAHO, 2000).
11. van Vuuran, W. et al., *The Development of an Incident Analysis Tool for the Medical Field*, Report EUT/BDK/85 (The Netherlands: Eindhoven University of Technology, Faculty of Technology Management, 1997).
12. Fahlbruch, B. et al., "Event Analysis as Problem Solving Process," in *After the Event: From Accident to Organizational Learning*, eds. A. Hale and B. Wilpert (Oxford: Pergamon, 1997).
13. Reason, J. T. *Human Error* (New York: Cambridge University Press, 1990).
14. Reason, J. T. *Managing the Risk of Organizational Accidents* (Aldershot: Ashgate, 1997).
15. Cullen, W. D. *The Public Inquiry into the Piper Alpha Disaster* (London: Department of Energy, HMSO, 1990).
16. Hughes, H. "The Offshore Industry's Response to Lord Cullen's Recommendations," *Petroleum Rev* Jan (1991):5–8.

17. Ferrow, M. "Offshore Safety: Formal Safety Assessments," *Petroleum Review* Jan. (1991):9–11.
18. Hale, A. R. et al., eds., *After the Event: From Accident to Organizational Learning* (Oxford: Pergamon, 1997).
19. Vincent, C. A. ed., *Clinical Risk Management Enhancing Patient Safety* (London: BMJ Publications, 2001).
20. Secker-Walker, J., and Donaldson, L. "Clinical Governance: The Context of Risk Management," in *Clinical Risk Management Enhancing Patient Safety*, ed. C. A. Vincent (London: BMJ Publications, 2001).

10

Applying Epidemiology to Patient Safety

Mark Keroack, MD, MPH and Emily Rhinehart, RN, MPH, CIC, CPHQ

Epidemiology is a relative newcomer among the medical sciences. Although its roots go back to Snow's studies of cholera in 19th-century London, its widespread application to the explanation of disease causation dates back only to the 1950s. Since that time, there has been a rapid growth of studies that have clarified the causes and risk factors of disease through careful observations of affected populations by methods that account for confounding clinical factors. Epidemiologic approaches have led to major breakthroughs in our understanding of cardiovascular diseases, cancer, and emerging infectious diseases, and their application to nosocomial infection control has led to systematic advances in prevention. However, epidemiologic tools have received little attention in advancing patient safety, largely because of concerns that underreporting of medical errors by clinicians will yield invalid data regarding the incidence of events that lead to patient harm.

The seminal chart review studies of Brennan and others that raised the consciousness of the medical community regarding medical error were epidemiologic in design, using surveillance by standardized chart review to estimate the incidence of errors and the deaths they caused.[1,2] The findings were highlighted in the Institute of Medicine report *To Err Is Human*, causing a national outcry for improvement and a renewed interest by governmental funding agencies in understanding and controlling medical error.[3] Although the report called for a 50% reduction in deaths from medical error by 2005, more than a decade after those original epidemiologic studies there has been little activity devoted to estimating the current rate using epidemiologic methods. Current approaches to understanding medical error have focused instead on intensive case reviews called root cause analyses, patterned after industries such as aviation and nuclear power, in which errors are relatively less common than in health care and much more dramatic in their manifestations. This method has proved its value for isolated events; however, approaches are also needed that enable quality and risk managers to learn from the numerous, more minor events that occur daily in modern hospitals and other healthcare settings. This chapter explores the ways in which the tools of epidemiology can answer this need, augmenting our understanding of medical error and complementing traditional case investigation approaches.

EPIDEMIOLOGY VERSUS CASE-BASED ANALYSIS: THE FOREST AND THE TREES

There is a long history of individual case analyses in medicine, evidenced by the tradition of clinicopathological conferences and morbidity and mortality rounds. Although some have dismissed these approaches as less than scientific when measured against the exacting standards of the controlled clinical trial, it is now clear that much progress has been made in advancing patient safety by in-depth analyses of isolated catastrophic events. The merits and shortcomings of this sort of "qualitative research" were well described by Runciman[4] nearly a decade ago and recently reviewed by Kaplan and Barach.[5] Over the years, root cause investigations have advanced by borrowing from the lessons learned by the aviation and nuclear power industries, shifting their focus from finding and blaming culprits to identifying systematic flaws in the processes of care that predispose clinicians to commit errors.[6]

The advantages of this approach are several. Root cause analysis can identify plausible causes of catastrophic events without requiring the standard of proof of a clinical trial. This means that an organization does not have to wait for recurrences of rare events, such as wrong-sided surgeries or infant abductions, in order to take corrective action. It allows the adoption of self-evident solutions, such as the removal of concentrated potassium chloride solutions from clinical wards to prevent fatal overdoses or the redesign of anesthesia tubing to prevent incorrect connections. When coupled with insight into human factors issues, it allows for a detailed, open-ended narrative that can lead to solutions not initially contemplated by the investigators. Lastly, by recounting a compelling story of care gone bad, case-based analysis can move the culture of an organization to face the existence of flaws in its systems. Because of these advantages, as well as its strong track record of accomplishment in disciplines such as anesthesia, root cause analysis will remain the preferred method for rare and catastrophic events.

However, the very elements that make the case-based investigative approach the methodology of choice for rare events make it a weaker method for events that occur commonly. Incident reports are usually selected for root cause analysis when there was considerable harm to the patient or the potential for considerable harm, but analysis of more minor events, such as missing laboratory tests or missed medication doses, may uncover system flaws every bit as serious as those uncovered through the investigation of rare, catastrophic events. In fact, reports of near misses have been shown to be valuable in improving safety in other industries.[6] If overall improvement of patient safety is the goal, one cannot afford to overlook the potential information from numerous event reports of common errors. However, if only the most serious events are selected for in-depth analysis, reporting of minor events will be discouraged and their potential importance discounted by staff.

An analysis focused on selected cases also will lead to conclusions that are weaker and narrower than cases analyzed as groups. The role of clinical or other contributing factors that would make the event more likely to occur is largely conjectural in an individual root cause analysis, because comparisons between the case being analyzed and other, similar cases are not performed. The potential contributions of such factors as age, comorbid conditions, site of care, and time of day cannot be discerned from an analysis focusing on a single case. A classic epidemiologic example will help illustrate this point.

Modern infection control traces its roots to the pioneering studies of Semmelweis on puerperal fever in the mid-1800s. His critical contribution was in discovering differences in rates of maternal death due to this common infection between different wards of the Allegemaines Krankenhaus in Vienna.[7] Although the disease occurred both in divisions attended by midwives and medical students, rates on the latter divisions were threefold higher. Semmelweis established the key risk factor of care by a medical student in the infection and hypothesized that the performance of autopsies by medical students led to cross-contamination of patients with contaminated materials. Institution of handwashing policies for the medical students led to a reduction of rates similar to those observed in the wards attended by midwives. It is unlikely that a detailed investigation of a single case of disease would have led to this insight; rather, noting differences in rates in clearly defined subpopulations at differential risk for disease led to a testable hypothesis regarding a key causal factor.

SURVEILLANCE SYSTEMS PAST AND PRESENT

The current management of patient safety in most healthcare organizations begins with incident reporting by front-line clinical staff. However, risk managers acknowledge that they are informed of most significant events not through incident reports, but via pages or urgent telephone calls from the staff. They may or may not eventually record the event on an incident report. Thus, incident reports are not actually used for their primary purpose—notifying the risk manager and triggering an investigation. Most are used for a secondary purpose—as a tool to document that proper procedures were followed after the occurrence of an adverse event.

Incident reports have been revised to capture more detailed data on a variety of events. This has resulted in several problems that hinder their use as a surveillance tool. For example, it is common to see forms that are lengthy and detailed, sometimes containing dozens of variables on a single page printed in a very small font. Alternatively, separate forms may exist for medication events, falls, behavioral events, and so forth. In addition, since the reports have evolved primarily to be a documentation tool, several sign-offs may be required before a report reaches the desk of the risk or quality manager. This often leads to weeks of delay while the report moves from one manager's desk to another, reducing the value of interviews based on recall for those events deserving further investigation. While the problem of underreporting of errors and adverse events is often ascribed to a culture of blame that exists in many organizations regarding error reporting,[8,9] the problem is made worse by tools and processes that are cumbersome and confusing.

Because of concerns regarding unreported events, many organizations have implemented changes in traditional incident reporting tools and processes. A few organizations have developed electronic event reporting systems that have the advantage of collapsing numerous paper forms into a single reporting tool and reducing the time lost in transferring paper between departments. Locally developed tools include the system at the University of Missouri at Columbia.[10] Systems that focus on a single type of error include the MedmaRx system developed by US Pharmacopoeia and the Medical Error Reporting System for Transfusion Medicine (MERS-TM) developed at Columbia University.[11,12] More broad-based tools include the products developed by Doctorquality.com and the University HealthSystem Consortium.[13,14] Experience with implementation of these latter products shows that lowering the barriers to reporting, when coupled with efforts to reduce blame and focus on system improvements, can lead to severalfold increases in reporting.[15,16] As numbers of reports increase, the average severity of a report tends to decrease. Indeed, a significant fraction of reports are of "close calls" or "near misses" in which chance or an active intervention prevented the error from reaching the patient. Encouraging this sort of reporting broadens the view of staff regarding the prevalence of human error in health care and its potential consequences.

If all event and near miss reports represent opportunities for learning about system flaws, how does a quality or risk manager come to grips with a growing number of reports in an organization that has made a commitment to patient safety? Prioritization methods have been suggested, including the VA Severity Assessment Matrix,[17] in which events that are most severe or most likely to recur receive priority for intensive investigation. This approach still tends to discard the majority of reports, however, some of which may herald future catastrophe. For example, the administration of a vitamin pill to the wrong patient may be dismissed as having no consequences, but it may provide clues to systematic flaws in the medication administration process that could lead to administering a far more toxic agent to the wrong patient in the future. Furthermore, the greatest disincentive to reporting for a frontline clinician is the message that nothing was done with the report filed. If one's only analytic tool is intensive case investigation, then a majority of reported events will be discarded in the current environment of limited analytic resources.

DEVELOPING SURVEILLANCE SYSTEMS FOR ERRORS AND ADVERSE EVENTS

An effective surveillance system should accomplish four main objectives. Monitoring the occurrence rate of a specific adverse event will allow the organization to (1) determine the overall magnitude of the problem relative to others, (2) decide whether it is increasing or decreasing in incidence, (3) identify which patient groups or care areas are most affected and therefore most in need of resources, and (4) decide whether efforts to improve are being effective. The term *surveillance* conjures up the image of a highly trained professional reviewing patient charts using strict case definitions or interviewing at-risk individuals using highly structured questionnaires. However, many forms of surveillance are far less exact. Aggregation of death certificate information was the first example of disease surveillance and is still used to track national trends in disease, in spite of its well-publicized shortcomings.[18,19] When legionnaire's disease and AIDS first came to attention, case definitions were rudimentary and inexact, but they nonetheless focused national attention on the emerging threats and allowed estimates of their magnitude and spread.[20,21] In each case, inferences made from tracking imperfect measures enabled the identification of specific risk factors that allowed investigators to focus more rigorous observation efforts in the areas where they would be the most fruitful. Such will likely be the case with the data sets on adverse events now being developed by pioneering organizations committed to a better understanding of patient safety.

Baylor Grapevine Hospital has implemented the Doctorquality.com computerized event reporting system and has coupled it with a senior leadership initiative to encourage reporting.[15] The leaders of the quality program found that simple trending of rates of adverse events could be accomplished by unit managers, allowing quality and risk staff to focus on priority areas. At the University of Wisconsin, hospital-wide implementation of the UHC Patient Safety Net, coupled with policies to encourage open reporting, has increased event reporting over the previous paper system by 260%.[16] The ability to select areas for more intensive review from these data is analogous to infection control programs in which routine infections are trended and interventions focused on areas of high severity or strategic importance, or instances when rates increase beyond preset limits. Note that in the individual case approach, cases merit investigation by virtue of the impact or potential impact on a single patient, whereas in the epidemiologic approach, groups of cases merit investigation by increases in overall rates or clustering in specific areas or patient groups.

The passive collection of adverse event reports must be augmented by a more structured and targeted approach to problem areas led by quality and risk managers. This may entail direct data collection through chart review, direct observation of clinical processes, or efforts to encourage front-line clinicians to focus their reporting on specific areas of interest. As these managers reevaluate and redesign their systems to focus on specific process errors and adverse events, they should first examine the basic principles of epidemiology and methods of disease surveillance. Surveillance is defined by the Centers for Disease Control and Prevention (CDC) as "the ongoing, systematic collection, analysis, and interpretation of health data essential to the planning, implementation, and evaluation of public health practice, closely integrated with the timely dissemination of these data to those who need to know."[20]

Going forward, systems for ongoing surveillance must be developed to focus on specific patients at risk, process errors, and adverse events and outcomes. Just as infection control abandoned the practice of total surveillance and the calculation of hospital-wide infection rates a number of years ago, risk management needs to hone its measurement approach and recognize, for example, that a hospital-wide medication error rate is not valid or useful in risk analysis or risk reduction. In approaching the collection and analysis of risk data, risk managers can successfully follow the recommended steps for developing a population-based surveillance system outlined in Table 10.1.[21]

Assessing the Population at Risk

First, the patient population should be assessed for the risk of specific errors or adverse events and outcomes. If the population at risk is defined too broadly, the resulting data will be crude and will not lead to identification of specific risks or contributing factors that can be remedied. Reporting should focus on those populations with the greatest risks, targeting either frequent errors or severe events. This will facilitate the use of the data

TABLE 10.1 Steps in Developing a Surveillance Program

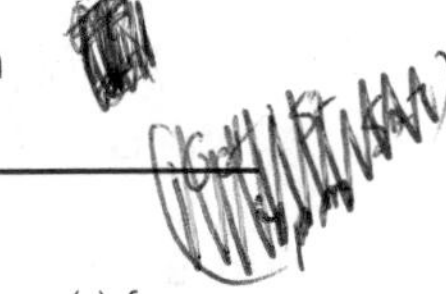

1. Assess the population at risk.
2. Select the process(es) and/or outcome(s) for surveillance.
3. Develop definitions.
4. Develop data collection methods and tools.
5. Calculate and analyze rates.
6. Apply risk stratification.
7. Report results on a regular schedule and use the data for the development of risk reduction strategies.

for further, more detailed study or the development of process improvements. Choosing the patient population on which to focus may be prompted by many considerations, including patients with high-mortality conditions or procedures, patients in strategically important programs (e.g., trauma patients in the region's only Level I trauma center), patients in new clinical programs, or patients in areas where baseline trends seem to indicate opportunities for improvement.

Selecting the Processes and Outcomes for Surveillance

As incident report forms have evolved, risk managers have included long lists of errors and events in very complex, difficult-to-read forms. Redesigning the incident reporting system provides an opportunity to focus on more specific errors and events. This may be accomplished by simplifying forms to allow for more free text, limiting the scope of the form to concentrate only on the most common or significant errors, or utilizing computer technology to tailor the questions being displayed to the event being reported. Limiting the list of events meriting the focus of risk and quality management staff will allow these professionals to (1) select more valid indicators of risk and related variables, (2) develop stable and accurate rates of incidence of the selected error or event, and (3) further refine the definitions of groups at risk and other risk factors. This will result in the development of more focused risk analysis studies that will more likely lead to valid conclusions and specific risk reduction strategies.

As part of a renewed approach to data collection, it is useful to determine which errors or adverse events should be captured and analyzed by considering the following factors:[20]

- Frequency of the event or error
- Negative impact (e.g., likelihood to lead to a claim or more serious outcome)
- Potential for prevention
- Specific risks within a patient population (e.g., obstetrics)
- Relationship of the adverse event to the process of care
- Resources available for reporting/surveillance

For the reasons mentioned earlier, most paper-based systems are not reliable guides for determining the incidence of adverse events. Computerized systems have shown promise in augmenting reporting substantially, often revealing potential areas of focus. Previous projects in which intensive measurement of specific processes or outcomes were conducted also may help guide the prioritization process. Lastly, the risk or quality manager's own experience in the organization may often serve as an accurate guide for those types of events most frequently associated with patient harm or liability risk exposure.

Because most areas of opportunity in systems of care require a team effort in order to improve them, it is advantageous to decide on priority areas in collaboration with other interested and involved individuals. This may include the participation of quality management staff as well as selected representatives from the nursing and medical staff. Input from clinicians who care for specific high-risk populations (e.g., obstetricians, emergency room staff) is valuable both in designing valid and relevant reporting tools and in gaining buy-in from those who will be involved in reporting and improvement initiatives.

Developing Definitions

Any surveillance system must include specific definitions for the data elements being collected. Taking the time to identify or develop definitions will contribute to more consistent, accurate, and reliable data. The first step in developing definitions is to search for existing definitions. For specific populations, definitions may have already been developed by professional organizations such as the American College of Obstetrics and Gynecology (e.g., delayed cesarean section), the American College of Surgeons (e.g., surgical wound classification), or the American Society for Anesthesiology (e.g., ASA score). Participation of clinicians from these specialty groups, as discussed earlier, will facilitate the identification of already existing definitions. For process errors or adverse events that may occur across multiple patient populations, such as medication errors or falls, a literature search should be conducted to find definitions already developed by others. Adoption of an existing definition may allow for external comparisons or benchmarking in the future. The Agency for Healthcare Research and Quality has funded research into the development of a national consensus classification system for medical errors and adverse events.

The proper criteria for determining the occurrence or category of events should be made available to those being encouraged to report, but because most events are observed by professionals trained in clinical care rather than data analysis, first-hand reports will have inaccuracies related to a misunderstanding of definitions. Areas of concern, determined by passive surveillance by untrained reporters, will require review by personnel well versed in the agreed-upon definitions. Ongoing staff education will sharpen the accuracy of reports by front-line clinicians with time, and it should be borne in mind that the first, crucial step in surveillance is the willingness of a clinician to come forward to share that an adverse event has occurred at all. Given the bias toward underreporting of errors and adverse events, inaccurate data are far better than no data at all.

Developing Data Collection Methods and Tools

Surveillance can be performed in a variety of ways. Incident reporting systems are usually passive surveillance systems that rely on staff members to recognize, report, and record events. In some cases, reports may be stimulated by making it clear that the organization is interested in specific types of events as part of a focused quality improvement project. Nosocomial infection surveillance, on the other hand, is a form of active surveillance focused on specific outcomes. This type of surveillance is easier to conduct than surveillance of other adverse events and errors because of the existence of objective corroborating microbiologic data. Active surveillance of error has been conducted in a few studies of medication errors in which trained observers scored errors as they occurred in clinical settings; however, this approach has not been adopted beyond research settings.[22] Given the long tradition of incident reporting, coupled with the difficulties of active surveillance by trained observers, it is likely that broad-based passive surveillance that relies on front-line staff reporting will remain the norm, with more active surveillance undertaken only in areas of focus suggested by the passive reports or mandated by regulatory and accrediting agencies.

In addition to being active or passive, surveillance may be concurrent or retrospective. Occurrence screening is a form of retrospective surveillance, with quality staff reviewing charts of patients at risk for a particular type of event. Surveillance of nosocomial infections, on the other hand, is concurrent in most cases, with infection control personnel reviewing microbiologic data on a daily basis to detect infections as they are diagnosed. The timeliness of reporting for errors and adverse events is determined largely by policies, procedures, and tools. Events associated with serious patient harm or serious error (e.g., maternal death or wrong-site surgery) tend to be reported by telephone to quality and risk personnel, whereas more routine events, such as minor falls or medication errors, may take weeks or months to come to the attention of quality and risk staff due to delays in processing paper reporting forms. Computer-based event reporting systems avoid these delays, but their adoption is just beginning.

Although they rely upon others to identify and report events, risk managers must determine what elements should be included on an incident report to characterize or describe the epidemiology of events in their organizations. Descriptive data for most incident reports should include the information listed in Table 10.2. In addition, some authors and risk management programs have categorized errors and adverse events by various types to allow for aggregate reporting.[23-26] The

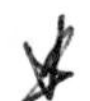

TABLE 10.2 Basic Data Elements for Event Reporting

Date and time of event
Patient identifier (i.e., name and/or record number if event involved a specific patient)
If patient involved, age and gender
Individual(s) involved in the event (if different from the one reporting)
Location where event occurred
Type of event (by category)
Harm to patient (by category)
Brief narrative description of circumstances that led to event
Suggestions for avoiding future occurrences of the event
Individual reporting the event (anonymous reporting optional)

major categories for adverse events utilized in the UHC Patient Safety Net reporting tool are listed in Table 10.3. It is also customary to categorize the extent of harm to the patient, using a system such as that developed by the National Coordinating Council for Medication Error and Prevention (NCC-MERP),[26] given in Table 10.4. The National Center for Patient Safety of the Veterans Administration has advocated a system in which severity is scored along with the observer's estimate of the likelihood of the recurrence of the event.[17] In addition to systems for categorizing types of events, there are emerging systems that seek to characterize medical error based on human factors analysis. These systems seek to provide a framework for understanding the underlying causes of error according to broad general types applicable to all complex organizations. Another suggested taxonomy for the underlying causes of error is the Einthoven classification system adapted for health care from error analysis in the nuclear power industry. Whatever classification system is used, one should be careful to distinguish the categories for actual events (the "what") from categories for factors that contributed to those events (the "why").

TABLE 10.3 Categories for Description of Errors and Events

Medication error
Adverse drug reaction
Fall
Equipment problem
Error related to procedure, treatment, or test
Complication related to procedure, treatment, or test
Transfusion event
Skin integrity problem
Behavioral problem (e.g., assault, elopement, etc.)
Other patient events
Visitor events
Staff events
Unsafe conditions with potential for harm

TABLE 10.4 Harm Scoring System for the National Coordinating Council for Medication Error Reporting and Prevention

No Error	
Category A:	Circumstances or events that have the capacity to cause error.
Error, No Harm	
Category B:	An error occurred but the error did not reach the patient. (An "error of omission" does reach the patient.)
Category C:	An error occurred that reached the patient, but did not cause patient harm.
Category D:	An error occurred that reached the patient and required monitoring to confirm that it resulted in no harm to the patient and/or required intervention to preclude harm.
Error, Harm	
Category E:	An error occurred that may have contributed to or resulted in temporary harm to the patient and required intervention.
Category F:	An error occurred that may have contributed to or resulted in temporary harm to the patient and required initial or prolonged hospitalization.
Category G:	An error occurred that may have contributed to or resulted in permanent patient harm.
Category H:	An error occurred that required intervention necessary to sustain life.
Error, Death	
Category I:	An error occurred that may have contributed to or resulted in the patient's death.

The goal of any classification system is to separate clearly distinct types of events, determine the frequency of each, and develop a common language for describing events that will allow comparisons between like organizations. Beyond providing meaningful rates, the data also must be informative enough for the risk manager to decide when to do additional analyses of an event through chart review or interviews. Because of this, incident reports also may include sections of free text in which the reporter gives contributing details regarding the event, an interpretation of why the event occurred, or suggestions for preventing recurrences. These additional details allows a triage function by managers, with some events meriting additional investigation through chart review or interview and others simply being aggregated in graphs or tables. This prioritization function has become critical in systems that have encouraged increased reporting through broad organizational initiatives to reduce blame and through implementation of electronic reporting tools.

Calculating Rates and Analyzing Data

As risk managers strive to improve event data for tracking, trending, benchmarking, and demonstrating risk reduction, they must employ rate-based measures. Although sentinel events should be counted one at a time, more common events should never be reported or counted using the number of events only. They should always be put into a rate in order to allow for trending or comparison between units or among organizations.

Incidence rates are the most commonly used and are very simple to apply to risk management data. The numerator of the rate is the number of times the specific event or error occurred in the observed population. The denominator includes the population at risk for the event of interest multiplied by the time the population was at risk (e.g., 50 patients at risk for 2 days each yields 100 patient-days of risk). A constant often is used to transform the result into a uniform quantity to allow for easier comparisons. Constants are usually multiples of 10 to ensure that the rate includes at least one integer (whole number) to the left of the decimal point. This avoids the need to manipulate awkward numbers: 4.3 errors per 1,000 patient-days is a preferable convention to 0.0043 medication errors per patient-day. When calculating incidence rates, it is important to remember the following:

1. Cases in the numerator must be taken from the population at risk, represented in the denominator.
2. Counts in the numerator and the denominator must be taken from the same period of observation.
3. Persons included in the denominator should be at risk for the event of interest in the numerator.[27]

The more one can narrow the population to those at actual risk, the more accurate the estimated frequency (i.e., incidence) and risk of the adverse event will be. For example, the use of the number of hospital admissions as a denominator to calculate medication error rates is crude and inaccurate. Patient-days would be an improvement as a denominator, since a patient with a 4-day admission would have on average twice the risk of exposure as one with a 2-day admission. Focusing measurement on a specific population receiving numerous medications (e.g., cardiology or oncology patients) will yield more meaningful data. The use of incidence rates allows for valid comparisons and identification of real differences in frequency, whereas the raw numerators alone may not. In the example in Table 10.5, focusing attention on the ward with the most falls (4 North) would divert attention from the ward with the highest rate of falls (6 East).

Rates also may be determined for the frequency with which a given procedure or trial results in the event of interest (because time is not specified, it is technically not an incidence rate). Examples would include 4 medication errors per 1,000 doses administered or 6 complications of anesthesia per 1,000 operative cases. Note that medication errors may

TABLE 10.5 Patient Falls by Inpatient Unit for April

Nursing Unit	Number of Falls	Patient-Days	Incidence
4 West	6	182	33 per 1,000 pt-days
4 North	12	720	16 per 1,000 pt-days
5 West	7	460	15 per 1,000 pt-days
5 North	2	900	2.2 per 1,000 pt-days
6 East	4	62	64 per 1,000 pt-days

be expressed either as an incidence rate (e.g., 4 errors per 100 patient-days) or as a rate per procedure (e.g., 4 errors per 1,000 doses).

Applying Risk Stratification and Subgroup Analysis

Calculating an overall incidence rate presumes that the rate remains constant over the time period of observation and across the population; however, that does not always reflect clinical realities. For example, adverse drug events are more common among neonates and among all patients in intensive care settings.[28,29] Heterogeneity of risk within the patient population or across the period of observation calls for risk stratification. Although this may sound like a complicated statistical approach, it is not. Stratification simply puts data into various categories to compare rates for one group or time period within the population to others.

For example, risk stratification may involve sorting the population at risk by a common variable, such as age, gender, or admitting diagnosis. More precise stratification can help to identify the groups within a population at greatest risk (e.g., patients on opiates, who are at greater risk for falls). The point of the analysis is to discern differences in rates for the subgroups in question that will further the understanding of the cause of the event being studied, in much the same way that Semmelweis advanced the understanding of handwashing by choosing to analyze rates among different types of caregivers. Whenever possible, one should use established clinical classification systems known to discriminate between populations at differential risk, such as the ASA score for anesthesia risk, or the American College of Surgery scoring system for risk of surgical site infection,[30] used to stratify risk of infection as shown in Table 10.6. The crude surgical site infection rate for this population is 6.8%, but because the population is heterogeneous in its risk, it is more meaningful to show the rate for each risk category. This would allow comparisons between institutions that cared for different proportions of patients in each category.

When stratification systems have not been established for the event being studied, selection of subpopulations for analysis represents a sort of hypothesis testing based on understanding of the event in question. For exam-

TABLE 10.6 Risk Stratification by Wound Class

Wound Class	Number of Infections	Number of Surgeries	Rate of Infection (%)
I. Clean	3	160	1.8
II. Clean contaminated	11	240	4.6
III. Contaminated	13	56	23.2
IV. Dirty	5	12	41.6

ple, one might analyze medication errors in medical patients boarding on surgical floors compared with those on medical floors to see if meaningful differences in rates emerged. Even a homogeneous population may be stratified if different periods during the time of observation are associated with different risks. For example, the time spent in intensive care versus a regular ward could be analyzed for differences in rates of medication error or pressure sore development in order to decide upon the design and scope of improvement initiatives.

Basic risk stratification as just described will improve risk analysis in most organizations, but as the measurement of patient safety data matures, more sophisticated methods will undoubtedly be applied. Statistical techniques to determine the statistical significance of one rate versus another can be applied (e.g., chi squared or Student's *t* tests). Logistic regression can be applied to a data set to analyze the circumstances where more than one stratification variable affects the rate. This would be used to calculate the relative contributions of variables such as age and opiate use on the rate of falls, for example. These more sophisticated strategies are more likely to be applied to clinical research studies seeking to understand the true causative factors for a given type of event in an environment where more active surveillance is performed.

In a stratified analysis, a single event is analyzed for different segments of the population at risk. This is different from an analysis of multiple endpoints, in which different types of events are analyzed for the same population. For example, analyzing the risk of stroke for patients with and without hypertension is an example of a stratified analysis. Analyzing the risk of stroke versus myocardial infarction in a group of patients with hypertension is an example of analysis of multiple endpoints. The distinction is an important one as we develop our understanding of distinct types of errors and adverse events. For example, rather than reporting a crude rate of medication administration errors, the errors may be sorted by the step in the medication administration process: prescribing, transcribing, dispensing, administration, and monitoring. These are not strata of risk for error, but rather different types of errors grouped under the broad heading of medication error. Reducing the overall medication error rate is impossible without understanding the relative frequency and causes of the relevant types. Even for a single type of error (administration), it is possible to perform a subtype analysis, as shown in Table 10.7.

Whether a given type of event deserves to be separated into a distinct category is more than a semantic exercise. The precision of a classification system, and the learning that can be gained by using it, is directly related to the extent to which it is free from redundancy (multiple names for the same type of event) and degeneracy (single name for different types of events).

Reporting Results and Using the Data for the Development of Risk Reduction Strategies

By applying epidemiologically sound techniques to define, collect, and analyze selected event data, the quality or risk manager should

TABLE 10.7 Errors While Administering Oral Medication, by Subgroup of Error

Type of Error	Number of Errors	Number of Doses	Prevalence
Wrong medication given	14	14,284	9.8 per 10,000 doses
Wrong dose	32	14,284	22.1 per 10,000 doses
Wrong patient	12	14,284	8.4 per 10,000 doses
Patient allergic	4	14,284	2.8 per 10,000 doses

realize a number of benefits. First, application of more rigorous measurement methods will allow a focus on the appropriate areas for risk reduction. It will also facilitate internal comparison across units and patient populations and demonstrate the impact of improvement initiatives. Valid benchmarking between organizations has come of age in areas such as nosocomial infection rates and adherence to national guidelines. This requires standardization of definitions and methods of measurement. Although this is not yet possible in the realm of medical error, it will become possible as national reporting systems and standards develop, as recommended by the IOM, and as the value of eliminating blame for error reporting becomes more widely appreciated. Even though meaningful cross-organizational comparisons are a thing of the future, organizations that begin a disciplined approach to measurement and data analysis will have a better understanding of their own risk epidemiology, allowing them to focus resources and evaluate the impact of interventions.

Reporting results of risk measurement and analysis is critical to the success of the patient safety program. Results should be presented to quality and safety oversight committees using visual methods such as tables, graphs, charts, and other displays. The type of display should be suitable to the data and the intended message. For example, a table is usually quite effective in demonstrating the characteristics of a population, a bar chart may demonstrate incidence within various strata of the population, and a line graph can show improvement over time. When presenting the same set of risk data over time to a committee or board, it is preferable to use the same type and format of charts and graphs each time. The group responsible for interpretation and risk management will be able to recognize significant changes more quickly. A suggested format for reports to the board or quality improvement committee is shown in Figure 10.1.

CONCERNS REGARDING AN EPIDEMIOLOGIC APPROACH TO PATIENT SAFETY

Numerous criticisms and caveats regarding a measurement-driven approach to patient safety management have been advanced, and most can be grouped into the following categories:

- Most events are underreported because of caregivers' fear, denial, or time constraints, so that conclusions based on rates cannot be meaningful.

FIGURE 10.1 Four sample reports from the UHC Patient Safety Net

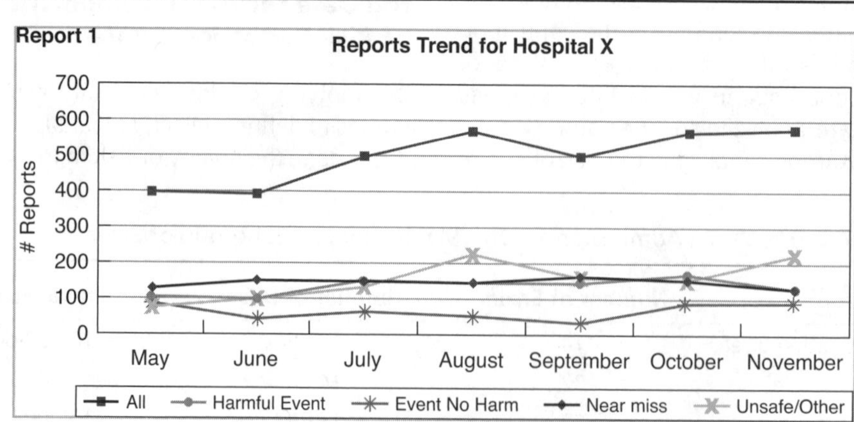

Source: University Health Consortium, 2003, Oak Brook, Illinois. Used with permission. *(continues)*

FIGURE 10.1 Four sample reports from the UHC Patient Safety Net (*Continued*)

Report 2 **Harm Score Distribution for Hospital X**

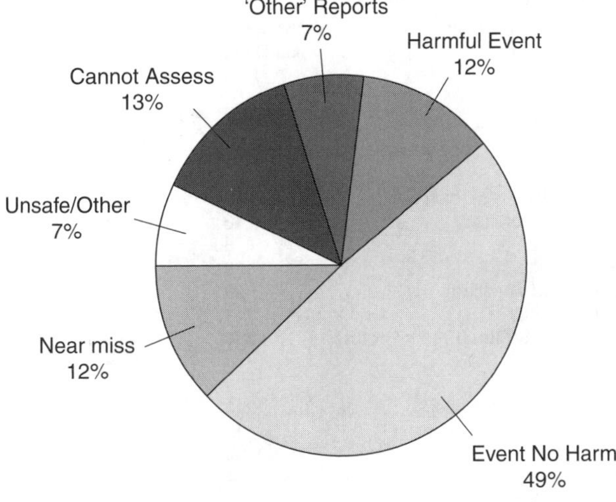

Report 3

Medication Error Subcategories		
	Count	**%**
Dose Omission	492	27%
Extra Dose	84	5%
Improper Dose/Overdosage	229	12%
Improper Dose/Underdosage	102	6%
Wrong Drug	160	9%
Wrong Dosage Form	44	2%
Wrong Duration	22	1%
Wrong Rate (IV)	57	3%
Wrong Route	22	1%
Wrong Strength/Concentration	61	3%
Wrong Technique	8	0%
Wrong Time	80	4%
Wrong Patient	66	4%
Monitoring Error	46	3%
Unauthorized Drug	13	1%
Narcotics Discrepancy	3	0%
Inadequate Pain Management	1	0%
Other Medication Error	222	12%
Blank	124	7%
Total	1,836	100%

(*continues*)

FIGURE 10.1 Four sample reports from the UHC Patient Safety Net (*Continued*)

Report 4

Contributing Factors Report for Hospital X

Organization Name: Hospital X
Time period: Jan-Dec 2002

		Manager Score	Pharmacist Score	Quality/Risk Score	Unique Reports with Factor
Team Factors					
	Communication problems	218	253	101	496
	Change of service	10	10	4	22
	Cross-coverage	8	14	5	26
	Shift change	28	79	19	113
	Unplanned workload	93	55	10	157
	Holiday	1	4	0	5
	Subtotal Team Factors	**358**	**415**	**139**	**819**
Work Environment					
	Distractions/Interruptions	213	173	46	414
	Limited access to patient info	17	7	4	27
	Poor lighting	4	2	4	8
	High noise level	64	3	2	69
	Equip malfunction				0
	Equip availability				0
	Subtotal Work Environment	**298**	**185**	**56**	**518**
Task Factors					
	Training issue	126	110	60	263
	Emergency	38	1	7	46
	Inexperienced staff	69	94	18	170
	Inadequate resident supervision	14	10	4	26
	Cardiac/respiratory arrest	4	0	4	6
	Order entry system problem				0
	Subtotal Task Factors	**251**	**215**	**93**	**511**
Staff Factors					
	Float staff	16	13	1	30
	Agency, temp or traveler	49	22	8	74
	Staff scheduling				0
	System for covering patient care	43	28	15	79
	Insufficient staffing	15	11	9	34
	Subtotal Staff Factors	**123**	**74**	**33**	**217**
Patient Characteristics					
	Patient compliance/adherence		3		3
	Patient understanding		1		1
	Language barrier				0
	Family member cooperation		8		8
	Subtotal Patient Characteristics	**0**	**12**	**0**	**12**
Organizational/Management					
	No 24hr pharmacy	6	1	0	7
	Bed availability				0
	Boarder pt/Different service	5	2	2	9
	Observation patient				0
	Policies/Procedures lacking	25	38	7	68
	Policies/Procedures unclear				0
	Subtotal Org/Mgmt	**36**	**41**	**9**	**84**

- Systems that rely on voluntary passive reporting by caregivers do not conform to standard definitions either of the events or the potential populations at risk, leading to misclassifications that invalidate the potential data set.
- The simple enumeration and aggregation of events fail to capture the richness of narrative detail from those involved in the process, detail that is essential to our learning about the events.

Each of these issues has been encountered in other disease surveillance systems, and there are lessons to be learned for the patient safety movement.

The bias of underreporting and underdetection has plagued the surveillance of newly recognized or emerging diseases for decades. In some instances, breakthroughs depended on technologic advances such as specialized culture media (e.g., legionnaire's disease) or specialized diagnostic techniques (e.g., hepatitis B). In other instances, when relying on reports from caregivers themselves, some underreporting continues to be a problem. The reluctance of operating surgeons to report delayed surgical wound infections may lead to underestimates of true wound infection rates, but it does not invalidate tracking established trends. Fear and shame are other potential causes of underreporting, which have affected the reporting of cases of AIDS or, in another era, of cancer. When biases remain constant over time, however, meaningful conclusions may still be drawn from imperfect data—conclusions that allow decision making in the allocation of resources to address specific problems.

When events occur to alter biases, dramatic changes in incidence may be seen, as in the implementation of anonymous reporting systems for AIDS or in the more scientific view of cancer that emerged in the 1960s. In the realm of patient safety, the rate at which reports are offered will depend greatly on how protected workers feel from repercussions for honest mistakes, the ease of the process of reporting, and the perceived role of reporting in making positive changes in the system of care. It has been observed that management initiatives to foster a blame-free approach to event reporting, sometimes coupled with novel electronic reporting tools, may lead to dramatic increases in reported events.[31,32] Efforts to improve the ease of reporting in a system of surveillance typically lead to a temporary inflection of the incidence rate, followed by a new trend line more accurate than the previous one. The lessons from other disease surveillance systems are that the growing pains associated with the attempts to bring systematic measurement to a new or newly appreciated disease or condition should not lead away from measurement; rather, patience and persistence are what reap ultimate rewards. Based on the lessons from these other surveillance systems, scientists and managers in the field of safety should remain open about the potential usefulness of trended rate data in advancing our learning.

An additional reservation regarding the epidemiologic approach to patient safety concerns the inaccuracy of events reported by front-line clinicians. The need for precision in interpreting definitions of nosocomial infections has given rise to the role of the modern infection control practitioner. Is a similar level of precision needed in patient safety? Clearly, many slips and lapses in everyday practice do not require specialized training to recognize or report. Thus, reports on falls, equipment failures, and most medication errors are more likely than not to be accurate with regard to the fact that an event has occurred. Furthermore, in the case of reporting near misses, it would be difficult to design a useful system for collecting data on events that do not require documentation in the medical record without relying on the willing and enthusiastic participation of those actually doing the work. Because of all of these reasons, improving accuracy in event reporting for patient safety will more likely require broad-based educational efforts than the establishment of a new class of professionals.

Although the risk or quality manager usually can place trust in the accurate reporting of the objective details of an event or near miss, interpretations of why it happened need to be approached with the skepticism of a skilled investigator. The input from those involved in the event is considered crucial, but it also should be borne in mind that causal theories abound during the initial recognition of breaches of safe care. A disciplined approach to the collection of data on putative causal or contributing factors will help the investigator avoid jumping to easy conclusions regarding root causes. The effective investigator will use aggregate reports of common events to help focus attention on those areas needing more intensive epidemiologic study, as detailed earlier in this chapter.

The last objection to epidemiologic approaches to patient safety is the fear that narrative detail will be lost, preventing investigators from thinking "outside the box" of a rigid classification system. Utilizing epidemiologic methods to trend adverse events and identify areas of high risk does not mean that one should abandon the tested method of detailed narrative and root cause investigation for selected cases. The latter approach has its greatest usefulness in events where one is inclined to ask "How could this happen?" Examples would include hundredfold overdoses, surgery on a wrong body part, or switching of one newborn for another. In each of these cases, the event occurs in spite of policies and procedures designed to prevent it. On the other hand, epidemiologic data analysis is a preferred approach for events that are subtler, frequent, and often accepted as part of the normal events in the care of patients, such as missed medication doses, minor falls, or delayed test results. While a single instance of the latter type of event may be considered to be within the bounds of acceptable practice, only an aggregate analysis demonstrating a high rate of event occurrence would suggest the need for more intensive scrutiny. In addition, a high rate or a rate at variance from an accepted standard may not be perceived or acknowledged by clinicians until careful analysis is performed. The iterative application of measurement and feedback serves to heighten awareness of the problem and strengthen the resolve to improve. This approach has also proved its value in the reduction of rates of nosocomial infection and surgical complications. In short, epidemiologic approaches and intensive reviews of individual cases should be seen as complementary, not antagonistic.

SUMMARY AND CONCLUSIONS

Major advances have been achieved in patient safety through attention to analysis of human factors and reduction of cultural barriers to reporting of events. As we succeed in learning more about the numerous everyday events that threaten patient safety, traditional methods for selecting certain cases for review (and ignoring the rest) will limit an organization's ability to achieve its goals for building safer systems of care.

Epidemiologic methods show promise in helping risk and quality managers to deal with the growing number of event reports by tracking rates and identifying groups at greater risks for events. The approach can add understanding to underlying causes of the events and allows for selection of those problems requiring focused review and intensive investigation. The bias inherent in passive reporting of errors and adverse events will make these initial determinations crude at best and will make comparisons between organizations uninformative. However, the history of disease surveillance provides us with several examples of the usefulness of aggregating and analyzing data on events that are only partially captured or incompletely understood. As the value of reporting becomes more widely appreciated and as systems for classifying events become standardized, comparing rates regionally and nationally will allow identification of innovative strategies that have successfully improved patient safety. Systematic measurement and epidemiologic analysis of events will then become the foundation of efforts to monitor trends, understand causes, and demonstrate improvements in patient safety.

References

1. Brennan, T. A., Leape, L. L., Laird, N. M. et al. Incidence of Adverse Events and Negligence in Hospitalized. *New Engl J Medicine* 1991;324:370–376.
2. Thomas, E. J., Studdert, D. M., Newhouse, J. P. et al. Costs of Medical Injuries in Utah and Colorado. *Inquiry* 1999;36:255–264.
3. Institute of Medicine. *To Err Is Human*. National Academy Press. 2000.
4. Runcinman, W. B. Qualitative versus quantitative research—balancing cost, yield and feasibility. *Anaesthesia and Intensive Care* 1993;21:502–505.
5. Kaplan, H., and Barach, P. Incident reporting: science or protoscience? Ten years later. *Quality and Safety in Health Care* 2002;11:144–145.
6. Barach, P., and Small, S. D. Reporting and preventing medical mishaps: lessons from non-medical near miss reporting systems. *British Medical J* 2000;320:759–763.
7. LaForce, F. M. The control of infections in hospitals: 1750–1950. In Wenzel, R. P., *Prevention and Control of Nosocomial Infections*. Baltimore: Williams and Wilkins, 1997, pp 3–18.
8. Antonow, J. A., Smith, A. B., and Silver, M. P. Medication error reporting: a survey of nursing staff. *J Nursing Care Quality* 2000:15:42–48.
9. Brewer, T., and Coldis, G. A. Postmarketing surveillance and adverse drug reactions: current perspectives and future needs. *JAMA* 1999;281:824–829.
10. Kivlahan, C., Sangster, W., Nelson, K. et al. Developing a comprehensive electronic adverse event reporting system in an academic medical center. *Joint Commission J Qual. Improvement* 2002;28:583–594.
11. MedMarx by US Pharmacopeia. www.medmarx.com.
12. Marx, D. The just culture. Published at www.mers-tm.net.
13. Adverse Event Reporting System. www.doctor quality.com.
14. University HealthSystem Consortium. UHC Patient Safety Net. www.uhc.edu.
15. The Quality Letter. November 2001, pp. 10–11.
16. Donna Sollenberger, CEO, University of Wisconsin Health System, personal communication.
17. Bagian, J. P., Lee, C., Gosbee, J. et al. Developing and deploying a patient safety program in a large health care delivery system. *Joint Commission J Qual. Improvement* 2001;27:522–532.
18. Buehler, J. W. Surveillance. In R. P. Wenzel, *Prevention and Control of Nosocomial Infections*. Baltimore: Williams and Wilkins, 1997, pp. 435–458.
19. Feinstein, A. R. *Clinical Epidemiology*. Philadelphia: Saunders 1985, pp. 581–587.
20. Fraser, D. W., Tsai, T., Orenstein, W. et al. Legionnaire's Disease: description of an epidemic of pneumonia. *New Engl J Medicine* 1977;297:89–97.
21. Centers for Disease Control and Prevention. Kaposi's sarcoma and *Pneumocystis* pneumonia among homosexual men—New York City and California. *Morbidity and Mortality Weekly Report* 1982;30:305–308.
22. Barker, K. N., Flynn, E. A., Pepper, G. A. et al. Medication error observed in 36 health care facilities. *Archives Int Med* 2002;162:1897–1903.
23. Frey, B., Kehrer, B., Losa, M. et al. Comprehensive critical incident monitoring in a neonatal-pediatric intensive care unit: experience with the system approach. *Intensive Care Med* 1999;26:69–74.
24. Dovey, S. M., Meyers, D. S., Phillips, R. L. et al. A preliminary taxonomy of medical errors in family practice. *Quality and Safety in Health Care* 2002;11:233–238.
25. Lesar, T. S., Briceland, L., and Stein, D. S. Factors related to errors in medication prescribing. *JAMA* 1997;277:312–317.
26. National Coordinating Council for Medication Error Reporting and Prevention. www.nccmerp.org.
27. Checko, P. J. Use of statistics for epidemiology. In R. Olmsted, *Infection control and applied epidemiology: principles and practice*. St. Louis, MO: Mosby-Year Book, Inc. 1996, pp. 11-1–11-5.
28. Kaushal, R., Bates, D. W., Landrigan, C. et al. Medication errors and adverse drug events in pediatric inpatients. *JAMA* 2001;285:2114–2120.
29. Cullen, D. J., Sweitzer, B. J., Bates, D. W. et al. Preventable adverse drug events in hospital-

ized patients: a comparative study of intensive care and general care units. *Critical Care Medicine* 1997;25:1289–1297.

30. Kluytmans, J. Surgical infections including burns. In R. P. Wenzel, *Prevention and Control of Nosocomial Infections*. Baltimore: Williams and Wilkins, 1997, pp. 841–865.
31. Davidoff, F. Shame: the elephant in the room. *Quality and Safety in Health Care* 2002;11:2–3.
32. Lawton, R., and Packer, D. Barriers to incident reporting in a healthcare system. *Quality and Safety in Health Care* 2002;11:15–18.

11

Patient Safety is an Organizational Systems Issue: Lessons From a Variety of Industries

Karlene H. Roberts, PhD, Kuo Yu, and Daved van Stralen, MD

The 1999 Institute of Medicine publication of *To Err Is Human: Building a Safer Health System* directed national attention to the issue of patient safety. Although its content is laudable in nailing the culprit behind the accident scene as being the organization or the system of organizations that together provide health care, its title is misleading. For years accident investigations and industrial psychological and human factors research on worker safety identified the worker/operator as the person behind the industrial accident. This perspective results in name-and-blame, then train-or-fire, cultures in industries concerned with safety.

For example, until quite recently investigations of U.S. Navy aviation accidents didn't look beyond the skin of the airplane for perpetrators. Once mechanical failure was ruled out, the investigation went on to look for operator failure, while failing to recognize that even when operators do fail, there is usually an organizational or systemic reason for failure. One might, for example, observe that the pilot was poorly trained. Is that the pilot's fault? Amount and kind of training are usually dictated by organizational policy. One might ask about the role of the commanding officer in the failure. Did he or she have a need to push his or her squadron beyond its capacity? Was the commanding officer under orders to deliver firepower to inaccessible places? How much pressure was brought to bear on him or her by his or her superior officers? One might also ask about the culture of the organization or system. Had the organization built a John Wayne–type individualistic macho culture when teamwork was required?

Over the last few decades, there has been a major shift in our social conception of the function of medical care.[1] Medicine has shifted from a disease-oriented to a health-oriented enterprise. That is, outcomes that are indicative of healthcare quality and safety have begun to include not only mortality and morbidity, but also the quality of life associated with illness and treatment. Physical functioning (e.g., pain, energy levels, sleep quality), cognitive functioning (e.g., memory, concentration), and emotional well-being (e.g., affective responses, suffering, anxiety, vitality) have all become part of the assessment of health-related quality of life.

This patient-centered ethic underscores the provider's obligation to inform the patient of potential adverse outcomes and solicit and take seriously the patient's self-report regarding unacceptable risks. In addition, such an ethic requires providers to be responsive to the patient's subjective experiences of the downside of care. Patient-centered care reminds us that healthcare excellence and safety not only concerns itself with technical excellence but also with the patient's experience of care. Patient-centered care encourages patients to communicate valuable information to their caretakers as well as mandates caretakers to take proactive approaches to elicit nuanced but valuable information that can improve patient safety. Patient-centered care parallels the shift from regarding patient safety as a human factors issue to a systems and organizational issue because, although it might take a single doctor to treat a disease, it takes a team of doctors, nurses, and other healthcare providers and administrators as well as an organization of safety culture and reliable operations to treat a person.

FOUNDATIONS OF RESEARCH THAT CAN INFORM SAFETY ISSUES

If the traditional industrial and human factors research on safety is largely unhelpful to us in teasing out the etiologies of medical error, is there any work that is more helpful? Engineers and statisticians, human factors researchers, psychologists, and sociologists have made forays into research issues concerned with reliability enhancement or risk reduction. The engineering perspective has, not surprisingly, centered on physical aspects of systems. Human factors researchers and psychologists are largely interested in individuals and groups, and sociologists take a more macro view of the social context in which people work. Here we will draw on both the psychological and sociological approaches.

Sociologists preceded psychologists in developing interests in risk mitigation through a side door, the study of catastrophe. At first these researchers were only interested in disaster aftermath, how the social fabric of a community regenerates itself after destruction.[2,3] In addition, what were originally viewed as individual-level constructs, such as panic, soon came to be seen more as socially driven.[4] In 1978 Barry Turner noted that until that time the only interest in disasters was in responses to them. He provided the first social psychological approach to accidents, looking at the socially driven components of causes.

Human factors and social psychological threads of activity regarding reduction of error merged in the aviation industry. The introduction of reliable jet transports in the airline industry and in the military in the 1950s brought with it a dramatic reduction in aircraft accidents. It became apparent that the remaining accident contributors had more to do with people than with technology. As in many other industries (for example, medicine and the commercial marine industry) it was often noted that 70% to 80% of the problems involved operator error.

Much of the social psychological research on crew resource management came from Robert Helmreich's laboratory at the University of Texas. One of his contributions is the Cockpit Management Attitudes Questionnaire (CMAQ), a 25-item Likert scale assessment of attitudes regarding crew coordination, flight deck management, and personal capabilities under conditions of fatigue and stress.[5] Helmreich adapted this questionnaire for operating room use in the medical industry. Dr. David Gaba at Stanford and the Veteran's Administration, Palo Alto, borrowed heavily from it in the development of his Survey of Patient Safety Cultures in Healthcare Organizations.[6] This is an example of applying research results obtained in one industry to the needs of another.

In 1984, Charles Perrow's seminal book *Normal Accidents: Living with High-Risk Technologies* was published (it was recently republished). Based on his experience as one of the few social scientists asked to contribute to the Three Mile Island investigation, Perrow analyzed a large number of industrial accidents. He concluded that some technologies, like commercial nuclear power plants and modern militaries, are so dangerous they should be shut down altogether because their technologies are both tightly coupled (one event follows immediately after another without mediation) and complexly coupled (events are so complexly linked that their causal relations cannot be deciphered).

HIGH-RELIABILITY ORGANIZATIONS RESEARCH

Simultaneously with the publication of Perrow's book, a group of researchers came together at the University of California, Berkeley. They were interested in the ways organizations achieve risk reduction and highly reliable operations in spite of the great odds against it as hypothesized by Charles Perrow. They focused their interests on what they called high-reliability organizations (HROs). Their contention was that while some technologies are indeed worrisome enough that in an ideal world they shouldn't exist, calling for their overthrow is unrealistic. Thus, we need to do the best we can to insure nearly error-free operation of these technologies. They also demonstrated that relatively low-technology organizations, such as banks, can cause similar degrees of devastation.[7]

Although the original researchers have dispersed, their concerns with risk mitigation were picked up by organizational scholars at other universities. These researchers have studied a diverse group of organizations, including those that should have avoided catastrophe and didn't and those that did. They work in parallel with people coming from the other traditions previously discussed. Thus, today there is considerable interest in risk mitigation that can be and is translated into patient safety issues in the medical industry. Although some of the HRO research is directly cited in *To Err Is Human*, a number of additional findings from it are alluded to without direct citation because of the nature of the testimony behind these kinds of reports.

Findings from HRO Research

Here we summarize some major findings from HRO research. We then discuss reliability-enhancing features that were missing in a failed organization and illustrate how a finely tuned HRO operated to avoid catastrophe. We then discuss an application of HRO findings in a healthcare setting and conclude with suggestions about the kind of research on reliability enhancement and patient safety that should be done in medical settings. HRO findings are divided into two sets: those having to do with major organizational processes, and those more appropriate to a category we call command and control. Some of these processes are more tractable than others. Managers may want to address the easy issues first.

Seven of the HRO research findings are organizational processes. First, HROs are flexibly *structured* so they can move rapidly from bureaucratic tight coupling to more flexible, malleable forms as conditions change. Thus, when an aircraft carrier is in port with little to do, its command can afford to be top-down bureaucratic. But when it is in air operations at sea, its command has to be far more flexible to meet the changing conditions or "fog of war."[8,9] Second, HROs must emphasize *reliability* over efficiency. In fact, reliability rivals productivity as the bottom line.[10] The *cultures* of HROs are heavily imbued with reliability and safety "musts."

Rewards are appropriately used in HROs.[7] They reward the behavior that is desired and avoid rewarding behavior A while hoping for behavior B.[11] HROs are characterized by the perception that *risk exists* and that strategies also exist to deal appropriately with it. Both appropriate attention and strategies must be in place.[7] In HROs, individuals must engage in valid and reliable *sense making*.[12] That is, they must come to the correct conclusions about the meaning of things that are happening around them.[13] Finally, the different senses or meanings people draw from their situation must be meaningfully worked together and integrated across the organization through the *heedfulness* of individual players. Managers try to maximize this integration when they talk about "making sure we're all on the same page." One doesn't have to see the totality of the situation (unless one is at the top of the organization), but should recognize how one's role fits into the roles of the rest of the people in the organization.[14,15] People do not, for example, attend just to the physiology of the situation, but rather to the integration of physiology with the teamwork to deal with it, the state of the patient's family, and so forth.

Although the next five findings are also concerned with organizational processes, we highlight them here as command-and-control issues. HROs are characterized by *migrating decision making*.[9,16] That is, decisions migrate to the part of the organization in which the expertise exists to make them. The highest-ranking person is not always the appropriate person to make a decision. Migrating decision making would be impossible in rigid organizational structures. In addition, in HROs the top management always has *the big picture*, or an overall sense of what is going on. HROs are characterized by *redundancy*. There needs to be sufficient slack so if one party doesn't catch a mistake, another will. In addition, there must be *formal rules and procedures* that are spelled out to and followed by all organizational participants. Finally, HROs are characterized by enormous amounts of *training*.

Departure from Safety

During the 1970s and early 1980s the two major shipping groups in the Baltic Sea began to lower prices, cut costs, and transform their ferries into floating hotels with casinos, night clubs, and shopping malls. Transforming ferries into palaces of entertainment doesn't remind passengers and crewmembers of the potential risks involved in sea travel. The crews were structured to focus on achieving high efficiency and economies of scale through standardization, specialization, and routinized decentralization.

Early one spring evening in 1994, the passenger ferry *Estonia* left its home port and steamed toward its next port, Stockholm, into the teeth of a Baltic Sea storm. Noises from the front of the ship were ignored. The captain headed the ship directly into the waves (3 to 4 meters high) and into an increasingly strong wind. The ship left port at 1915 hours and sailed normally until about 0100 hours. On the bridge the master noted that she was rolling and that they were 1 hour behind schedule despite having all engines running. Shortly before 0100, during his scheduled rounds on the car deck, the seaman on watch heard a metallic bang. The master attempted to find the sound, but none of the orders given or actions taken by him or the crew was out of the ordinary.

Further observations of the noise were made at about 0105 by passengers and off-duty crewmembers. When a seaman reported water on the deck, it was news to the bridge. At 0115 the third engineer saw an enormous inflow on his monitor. He didn't report this to the bridge because he assumed the bridge had the same picture. And he didn't slow the ship down because he was waiting for orders from the bridge. In fact, the engines automatically shut down, and he tried to restart them. The officers on the bridge probably didn't look at the monitor.

The visor (top half of the double doors) separated from the bow at about 0115. As a result, the ramp was pulled fully open, allowing water to rush in. The distress message traffic from *Estonia* began at 0122 hours; the last one was at 01:29:27. The ship disappeared from the radar screens of other ships in the area at about 0150 hours.

The *Estonia* was one of a class of ferries with very large bows, and experience with similar designs was limited. The crew work schedule was 2 weeks on and 2 weeks off. This crew was in the 13th day of a 14-day cycle. It was relatively inexperienced. That night, except for the short time the captain was on the bridge and during the time the storm was increasing, the ship's responsibility was in the hands of the first through the fourth mates. The shift from 0100 to 0600 was in the hands of the second and fourth mates, with respectively 2.5 and 1.5 years of experience. These men were not trained to deal with heavy weather. The life boat orders were not given until 5 minutes after the list developed, and the time available for evacuation was between 10 and 20 minutes.

In this case the organizational structural problem is clear. Although standardization, specialization, and routinization are good strategies for operating organizations faced with benign and unchanging circumstances, they are very poor strategies if the organizations must face new, unexpected contingencies. This is well illustrated by the fact that the engineer failed to report the water on the deck to the bridge and failed to turn the engines off. Under routinization, it was appropriate for him to think the captain would tell him what to do. The industry's decision to change their ships into travel playgrounds was a system characteristic within which ships had to operate with no increased attention to structural safety enhancements.

The emphasis on efficiency over reliability is also clear. The new structure, with its focus on such things as shopping malls, directed attention away from reliability as a primary goal. It also changed the culture from one of seagoing wariness to one of having fun. That the reward system was out of kilter is clear. The master was concerned about schedules and therefore pushed his ship into rough seas. There was no reward system for other crewmembers to report activities that could put the ship in harm's way. It is unclear from evidence available to us whether the ship saw itself as experiencing risky situations. What is clear is that if the crew did so, they did nothing about it.

Sense making was not done in an appropriate way. Vigilance was entirely lacking on the bridge. It is probable that a bridge monitor showed exactly what was happening, but the crew failed to see it. The master had exactly the wrong picture of what was transpiring. Even when evidence of danger was clearly on the bridge's monitors, he and his crew failed to perceive it. The situation with the engineer shows even more clearly the absence of appropriate sense making. He *had pictures* of water. Despite that information, he tried to override an automatic engine shutdown. In every case, representation of the situation was incorrect. The decisions made on the bridge appear to have been rational responses to a situation that didn't exist. Without appropriate sense making, it was impossible to engage in heedful interaction.

Migrating decision making failed to occur, as in the case of the engineer failing to make a decision he was supposedly qualified to make, and waiting for the captain to give him orders. Clearly, the captain failed to have the big picture. Redundancy didn't exist, or someone would have said "why are we doing this?" Although we have no evidence of this, it appears that formal rules of safety didn't exist, weren't practiced, or weren't considered important. The case includes several references to lack of experience or training.

A Safe Landing

Following is an incident that could have turned into a disaster. In fact, it started as a disaster. One night in the summer of 1999, an F/A 18 Hornet (fighter/attack aircraft) was first in the launch cycle aboard the U.S.S. *Constellation*, awaiting launch from catapult 1. Upon launch the aircraft ingested rubber catapult covers that someone failed to remove from the catapult. The pilot (call sign "Oyster") could only manage his plane in full afterburner and at low altitude. He needed to land by trapping with the hook of the aircraft one of the wires at the rear end of the ship, preferably number 3. A number of people are involved in the story, including the landing signal officer, called Paddles. (Paddles he was in World War II movies, and Paddles he is today.) During flight operations the carrier is always followed by an escort (picket) ship and flies its helicopter as safety precautions. Here's the incident, as told by the pilot:

> There I was. Manned up in the hot seat for the 2030 launch about 500 miles north of Hawaii (insert visions of "The Shore Bird" and many mai tais here). I was positioned to be first off of cat one (insert foreboding music here) in the launch cycle. As the cat fires, I stage the blowers and am along for the ride. Just prior to the end of the stroke there's a huge flash and a simultaneous boom! and my world is in turmoil. My little pink body is doing 145 knots or so and is 100 feet above the Black Pacific. And there it stays—except for the knot package, which decreases to 140 knots. The throttles aren't going any farther forward despite my Schwarzzeneggerian efforts to make them do so.
>
> From out of the ether I hear a voice say one word: "Jettison." Roger that! A nanosecond later my two drop tanks are Black Pacific bound. The airplane leapt up a bit but not enough. I'm now about a mile in front of the boat at 160 feet and fluctuating from 135 to 140 knots. The next comment that comes out of the ether is another one worder: "Eject!" I'm still flying so I respond, "Not yet, I've still got it." Finally, at 4 miles from the ship I take a peek at my engine instruments and notice my left engine doesn't match the right (funny how quick glimpses at instruments get burned into your brain). About now I get another "Eject!" call. "Nope, still flying." At 5½ miles I asked the tower to please get the helo headed my way as I truly thought I was going to be shelling out. At some point I thought it would probably be a good idea to start dumping some gas. At 7 miles I eventually started a (very slight) climb. A little breathing room.
>
> Air Traffic Control chimes in with a downwind heading and I'm like: "Ooh. Good idea and throw down my hook." Eventually I get headed downwind at 900 feet and ask for a squadron representative on the radio. While waiting I shut down the left engine. In short order I hear his voice. I tell him the following: "OK, my gear's up, my left motor's off and I'm only able to stay level with minimum blower." At ten miles or so I'm down to 5000 pounds of gas and start a turn back toward the ship. Don't intend to land but don't want to get too far away. Of course as soon as I start in an angle of bank I start dropping like a stone so I end up doing a five mile circle around the ship. Air Traffic Control is reading me the single engine rate of climb numbers based on temperature, etc. It doesn't take us long to figure out that things aren't adding up. One of the things I learned in the training group was that the Hornet is a perfectly good single engine aircraft. It flies great on one motor. So why do I need blower to stay level!?
>
> By this time I'm talking to air traffic control, the Deputy Air Group Commander (who's on the flight deck) and the Air Group Commander (who's on the bridge with the Captain). We decide that the thing to do is climb to three thousand feet to see if I'm going to have any excess power and will be able to shoot an approach. I get headed downwind, go full burner on my remaining motor and eventually make it to 2000 feet before leveling out. Start a turn back toward

the ship and when I get pointed in the right direction I throw the gear down and pull the throttle out of AB. Remember that flash/boom! that started this little tale? Repeat it here.

I jam it back into after burner and after three or four huge compressor stalls and accompanying deceleration the right motor comes back. I'm thinking my blood pressure was probably up there about now and for the first time I notice that my mouth feels like a San Joaquin summer. (That would be hot and dusty.)

This next part is great. You know those stories about guys who deadstick crippled airplanes away from orphanages and puppy stores and stuff and get all this great media attention? Well, at this point I'm looking at the picket ship at my left at about two miles and I say on departure freq to no one in particular, "You need to have the picket ship hang a left right now. I think I'm gonna be outta here in a second." I said it very calmly but with meaning. Paddles said the picket immediately started pitching out of the fight. Ha! I scored major points with the heavies afterwards for this. Anyway, it's funny how your mind works in these situations.

OK, so I get it back level and pass a couple miles up the starboard side of the ship. I'm still in min blower and my (fuel) state is now about 2500 pounds. Hmmm. I hadn't really thought about running out of gas. I pull it out of blower again and sure enough . . . flash, BOOM! I'm thinking that I'm gonna end up punching out.

Eventually discover that even the tiniest throttle movements cause the flash/boom thing to happen so I'm trying to be as smooth as I can. I'm downwind a couple miles when the Air Group Commander comes up and says "Oyster, we're going to rig the barricade." Remember, he's up on the bridge watching me fly around and he's thinking I'm gonna run outta fuel too. By now I've told everyone who's listening that there is a better than average chance that I'm going to be ejecting—the helo bubbas, god bless 'em, have been following me around this entire time. I continue downwind and again, sounding calmer than I probably was, call Paddles. "Paddles, you up?" "Go ahead," he replied. "I probably know most of it but you wanna shoot me the barricade brief?" (He was awesome on the radio, just the kind of voice you'd want to hear in this situation.) He gives me the brief and at nine miles I say, "If I turn now will it be up when I get there? I don't want to have to go around again." "It's going up now Oyster, go ahead and turn." "Turning in, say final bearing." "063" replies the voice in air traffic control (another number I remember—go figure).

I intercept glideslope at about a mile and three quarters and pull power. Flash/boom. Add power out of fear. Going high. Pull power. Flash/boom. Add power out of fear. Going higher. (Flashback to LSO school. . . . "All right class, today's lecture will be on the single engine barricade approach. Remember, the one place you really, really don't want to be is high. Are there any questions? Yes, you can go play golf now.")

Another landing signal officer is backing up Paddles and as I start to set up a higher than desired sink rate he hits the abort light. Very timely too. No worries. I cleared the deck by at least ten feet. As I slowly climb out I say, again to no one in particular, "I can do this." I'm in blower still and the Air Group Commander says, "Turn downwind." Again, good idea. After I get turned around he says, "Oyster, this is gonna be your last look so turn in again as soon as you're comfortable."

I lose about 200 feet in the turn and like a total dumbshit I look out as I get on centerline and that night thing about feeling high gets me and I descend further to 400 feet. Flash/boom every several seconds all the way down. Last look at my gas was 600-and-some pounds at mile and a half. "Where am I on the glideslope?" I ask Paddles and hear a calm "Roger Ball." Now the ball's shooting up from the depths. I start flying it and before I get a chance to spot the deck, I hear "Cut, cut, cut!" I'm really glad I was a Paddles for so long because my mind said to me "Do what he says Oyster" and I pulled it back to idle. (My hook hit 11 Oyster paces from the ramp.) The rest is pretty tame. I hit the deck, skipped the one, the two and snagged the three wire [and] rolled into the barricade about a foot right of the centerline. Once stopped my vocal chords involuntarily yelled "Victory!" on the radio. (The 14 guys who were listening in air traffic control said it was pretty cool. After the fact I wish I had done the Austin Powers' "Yeah Baby!" thing.) The lights came up and off to my right there must have been a gazillion people. Paddles said that with my shutdown you could hear a huge cheer across the flight deck.

I open the canopy and start putting my stuff in my helmet bag. I climb down and people are gathering around patting me on the back when one of the boat's crusty yellow-shirt Chiefs interrupts and says, "Gentlemen, great job but fourteen of your good buddies are still up there and we need to get them aboard." Here I sit with my little pink body in a ready room chair on the same ship I did my first cruise in 10 years and 7 months ago. And I thought it was exciting back then. By the way, I had 380 pounds of fuel when I shut down. Again, remember this number as in ten years it will surely be *fumes man, fumes I tell you!**

Although militaries are hierarchically structured, notice how in this case the structure was sufficiently elastic to allow many parts of the ship to help Oyster: the captain and air group commander on the bridge, the deputy air group commander and Paddles on the flight deck, the squadron representative in the tower, and the air traffic controller in the air traffic control center on the third deck. If efficiency had ruled over reliability, many things might have occurred differently. Perhaps the order to eject would not have gone out as soon as it did or the drop tanks would have not have been dropped as early as they were. The culture of reliability is illustrated by the several "must do's" Oyster engaged in that clearly came from his training.

The rewards for Oyster were clearly in the right place. In the first place, it was assumed by his superiors on the ship that he knew what he was doing, particularly when he refused to eject. Second, he was rewarded for getting the picket ship out of harm's way. Everyone perceived that risk existed, and appropriate strategies were in place to handle the risk. Valid and reliable sense making was surely characteristic of Oyster, and information from air traffic control and the squadron representative helped him to make appropriate sense of his situation. He needed the heedfulness of

*This account has been widely discussed in the Navy, and is in the public domain. There is no known published source.

the air group commander, the deputy commander, Paddles, the squadron representative, and air traffic control, each of whom saw his own role in the situation and helped keep it knit together.

Migrating decision making was also apparent. Oyster, not his superiors, made the decision about what to do. When he landed, a lower-level chief (aviators are officers) ordered him from the deck. Although we don't know this from the case, it is likely the captain of the ship had the big picture. We have some evidence that the air group commander did. We certainly know that redundancy was at work when Oyster and the air group commander simultaneously thought about the plane's fuel state. Formal rules and procedures guided Oyster's activities and were clearly evident when Paddles gave Oyster the barricade brief. Training was evident throughout (Oyster had over 10 years' experience flying off ships), and he mentions it with regard to the characteristics of the Hornet and the class on barricade approaches. Hopefully, every evolution a ship does is a training evolution.

A BROADER STORY

A number of researchers have confirmed that these and other organizational processes are necessary for reliability enhancement, which broadly includes safety. The information was obtained through analyses of accidents as well as systematic research in HROs. Work was done in the commercial nuclear power industry,[17] the commercial airlines,[18,19] primary school education,[20] wildland fire authorities,[12] community fire authorities,[9] the U.S. Navy,[8,21] offshore oil and gas platforms,[22] offshore pipeline operations,[23] commercial shipping,[24] and other aspects of the commercial marine industry.[25]

A number of organizations have applied some of the findings of the work in a variety of different ways. It was used to develop training programs in community policing.[26] The U.S. Coast Guard used it as a basis for their comprehensive Prevention Through People program, the only management program the Coast Guard developed to reduce mishaps and errors. The Society for Worldwide Interbank Financial Telecommunications (SWIFT) used various aspects of the work to develop what it calls its Failure Is Not an Option program. SWIFT moves 97 % of the money that is moved worldwide and very successfully progressed through both the European move to the euro and Y2K.

Findings from this research are behind a recently conceived program for the U.S. Navy. After the fatal crashes of three F-14 aircraft in 1996, the Navy developed a Human Factors Quality Management Board to review its safety-related activities in carrier aviation. At the request of the board, the Navy developed what is now called the aviation Command Safety Assessment. This is a device to help aircraft squadron commanding officers assess the safety readiness of their squadrons in comparison with all squadrons in the database, squadrons of the same type, squadrons at sea or on land, and so forth. The program is on the Web at safetyclimatesurveys.org. To date it has been used by about a third of the naval aviation squadrons and some aviation maintenance squadrons.[6] The Marine Corps ground forces are beginning a special project to adapt the instrument to their specific needs. The commercial aviation community is showing considerable interest in this approach.

Some aspects of the approach, including specific items, were borrowed by David Gaba at the Palo Alto Veteran's Administration Hospital for use in the Patient Safety Center of Inquiry's development of a safety assessment for the Veteran's Administration.[6]

AN APPLICATION IN THE HEALTH INDUSTRY

Loma Linda University Children's Hospital (LLUCH) is the tertiary children's hospital for a geographic area more than three times the size of the state of Vermont. The population is 2.5 million people, with 500,000 younger than 15 years. The catchment area includes urban, rural, and wilderness areas, with a large number of desert and mountain communities. The LLUCH pediatric intensive care unit (PICU) has 25 beds with an average daily census of 21 patients, 9 on ventilators. One hundred and five registered nurses are assigned to the PICU, with 14 on duty at any one time. There are 20 respiratory care practitioners, with 4 working at any one time. Four residents rotate through the PICU for 1 month at a time, one from emergency medicine and three from pediatrics. Pollack, Cuerdon, and Getson report mortality rates of 7.8 ± 0.8% for PICUs with more than 18 beds.[27] The PICU at LLUCH had a 5.2% mortality rate in 1996. About half of the admissions come through LLUCH's pediatric critical care transport system, now one of the larger transport services in the country.[28]

In an environment that has numerous social and psychological hazards, particularly for the nurses, the PICU philosophy is to support the bedside caregiver with an organizational culture of safety that encourages learning from mistakes in collaborative teams. Teamwork and team formation are fostered. Shaming, naming, and blaming, particularly after a bad outcome, are not accepted. There are many ways to approach care in the PICU; no one method is touted above the rest. The center of care is the team and support for the team leader and bedside caregiver. During rounds the patient is presented to the group for discussion of the diagnosis, general treatment plan, potential problems that may develop, and the family's response to the situation. All participants have an opportunity to present their perceptions, and ideas and questions are solicited. As a general rule, the team doesn't move on until all caregivers feel comfortable with the plan. Doctors, pharmacists, respiratory care practitioners, nurses, and a clinical dietitian make rounds presentations.

The Loma Linda University PICU can be described in the context of the good organizational processes and command-and-control mechanisms identified in HROs. The HRO concepts adopted by Drs. Daved van Stralen and Ronald Perkin include risk awareness, process auditing, quality review, appropriate rewards, and command and control.

Risk awareness increased over the first several years, with the goal of identifying a child who is in a state of covert compensated physiologic dysfunction. Van Stralen and Perkin began a program of in-service lectures specific to the various disciplines (nursing, respiratory care, resident physicians). They also developed two regularly scheduled conferences, one directed to emergency medical service providers and the other directed to nurses in emergency departments and intensive care units. Today it is rare for a patient to unexpectedly deteriorate in the PICU.

Process auditing in the PICU includes systematic checks and formal audits to inspect for problems in the "process." For LLUCH, the process is providing critical care medicine in an environment of physiologic uncertainty and instability. The unit constantly entertains the thought that it has missed something. It encourages questioning and the presentation of data that support or refute the working hypothesis. Quality review is performed to ensure that the PICU has the lowest rate of potentially preventable mortalities and morbidities. Quality improvement reviews are made by formal standing committees of the institution. Referent levels for quality improvement are adopted from nationally accepted norms and the medical, respiratory care, and nursing literature.

Appropriate rewards are made to encourage participation in patient care. Through participation of all disciplines, the PICU seeks to reduce accidents and the level of stress on caregivers while improving morale. The team is composed of members who respond quite well to symbolic rewards. As members demonstrate knowledge, insight, and discretion in care of patients, they tend to play a larger role in tactical and strategic management. Their opinions are more frequently sought and incorporated into care plans.

Command and control plays a major part of care and has given the unit its greatest successes. In the PICU this concept includes decision migration, authority gradient, situational awareness, redundancy, rules and procedures, and training.

The PICU fosters decision migration to the best-qualified caregiver (recognizing the limits to caregiver decision making). At the interface with a patient emergency, the most qualified person to make or guide decisions is the bedside caregiver. Frequently, team members can't predict what will work in a specific situation. However, quick decisions can bring stability to a rapidly changing situation during crisis situations. The authority difference that can occur between the physician or surgeon and other team members can lead to tragedy; this is especially likely if authority differences inhibit low-status members from offering valuable information that disagrees with the judgments of high-status members. In the past few years, nursing staff has made use of a form for professional interactions. These forms follow up the chain of command from the nurse to administration. It then moves downward to the physician involved through his or her chain of command. This insulates the nurse from reprisal.

Situational awareness comes both with experience in the PICU and experience as a supervisor. Experienced staff almost always teaches new staff. This is of major importance because residents come to the unit with limited experience in critical care. Van Stralen and Perkin rely on experienced nurses and respiratory therapists to teach the residents. Redundancy ensures thoroughness in evaluating the patient and in choosing a therapy. Many of the signs they monitor are measured by two methods; furthermore, during resuscitations, several team members will monitor the same vital sign.

Rules and procedures have allowed respiratory therapists and nurses to influence medical care to a greater degree and with a quicker response to change. As a teaching institution and one that develops new therapies, the PICU has the goal of always considering itself in training. Consequently, its members watch each other's performance and give assistance through mutual teaching and learning.

CONCLUSIONS

While van Stralen and Perkins have demonstrated at Loma Linda the effective application of HRO research findings to reduce errors in the PICU, much research remains to be done. Researchers must view health care from a systems perspective as well as from the perspective of a single unit. Errors are made in units and errors are made across units. Policies and procedures developed in one unit influence errors that develop in adjacent or distant units.

As complexity theory suggests, systems that consist of independent actors whose interactions are governed by a system of recursively applied rules naturally generate stable structure.[29] Here, we suggest that some good HRO practices or potentially good "rules," once applied to organizational systems, might generate increasingly safer and stable structures because the output of one application of rules becomes the input for the next round. That is, positive feedback loops that result from the interactions of a large number of components eventually simplify structures and give clarity to operations that enhance safety, crowding out irregular or nonstandard microscopic behavior and structures.

Research into how healthcare systems structure themselves would help us develop concepts of adaptability and flexibility useful in the medical industry. Medical practitioners need to know the conditions under which complex, tightly tied medical units and systems must incorporate flexibility. We also need to examine closely how roles should be interrelated in and across healthcare units. The imbalance of power held by physicians is probably dysfunctional to the delivery of safe health care. Once we know what appears to be appropriate role inter-relationship, we need to address the issue of how training institutions should deal with this knowledge. We need also to develop ideas about training mechanisms to disseminate such research findings and encourage their application. Last, we need to observe empirically how intervention of any kind affects the interdependence of the system, as well as how interventions of several kinds can combine and integrate to create larger systematic changes. These are tough nuts to crack!

Although David Gaba has begun to develop a culture assessment along HRO lines for the Veteran's Administration, more work needs to be done on this issue. The concept development work is far from complete and needs to be carried on in medical settings. Although constructs such as command and control seem useful, these constructs have not been sufficiently fleshed out. Nor does the instrument derived from these constructs have adequate psychometric properties. We need a good way to assess culture in medical settings that clearly follows from theoretical development. The cultures of various continuous medical units need to be examined together to see how one influences the other. Training needs can be identified from cultural phenomena.

As we saw from our examples, reward systems are extremely important to the adequate management of HROs. However, appropriate rewards are often specific to their situations. We need to develop a taxonomy of appropriate rewards for medical systems. We suspect that current policies in many medical units foster the use of the wrong rewards, if for no other reason than the requirements of managed care.

One of the most difficult research issues will be the investigation of sense making within and across units. Understanding the cognitive functioning of a single individual is difficult. But the characteristics of HRO operations require the integration of cognitions across many individuals. Mapping this integration to develop a picture of the heedfulness of a unit is challenging. Mapping the integration of units constituting a system is even more challenging.

References

1. Sharp, V., and Faden, A. *Medical Harm: Historical, Conceptual, and Ethical Dimensions of Iatrogenic Illness* (New York: Cambridge University Press, 1998).
2. Quarentelli, E. L. ed., *What Is a Disaster?* (London: Routledge, 1998).
3. Turner, B. M. *Man Made Disasters* (London: Wykeham Press, 1978).
4. Quarentelli, E. L. "The Nature and Conditions of Panic," *American Journal of Sociology* 60 (1954):267–275.
5. Helmreich, R. L. et al., *Revised Versions of the Cockpit Management Attitudes Questionnaire (CMAQ) and CRM Seminar Evaluation Form*, NASA University of Texas Technical Report 88–3 (Austin, TX: University of Texas, 1991).
6. Singer, S. J., Gaba, D. M., Geppert, J. J., Sinaiko, J. D., Howard, S. K., and Park, K. C. (2003). "The culture of safety: Results of an organization-wide survey in 15 California hospitals." *Qual Saf Health Care* 12(2003):112–118.
7. Libuser, C. "Organizational Structure and Risk Mitigation," PhD diss., University of California, Los Angeles, 1994.
8. Roberts, K. H. "Some Characteristics of One Type of High Reliability Organization," *Organizational Science* 1 (1990):160–176.
9. Bigley, G. A., and Roberts, K. H. "Structuring Temporary Systems for High Reliability," *Academy of Management Journal* (in press).
10. La Porte, T. R., and Consolini, P. "Working in Theory but Not in Practice: Theoretical Challenges in High Reliability Organizations," *Journal of Public Administration Research and Theory* 1 (1991):19–47.
11. Kerr, S. "On the Folly of Rewarding A While Hoping for B," *Academy of Management Journal* 47 (1975):469–483.
12. Weick, K. E. "South Canyon Revisited: Lessons from High Reliability Organizations," working paper, University of Michigan, 1995.
13. Weick, K. E. *Sense Making in Organizations* (Thousand Oaks, CA: Sage, 1995).
14. Weick, K. E., and Roberts, K. H. "Collective Mind and Organizational Reliability: The Case of Flight Operations on an Aircraft Carrier Deck," *Administrative Science Quarterly* 38 (1993):357–381.

15. Roberts, K. H., and Bea, R. "When Systems Fail," *Organizational Dynamics* (2001).
16. Roberts, K. H. et al., "Decision Dynamics in Two High Reliability Military Organizations," *Management Science* 40 (1994):614–624.
17. Schulman, P. "The Analysis of High Reliability Organizations," in *New Challenges to Understanding Organizations*, ed. K. H. Roberts (New York: Macmillan, 1993), 33–54.
18. Tamuz, M. "Developing Organizational Safety Information Systems for Monitoring Potential Dangers," in *Proceedings of PSAM II* 2, eds. G. E. Apostolakis and T. S. Win (Los Angeles: University of California, 1994), 7–12.
19. Weick, K. E. "The Vulnerable System: An Analysis of the Tenerife Air Disaster," *Journal of Management* 16 (1990):571–593.
20. Stringfield, S. "Attempting to Enhance Students' Learning Through Innovative Programs: The Case for Schools Evolving into High Reliability Organizations," *School Effectiveness and School Improvement* 6 (1995):67–90.
21. Bierly, P. E., and Spender, J. C. "Culture and High Reliability Organizations: The Case of the Nuclear Submarine," *Journal of Management* 21 (1995):639–656.
22. Hee, D. D. et al., "Safety Management Assessment System (SMAS): A Process for Identifying and Evaluating Human and Organization Factors in Marine System Operations with Field Test Results," *Reliability Engineering and System Safety* 65 (1999):125–140.
23. Bea, R. G. "Risk Based Engineering Design of Marine Systems: The Human and Organizational Factors (HOF)," Paper presented at the State of the Art Pipeline Risk Management Conference, Perth, Western Australia, November 11, 1999.
24. Boniface, D., and Bea, R. G. "A Decision Analysis Framework for Assessing Human and Organizational Error in the Marine Industries," Paper presented at the Symposium on Human and Organizational Error in Marine Structures, Ship Structure Committee, Society of Naval Architects and Marine Engineers, Arlington, VA, November 1996.
25. Grabowski, M. et al., "Decision Support and Organizational Forms in a High Velocity Environment: Responses to Catastrophic Oil Spills," in *Advances in Expert Systems for Management: Evaluation and Value in Knowledge Based Systems*, eds. M. Grabowski and W. A. Wallace (Greenwich, CT: JAI Press, 1997).
26. Sarna, P. C. "Sense Making in the Incident Command: Developing and Maintaining the 'Big Picture,' " Paper presented at IDER/IEPC Conference, The Hague, October 12–14, 1999.
27. Pollack, M. et al., "Pediatric Intensive Care Units: Results of a National Study," *Critical Care Medicine* 21 (1993):607–611.
28. McCloskey, K. A., and Johnston, C. "Critical Care Interhospital Transports: Predictability of the Need for a Pediatrician," *Pediatric Emergency Care* 6 (1990):89–92.
29. Drazin, R., and Sandelands, L. "Autogenesis: A Perspective on the Process of Organizing," *Organization Science* 19, no. 3 (1992).

12

Admitting Imperfection: Revelations From the Cockpit For the World of Medicine

John J. Nance, JD

The proverbial hush falls over the crowd as the Olympic athlete pauses at the starting point, focusing his mind and preparing to do battle with gravity, the record book, his fellow competitors, and himself. At last the seminal moment arrives and the contestant explodes into motion. Thousands of spectators watch in person along with millions more before TV sets around the world, each of the spectators drawn onto the razor edge of the moment as the uncertain outcome unfolds.

The task before the athlete is nothing less than to push hard at the envelope of human endurance and dexterity, forcing his body to perform better, faster, with greater accuracy, and closer to the ideal of flawlessness than anyone who has dared this competition before.

But as we watch him struggle, the element that rivets us so—the element that suspends time and space with unbearable suspense—is the absolute knowledge that failure is not only a possibility, it is, in fact, a distinct likelihood.

This we understand as a species: The possibility of human failure makes success all the sweeter, and not just in sports. Philosophers and poets alike have long extolled the incalculable value of the struggle against the possibility or probability of failure as an element that defines us and elevates us to achieve more than what we are. "A man's reach should exceed his grasp," wrote Robert Browning, "or what's a heaven for?"

Moreover, we understand that little if anything in human existence is guaranteed, including our own continued existence. "Civilization," wrote Will and Ariel Durant, "exists by geological consent, subject to change without notice," and as we live with uncertain geology and uncertain physiology, we face on a daily basis the evidence that life can end in a heartbeat.

Yet, whether by operation of an eternal optimism inextricably inherent in the human species or by a need for institutional denial, we humans not only reach routinely beyond our grasp, but we also elevate certain members and *classes* within our own species to an eternally unachievable status: infallibility. We assume that with enough years of practice and instruction, we can perform perfectly all of the time. This is nothing less than a classic contradiction, a dichotomy of immense proportions. The same race of beings, in other words, that can fully understand the propensity for human imperfection in one class of human endeavors refuses to accept that propensity in others. Yet the propensity for human failure is not a variable characteristic. It is universal.

Throughout the ages, humans have invested those trained to fulfill higher callings with the presumption of omnipotence and perfection. Kings and prelates, for instance—both presumed to be the invested representatives of God—not only dominated Western humanity from the first century after Christ through the Middle Ages, but were presumed *by definition* to be incapable of error. With a great and staggering gulf between the common man and those in control (based on education and position), that primal investiture of assumed perfection was one that served the convenience and comfort of the people as much as it sprang from faith or the actual perceived performance of the nobility. One *wanted* one's king to be infallible, since life and prosperity in whatever form depended on his protection, his judgment, and his performance as leader and defender of the state. Correspondingly, the head of a church *needed* to be presumed infallible in order to be given the authority to translate for the common man the will of the deity. So, too, the rising class of masters of various crafts and professions were afforded the presumption of perfection by those of lesser position, experience, and ability, and to such ranks were added the presumed intellectual infallibility of senior scientists and professors of the nobility, especially as we rounded the end of the eighteenth century and built a foundation of technological achievements on which would be raised the industrial revolution.

The late nineteenth century brought with it a further expansion of this expectation of human perfection, but this version—inasmuch as it encompassed the practitioners of professions and trades without reference to station of birth, royalty, or inherited position—was testimony to the need of society to *depend* on the performance of these venerated practitioners (of whatever profession) precisely because their performance had become so critical to society.

A captain of the British navy or any other great navy, for instance, was charged with the responsibility and presumption of possessing perfect judgment by the time he had acceded to that rank. After all, Britain, for one, granted its captains godlike authority over their human charges, including the power to order any crew member executed at any time for any reason. Although the Lords of the Admiralty passed judgment on just how perfect their captains' performance might be, no one else was afforded the right to question a commander. There was an enforced presumption, held dear by ordinary seamen and junior officers alike, that the captain was, in fact, incapable of error. Yet, in the last moments of his life, many a seaman must have flailed as much against the reality that his captain had been wrong as against the waters of a shipwreck that were about to engulf him. And, of course, for a seaman to *question* the judgment of his captain was a capital offense punishable by death in whatever gruesome form the captain chose.

So, too, in the nineteenth century was the physician raised from the status of benevolent medicine man and healer to the practitioner of a profession that, insofar as it incorporated ways and means mysterious to the average citizen, required the presumption of perfection. One had to trust that a physician knew what to do and how to do it, and that trust came hard in the ages before anesthesia, microbiology, antibiotics, and the abilities to heal and soothe granted by modern pharmacology became available. One has only to examine the history of the field physicians of the Union and Confederate armies during the American Civil War to understand the required level of blind trust. It was the physician who pronounced the need to saw off damaged limbs, inflict horrible pain in attempts to reassemble broken bodies, or consign the wounded to death. To the recipients of such emergency/

trauma medicine, trust was enabled by the comforting belief that the process of medical training had transformed these healers from mere mortals to something more, and that added element was infallibility. The dead could be mourned more easily, the broken and sick resigned more benevolently on the advice of a medical man whose word could be trusted absolutely. We, as a species, wanted and needed the inherent comfort of that presumption, despite its terrible predations on the very practitioners it sought to sanctify.

Now, in the third millennium of Western time-keeping, the ranks of those who must be presumed infallible have expanded yet again. At their core, they still encompass the healer, the physician, and all those arrayed with the physician in providing professional health care. But they also encompass those whose fingers hover over nuclear triggers and those in control of various machines and systems on which our lives periodically depend, such as airline pilots, civilian ship captains, and even railroad engineers. Whenever we place our lives and physical well-being (or those of our loved ones) in the skilled hands of other humans, we try hard to convince ourselves that those so trusted have been trained to a standard that allows them to perform without flaw and without error. We make these presumptions, yet react with institutional fury when someone so anointed has the temerity to prove less than perfect. We have as humans, in other words, created a systemic presumption of the possibility of human perfection and assigned that presumption to mere mortals engaged in a wide array of pursuits, the expertise for which has been granted by training and experience, not birth. It is an endemic expectation, and it is a myth. But the most dastardly element of the expectation of professional perfection is that *we professionals* have been trained to believe it!

Although a major point of this chapter is transference to health care of some of the revolutionary lessons recently learned by aviation about dealing with human failures and human nature, the inescapable truth is that the very same challenges of human imperfection causing injuries and deaths are faced by medical professionals every day. What's new is the perspective developed by aviation, the unique approach to handling fallible humans in a human system demanding critical performance at near-perfection levels. Yet there are basics that apply to all of us in any human endeavor, and before taking you into aviation's revelatory experiences, this bedrock element of commonality should be discussed.

Pilots, military commanders, operators of nuclear power plants, and tens of thousands of other highly trained, highly skilled, highly motivated people learn their professions with the understanding that they will be expected to rise to the level of operational perfection and will be dealt with harshly if they fail. Indeed, the security of their job, they are told (by word and by deed), depends on making no mistakes (or at least on making no large, costly mistakes that must be explained). So, too, are physicians and nurses trained to believe they can become infallible, and those who train them browbeat that expectation into their students with such effectiveness that the majority of medical practitioners are launched with a severely dysfunctional contradiction ticking away inside their psyches like a bomb: "I must be perfect. My teachers and my peers are perfect. People will think much less of me if I'm not perfect. Yet, I see increasing evidence that I am not perfect and may never achieve that status, and I must hide that possibility at all costs."

THE MYTH OF MEDICAL INFALLIBILITY

The practice of medicine and the very operation of the healthcare industry have been built on the foundation of the mythological assumption that professionals can achieve perfection. Aviation built its citadel of operational safety on the very same assumption. Using that precept eliminates the need to build safety systems to absorb human mistakes, because there should *be* no human mistakes to absorb. Yet, medical mistakes are, by definition, human mistakes, and that fact becomes immediately offensive to the system and all within it. Thus, a human practitioner who commits an imperfect act by making a mistake does nothing less than offend and assault the belief system upon which health care as an industry and a profession has been built.

There are only two major pathways to use in dealing with human mistakes. One is to get rid of (or sanction and retrain) the flawed human. The other is to massively alter the expectations and structure of the system to accept and anticipate the existence of human imperfection. Historically, both health care and aviation have always chosen the former.

Traditionally, firing the person or persons who are determined to have committed a medical error enabled the system to maintain the facade of normalcy. The system could thus proclaim that the *expectation* of human perfection was still valid, but that the *system's* only mistake was picking the wrong human.

Yet human mistakes—medical mistakes—never occur in a vacuum as a singular, unsupported event. It is axiomatic that there is always a chain of acts or omissions that surrounds the triggering human mistake and enables it, just as it is axiomatic that there is never a single, isolated cause for an airline accident.

Take the classic example of a nurse who accidentally prepares a solution of undiluted potassium chloride for IV infusion instead of the heavily diluted solution ordered by the attending physician. When the patient's heart stops in chemical obedience to the expected physiologic reaction, there is no question that the nurse's mistake was the triggering element. But what of the *enabling* elements that were undisputedly under the control of the *system*? Why was undiluted potassium chloride available outside the confines of the pharmacy? Where was the special training to warn the nurse of the dangers of any potassium chloride infusion? Where were the established procedures or forcing functions that would have made such a mistake impossible?

When we proceed from the assumption that nurses, doctors, and pharmacists (and all other healthcare professionals) will never be able to completely expunge mistakes from their professional performance, it becomes obvious that simply firing or disciplining (or even retraining) the nurse who makes a medical mistake does absolutely nothing to repair the safety gaps in the delivery system itself. Only by building safety buffers—emergency backups, if you will—can the system safely and routinely absorb future human mistakes short of patient impact. Certainly, firing a nurse assures that *that* nurse will never make *that* mistake in *that* facility again, but the next nurse hired to replace him or her may, especially if the surrounding environment is not restructured. Clearly, simply firing or eliminating flawed humans and replacing them with others does virtually nothing to correct the system's vulnerability. The system itself must be changed.

That is precisely where we are in American health care at the dawn of the third millennium: possessed of a system that, despite its stunning successes in delivering the best health care in history to the largest number of people, nevertheless enables and sometimes facilitates a staggering number of patient injuries and deaths each year.* This happens not because the system employs "bad" humans who should never have been trusted to be perfect. It happens because the system employs humans who are generically incapable of absolute perfection, yet wrongly expects precisely what they generically can never provide: continuous flawless performance. In so doing, it reflects not just the self-generated expecta-

*Dr. Lucian Leape in February 2001 prepared a graphic comparing health care to numerous other publicly trusted professions, trades, and activities, showing that those admitted to hospitals were taking only a slightly lesser risk than bungee jumping from a bridge or other high precipice, and a slightly *more* hazardous one than mountain climbing, with mortality rates from medical accidents (medical mistakes) at approximately 1 per 1,000 patients.

tions of medical professionals, but the misguided expectations of an entire population who dearly wants to believe that their physicians, nurses, and healthcare providers have been somehow elevated to a status of perfect judgment, knowledge, and performance.

That popular expectation of perfection has been a part of the airline industry for the past 40 years. As startling as it may seem, one of the first major steps in improving airline safety was to lower the expectations of airline customers, urging them to accept the reality that pilots, as humans, are not perfect, but that integrated safety systems that fully anticipate human fallibility can and do approach perfection.

When any of us approach an airline's ticket counter these days with the intent to fly, we are well aware of several realities: (1) Commercial aviation is not 100% safe and sometimes does end in crashes and tragedy, and (2) the safety record of commercial aviation has not only continued to improve, but flying is without question the safest method of travel.

But if airlines and their personnel are not perfect, why do we climb aboard? Because the airline industry and the media have done an effective job of educating the population about the methods the airlines use to achieve such incredible safety records: simulators, intensive training, checkrides, high standards, checklists, backup systems backing up backup systems, and within the last decade, increasing public exposure to the seismic change in the culture of the airline cockpits.

Aiding this process have been the open and continuously visible investigations of the National Transportation Safety Board (NTSB). Although much of the public still mistakenly views the process of accident investigation as a process designed to lay blame, an increasing number of Americans understand that the NTSB is not interested in blame, but in uncovering all the contributing causes to an accident so that the system may be adjusted appropriately in time to prevent a new accident from similar causal factors. This constant public exposure of the process has slowly but profoundly changed the role of airline pilots from that of an arcane priesthood whose ways were too mysterious to know to that of a cadre of highly trained professionals who, though imperfect and thoroughly human, utilize advanced methods of teamwork and technical ability to achieve what few thought possible a half century ago: almost perfect systemic performance.

AVIATION AS A CAUTIONARY EXAMPLE FOR HEALTH CARE

The road to this status, however, has been rough. Since 1977, aviation has lived through a revolution that health care is now entering, a painful redefining of reasonable expectations of human performance in a human system and how to minimize the effects of human failure. The scope of the changes has been vast, and it has taken fully 20 years to reach the threshold of maturity. In short, aviation as a community has embraced the reality of human imperfection and altered its training courses and its systemic structures to do two things: work to minimize human errors, and prepare aviation systems to safely absorb those errors that cannot be fully eliminated. The results have been demonstrable and impressive gains in flight safety through the process of building systems that are redundant enough to safely absorb not only mechanical failures, but human failures as well.

Why is this a process health care should study closely? Because the lessons that aviation purchased with the blood of lost passengers and crew members have direct applicability to the medical community.

Airline pilots, and pilots in general who fly for compensation or for the military, are traditionally charged with the same expectation of perfect performance as doctors, nurses, pharmacists, and other healthcare professionals. Historically, aviation has built its systems and organizations on the very same myth that there will be no dangerous human errors that the system from time to time must be able to safely absorb. Unlike health care, however, the aviation industry has been forced by the very public nature of its mistakes to come to grips with human failure at a much earlier time. Specifically, aviation safety leaders were forced by the terrible drumbeat of accidents in the 1970s to face four major systemic flaws that were preventing the aviation safety system from improving further:

1. Aviation's historic refusal to fully accept the inevitability of human failure and readjust the safety system to both minimize their causes (such as fatigue, distraction, anger, and lack of standardization) while safely absorbing those human mistakes that remain
2. The presence of massive barriers to communication among crew members and associated members of the operational team (such as dispatchers, mechanics, pilots, and flight attendants), which too often prevented the passage of vital information at critical times
3. The traditional method of grading the worth of cockpit leadership based on omnipotence and infallibility rather than on the most interactive and effective use of human resources
4. The inability to appropriately utilize teams and teamwork

Similarities between Aviation and Health Care

Aviation and health care share a staggering commonality, which means that each can learn from the other. Both fit the description coined by Dr. James Reason of Britain of a "sharp end" industry, in which the extensive infrastructure of knowledge, investment, performance history, and invested capital (the so-called blunt end of the organization) can be instantly imperiled by the human mistake of someone working at the so-called sharp end. The sharp end is the place where the entire collective professional capabilities of the organization rest in the hands of one or more practitioners working in a highly dynamic and changeable environment in which successful outcomes may be routine, but cannot be assured.

In other words, one slip in aviation, and an airliner may be lost. One slip in the operating room, and a patient may be lost. In fact, the following definition fits both professions:

> Highly trained, highly motivated professionals working in a real-time, high-pressure environment, using very sophisticated implements and tools under great public and regulatory scrutiny, where the penalties for failure are potentially very great in both human and monetary terms.

Certainly, the penalties for crashing an airliner are very great in "both human and monetary terms," just as the potential penalties for losing a patient to a medical mistake include not only the nightmare of lawsuits and diminished stature, but also the specter of intense professional self-doubt, deep remorse, and, typically, the weight of undeserved shame and blame exacerbated by an archaic system of disciplining humans for the offense of being human.

This, too, is an element of historic commonality—the propensity when something goes wrong to ask the question "Who's wrong?" versus the correct systemic question, "What's wrong?"

Aviation is replete with stories of pilots and mechanics fired for making a mistake that, in fact, would have been impossible without extensive "help" from the system in which that professional worked. Although professionals in health care and aviation must have professional performance standards and disciplinary systems to enforce them, using discipline to address a purely human failure is a useless, counterproductive exercise rooted more in tradition than logic.

Take the example of a Delta Airlines Boeing 727 crew of three highly trained and experienced pilots who crashed on takeoff in 1985 at Dallas–Fort Worth airport because they forgot to position the flaps correctly. All three men not only responded to the checklist, but looked in the direction of the gauges that would have told them the true position of the flaps (extendable panels on the back of the wing that enable a jet to take off and land at slow airspeeds). As heard on the cockpit voice recorder, all three responded "Fifteen, fifteen, green," meaning the flaps were in the correct position for takeoff. The flaps, however, were in the zero position, as clearly indicated on the gauges that all three men looked at and all three men misinterpreted.

How could that happen? Because, as human beings, we sometimes see and hear what we expect to see and hear, even though that may be at variance with what's actually there. This was, in other words, a mistake that resulted simply from the status of being human. There were no rules about how to look at the forward panel that were violated, no missed checklists, and no intent by any of the pilots to ignore procedures. All three simply failed as human beings.

The pilots all survived the crash, though some of their passengers did not. Delta, acting in accordance with the tradition of aviation and health care (a tradition that dictates that the responsible parties pay an appropriate price for failure), fired the pilots. They did so in part to send a message to all other Delta pilots: "If you fail like these men did, you, too, will be terminated."

But the failure was a *human* failure, a *human* vulnerability. So the actual message sent by Delta was utter nonsense: "If you make a human mistake that you neither intended to make nor had any control over, we will fire you. Therefore, don't you dare be human."

It is impossible to find any corrective value in that message, other than to let the rest of the pilot force know that their jobs depended precariously on the fickle element of fate. Such a misuse of discipline does violence to the goal of understanding our human failure potentials so that we can design better systems to prevent those human potentials from resulting in dangerous situations like inadvertent no-flap takeoffs.

In other words, firing a pilot or a nurse to address an inadvertent human error and thus leaving the important systemic questions of what nurtured the error into a disaster unanswered and unaddressed becomes a form of organizational narcotic: It makes the system feel good at the same time as it guarantees addiction to more repetitions of that and other mistakes.

The Safety Hazards of the Isolated Omnipotent Leader: Firing Captain Kirk

The four major mistakes aviation was making, listed earlier, are all facets of the same basic malady: the presumption of human infallibility. But once airlines began institutionally admitting that its crews could make mistakes, a renaissance was triggered in method and outlook that began leading to the elimination of the most serious barriers to communication among crew members. At the same time, aviation began redefining what constituted a good leader and working to invigorate true teamwork in the cockpit and the cabin.

The vast majority of healthcare professionals recognize the name James T. Kirk as the fictional captain of the United Federation Starship *Enterprise* from the 1966–1969 vintage NBC/Paramount science-fiction television series *Star Trek*. Kirk (played by actor William Shatner) was largely representative of the way leaders were supposed to think and act, whether in health care, aviation, the military, or business in general. They were expected to be strong-willed, technically competent, highly innovative individuals who needed no one's advice and who were extremely careful to maintain the image of command.

Specifically, Jim Kirk was ready to fire off orders at any time with a firm air of infallibility in reaction to any problem. Other than the reports and responses he requested from his crew, Kirk neither needed nor wanted anyone's advice, because (1) he already had the perfect answers, and (2) the act of requesting or accepting a subordinate's recommendation might somehow suggest to the crew that he was less than omnipotent.

Kirk, in other words, embodied the accepted model of a modern physician, and too often the resultant model of a leader in nursing, pharmacy, and any other position of management in medical practice. And, of course, the Kirk method was the very essence of what airline captains and military commanders alike were supposed to be: omnipotent, perfect, and endlessly effective.

The problem, of course, was not that healthcare professionals or airline professionals had begun spending time studying the *Star Trek* school of command as portrayed by Kirk and then emulating him, but rather that the writers of the show had effectively captured our model of leadership without a corresponding portrayal of the fact that the Kirk command style was demonstrably hazardous to human health.

Kirk, like healthcare professionals and pilots alike, was surrounded by subordinates, the vast majority of whom fit the definition of being "highly trained, highly motivated professionals." Those professionals were there to contribute their intellect, training, and human compassion to the job at hand, which was always to serve the best interests of the common goal. So, too, are subordinate pilots paid salaries and given expensive training to provide something more than companionship and blind obedience in an airliner cockpit. Yet in health care, aviation, and the USS *Enterprise*, subordinates were not free to contribute their professional abilities without severe constraints.

In the case of the airline industry, a long string of galvanizing disasters in the 1970s served to force a seminal change in attitude and culture. It was impossible, for instance, to ignore the fact that the information that could have saved 583 lives on a foggy runway in the Canary Islands in 1977 resided in the minds of two subordinate pilots. The chief pilot of KLM Royal Dutch Airlines had begun a hurried takeoff without the proper clearance, but that information could not be passed to the captain simply because the copilot and flight engineer could not bring themselves to question or override a man in whom they had such confidence and held in such respect.

The location was the airport at Tenerife in the Canaries, and the problem was the sudden arrival of several jumbo jets diverting into the normally sleepy airport because the main island airport of Las Palmas had been temporarily closed by a bomb threat. The KLM flight carried a charter group inbound from Amsterdam, and the crew was supposed to pick up an outbound charter group and return to Amsterdam on schedule. After a frustrating several hours trying to get refueled and get under way, the KLM captain was in a state of agitation by the time he turned his huge aircraft into position at the end of the foggy runway and began pushing the throttles forward to go.

"Wait a minute, sir," the first officer/copilot had said, "We don't have the clearance yet."

Captain Jacob van Zanten had pulled the throttles back in embarrassment, yet, like all senior leaders, admitting embarrassment or mistake was not an option. "I knew that," the captain said. "Get the clearance." Time was passing, and van Zanten had only a few minutes left to get off the ground before running past his maximum projected crew duty time limits. Were he to exceed those limits, the entire charter flight would have to be stopped for 12 hours of crew rest, costing the airline over $30,000 dollars and costing Jacob van Zanten considerable embarrassment. This captain, in other words, wanted to get airborne as fast as possible.

The tower controller issued the first of the two required clearances, but van Zanten, mistakenly believing that both the air traffic control clearance *and* the takeoff clearance had been issued, pushed the throttles up again to start the takeoff roll.

Suddenly, the experienced copilot was thrown into an incredible diplomatic dilemma. He had already corrected—and embarrassed—his senior commander once. He did not want to do it again! Unable to force himself to point out that the captain was, for a second time, attempting takeoff without a clearance, he tried clearing them for takeoff by simply announcing the fact to the tower, hoping the tower controller would order them to hold position, and thus solve the problem.

This was, after all, his boss in the left seat, and one of the most beloved men at KLM. Van Zanten was the chief pilot. He was the director of safety, an important post. He was also the man whose face was all over the world in a two-page slick magazine ad for KLM, the very spokesman for the safety and performance excellence of Dutch aviation. The bright halo over van Zanten's head—his assumed status of infallibility and omnipotence—was too powerful to allow the other two officers in the cockpit unfettered communication of the extremely vital fact that the takeoff clearance had not yet been issued and other aircraft were moving around in unknown locations on the airport surface in the foggy conditions.

The copilot's garbled statement to the unseen tower controller that "We are . . . at . . . takeoff, KLM," a puzzling nonstandard transmission, led to a mistaken reply by the tower controller: "Okay. . . . stand by, I will call you."

Unfortunately, another aircraft, puzzled at the meaning of the strange phrase uttered by the copilot, pressed its transmit button milliseconds after the tower controller had spoken the word "Okay." The new transmission blocked the tower controller's following order to stand by, and suddenly the KLM first officer was left with the impression that the tower had approved the self-announced takeoff roll.

"Set power," ordered Captain van Zanten. "We go."

Approximately 30 seconds later, at 112 knots, which was well below flying speed, the huge Boeing 747-200 rolled out of the clouds that had been obscuring ground visibility and slammed into a Pan American 747 that had missed a turn and was sitting sideways on the runway. The ensuing fireball led to the worst loss of life in airline history to that date.

Similarly, a United Airlines crew ran a huge four-engine DC-8 out of fuel and crashed 7 miles short of the Portland, Oregon, airport one December night in 1978 because the two experienced subordinate pilots were so used to being overruled by an autocratic captain that they'd given up trying to communicate with him. They couldn't even tell him that they were about to flame out after an hour and twelve minutes of preparations for a relatively routine emergency landing.

In 1982, a situationally disconnected Boeing 737 captain disregarded four warnings from his vastly more qualified young copilot and tried to haul their ice-encrusted Air Florida jet into the air with only three quarters normal power. Instead of sustaining flight, they thundered into the nearby 14th Street Bridge over the Potomac River in Washington, DC, killing all but five, and most Americans watched the amazing helicopter rescue of those five from the icy river on live TV.

Blockages of critical cockpit communication were occurring for many reasons and causing crash after crash, but the ultimate cause of this lack of communication was the dysfunctional cockpit culture. More specifically, it was the utter absence of *teamwork*.

Aviation professionals had collectively thought of airline cockpit crews as exemplifying the best aspects of teamwork. But teamwork requires a team, and a team does not consist merely of one giving orders and others carrying out those orders—which was essentially the way airliners were flown. By the early 1980s, it had become obvious that somehow in the maturation of the airline business, airline cockpits had been allowed to develop a culture that was essentially and dangerously dependent on the captain's skill and judgment to the exclusion of all other influence. Although there were certainly large numbers of captains who sought the advice and participation of their subordinate pilots, the model—the norm—was the autocratic captain essentially flying solo in a multiplace aircraft with other qualified pilots who were very careful about countering him, making suggestions, or ever attempting to override his decision. In other words, the Captain Kirk model of leadership was the norm.

The word *culture* is important here, because when a dysfunctional human culture develops, the culture itself often does not recognize its own dysfunctionality. Thus, even subordinate pilots who were well aware of their inability to influence a headstrong captain would adopt the same autocratic methods when they became captains, thus perpetuating the problem. The phrase "This is the way we've always done it" was too often used to justify the continuation of a demonstrably dangerous environment, just as tradition and training too often serve to perpetuate the same sort of autocratic, noncommunicative environment among physicians, nurses, and healthcare workers.

Although a surgical operating room (OR) provides a close parallel to the crucible of an airline cockpit in many ways, there are numerous dissimilarities. For example, the OR involves numerous variances in professional training and people working for different entities coming together to practice under the same roof, whereas an airline crew works for the same entity and is trained to the same standards. Nevertheless, in terms of whether vital information can flow in unfettered fashion between members of a true team, the OR, the intensive care unit (ICU), and the emergency department (ED) present high-pressure parallels to the cockpit. In all cases, blocked communication, excessive hierarchies, poor leadership techniques, and the absence of a common vision (i.e., patient safety) involve the same principles.

But these principles apply far beyond the ED, the ICU, and the OR. These principles apply wherever two or more medical professionals are engaged in a common purpose and need to cooperate and communicate for the good of the patient and the good of the mission.

The leadership style traditionally taught by example in most medical and nursing schools matches the leadership style traditionally expected of pilots in command in that we were all essentially trained to emulate the command style of Captain Kirk.

In medical practice as well as in aviation, the concurrent need to keep up the *appearance* of infallibility, firm control, absolute knowledge, and self-sufficiency is beyond well established—it's endemic. Newer nurses are careful about questioning or challenging more experienced nurses or management nurses, who in turn are often loathe to question or challenge strong-willed doctors, who in turn are careful about challenging or countering stronger-willed, better-established doctors. Senior people are afforded such high levels of respect that subordinates will routinely question their own judgment or professional knowledge rather than quickly accept the idea that a respected leader might be making a mistake. In addition, even when a senior leader invites full participatory critique and open communication, the subordinates—in the absence of specific training and tangible cultural change—are too often unwilling to speak up.

The airline cockpit held precisely the same problems: captains whose mere level of experience or status as a captain retarded or eliminated critique, questioning, or even professional oversight by the other pilots in the same cockpit; and subordinate pilots who felt constrained and refused to speak up, even when invited to do so by a fully participatory captain. These are serious barriers to communication that prevent those with critical knowledge from passing that knowledge to a leader in timely fashion. In airline cockpits this communication malady was regularly permitting the failure of a single human being—the captain—to metastasize into a fatal accident even though one or more of his or her crewmembers had timely knowledge that the captain's chosen course of action was dangerous. So, too, have countless patients been injured or killed by medical mistakes made by experienced practitioners in the presence of other healthcare professionals who knew something was wrong, but could not or would not speak up.

How Aviation Addressed Teamwork Problems

It took more than 5 years after the Tenerife disaster before the beginnings of a solution surfaced to address the problem of retraining or firing the Captain Kirks in airline cockpits. United Airlines, which had suffered the embarrassment of the Portland crash and one other near Salt Lake City resulting from poor-to-no cockpit communication and coordination, identified the problem not as a need for democracy in the cockpit (an oft-heard criticism), but as a need to invest the leader—the captain—with a new charge: the responsibility to appropriately utilize all the resources entrusted to him, *inclusive* of the human crewmembers. In order to train United's pilots how to discharge this strange new responsibility, United created a new FAA-approved course called CLRM, cockpit leadership resource management, later shortened to cockpit resource management (CRM), and finally changed to *crew* resource management to reflect the growing realization that the crew—the team—included the flight attendants, the mechanics, the dispatchers, and everyone else operationally involved.

In principle, CRM is a fairly simple process of training captains to accept their fallibility as humans and accept the concept that their worth as leaders is measured by how well they can consistently invite, extract, and utilize the full intellectual and professional capabilities of the other pilots and crewmembers—their "resources"—by invigorating and perpetuating an atmosphere of unfettered communication.

At the same time, it became vitally important to train the copilots and flight engineers as well as flight attendants (in later versions of the courses) that they had an unshakable responsibility to speak up assertively and not keep silent when something needed to be said. Certain additional procedures were coined, such as the "two challenge" rule, which dictated that when a subordinate pilot realized professionally that something had to be done, he or she was to challenge the captain and the copilot twice, and even if not listened to, was to make it happen.

In February 1989, United Airlines Flight 811 was on climbout some 60 miles from Honolulu, southbound for New Zealand, when the incompletely closed forward cargo door blew out, killing nine passengers and seriously damaging the fully loaded 747. Using the newly trained principles of CRM and full communication, the three pilots successfully returned the jet to Honolulu International during a harried emergency in which the flight engineer twice saved the aircraft: first, by dumping fuel before being directed to do so, and second, by speaking up when the captain was about to mistakenly ditch the aircraft, an act that would have killed all aboard given the extensive damage to the airframe.

CRM, even though never mandated by the Federal Aviation Administration, has become the gold standard in crew training in aviation. By the mid-1990s no U.S.-based airline could qualify for decent insurance rates without adopting both the CRM course and the CRM philosophy. There are many versions and variations of CRM courses, but they all have in common the basic philosophy of "leadership with participation, and [subordinate] assertiveness with respect."

CRM courses are not adaptable to health care without significant modification. Airlines learned by trial and error that psychologists teaching pilots didn't work, but that when pilots and flight attendants were trained as facilitators and became the teachers to their own people, the effectiveness of the CRM courses soared.

So, too, CRM must not only be adapted in health care, but equivalent teaching of the concepts of teamwork must be taught by medical professionals to medical professionals. This is an evolving science, but the benefits from altering the way the community looks at communication, teamwork, leadership, and the willingness to ask for advice and assistance with no hesitation or shame are critical to improving patient safety and significantly decreasing the opportunity for human mistake to metastasize into patient impact.

The Picard Method

The citing of *Star Trek* in a serious work may seem strange, but in fact the writers of all versions of the show have given both health care and aviation some highly useful examples of the extremes of leadership style and have crystallized those styles in the command personalities of Captain Kirk (of the original series) and Captain Jean-Luc Picard (of *Star Trek: The Next Generation*, which appeared some 25 years later).

Consider, for instance, the remarkable difference between those command styles. Where Kirk, under fire, would rattle off orders and ignore contrary advice (as well as belittle the would-be adviser), Picard would almost immediately call his senior officers into an emergency staff meeting, a move that enabled him to extract in the shortest period of time the maximum intellect from his highly trained, highly motivated crew. Thus equipped with a better array of advice and options than he could have generated by himself, Picard would then use his cognitive intellect and command abilities to come up with better decisions. Picard made sure his crew understood that, while he was an excellent commander, he was also an imperfect human and thus needed to utilize all his people to improve the effectiveness of his leadership. That command style, as ably portrayed by Shakespearean actor Patrick Stewart, was never one of weakness. Picard retained virtually all of his crew's respect and his leadership and command authority. But by utilizing all the human resources at his command, he was a far better commander and the very model of what the airline industry has come to expect of its airline captains.

The Picard method is the correct one for health care as well. Dr. Picard, Nurse Picard, pharmacist Picard, administrator Picard—the list of positions for which this method of interactive leadership is the correct one is endless. The best leaders must be redefined as men and women who are virtually unafraid of asking for the advice and counsel of the professionals and subordinates around them, and who are skillful in extracting the last ounce of intellect and participation from such people in order to facilitate better decisions. That takes a substantial change in the way leaders view themselves. It takes self-confidence, development of new communication skills and techniques, the virtual abandonment of the traditional tendency to compete with one's eager subordinates, and the comfortable willingness to say in word and deed, "I am human, I am imperfect, and that very recognition makes me a strong and reliable leader who knows how to work safely within my own limitations."

CONCLUSION

The worth of the airline experience to health care is quite simple: The new definition of what it takes to lead has been forged in the fires of airline disasters and the extensive renaissance in teamwork and communication methods that resulted from those accident investigations. No longer are dangerously impossible claims of human infallibility acceptable. No longer is autocratic, noncommunicative leadership tolerable. No longer are healthcare participants given the false luxury of silence, or the challenge of using excessive diplomacy as a license to remain silent.

From the smallest clinic to the largest hospital, this massive change in the way we view teamwork, communication, leadership, and human fallibility is the basic formula needed to change the structure of health care's approach to the very real patient safety issues before it. The vast majority of human errors that metastasize into patient injury or death, whether involving medication errors or otherwise, can be prevented by attacking and improving bad systems, not assuming the presence of bad people. And the necessary changes in health care are the very same ones made over the last 20 years in aviation.

13

Creating a Just Culture: A Nonpunitive Approach to Medical Errors

Laura Ashpole

INTRODUCTION

The concept of "just culture," developed by David Marx and colleagues, is predicated on the notion that a disciplinary system in which medical professionals are punished for making mistakes fails to improve patient safety.[1] The healthcare industry as it exists today literally prohibits human error.[1] Medical professionals are blamed and punished for their mistakes, which are often unintended.[1] This intolerance for error serves as a disincentive to providers sharing their mistakes with the medical community.[1] Furthermore, this punitive approach to medical errors discourages transparency, presenting a significant roadblock to the improvement of patient safety. In essence, such a model focuses exclusively on the people and very little on the system in which those people work.

In a just culture, weaknesses are openly identified and examined.[2] This concentration has the important effect of making providers feel supported and safe when voicing their concerns about errors in the workplace.[2] The most important goal of a just culture is to maintain safety and reliability, and medical professionals should be made to feel accountable in achieving that goal.[2] Given that a successful just culture depends on transparency and accountability, it is essential that strong leadership be developed in organizations effectuating a just culture, such that the concerns of all individuals in the organization are considered and evaluated.[2] Furthermore, the departments of quality, safety, and risk management must be involved in addressing the concerns and comments of the organization's employees so that proper oversight is provided and opportunities for process improvement are identified.[2] Finally, and most importantly, medical errors must be evaluated based on their quality, such that human error is consoled, at-risk behavior is coached, and reckless behavior is punished.[3] In brief, the just culture concept shifts attention from the retrospective judgment of individual behaviors and the severity of outcomes to a real-time assessment of behavioral decisions in a rational and organized way.[4]

The aim of this text is to analyze the features of a just culture and the practical implications for implementation of just culture principles in a healthcare organization. The first part contains an explanation of the just culture model and examines how medical error is responded to under such a model. The second part deals with how a healthcare organization might build the foundation for establishment of a just culture. The third part provides three illustrations of the implementation of just culture principles, both at the level of the individual hospital and at the statewide level. The fourth and final part includes recommendations for practical strategies and tools a healthcare organization should pursue in implementing a just culture.

WHAT IS A JUST CULTURE?

Put simply, a just culture is a values-supportive model of shared accountability.[5] Under the just culture model, a systems focus exists; however, all individuals within the system are accountable for the quality of their choices and are expected to report their individual errors, as well as system vulnerabilities.[5] A just and fair organization not only responds to these reports to prevent future adverse outcomes, but also utilizes these reports to assess the daily risks inherent to its operations.[5] In performing these related tasks, a just culture organization works to improve individual behaviors, as well as system design and related processes.[5] This combined focus is what makes the just culture model as successful and effective as it is.

Another important facet of the just culture model is its emphasis on a defined set of values, which include learning, openness, fairness, and safety.[5] Providers are encouraged to learn to understand risk and how system design directly affects patient safety.[5] Additionally, providers are incentivized to take part in the honest reporting of medical errors.[5] Identified mistakes are subsequently addressed fairly and justice is administered.[5] A just culture organization, although not blame free, ensures that discipline is employed only when the quality of a person's choice requires it; for example, if a provider engages in reckless conduct or knowingly violates a rule.[5] Moreover, a focus on patient safety remains the primary aim of a just culture. Instead of concentrating solely on undesired outcomes, a just culture scrutinizes the intent accompanying individual choices.[5] A just culture organization importantly recognizes that at-risk or reckless behavior may have been engaged in without a resulting bad outcome but still requires attention and that, alternatively, human error can in some instances cause serious, although unintended, harm.

The just culture model can also be conceptualized as the balancing of organizational and individual values with three specific duties.[3] The first of these duties is to avoid causing unjustified risk or harm.[3] The second duty is to produce an outcome, and the third duty is to follow a procedural rule.[3] Organizational and individual values, namely safety, cost, effectiveness, equity, and dignity, are then balanced against these three duties.[3]

Although the just culture model is primarily focused on improving patient safety, the implementation of just culture principles has many additional benefits. One such benefit is the advancement of increased trust within an organization. In health care, greater transparency and disclosure builds trust[6] not only between providers and patients but also between medical professionals. Furthermore, establishment of a just culture necessitates the regular assessment and evaluation of medical error. Reporting systems provide healthcare organizations with a consistent method for keeping informed of medical errors and responding to errors on a regular basis. Further, the just culture model requires inquiry into the kind of errors made. Understanding the character of medical errors provides for more productive responses to such errors, ensuring that an organization resolves issues and cures deficiencies that extend beyond the individual actor.

EVALUATING AND RESPONDING TO MEDICAL ERRORS

Establishing a just culture requires proper categorization of behaviors. David Marx's model of a just culture divides behavior into the following three categories: human error, at-risk behavior, and reckless behavior.[3] Human error is defined as inadvertent action, or a slip, lapse in judgment, or mistake.[3] In contrast, at-risk behavior involves a choice in which the risk is either not realized or believed to be justified.[3] Finally, the conscious disregard of an unreasonable risk constitutes reckless behavior.[3]

Behaviors can also be divided into four categories under the just culture model. This alternative system of categorization is often referred to as the "four evils," consisting of human error, negligent conduct, intentional rule violations, and reckless conduct.[1] Conceptions of human error and reckless conduct are the same as in the first model. However, an important distinction is made between negligent behavior and intentional rule violations under this model. Negligent conduct is conduct subjectively more culpable than human error.[1] In the healthcare context, negligence is defined as the failure to exercise the skill, care, and learning expected of a reasonably prudent healthcare provider.[1] Intentional rule violations, on the other hand, occur when an individual knowingly violates a rule, procedure, or duty in the course of performing a task.[1]

Depending on the categorization to which a particular behavior belongs, that behavior is addressed. First, human error is consoled under the just culture model.[3] The concept of just culture recognizes that human error is unintentional and inadvertent but unfortunately can have catastrophic outcomes.[1] At-risk behavior is instead coached.[3] Specifically, the just culture model dictates that incentives for at-risk behaviors are removed, incentives for healthy behaviors are created, and situational awareness is increased.[3] Conversely, reckless behavior is punished.[3] Although in general, the just culture model discourages the use of blaming behavior, it distinguishes behavior based on its underlying intent. The resulting schematic requires that behavior having bad intentions or exhibiting conscious disregard for the consequences receives adequate punishment to effectively extinguish similar future conduct. Often in a just culture, reckless behavior is managed using a combination of both remedial and punitive action.[3]

BUILDING THE FOUNDATION FOR THE INTRODUCTION OF JUST CULTURE PRINCIPLES

Due to the fact that establishment of a just culture is a fairly complicated endeavor, it is essential that a healthcare organization planning to make such a change lay the appropriate foundation for the adoption of just culture principles. The first step to be taken is the elimination of policies that are either contrary to just culture principles or practically prevent the implementation of a just culture model.[4] Policies that mandate punishment, for example, are contrary to just culture principles and therefore must be extinguished.[4] Additionally, policies that focus solely on systems and leave little room for the consideration of individual human behaviors will be incompatible with the just culture model.[4] After successful removal of policies obstructing the development of a just culture, policies that advance just culture principles can be created and effectuated.

Policies that outline expectations and consequences with regard to behavior and promote event investigation support just culture principles.[4] These values should be incorporated into a healthcare organization's bylaws and codes of conduct.[4] Efforts to explicitly specify these principles in the policies and laws governing an institution will help to change the mentality of an organization and its employees.

Just as physical policies have much to do with the business of an organization, so do the administration and leadership managing that organization. Therefore, effective implementation of just culture principles necessitates the active involvement of those operating the organization. The leaders of a healthcare organization must buy into the concept of just culture and begin to incorporate its principles in the work they perform on a daily basis.[4] To this point, healthcare administrators and employees in leadership positions must not present the concept of just culture as an initiative or a temporary program but rather as a change in mindset that should be applied situationally.[4] This practice should begin with the provision of education to medical staff about which behaviors are considered reckless and therefore punishable.[4] Furthermore, informing medical staff about the range of behaviors that occur in the workplace and the relative degrees of severity of those behaviors is important.[4] In this context, simulation activities can be very useful in enabling employees to better understand the practical application of just culture principles. Finally, requiring departments to work together to achieve specified goals with regard to just culture principles can be a productive way to foster and reward desirable behavior.

Under the just culture model, every effort at preventing medical errors should be made.[7] In health care, one of the most effective ways to decrease the occurrence of preventable medical errors is to build redundancy into processes, particularly high-risk procedures.[7] Creating checks and rechecks both prior to and during medical procedures both in the office and operating room can prevent most honest mistakes.[7] Standardizing protocols can help to mitigate risk, such as fatigue, distractions, overload, and complexity.[7] Unfortunately, however, the causes of many medical errors are unpredictable.[7] But greater insight into such causes can be gained through increased investigation of weaknesses and mistakes.[7] Investigation must also be made into the processes and systems that may have contributed to such medical errors.[7] Efforts of this kind can be accomplished through the establishment of reporting systems, for example.

The aforementioned strategies can be better understood by examining the experiences individual healthcare organizations have had in attempting to implement just culture principles.

ONE ORGANIZATION'S APPROACH TO ESTABLISHMENT OF A JUST CULTURE

In 2001, Fairview Health Services (Fairview) discovered, from an assessment of patient safety, that its culture needed to change.[4] Specifically, Fairview set about to transform its leadership culture, which sets the tone for the behavior of others, in addition to its team culture, or culture at the point of care.[4] Since Fairview is a large, integrated healthcare delivery system, it decided to team up with the Minnesota Alliance for Patient Safety (MAPS) in its attempt to establish a unified just culture.[4] MAPS is a multistakeholder group founded by the Minnesota Hospital Association, the Minnesota Department of Health, and the Minnesota Medical Association.[4]

The organization found that establishing a just culture requires action on the following three fronts: raising awareness, implementing just culture policies, and building just culture principles into the organization's practices.[4] In beginning its efforts, the organization sought to build awareness. With help from David Marx, one of the founders of the just culture model and the president of Outcome Engineering, the organization conducted a survey of its administration, leadership, medical staff, and managers concerning the organization's response to harm.[4] The organization was somewhat astounded by the results of the survey, which found that members of the organization were largely unaware of how the organization would respond when the wrong behavioral choice was made by an employee or provider.[4] Furthermore, the survey revealed that if the wrong behavioral choice was made, members of the organization were much more likely to judge that behavior harshly.[4]

After completion of this survey, the organization raised awareness by educating the members of its organization. Organization leadership attended a daylong session with David Marx, which informed attendees about how they could implement just culture principles both within their organizations and at a larger level throughout the state.[4] After this session, 60 Minnesota healthcare leaders attended a two-day summit sponsored by MAPS, focused on helping healthcare professionals better understand the just culture concepts.[4] Following these separate sessions, a large-scale educational session was provided for operational and clinical leaders throughout the system, where individuals were educated on the use of a set of algorithms aimed at guiding them through practical application of the just culture principles.[4] Participants in the training session were also given opportunities to practice applying these algorithms to real-life scenarios.[4]

Following its efforts related to raising awareness and providing education, Fairview was able to begin practical application of just culture principles to the delivery of health care. Fairview implemented clear policies and behavior expectations relating to just culture principles in the hopes of changing individual behaviors.[4] Furthermore, Fairview integrated just culture principles into two of its performance improvement initiatives related to patient identification and hand-washing procedures specifically.[4] Fairview also made efforts to incorporate just culture principles into its team training activities.[4]

In summary, Fairview's approach to implementation of the just culture model was quite strategic. Due to the sheer size of the organization, Fairview made the wise decision to team up with a state sponsor, namely MAPS, to ensure consistency within its large delivery system. Additionally, Fairview acquired the participation of David Marx, the father of the just culture concept, likely in an effort to increase buy in from members of the organization. Moreover, the involvement of David Marx brought significant legitimacy to Fairview's efforts, suggesting to its staff and neighboring healthcare organizations the importance of just culture concepts in the delivery of safe and effective health care.

THE DANA-FARBER CANCER INSTITUTE'S "PRINCIPLES OF A FAIR AND JUST CULTURE"

The Dana-Farber Cancer Institute (DFCI), in Boston, Massachusetts, provides another important example of the implementation of just culture principles within a healthcare organization. After finding itself in the media spotlight following two tragic incidents involving chemotherapy overdoses, DFCI created its own "Principles for a Fair and Just Culture."[8] These principles define the behavioral expectations of the Institute's staff and managers when a medical error occurs.[8] Moreover, the principles created by DFCI apply to all departments of the medical center, including the clinical, research, and administrative arenas.[8]

Unfortunately the development of just culture principles at DFCI was driven in part by the occurrence of two very serious chemotherapy overdoses in 1995 that resulted in the death of one patient and the cardiac toxicity of another.[8] Following these events, DFCI began an investigation and eventually discovered that significant problems existed with some its major systems and their functioning.[8] DFCI subsequently lost deemed status with Medicare and was placed on conditional accreditation by The Joint Commission.[8] As a result of what had transpired, DFCI began to incorporate the use of root cause analysis (RCA) into its medical error evaluation processes to more thoroughly examine errors in the context of the systems in which they occurred.[8] This change in the way DFCI did business resulted in an accompanying change in mindset. The organization began to realize the importance of transparency, accountability, and learning in the delivery of quality health care.[8]

Soon thereafter, the organization decided to formally articulate its belief in such ideals by creating the now-existing "Principles of a Fair and Just Culture."[8] In drafting these principles, DFCI was guided by three organizational needs, the first being that staff seemed unaware of what a nonpunitive reporting system entailed.[8] The second organizational need identified was that supervisory staff was unequipped to address errors in a nonpunitive way because most of the staff was socialized using the old method of error management and reporting.[8] Finally, the human resources department at DFCI learned that most employees were being disciplined using a punitive approach and were generally unfamiliar with a systems analysis.[8]

With these needs in mind, the organization gathered employees and medical staff from a variety of departments to draft just culture principles specifically tailored to its organization.[8] Individuals from the following departments were involved: management, pharmacy, nursing, human resources, quality improvement, and legal.[8] Charged with heading the committee were the vice president of patient care services and the chief nursing officer.[8] Appointing such individuals in leadership roles was a strategic decision on the part of DFCI, likely intended to ensure that whatever decisions made were feasible in terms of implementation.

After meeting several times, the group quickly realized that its members had varying degrees of knowledge of the principles of nonpunitive reporting.[8] However, human resources employees were identified as being the most familiar with a systems approach; therefore, those individuals were given a leadership role within the group.[8] Within a relatively short period of time the members of the group agreed that one defining principle should guide their work—that it is safe to talk about mistakes.[8] After agreeing on this central principle, the team added a physician researcher and the director of environmental health and safety to its team.[8] The team worked together in making the first draft of just culture principles, which was eventually presented to a series of executive committees at DFCI in 2003.[8] A number of revisions resulted.[8] Medical staff and administrators who took issue with some of the concepts and details of the principles proposed were able to make suggestions and recommend specific changes.[8] This process therefore involved a large percentage of DFCI staff. Eventually, the revised set of principles was presented to the organization's board of trustees and was granted unanimous approval.[8]

The team's seven principles were approved and titled "Principles of a Fair and Just Culture."[8] The first principle set out the organization's core values of impact, excellence, respect, compassion, and discovery in the workplace.[8] DFCI's second principle established its standards for transparency and accountability and for understanding and recognizing errors made.[8] The third principle specified that individuals were to be held accountable for only their own performance flaws and not for system failures.[8] DFCI's fourth principle promoted an open discussion between disciplines within the organization, and DFCI's fifth principle aimed to improve all areas of the workplace by implementing changes based on analysis of existing problems having the potential to cause harm.[8] DFCI's sixth principle committed the organization to a culture of inclusion and education, and DFCI's seventh and final principle required that the organization continually monitor and assess its attitudes and actions in furthering these goals intended to create a culture of safety and support.[8]

Following receipt of approval, the team was able to begin working toward implementation of these principles.[8] DFCI was realistic in beginning this phase, recognizing that changing the organizational culture would be a multiyear process.[8] The organization began the implementation phase by instilling the agreed-on principles with its senior leadership and diversity council.[8] This aim was achieved by having said individuals attend two full-day retreats.[8] Those involved in creating the principles actively participated in these retreats to aid in learning.[8]

Next, the principles were presented to midlevel managers and staff in various departments of DFCI.[8] The team developed a train-the-trainer module that was provided to midlevel managers to use to train their staff with regard to these principles.[8] The module also helped staff to understand how to practically apply these principles on a daily basis.[8] The organization also added an introduction to the principles to its orientation for new staff so that those entering the organization could make a seamless transition.[8]

Although the process is ongoing, DFCI noticed a few rather immediate changes in its systems as a result of implementation of just culture principles. For example, when an adverse event does occur, managers now refer the incident to the risk management department, where the case is studied, reviewed, and an RCA is performed if necessary.[8] In the past, when an adverse event occurred, a disciplinary process was immediately activated and although an individual might have learned something, the organization failed to better understand potential deficiencies in its processes.[8]

As this case study demonstrates, achieving a just culture in the healthcare setting is an involved process. Moreover, effective implementation of just culture principles and policies requires coordinated efforts by leadership, managers, medical staff, and all other employees of a healthcare organization. If administration and those in leadership positions on the organization's staff are not fully committed to the ideals of the just culture model, behaviors are unlikely to change and mistakes are likely to be repeated.

Much can be learned from the trials and tribulations other healthcare organizations have experienced in their attempts to create a just and fair culture. In reviewing its own process, DFCI proffered five tips for organizations that decide to embark on a similar journey. DFCI's first recommendation is to develop an understanding on the part of employees that a blame-free culture does not absolve individuals of accountability.[8] Second, DFCI suggests that organizations include the value of respect in their founding principles for achieving a just culture.[8] Third, DFCI advises that executive leaders and board members both understand and support the principles ultimately adopted.[8] Finally, DFCI advocates for the measurement of the effects implementation of just culture principles have on the organization's delivery of health care.[8] As these suggestions indicate, an organization's employees need to be thoroughly educated about the practical implications of just culture principles, as well as their founding ideals, if they are expected to put them into action. Furthermore, employees of a healthcare organization seeking to implement a just culture must be made cognizant of the important role each individual plays in achieving the aims of these ideals.

Even larger scale initiatives than those made by Fairview and DFCI have been affected in an effort to successfully incorporate just culture principles into the delivery of safe and effective health care. One such collaboration is explored in the section that follows. Specifically, a statewide effort was made that involved not only healthcare administrators and providers but also regulators and educators. Efforts of this kind suggest the importance of coordination and learning in the implementation of just culture principles within the healthcare environment.

A STATEWIDE EFFORT TO IMPLEMENT THE JUST CULTURE MODEL

In Missouri, the Missouri Center for Patient Safety (MOCPS) engaged 67 organizations in the Missouri Just Culture Collaborative.[9] The collaborative consisted of healthcare systems, acute-care and critical-access hospitals, physician practices, regulators, nursing homes, professional schools, and nursing associations.[9] By combining these groups, the collaborative was able to help more than 4,000 individuals in their efforts to implement a just culture.[9] Specifically, the collaborative helped to integrate just culture concepts into provider and regulatory agency daily activities, to improve understanding among healthcare leaders of constructive perceptions of safety, and to cultivate statewide interest in the just culture concepts.[9]

After holding a statewide leadership meeting, the collaborative had successfully convinced 67 healthcare organizations to join them.[9] To join the collaborative, organizations were required to complete an online training program, participate in on-site educational training sessions, and implement learning acquired through the collaborative in their respective institutions.[9] Furthermore, after receiving approval from the Institutional Review Board (IRB), the collaborative was able to measure the performance of these 67 organizations in implementing just culture principles.[9]

The findings yielded from the study are both encouraging and informative. First, the collaborative provided participants with a clearer understanding of just culture concepts and their application to healthcare delivery.[9] Second, the collaborative helped regulators better understand their role in implementation of a just culture, namely, support of healthcare organizations working to implement such principles.[9] Moreover, the study uncovered some of the legislative and regulatory barriers to implementation of just culture principles, which include the need regulators experience to take disciplinary action against individuals involved in adverse events.[9] Furthermore, regulators reported gaining an increased understanding of how the implementation of just culture principles can improve patient safety by encouraging organizations to uncover the root causes of adverse events and learn from mistakes made.[9] Finally, regulators suggested further coordination and cooperation among regulators, agencies, and healthcare organizations in an effort to create a stronger learning environment.[9]

The Missouri Just Culture Collaborative illustrates the benefits of working toward implementation of just culture principles at a large scale. Although coordinated action at a statewide level can be difficult and involves significant resources, the learning fostered by such efforts is tremendous. However, regardless of the size of an organization's efforts, it is essential that any healthcare organization attempting to establish a just culture take certain steps in achieving that aim.

THE TOOLS NECESSARY FOR EFFECTUATION OF A JUST CULTURE

Implementation of just culture principles in a chaotic healthcare organization is undoubtedly a complicated undertaking. Not only can practical application of just culture principles be difficult, but this transformation of mentality with regard to medical errors also takes time. Therefore, it is necessary to apply certain practical tools that aid in effectuating the process.

The first important tool is the clear articulation of just culture principles intended to be implemented.[2] Specifically, experts recommend that an organization setting out to achieve a just culture develop a just culture strategic vision document or a set of specific principles that is drafted and signed by all interested and affected parties.[2]

Another important tool for use in implementation of a just culture is the unsafe acts algorithm.[2] This algorithm provides a practical method of ensuring a just assessment of individual acts, imparting hospital managers with a list of questions to investigate when determining the appropriate course of action required following a medical error.[2]

A third tool that can be used to support the development of a just culture is open commitment to "just citizenship."[2] In other words, providers and staff should be expected to support transparency and open communication, such that the just culture principles are reinforced in practice.[2]

Safety concepts should also be incorporated in training and evaluation of hospital staff to establish a just culture. Concepts of safety should be an integral part of new employee orientation, nursing competencies, and physician credentialing, for example.[2] Successful incorporation of concepts of safety in these processes will ensure that employees and providers are reminded of their ultimate goal in adopting just culture principles, which is the improvement of patient safety.

Another productive tool for the development of a just culture is the engagement of hospital leadership.[2] Leadership oversight can afford further coordination among quality, safety, and risk management departments, managing these relationships and promoting open communication.[2] The WalkRounds concept illustrates the role leadership can play in the achievement of a just culture.[2] During WalkRounds, hospital leadership essentially walks around the hospital premises and has somewhat informal conversations with healthcare providers.[2] WalkRounds not only elicit useful information for use by leadership but also foster transparency and openness within an organization.[2] Provided information yielded by a program such as WalkRounds is used to make changes in the physical work environment, leadership has accomplished the goal of engaging its organization in the quest for a more just culture.

Related to the proper engagement of leadership in the formation of a just culture is the advancement of teamwork. It is absolutely critical in this changing healthcare environment that clinicians work as a team. As the dependence on technology in healthcare delivery grows, barriers to effective teamwork among clinicians perpetuate.[2] Therefore, critical tools must be applied to encourage collaborative work.[2] Namely, education and simulation can present helpful practices in stimulating teamwork in the healthcare environment.[2]

The basic core skills of effective teamwork include structured language (or SBAR, which stands for situation, background, assessment, and recommendation), critical language, and psychological safety.[2] Structured language, such as the use of SBAR, provides a common template for communication.[2] Due to the variance in personal communication styles, structured language can ease the achievement of successful communication, particularly in the hectic healthcare environment.[2] Critical language, or assertion language, is similar, in that it provides yet another mechanism for increased communication.[2] Critical language can enable providers to more simply voice their concerns.[2] Finally, psychological safety ensures that people can voice their concerns without fear of judgment.[2] This tool effectively curbs avoidable harm by encouraging providers to recognize and report on opportunities for improvement.[2]

Simulation models afford a final tool for effective implementation of just culture principles.[2] Although restrictions exist on the complexity of simulation that can be attempted, such efforts are both flexible and cost effective.[2] Simulation can be done using computerized mannequins or can be performed within clinical units where care is actually delivered.[2] Although simulation demands a significant amount of resources, it can be very realistic and therefore can provide an incredibly useful learning tool.[2] Interactive classroom training can also be attempted as a sort of simplistic simulation tool. The benefit of interactive classroom training is that many more individuals can be incorporated in a single session.[2] In the context of teamwork training, simulation can help individuals communicate more effectively and collaborate with one another when useful.[2] These trainings help individuals develop an entirely new set of skills that will prove extremely helpful in solving clinical problems that require much more than just clinical knowledge.[2]

In conclusion, a healthcare organization seeking to implement the just culture model should begin by articulating the just culture principles it hopes to advance in writing and explaining to its staff what these principles explicitly mean in practice. Then, the organization should engage leadership in implementation of just culture principles. Finally, the organization should provide its staff with opportunities for practicing implementation of these principles by having staff participate in simulation activities, for example. While all of these tools and practices are advantageous in the development of a just culture organization, leadership is especially critical in fostering values and driving behaviors that reflect accountability, enhanced communication, and a preoccupation with safety.

CONCLUSION

Since the Institute of Medicine (IOM) released the *To Err Is Human: Building a Safer Health System* report in 1999, patient safety has become an area of increasing concern within the healthcare industry.[6] Moreover, the IOM report importantly revealed that the majority of medical errors result due to failings in systems and processes, not in people.[6] The revelations contained in the IOM report have significantly affected the just culture movement, stimulating healthcare organizations across the country to assess their work environments and remove punitive approaches to medical error assessment and management.

The just culture model fosters increased safety in the delivery of health care by promoting transparency, fairness, communication, and learning.[6] Unfortunately, changes in the healthcare environment cannot be achieved overnight. However, the just culture model provides regulators, leadership, providers, and healthcare organization employees with practical tools and tips for the successful implementation of principles specifically focused on improving patient safety. With defined just culture principles, involved leadership, informed staff, and opportunities for training and practice, an organization can achieve a just culture environment in which errors are openly disclosed, deficiencies in systems and processes are appropriately addressed, and patient safety is made the number one priority.

References

1. Marx D. (2001). *Patient safety and the "just culture": A primer for health care executives*. New York, NY: Columbia University. Retrieved from http://www.unmc.edu/rural/patient-safety/tools/Marx%20Patient%20Safety%20and%20Just%20Culture.pdf.
2. Frankel, A. S., Leonard, M. W., & Denham, C. R. (2006). Fair and just culture, team behavior, and leadership engagement: The tools to achieve high reliability. *Health Services Research, 41*, 1690–1709.
3. Marx, D. (2007). *Patient safety and the "just culture."* Retrieved from http://www.health.ny.gov/professionals/patients/patient_safety/conference/2007/docs/patient_safety_and_the_just_culture.pdf.
4. Page, A. H. (2007). *Making just culture a reality: one organization's approach*. U.S. Department of Health and Human Services, Agency for Healthcare Research and Quality. Retrieved from http://webmm.ahrq.gov/perspective.aspx?perspectiveID=50.
5. Griffith, K. S. (2009). Column: The growth of just culture. *The Joint Commission Perspectives on Patient Safety, 9*(12), 8–9. Retrieved from http://www.justculture.org/media/Joint_Commission-Just_Culture.pdf.
6. Vogelsmeier, A., & Scott-Cawiezell, J. (2007). A just culture: The role of nursing leadership. *Journal of Nursing Care Quality, 22*(3), 210–212. Retrieved from http://www.sjsu.edu/people/phyllis.connolly/courses/c17/s1/Volegjustcult25551475.pdf.
7. Pastorius, D. (2007). Crime in the workplace, part 1. *Nursing Management, 38*(10), 18, 20, 22, 24, 26–27. Retrieved from http://www.nursingcenter.com/pdf.asp?AID=746042.
8. Connor, M., Duncombe, D., Barclay, E., Bartel, S., Borden, C., Gross, E., . . . Reid Ponte, P. (2007). Creating a fair and just culture: One institution's path toward organizational change. *The Joint Commission Journal on Quality and Patient Safety, 33*(10), 617–624. Retrieved from http://psnet.ahrq.gov/public/Connor_JtCommJQualPatientSaf_2007.pdf.
9. Miller, R., Griffith, S., & Vogelsmeier A. (2011). A statewide approach to a just culture for patient safety: The Missouri story. *Journal of Nursing Regulation, 1*(1), 52–57. Retrieved from http://www.mocps.org/wp-content/uploads/2011/05/JNR0410_Miller_Final.pdf.

14

Addressing Clinician Performance Problems as a Systems Issue

John A. Fromson, MD

Systems issues can contribute to addressing clinical performance problems. Suboptimal clinical performance can be related to knowledge and skill deficits or be the result of health-related issues. Barring an underlying organic etiology to the problem, such as dementia, various knowledge and skill deficits can usually be addressed with educational or remediation activities. Yet, like the general population, practitioners are also susceptible to psychoactive substance use disorders, mental health issues, and physical illness and disability. Left untreated, these conditions can interfere with professional performance. Knowledge and skill deficits, as well as a clinician's illness, can be mediated or influenced by the context or system in which they take place.

Practice setting systems, from major academic teaching centers to private office venues, are sometimes unable to respond to suboptimal performance in a proactive, timely, and decisive way. The reasons for this are multifold. The practitioner's problem may be difficult to detect at an early stage when the ability to practice is not affected. In addition, the institution may have organizational, supervisory, and economic issues that serve as barriers to an effective administrative response to the problem. This chapter looks at how addressing substandard performance can be influenced by systems issues.

In institutional settings, deficits in knowledge or in specific skills are usually identified by clinical supervisors or by risk managers utilizing quality improvement thresholds. When administrative procedural thresholds, such as timely dictation, or clinical thresholds, such as mortality, have not been met, the data can be de-identified and shared in a group setting, or outliers can be given feedback on an individual basis. Because of the difficulty of giving constructive feedback to a colleague, this process is one of the more administratively challenging tasks that a chief of service or a department head faces. However, a factor that helps facilitate the process is that there is usually a staff person at the institution whose responsibility is to monitor these indices. It is also required by The Joint Commission and other certifying organizations, so that the institutionalization of this process has been going on for decades.

Constructive feedback is usually enough to engage the practitioner to take corrective action. If a specific clinical procedure or outcome measure such as infection rate persists, the institution can recommend specific educational programs with the hopes that outcomes will improve. If these fail, the institution then has the option of engaging assessment and remediation programs.[1] Using psychometric testing, chart reviews, observed clinical examinations of standardized patients, and fund-of-knowledge testing, the assessments are designed to ascertain the etiology of the problem. If it is due to knowledge or skill deficits, a remediation plan is devised. If the problem is found to be secondary to an illness, appropriate treatment or counseling the clinician out of the field may take place. When a physician does not comply with recommendations for performance enhancement, administrative sanctions such as restriction or suspension of clinical privileges may be necessary.

Currently, the Federation of State Medical Boards and the National Board of Medical Examiners have instituted a testing protocol, the Special Purpose Examination (SPEX). If the physician in question fails the exam, he or she is referred to the Colorado Personalized Education Program (CPEP) at the Institute for Physician Evaluation for a comprehensive assessment. Physicians can also go to the CPEP program without taking this test or having their respective state medical board involvement. If deficits are detected, an educational remediation program can then be recommended.

A much more complex and difficult situation arises when a practitioner, such as a physician, is not falling short of quality improvement thresholds, but manifests aberrant behavior that has the *potential* to place patients and other staff at risk for harm. While most medical staff bylaws are written in such a way as to give wide latitude towards interpreting the seriousness of these kinds of behaviors, the lack of clear thresholds makes it much more difficult for an administrative response to be initiated. Thus, it may be easier for a system to respond to a healthcare professional who clearly crosses thresholds of performance based on knowledge or skill, than it is to respond to one who has subtle manifestations of a substance use disorder, mental or physical illness, or behavioral problem.

Psychoactive substance use disorders occur generally at the same rate in healthcare professionals as they do in the general population.[2] Interestingly enough, for physicians, problems associated with alcohol use actually increase with age, as opposed to the general population, where they decrease.[3] Why this is so is not clear. Yet, throughout a physician's active professional life, a significant amount of time and energy is directed toward developing clinical competence, savvy, and acumen. This can come at the exclusion of cultivating and nurturing interpersonal relationships. If one enters middle and late adulthood and begins to limit the number of hours practicing medicine, it can be hypothesized that there is more time for intimacy, especially with a significant other. The very short-term disinhibiting effect of alcohol may be used to facilitate closeness with a loved one. Conversely, the longer term sedating effects may contribute to avoiding intimacy altogether. Perhaps this contributes to the age-related increase in alcohol-related problems among physicians.

In active clinical practice, stress, isolation, accessibility, family history, and chronic medical conditions such as ongoing pain, contribute to drug and alcohol use.[4] As one becomes more addicted and physiologically dependent on psychoactive substances, relationships and activities begin to become impaired. First, spousal or significant other relationships deteriorate, followed in turn by nuclear family member relationships, extended family member relationships, friends, extracurricular-type activities, community and religious involvement, and the last area to be affected is professional practice. The drug of choice may determine the timeframe for identification. For example, a short-acting synthetic narcotic analgesic such as sufentanil may take weeks to months before impairing the ability to practice. At the other end of the spectrum, detection in the workplace of alcohol use could take years.

In the practice setting, avoidance in confronting or reporting a colleague can also be secondary to denial of observing colleagues or to over-identification with the physician who has a problem. In the latter case, peers are reluctant to intervene as they are all too familiar with the rigors associated with achieving professional credentials and subsequent success and feel they do not want to "punish" their flailing colleague. They also feel doing it would be too emotionally painful for them, at once mindful that inactivity in the face of the risk of harm to patients is inexcusable.

Illustrating this point is a 42-year-old cardiologist[5] found to have alcohol on her breath while engaging in an office-based practice. While her practice partner acknowledged the problem after it was brought to his attention by office staff, it took two more episodes and an inquiry by a patient before she was referred to the state's physician health program. During the referral process, the practice partner acknowledged that he was fearful to do anything, even as he was mindful of the risk to patients, because he had had trouble successfully hiring for his partner's position. He also depended on the practice partner for coverage and handling the large caseload of referred patients with cardiac problems. He was given positive reinforcement for trying to get help for his colleague. However, he had a difficult time appreciating that loss of revenue and the added stress of not having full coverage paled in comparison to a bad outcome with harm to a patient due to his ambivalence in referring the physician for help.

The changes that take place with drug or alcohol use over time are subtle. There seems to be a very thin line that is crossed between being a productive practitioner and one that is beginning to go down the slippery slope of addiction. It takes an astute observer to pick out these subtle changes in their early stages. Finally, when the point is reached where there are overt manifestations of impairment in terms of the ability to practice medicine, interventions are usually made. These manifestations can occur on many levels:

- *Personal:* Deteriorating hygiene, accidents, inappropriate behavior, excessive prescriptions for self and family members, and escalating emotional crises
- *In home and family:* Behavior excused by family and friends, drinking activities given priority, arguments, violent outbursts, sexual problems, withdrawal from family, fragmentation, neglect of children, financial crises, separation or divorce, unexplained absences at home
- *With friends and community:* Personal isolation, embarrassing behavior, drunk driving arrests, legal problems, neglect of social commitments, inappropriate spending
- *In the office:* Workaholic behavior (which may be seen as role modeling by colleagues), disorganized scheduling, unreasonable behavior with patients and staff, frequent absences, excessive prescriptions for drugs, excessive ordering of drug supplies, frequent complaints, prolonged breaks, and alcohol on the breath[6]

It is only when these later signs are manifested and patients are placed at risk that colleagues are mobilized into action to intervene.

Psychiatric and physical illness may present in a similar fashion and engender the same reluctance on the part of colleagues to intervene. Often the only early signs are mental status and physical changes that slowly manifest and progressively worsen over time, as illustrated by the following case.

A 54-year-old surgeon began making negativistic and inappropriate comments to the hospital staff. At the same time, he initiated "midnight rounds," claiming, "I'm not tired, so we should see the patients now and I can get started early with surgery." Inability to fall asleep, agitation, negativistic behavior, and later lewd and problematic comments to patients were the early signs of a manic phase of bipolar illness. Despite the knowledge by the chief of his department of these overt stigmata of a mood disorder, there was no attempt to confront this physician until he was pulled over for speeding and arrested after assaulting a police officer. After inpatient hospitalization, outpatient treatment is now monitored by the state physician health program. When questioned, the department chief commented that at his community hospital he had taken on the administrative role of chief on a voluntary, unpaid, rotating basis. He felt he had no real supervisory authority over this physician since the physician was not an employee of the hospital but "just" had attending privileges there. He also commented that he and others were willing to give the physician in question the "benefit of the doubt" because the revenue the affected physician generated for the hospital was crucial during a particularly trying financial time the institution was experiencing.

Also difficult to stop or prevent in its early stages are repetitive verbalizations, deeds, or actions that are not the result of what one would usually refer to as easily recognizable mental illness, but have the potential to be a detriment to patient care. These physicians are often referred to as "disruptive" and manifest inappropriate anger, blaming, threatening, uncooperative, and unprofessional behavior. They often have an underlying personality disorder and see themselves as always "right" and the rest of the world as "wrong."

An example is a 72-year-old obstetrician-gynecologist with a large and lucrative practice who would use profanity when under stress during routine or difficult hospital procedures. When told that his words were negatively affecting the work environment, he responded by saying that the lack of staff support was responsible for the undue stress he was experiencing and that he had to say what he did to get the operating team to respond to critical situations. In essence, he felt he behaved the way he did in the interest of patient care. Only when nurse retention was at stake did the administration take action and require him to attend a physician health program–sponsored anger management course. He also voluntarily entered into psychotherapy.

Whether clinical performance problems arise from knowledge or skill deficits, health concerns such as psychoactive substance use disorders, mental or physical illness, or a behavioral issue, early intervention that can result in treatment and recovery are difficult to initiate because of the subtle signs and symptoms of the underlying problem and by systems barriers. The latter can range from administrative inactivity due to denial and over-identification with the affected professional, to over-reliance on formal professional relationships such as partnership and the need to provide patients with coverage. Administrative barriers at this level may also include an open staff model where there is a paucity of direct supervision and accountability. This can be seen when there is a voluntary, rotating, supervisory administrative position such as a chief of a department, who may be dependent on the physician in crisis. Economic dependency may also contribute to inactivity.

A model for identifying the source of professional performance problems and the strategy to correct them is similar to the various proposed confidential near miss reporting systems used for medical errors. However, instead of looking at a specific error or harmful event, the focus can be placed on the healthcare professional such as a physician. There are physician health programs in all 50 states. There are also similar programs for nurses and other healthcare professionals as well. Most physician programs are designed to help identify, refer to treatment, guide, and monitor physicians with psychoactive substance use disorders. Most also deal with physicians who have mental or physical illness, or behavior issues. Where there has been no risk of harm to patients, many state licensing boards of registration in medicine allow physicians to be referred to these peer review protected (and hence confidential) programs in lieu of a board administrative response. In essence, this is very similar to a voluntary near miss medical error reporting system, where medical errors that do no harm are reported to a confidential data repository. Where there is patient harm, those reports are made to a governmental regulatory agency. The difference here is that instead of reporting a specific error or harmful event, it is a physician who is the entity being referred. Not only is the physician referred to appropriate treatment and monitored so he or she can return to practice, but de-identified data are compiled and shared among physician health programs for educational and preventative purposes.[7]

Effective January 1, 2001, The Joint Commission has required that hospital organizations have their medical staff implement a process to identify and manage matters of individual physician health, which is separate from the medical and staff disciplinary function. The intent of the The Joint Commission's requirement (Physician Health MS.2.6) is consistent in many aspects to the mission of most physician health programs, which is to assist physicians with health concerns and therefore provide protections to patients. In this regard, The Joint Commission requires medical staff and organization leaders to design a process that provides education about physician health, addresses prevention of physical, psychiatric, or emotional illness, and facilitates confidential diagnosis, treatment, and rehabilitation of physicians from a potentially impairing condition.

As The Joint Commission provides, the purpose of the process is assistance and rehabilitation, rather than discipline, to aid a physician in retaining or regaining optimal professional functioning, consistent with protection of patients. If at any time during the diagnosis, treatment, or rehabilitation phase of the process it is determined that a physician is unable to safely perform the privileges he or she has been granted, the matter is forwarded to medical staff leadership for appropriate corrective action, which includes strict adherence to any state or federally mandated reporting requirements.

The process design should include:

- Education of the medical staff and other organization staff about illness and impairment recognition issues specific to physicians;
- Self-referral by a physician and referral by other organization staff;
- Referral of the affected physician to the appropriate professional internal or external resources for diagnosis and treatment of the condition or concern;
- Maintenance of the confidentiality of the physician seeking referral or referred for assistance, except as limited by law, ethical obligation, or when the safety of a patient is threatened;
- Evaluation of the credibility of a complaint, allegation, or concern;
- Monitoring of the affected physician and the safety of patients until the rehabilitation or any disciplinary process is complete; and
- Reporting to the medical staff leadership instances in which a physician is providing unsafe treatment.[8]

Physicians' performance problems can be the result of knowledge and skill deficits, psychoactive substance use disorders, mental and physical illness, or behavioral problems. Barriers to taking early and decisive intervention leading to referral for remediation or assessment, treatment, and monitoring can be related to systems issues. These include practice setting, supervisory and collegial relationships, and economic associations. Assessment and physician health programs can assist both the individual physician and systems experiencing these difficulties.

References

1. Physician Prescribed Educational Program (PPEP) Syracuse, NY (315) 464-6997. Colorado Personalized Education for Physicians (CPEP), Denver, CO (303) 750-7150.
2. Flaherty, J.A., Richman, J.A. 1993. Substance use and addiction among medical students, residents and physicians. *Psychiatric Clinics of North America. 16*(1): 189–97.
3. Ibid.
4. Farley, W.J. 1992. Addiction and the anaesthesia resident. *Can Journal Anaesth. 39* (5) R11.
5. Cases have been de-identified to protect confidentiality.
6. Physicians Recovery Network—Alabama Physicians Health Program.
7. To access more information about state physician health programs, contact the Federation of State Physician Health Programs at www.amaassn.org.
8. Physician Health Services, Inc., a Massachusetts Medical Society subsidiary, at www.physicianhealth.org.

15

IMPROVING HEALTH LITERACY TO ADVANCE PATIENT SAFETY

Caroline Chapman, JD

INTRODUCTION

More than 300 studies have shown that health information cannot be understood by most of the people for whom it is intended, suggesting that the assumptions regarding the recipient's level of health literacy made by the creators of this information are often incorrect.[1] Almost 83 million adults in the United States struggle to understand basic information about their health and medical care. According to the 2003 National Assessment of Adult Literacy, conducted by the U.S. Department of Education, 36% of adults have below basic or only basic health literacy.[2] This means that more than a third of adults in the United States cannot read a prescription drug label well enough to determine what time to take the medication with regard to eating. More than one-third of adults in the United States cannot find the age range in which a child should receive a vaccine using a table or understand a body mass index chart. More than one-third of adults cannot read an over-the-counter drug label well enough to identify substances that may interact badly with the drug.[2] Perhaps an even more disturbing trend revealed by the study is the populations for whom health literacy limits are endemic: elderly patients, nonnative English speakers, and the poor. For these patients, many of whom already face barriers to getting medical care, limited health literacy creates yet another obstacle to accessing meaningful, appropriate, and safe care.

On the other side of the equation, only about 12% of adults in this country are proficient with health information.[2] In other words, just over one in 10 adult patients possess the reading and quantitative skills needed to process the full range of information about their health. Lest we feel confident with this 12%, even these numbers may deceive because study participants answered questions under optimal conditions, none experiencing the stress of acute illness or the fear that accompanies a life-threatening diagnosis. Physicians, nurses, pharmaceutical companies, and public health agencies are all talking to Americans, but the data show that they are simply not being understood.

That healthcare providers and patient safety experts concern themselves at all with patients' health literacy is in large part a reflection of the changing role of patients in recent decades. The current U.S. healthcare system is undergoing a revolution in perspective by being challenged to become patient centered and to ask individuals to take an active role in medical decision making, choosing quality providers, disease self-management, and in safety efforts.[1] The simultaneous proliferation of pharmaceuticals and the increasingly complex web of health insurance have significantly complicated patients' roles in their own care. The degree to which patients have the capacity to obtain, process, and understand the information required for good medical decision making in all these arenas will directly affect how safe and effective their health care is. Never before have successful outcomes depended so directly on the skills not just of caregivers but also of patients themselves. Upon this schematic, we must now impose the stark National Assessment of Adult Literacy (NAAL)[2] data demonstrating that only about one in 10 patients has the skills for the task.

Even this brief introduction to the concept of health literacy evokes the obvious practical link between the ability of patients to understand and process health information and patient safety. When communication between patients and providers is derailed by the patient's inability to meaningfully comprehend what he or she is reading or being told, opportunities for adverse events abound. After analyzing its extensive data on sentinel events, The Joint Commission concluded that the failures of communication are the root cause of nearly every reported unexpected death and catastrophic injury.[3] Similarly, studies reviewed by the Institute of Medicine (IOM) in its landmark report, *To Err Is Human*, reveal that as many as 10% of adverse drug events arise from communication errors.[4] Patients who cannot accurately identify their medications or fill out medical history forms or who nod yes to any question asked because of limited English are at risk for a panoply of errors with each and every medical encounter. To make sure those encounters are safe, providers must make meaningful reciprocal communication of health information one of their highest priorities.

HEALTH LITERACY DEFINITION

The definition of health literacy proposed by the National Library of Medicine and used in *Healthy People 2010*[5] has been adopted by the Institute of Medicine in its recently published seminal report on health literacy, *Health Literacy: A Prescription to End Confusion*, and has since become widely used.[1] Under this definition, health literacy is, at its most basic, "the degree to which individuals have the capacity to obtain, process, and understand basic health information and services needed to make appropriate health decisions."[1]

Beyond its most basic definition, health literacy has also been defined in more functional terms. Functional health literacy has been noted to include "the ability to understand instructions on prescription drug bottles, appointment slips, medical education brochures, doctor's directions and consent forms, and the ability to negotiate complex health care systems."[6] To be fully functional, health literacy also requires oral communication skills, such as being able to articulate symptoms, to formulate relevant questions, and to convey health history and current treatment.[1] In addition, health literacy in the information age requires quantitative literacy, or numeracy: the ability to perform computations and reason numerically. Health literate patients thus need to be able to calculate dosages, interpret test results, weigh risks and benefits, and evaluate health information for quality and accuracy.[1] Notably, patients need to implement their health literacy skills under less than ideal circumstances, generally, when they are sick or under the stress of discovering that they or a loved one has an illness.

These definitions of health literacy are multifaceted, and providers may see themselves as ill equipped to improve the demonstrably poor skills of so many U.S. patients. This has led to a number of efforts to incorporate health literacy building into the U.S. education system and even to a legislative proposal to fund the development of curricula for health literacy to be implemented in schools and colleges and through agencies such as the Centers for Medicare & Medicaid Services (CMS) and public health departments.[7] However, a shift in perspective from the needs of the patients to what might be called the health literacy quotient of providers shows what the latter group can do to ensure meaningful communication of health information. When seen from the perspective of providers, health literacy means the ability to speak and write clearly when addressing patients. Later in this chapter, the components of clear communication will be discussed in detail, but to begin, they include the ability to speak and write plainly about health information; to effectively use visual aids, pictograms, and videos; to implement teach-back techniques in which patients' true comprehension is tested; to provide interpreter services when required; and to provide culturally competent care to all patients. Providers have available to them a variety of fairly simple tools that can be universally applied to facilitate a meaningful exchange with patients seeking care.

HEALTH LITERACY AND PATIENT SAFETY

The literature is replete with anecdotal evidence of a strong link between health literacy and patient safety. From the illiterate patient who nearly bleeds out after misunderstanding his doctor's instructions about taking a blood thinner, to the mother who pours an oral antibiotic into her child's infected ear, to the Spanish-speaking patient who receives another man's medication because he incorrectly nods in response to an identification question asked in English, these stories illustrate the concrete and commonplace medical errors that result from a failure to implement health literacy initiatives.[1,3] A strong logical connection exists between a patient with limited health literacy or limited English proficiency and an increased risk that a communication error with this patient will cause harm.

With this logical starting point, providers have gone to their own data for an evidence-based confirmation of their concerns. One hospital reported to The Joint Commission that they categorized their adverse events by native language of the patient and found "clusters of adverse events in patients with English as a second language."[3] According to the Center for Health Care Strategies, low-literacy patients at 659 public hospitals were five times more likely to misinterpret prescription information.[8] Low literacy also affected the proper use of a metered-dose asthma inhaler and medication compliance among HIV-positive adults.[8] As the field of health literacy has grown over the past decade, so have efforts to study and quantify this link on a broader scale. As the IOM report *Health Literacy: A Prescription to End Confusion* noted, limited health literacy has already been linked to problems with chronic illness management, patient involvement in decision making about treatment, lower adherence to certain therapy regimes, and lower self-reported health status.[1]

The Agency for Healthcare Research and Quality (AHRQ) recently undertook a literature review regarding existing studies of the nexus between health literacy and health outcomes. The authors concluded that low reading skill and poor health were demonstrably related. Additionally, the review confirmed anecdotal evidence that low health literacy does correlate with "a range of adverse health outcomes."[9]

Low numeracy has also been linked to poor outcomes. One study linked low numeracy with poorer anticoagulation control among patients taking warfarin to reduce stroke risk.[10] Another study found that less-numerate women aged 40 to 49 could not accurately assess the risks and benefits of screening for breast cancer although the National Institutes of Health (NIH) advises women in this age group to decide whether to have mammography based on a discussion of the risks and benefits with their physicians.[10] Although the IOM and the AHRQ have both noted that the causal connection between low health literacy and adverse events requires additional study, they concur that existing studies and clinical experience demonstrate a strong connection between the two.

A link has also been demonstrated between low-literacy patients and increased medical expense. Although it is hardly surprising that poor management of chronic illness or failure to adhere to therapy plans creates additional expense for the healthcare system, the IOM report and others have suggested that low-literacy patients have higher hospital utilization rates, higher use of emergency services, and higher inpatient spending rates.[1] The National Academy on an Aging Society estimates that the additional healthcare expenditures due to low health literacy were approximately $73 billion in 1998 healthcare dollars.[11] Money spent to address poor outcomes, increased emergency department use, and longer inpatient stays could be redirected to health literacy programs and education for providers and has the potential to improve outcomes and reduce communication-related errors for patients.

HEALTH LITERACY DATA

It is not always easy to determine which patients have low literacy. These patients may have spent years developing sophisticated masking and coping strategies. They may be articulate and present well. One study of low-literacy patients suggested that low-literacy patients are not likely to share this information with healthcare providers.[12] The study revealed that 85% had not revealed their limited literacy to coworkers and 67% had not even told their spouses. Fifteen percent had told no one. Another study revealed that clinic physicians accurately identified only 20% of their low-literacy patients.[8] Patients themselves may think that their health literacy skills are adequate, but they may simply not be.

The lesson from these studies is twofold. First, health literacy efforts must be implemented universally and contain behavioral and communication changes that improve clarity of communication regardless of the literacy level of the patient or the accuracy of the perceptions of the provider. Second, specific data about populations that may be particularly vulnerable to low health literacy can help providers focus their self-assessment of patient safety issues on those patient's at highest risk for communication-related errors.

Where might this data come from? Providers now have an up-to-date and comprehensive resource in the 2003 National Assessment of Adult Literacy (NAAL). The NAAL was administered to more than 19,000 adults and, for the first time, contained a specific health literacy component.[2] The assessment measured literacy by asking participants to complete literacy tasks, as opposed to self-reporting literacy, drawn from actual health-related materials. The assessment was thus designed to capture the true functional literacy of participants in real-life contexts. The assessment was also designed to measure different types of literacy, each of which reflected skills required to comprehend and properly process health information. The assessment measured prose literacy (basic reading and comprehension), document literacy (the ability to search and read through longer, noncontinuous text), and quantitative literacy (the ability to perform computations using numbers embedded in print materials). The specific tasks focused on three areas of health information: clinical and preventive information and navigation of the healthcare system. None of the tasks required special knowledge of health-related vocabulary. The assessment defined four categories of health literacy. "Below Basic" represents those individuals who range from nonliterate in English to those able to locate easily identifiable information in a short prose text; to locate easily identifiable information and follow simple instructions in charts or forms; and to perform simple computations (such as addition) with concrete and familiar numerical information. Fourteen percent of U.S. adults' health literacy is limited to this level. "Basic" represents those individuals who could read and understand short prose text and simple documents and who could locate numerical information and use it to solve simple, one-step arithmetic operations. Twenty-two percent of adults have only basic health literacy.[2]

"Intermediate" represents the individuals who could read and comprehend moderately complex prose and make simple inferences from it, locate information in dense documents and make simple inferences from it, and locate less familiar quantitative information and use it to solve arithmetic operations not previously specified. Just over half of adults have intermediate health literacy levels. "Proficient" included individuals who could read and comprehend lengthy and abstract prose, integrate and synthesize multiple pieces of information, and locate abstract numerical information and solve multistep problems. Twelve percent of adults are proficient.[2]

Certainly, these numbers are not all discouraging. About two-thirds of adults have intermediate health literacy or higher.[2] Although the skills required for intermediate health literacy may not include the full panoply of skills necessary to reliably navigate all medical encounters, there does appear to be a reasonable cohort of adults who have a degree of competency with medical information. However, a word of caution must be noted regarding this group: health literacy is contextual. The NAAL did not measure the literacy skills of these individuals under the extreme stress of a health crisis. As the U.S. Department of Health and Human Services has aptly noted, "[T]he health literacy capacities of a 50-ish English-speaking woman with 2 years of college and a head cold who is buying a familiar over-the-counter medicine *are different in that moment* from the capacities of that same woman when she undergoes diagnostic tests, learns she has breast cancer, and has two different treatment options, neither of which she really understands."[13] It is important to remember that, although demographic information is unquestionably useful to providers, the benefit of applying health literacy principles universally is the benefit to anyone whose skills in a particular moment are affected by external factors such as extreme stress or physical illness.

Not all the news from the study was good. Just over one-third of adults in the study had only Basic or Below Basic health literacy skills.[2] These individuals cannot consistently read and follow directions on prescription bottles and may have difficulty reading and completing a medical history form or reporting what medications they are currently taking.[2] Although this news is disturbing, the good news is that as a result of the NAAL study, health-care providers are now armed with the relevant data to begin addressing the problem. Although many of the programs discussed in the latter part of this essay would be appropriate to implement for all patients, knowing the depth and breadth of the literacy crisis and which subpopulations may face the greatest health literacy challenges allows providers to target those groups whose literacy limitations may place them at the greatest risk for communication-related adverse events.

On average, women were more health literate than were men, with men representing a higher percentage of the Below Basic population by four percentage points.[2] Breakdowns by race and ethnicity were even more marked. Only 9% of Caucasians had Below Basic health literacy and only another 19% had basic health literacy, whereas 24% of African American adults had Below Basic health literacy and an additional 34% had Basic health literacy.[2] In total, more than one-half of African American adults had not more than Basic health literacy. The study also revealed that 41% of Hispanic adults had Below Basic health literacy in English.[2] This means that almost one-half of the adult Hispanic population in this county is trying to navigate medical encounters with a very limited English literacy skill set. Another 25% of Hispanic adults had only Basic health literacy.

When totaled, two-thirds of Hispanic adults have health literacy limitations.[2] The implications for providers from the race and ethnicity data in the study are profound. Depending on the racial and ethnic makeup of an institution's patient population, significant numbers of patients may need health literacy assistance to ensure safe and appropriate care.

Disparities extended beyond race and ethnicity. Adults 65 and older had the lowest average health literacy score of any other adult age group. Twenty-nine percent of older adults had Below Basic skills and another 30% had only Basic skills.[2] Among seniors, 59% had no more than basic skills.[2] The implications of this measure are significant. We are an aging society, and older adults consume more health services and products than does any other single group.[8] As of 2003, the year the NAAL was conducted, 78% of the Medicare population (those over 65 and some disabled individuals under 65) "suffer from one or more chronic conditions that require ongoing medical management."[14] Strikingly, 20% of the older adult Medicare population has at least five chronic conditions.[14]

The NAAL did not measure the objective health condition of its participants; however, self-reports were taken from participants. Notably, of those who reported their health conditions as poor, 42% had Below Basic health literacy and another 27% had only Basic health literacy. Of those who consider themselves in excellent health, 57% had intermediate health literacy and 19% had Proficient health literacy.[14] Although some consideration must be made for personal perception of health, the numbers strongly suggest that poor health and poor health literacy are at least coincident if not causally related.

Finally, the NAAL established that economic status had an effect on a group's health literacy. Adults living in poverty had a lower health literacy score than did non-poor adults. Thirty-five percent of this group had Below Basic literacy skills and another 27% had only Basic skills.[14] Critical to providers serving a poor patient population is the knowledge that well over half of these patients have very limited skills for comprehending medical information.

The NAAL data have obvious relevance in several areas. First, the data highlight that those populations already at risk for healthcare provision disparities, people of color and the poor, are also burdened by more-limited skills for obtaining meaningful information about that care. To ensure that these patients get safe care and can participate in medical decision making, providers must evaluate the way that health information is provided. As the U.S. Department of Health and Human Services has poignantly noted, "Closing the gap in health literacy is an issue of fundamental fairness and equity and is essential to reduce health disparities."[5] Second, the data indicate that a substantial percentage of the adult population has health literacy limitations. Implementing system wide health literacy measures has the potential to aid a significant portion of the patient population. Finally, providers now have the basic data needed to conduct analysis of their adverse event data with an eye toward populations known to have health literacy issues. If these populations are demonstrably more vulnerable to error than others, then health literacy–oriented responses may lead to a more targeted error reduction response.

SAFE CARE FOR NON-ENGLISH SPEAKERS

According to a national survey conducted by the Health Research and Educational Trust, 63% of hospitals treat Limited English Proficiency (LEP) patients either daily or weekly.[15] In analyzing its data on adverse events, The Joint Commission found that, although only about 30% of English speakers suffered physical harm from reported adverse events, almost 50% of LEP patients were harmed by the adverse events they suffered.[3] As the NAAL study profoundly highlighted, the English health literacy skills of the Hispanic population, many of whom are not native English speakers, is an area that merits significant attention from providers. The NAAL study revealed that 67% have only Basic health literacy in English or lower.[2] These statistics starkly indicate how critical health literacy efforts targeted at LEP patients are to addressing potential safety issues.

Although a fundamental concern for the safety of all patients undoubtedly underlies providers' interest in tackling the health literacy obstacles for LEP patients, Title VI of the federal Civil Rights Act also mandates that providers take action. Under Title VI, providers must provide interpretation services to their LEP patients. Title VI has also been interpreted by the Office of Civil Rights to demand that all vital written materials be translated, including consent and complaint forms; information about free translation programs; notices of eligibility criteria, rights, denial, loss, or decreases in benefits or services; and intake forms.[16] In addition, a Presidential Executive Order issued in 2000 mandates that all recipients of federal financial assistance (in other words, providers who receive Medicare or Medicaid funds) provide "meaningful access" to services to their LEP beneficiaries.[17] Under this mandate, the Centers for Medicare & Medicaid Services (CMS) has taken an aggressive position on LEP, mandating that all of its beneficiaries have access to interpreters. All of these legal requirements, however, beg the question of what exactly these translation and interpreter services will be at any given institution.

Interpreters

Who will be the interpreters that a medical institution provides? At what kind of encounter will those services be available? What, if any, training will be provided to these interpreters? Although the ease of using family members or friends as interpreters for LEP patients is undeniable, reliance on these individuals creates risks for the institution. A 2003 study on the error rates of medical interpretation provides a cautionary tale for the safety minded health literacy advocate. The study found an error rate of 31 interpretation errors per medical encounter.[3] The interpreters in the study included hospital-provided interpreters and ad hoc interpreters, with the latter making significantly more errors than the former. Generally, the errors ranged from omissions, substitutions, editorializing, and additions and included instructing a parent to put an oral antibiotic in a child's ear.

The results of this study highlight two important points. First, that the use of family members, friends, and other ad hoc interpreters risks the miscommunication of vital health information. Because federal law mandates the provision of interpretation services, an error of this kind not only puts patients at risk but creates potential liability for hospitals. Whenever a provider is attempting to convey to or obtain from an LEP patient meaningful medical information, an ad hoc interpreter is a poor choice. Second, even using institution staff as interpreters can present risks if those staff members have not been trained as medical interpreters. Again, relying on the accuracy of interpretation by a fluent bilingual staff member may not shield an institution from liability if that interpreter was not qualified for the task. The Joint Commission recommends that providers should evaluate the proficiency of their interpreters with regard to communicating medical information, guidance for which is available through the National Council on Interpreting in Health Care.[16]

Translation

In addition to using appropriately trained medical interpreters and weaning providers off the use of ad hoc interpreters, the provision of translated written materials can reinforce the communication of vital medical information. Translated written materials may be critical in informed consent contexts and may provide a critical backup for oral communication under certain circumstances. Direct translation must be avoided because it is likely to produce materials that are confusing or even nonsensical in the second language. As the U.S. Department of Health and Human Services found when translating its *Five Steps to Safer Health Care* fact sheet, the metaphor of stairs evoking progression had to be entirely reworked because it had no meaning in Spanish.[18] Providers also need to be reviewing translated documents to check their clinical and cultural accuracy and can use focus groups, translation services, or their own trained medical interpreters for this review. The Joint Commission recommends that providers consider pooling resources for translating critical and broadly used written materials.[3] Also important to the creation of appropriately translated materials is the health literacy level of LEP patients in their native language. As CMS discovered when surveying Medicare beneficiaries, Spanish-dominant persons were unfamiliar with words such as *ibuprophen* or *heart bypass surgery* in either language.[18] Although providing translation services for these individuals is crucial, those written materials must be written in appropriately plain language that will communicate effectively to those at even the lowest literacy levels.

Cultural Competency

Another critical component to providing safe care to non-English or limited-English speakers involves the concept of cultural competency. The Joint Commission defines cultural competency as "the ability of health care providers and organizations to understand and respond effectively to the cultural and language needs brought by the patient to the health care encounter."[19] "Cultural competence requires organizations and their personnel to: 1) value diversity; 2) assess themselves; 3) manage the dynamics of difference; 4) acquire and institutionalize cultural knowledge; and 5) adapt to diversity and the cultural contexts of individuals and communities served."[16] Just as important as making your words understood is the concept of communicating with patients in a way that is most likely to achieve their desired outcome.

If, as did a provider in one well-documented case, a provider explains to a family that their child is dying and that family is from a culture that interprets this as threatening and offensive, the family might remove that child from the provider's care in a way that puts the family and the child in unnecessary peril.[3] The chances of noncompliance, treatment refusal, and withholding of crucial information rise when the provider is unaware of the cultural forces shaping patients' decisions. As the IOM has stated, "A principle of patient safety is to include patients in safety designs and the processes of care."[1] To do so, it is essential to understand cultural nuances of what patient safety means to different people and what beliefs, values, and actions inform people's understanding of safe care come into play."[1]

The Joint Commission has issued two reports directly confronting cultural competency issues for medical care providers.[16,19] These reports outline best practices for dealing with LEP patients and cultural competency issues and highlight the current work being done by specific institutions to address these issues. The reports also indicate the emphasis that The Joint Commission as an accrediting body is placing on monitoring institutions' efforts in these areas. Also in recognition of the importance of cultural competency, the Department of Health and Human Services (HHS) has created National Standards for Culturally and Linguistically Appropriate Services (CLAS) in Health Care. The CLAS dictates not only that "health care organizations must make available easily understood patient-related materials ... in the languages of commonly encountered groups" but that these materials must be culturally responsive as well.[3] The Joint Commission's accreditation standards mirror the CLAS dictates, and that organization has published a self-assessment tool for institutions to evaluate their cultural competence.[20]

For healthcare providers to better understand the potential health literacy obstacles facing their LEP patient population, the National Patient Safety Foundation (NPSF) recommends that they conduct an audit of all written, visual, and verbal patient points of contact.[21] They should ask questions about the accessibility of written materials, the ability to navigate the physical layout of the hospital, and the reading level of items such as medication instructions and responses to patient questions. Understanding and responding to patient needs in this way not only can improve patient safety but can also help keep the institution from facing unfortunate legal consequences.

THE LAW AND HEALTH LITERACY

The legal system both though regulation and court opinions has also provided a framework for addressing literacy particularly as it relates to issues in health care where effective communication is paramount.

Informed Consent

The safety implications for effective communication between providers and patients is unquestionably a key force driving the health literacy movement. However, important liability issues underlie the question of whether patients understand information presented to them concerning their medical care. First is the issue of informed consent. Although specific laws vary from state to state, according to the American Medical Association's (AMA) general principles, to give informed consent to medical care, a patient should be informed of his or her diagnosis, if known; the nature and purpose of a proposed treatment or procedure; the benefits and particularly the risks of a proposed treatment or procedure; alternatives and their risks and benefits; and the risks and benefits of undergoing no treatment.[22] The adequacy of the communication is judged by what a reasonable person would need to know to make an informed choice about the proposed treatment. Failure to obtain informed consent before treating a patient opens a provider to a malpractice claim. Obtaining a meaningful informed consent from patients, understanding that for every institution significant numbers of those patients have limited health literacy, presents its own challenges.

Anecdotal evidence about the cryptic nature of informed consent forms abounds, and the literature is replete with quotes from these forms that are unreadable by anyone who does not possess both a medical and a legal education. A brief literature review conducted by the Agency for Healthcare Research and Quality (AHRQ) revealed the incompleteness and inadequacies of the majority of the informed consent interactions studied.[23] From omissions of central aspects of the informed consent components to level of satisfaction by patients with the amount of information they had prior to undergoing a treatment, to the readability of written consent forms, the studies all highlighted the health literacy challenges presented by typical informed consent procedures.

This literature review also included studies of the effectiveness of several approaches to improving the communication effort in informed consent processes. Although the AHRQ authors concluded that additional study into the most effective means for conveying the information required for a truly informed consent is needed, they recommended several evidence-based steps providers can take to improve their informed consent process. First, consent forms should be revised for increased readability and written at a reading level that more accurately reflects the skills of a provider's average patients. Second, informed consent discussions should be highly structured teaching sessions rather than ad hoc discussions between providers and patients. Third, the teach-back method significantly improved patient recall of risks. Finally, the use of visual or auditory learning aids assisted patients in recalling information about the proposed treatment. With these relatively simple steps, the AHRQ authors concluded that institutions could communicate far more effectively with not only low health literacy patients but with the patient population generally.

An important subset of the informed consent dialogue is providing patients information about the risks of the treatment or procedure. Because risk information is generally gathered in the aggregate, understanding risk and applying that information to oneself as an individual patient requires numeracy or quantitative literacy. Understanding risk requires weighing benefits and interpreting percentages, ratios, risk magnitude, and statistical information. The NAAL study revealed that a substantial percentage of patients have limited quantitative literacy, with many able to do no more than simple arithmetic computations when identified for them. It is critical, then, that institutions meet their obligation to inform patients about risks and benefits by finding effective ways to communicate quantitative risk information. Suggestions for communicating quantitative information effectively include providing smaller amounts of data at any given interaction, reducing the calculations and inferences from data required by the patient by providing more analysis and conclusions within the communication, and using visual displays.

LEP and Cultural Competency

The earlier discussion of the challenges and requirements of providing information to LEP patients maps equally well onto the process of obtaining informed consent from these patients. Again, a successful approach must be comprehensive and unified. Translating an informed consent form into another language has limited value without an interpreter to facilitate questions and answers between providers and patients and almost no value if the patient has limited literacy in his or her native language. Likewise, issues of cultural competency do arise in the informed consent context. As The Joint Commission has noted, a patient's cultural belief may have an impact on his or her decisions about care.[16] "Cultural brokers" can help providers communicate the importance of care that may be the subject of a cultural barrier with a patient by creating an environment of trust that allows the wishes of the patient and the provider to more likely align.

Advanced Directives

A corollary to the issue of informed consent is the advanced directives issue. Advanced directive can be a powerful tool in helping providers act on the wishes of their patients, but the forms used for these directives may be unreadable and not comprehensible for low-literacy patients. Considering that the NAAL census found consistently lower health literacy rates among the elderly, critical advance directive users, this area requires additional focus by providers. As the IOM noted in its report, one institutional provider developed a form written at a fifth-grade reading level that gave simple, step-by-step instructions for completing it and included text-enhancing graphics for low-literacy users. Because the provider had a significant Spanish-speaking patient cohort, the form was also translated into Spanish.

Accreditation

In addition to federal requirements, accreditation bodies such as The Joint Commission are becoming increasingly focused on health literacy efforts at accredited institutions. The Joint Commission has directed a number of its National Patient Safety Goals to health literacy–related subjects.[3] Institutions seeking to obtain or retain accreditation from The Joint Commission are expected to be in compliance with these goals. Similarly, the AHRQ is developing a new module for its Consumer Assessment of Healthcare Providers and Systems (CAHPS) survey that will measure patients' satisfaction with communication from providers.[9] The module will assess the clarity of communications concerning treatment, test results, and medications among others.

HEALTH LITERACY PRINCIPLES AND PROGRAMS

As the previous section stressed, adopting an institution-wide health literacy program is a promising option for staying in compliance with the many legal and regulatory requirements that dot the current healthcare landscape. This is particularly true in light of the evidence that a provider cannot assess a patient's health literacy "just by looking." Making providers aware of the problem of low health literacy is only one part of the solution. Institution-wide health literacy best practices can provide an important degree of protection against provider–patient miscommunication-based adverse events and, unlike the literacy level the average patient presents with, is under providers' control.

Although a number of programs now exist, and will be discussed shortly, one of the most important steps providers can take is to analyze their own patient population and keep current with the demographics of those they serve. Staying aware of the number of non-native English speakers, the languages they speak, and the cultural issues that they bring with them when seeking care is vital to addressing health literacy issues they may have. Maintaining current data on the number of senior patients at the institution will assist in addressing the particular health literacy needs of this population. Institutions serving a large number of patients at or below federal poverty levels will need to carefully examine their patient communications as well. Having staff members who reflect the population that the institution serves is another technique to address health literacy at an organic level. Staff members who speak patients' native tongues, understand their cultural preferences, and are familiar with the obstacles that influences such as poverty and age have on literacy can help integrate institutions' efforts to ensure that literacy limits do not lead to adverse events.[16]

Institutions are also their own best repositories for their particular risks related to health literacy. Examining adverse events and near misses for any components that can be attributed to patients' abilities to understand and communicate health-related information provides a starting place for an institution to identify and address the particular needs facing its patient population. As an example, a hospital serving a large population of Navajos with limited English proficiency had concerns about the safety of its medication self-administration program.[16] The hospital used sun and moon stickers to help patients understand when to take the medicines and dots to indicate how much medication to take. Implementing such an idea and then gathering data about adverse events in the medication self-administration program could provide an institution with specific patient safety initiatives tailored to that institution's particular needs.

Health Literacy Programs

Although relying on its own data to pinpoint problems and test solutions is critical for institutions trying to staunch health literacy–related adverse events, there will also be efficiencies in adopting programs created by the many groups that have been studying health literacy over the past decade. The AMA, the NPSF, and even the federal government have created health literacy programs for healthcare providers.

The NPSF's Ask Me 3 program centers around encouraging patients to understand three questions: 1. What is my main problem? 2. What do I need to do? 3. Why is it important for me to do this?[21] The Ask Me 3 program provides posters and brochures aimed at patients and providers. Providers are encouraged to understand the demographics and potential health literacy issues of their patients, to use the program's tools to conduct in-service trainings for practitioners, and to audit their points of contact with patients for clarity and opportunities to assess patients' true understanding of what they are being told. Additionally, the AMA offers providers a Health Literacy Kit, a clinician-oriented program designed to "define the scope of the health literacy problem; recognize health system barriers faced by patients with low health literacy; implement improved methods of verbal and written communication;

and incorporate practical strategies to create a shame-free environment."[24] Also available are videos for clinicians to use with patients describing barriers to their understanding of medical information.

Although much attention has been paid to the oral communication between providers and patients and the opportunity these moments create for providers to tailor their words to the specific skills of a specific patient, attention must also be paid to written communication. The federal government has initiated a "plain language" strategy to improve the clarity of written communication.[13] The strategy proposes techniques for plain writing, including putting the most important information first, breaking information into accessible chunks, using simple language or defining important technical terms, and providing enough white space to make pages easy to read. Plain language strategies also include speaking tips, including the teach-back method whereby patients restate the information they have gotten from providers in their own words so providers can assess their comprehension. The information is repeated until the patient comprehends it well enough to restate it accurately. Demonstration techniques also assist with oral communication—showing patients how to do something and then watching them do it themselves.

As important as knowing the capabilities of your patient base is, it is also important to know the readability of your own materials. Several basic principles of clear writing have been generally adopted. Using common words and eliminating jargon help to clarify text for limited literacy readers. Several groups have created thesauri translating complex words and medical terms in to plain language that will be accessible to more readers. Other tips include writing in conversational sentences, limiting one idea to each paragraph, leaving white space on the page, emphasizing desired behaviors instead of medical facts, using headers and bullets as road signs for readers, and using only short sentences. Field testing materials and then revising them based on comments can also help ensure that the materials accomplish their goals. Even providing surrogate readers may help some patients whose skills are the most limited.

The Group Health Research Institute provides a readability toolkit to help providers evaluate their written materials.[25] Also available is the Simple Measure of Gobbledygook tool, which estimates the reading level required to understand a given text.[26] The Maximus Center for Health Literacy offers *The Health Literacy Style Manual* online to provide style manuals, translation services, and other readability services to state governments and other organizations.[27] Finally, Harvard School of Public Health's Health Literacy Studies Department provides a variety of Web-based resources for organizations seeking to provide readable materials and to address other health literacy challenges facing them.[28]

Health Literacy Case Study

Recent efforts by the Iowa Health System (IHS) provide an example of an institution using many of these resources to address health literacy head on. After assessing its own patient population and recognizing that half of its patients were at risk for low health literacy, the IHS created a Health Literacy Collaborative to coordinate a literacy initiative.[29] The Collaborative conducted staff workshops, implemented the AMA's Health Literacy Toolkit and the Ask Me 3 program, and evaluated their efforts based on patient feedback. The Collaborative had as its goals improving communication between providers and patients using specific tools to help ensure patients' comprehension of health information and simplifying paperwork, materials, referrals, and check-in. After implementing the program the IHS saw an increase in the comprehension and retention of information by patients, and although the study did not specifically examine adverse events, the system met its primary goal of facilitating better informed patients.

Health Literacy Tests

Several tests have been developed for measuring an individual's health literacy. The most widely known are the Rapid Estimate of Adult Literacy in Medicine (REALM) and the Test of Functional Health Literacy in Adults (TOFHLA). The REALM assessment takes about three minutes and tests a person's ability to recognize and pronounce medical words.[9] The TOFHLA tests numerical ability and reading comprehension and takes about 20 minutes to administer.[9] Both tests have proved highly valuable to those conducting research into specific areas of health literacy. However, the formality of both tests and the limitations in what they can tell providers about a patient's true ability to process and evaluate medical information in the actual moment of treatment make them cumbersome and of limited value to providers on a day-to-day basis. These limitations indicate that the health literacy techniques discussed above and those that will be coming out of ongoing research into the area should be applied as universally as possible. Using simple language, teach-backs, visual aids, trained interpreters, and culturally competent communication methods should become the best practice for all patients.

CONCLUSION

Although this book examines patient safety from the perspective of its myriad components, the nexus between good communication and safety resounds in each chapter. For more than a decade, increasing attention has been paid to the provider–patient communication dyad, and the concept of health literacy and the role it plays in patient safety have been developed. Although the starting point may appear to be the capabilities of patients to comprehend medical information, the IOM has recognized that "[e]qually important are the communication and assessment skills of the people with whom individuals interact regarding health."[1] Although the issues underlying patients' limited literacy reach well beyond the control of providers, providers can take a lead role in combating the effects of limited health literacy on patient outcomes. As the *Healthy People 2010* authors noted, "[d]iagnoses and treatments require doctors to negotiate a common understanding with patients about what is to be done. The quality of provider-patient communication can affect numerous outcomes [and] [a]ppropriate information and communication with a provider not only can relieve patients' anxieties but also can help patients understand their choices, allow them to participate in informed decision making and better manage their own health concerns."[5]

The IOM has articulated 12 principles of health literacy that sum up the vision for the future of patient–provider communication:

1. Everyone has the opportunity to improve his or her health literacy.
2. Everyone has the opportunity to use reliable, understandable information that could make a difference in his or her overall well-being, including everyday behaviors such as how he or she eats, whether he or she exercises, and whether he or she gets checkups.
3. Health and science content would be basic parts of K–12 curricula.
4. People are able to accurately assess the credibility of health information presented by health advocates, commercials, and new media sources.
5. There is monitoring and accountability for health literacy policies and practices.
6. Public health alerts, vital to the health of the nation, are presented in everyday terms so that people can take needed action.
7. The cultural contexts of diverse peoples, including those from various cultural groups and non-English-speaking peoples, are integrated into all health information.
8. Health practitioners communicate clearly during all interactions with their patients, using everyday vocabulary.

9. There is ample time for discussions between patients and healthcare providers.
10. Patients feel free and comfortable to ask questions as part of the healing relationship.
11. Rights and responsibilities in relation to health and health care are presented or written in clear, everyday terms so that people can take needed action.
12. Informed consent documents used in health care are developed so that all people can give or withhold consent based on information they need and understand.[1]

References

1. Nielsen-Bohlman, L., Panzer, A. M., & Kindig, D. A. (Eds.). (2004). *Health literacy: A prescription to end confusion*. Washington, DC: National Academies Press.
2. Kutner, M., Greenberg, E., Jin, Y., & Paulsen, C. (2006). *The health literacy of America's adults: Results from the 2003 National Assessment of Adult Literacy*. U.S. Department of Education, Institute of Education Sciences, National Center for Education Statistics. Retrieved from http://nces.ed.gov/pubsearch/pubsinfo.asp?pubid=2006483.
3. U.S. Department of Health and Human Services, Agency for Healthcare Research and Quality. (2007). *"What did the doctor say?": Improving health literacy to protect patient safety*. Oakbrook Terrace, IL: The Joint Commission. Retrieved from http://minorityhealth.hhs.gov/assets/pdf/checked/finalreport.pdf.
4. Kohn, L. T., Corrigan, J. M., & Donaldson, M. S. (Eds.). (2000). *To err is human: Building a safer health system*. Washington, DC: National Academies Press.
5. U.S. Department of Health and Human Services, Office of Disease Prevention and Health Promotion. (2000). *Healthy People 2010*, Chapter 11: Health Communication. Retrieved from http://www.healthypeople.gov/2010/document/html/volume1/11healthcom.htm.
6. Department of Health and Human Services, National Institutes of Health, National Library of Medicine, National Network of Libraries of Medicine. (2011). *Health literacy*. Retrieved from http://nnlm.gov/outreach/consumer/hlthlit.html.
7. 110th Congress (2007–2008). S.2424 National Health Literacy Act of 2007. Retrieved from http://thomas.loc.gov/cgi-bin/query/z?c110:S.2424:.
8. Potter, L., & Martin, C. (2005). *Health literacy fact sheets*. Retrieved from http://www.chcs.org/usr_doc/Health_Literacy_Fact_Sheets.pdf.
9. Berkman, N. D., DeWalt, D. A., Pignone, M. P., Sheridan, S. L., Lohr, K. N.,
10. Lux, L., ... Bonito, A. J. (2004). *Literacy and health outcomes*. Rockville, MD: Agency for Healthcare Research and Quality. Retrieved from http://www.ncbi.nlm.nih.gov/books/NBK37134/.
11. Peters, E., Hibbard, J., Slovic, P., & Diekmann, N. (2007). Numeracy skill and the communication, comprehension, and use of risk-benefit information. *Health Affairs, 26*(3), 741–748.
12. National Academy on an Aging Society. *Fact sheet: Low health literacy skills increase annual health care expenditures by $73 billion*. Retrieved from http://www.agingsociety.org/agingsociety/publications/fact/fact_low.html.
13. Parikh, N. S., Parker, R. M., Nurss, J. R., Baker, D. W., & Williams, M. V. (1996). Shame and health literacy: The unspoken connection. *Patient Education and Counseling, 27*(1), 33–39.
14. U.S. Department of Health and Human Services, Office of Disease Prevention and Health Promotion. *Plain language: A promising strategy for clearly communicating health information and improving health literacy*. Retrieved from http://www.health.gov/communication/literacy/plainlanguage/PlainLanguage.htm.

15. Medicare Rights Center. (2005). *Medicare statistics: The Medicare population*. Retrieved from http://www.guidestar.org/PartnerReport.aspx?partner=justgivews&ein=13-3505372.
16. The Commonwealth Fund. (2006). Quality Matters: Health Literacy (Vol 21). Retrieved from http://www.commonwealthfund.org/Newsletters/Quality-Matters/2006/November-December/Issue-of-the-Month-Health-Literacy-A-Quality.
17. Wilson-Stronks, A., Lee, K. K., Cordero, C. L., Kopp, A. L., & Galvez, E. (2008). *One size does not fit all: Meeting the health care needs of diverse populations*. Oakbrook Terrace, IL: The Joint Commission. Retrieved from http://www.jointcommission.org/assets/1/6/HLCOneSizeFinal.pdf.
18. Presidential Executive Order 13166. Improving Access to Services for Persons with Limited English Proficiency. (2000). Retrieved from http://www.usdoj.gov/crt/cor/Pubs/eolep.php.
19. Miranda, D. J., Zeller, P. K., Lee, R., Koepke, C. P., Holland, H. E., Englert, F., & Swift, E. K. Speaking plainly: Communicating the patient's role in health care safety. In K. Henriksen, J. B. Battles, E. S. Marks, & D. I. Lewin (eds.), *Advances in patient safety: From research to implementation* (Vol. 4). Rockville, MD: Agency for Healthcare Research and Quality. Retrieved from www.ahrq.gov/downloads/pub/advances/vol4/Miranda.pdf.
20. Wilson-Stronks, A., & Galvez, E. (2008). *Exploring cultural and linguistic services in the nation's hospitals: A report of findings*. Oakbrook Terrace, IL: The Joint Commission. Retrieved from http://www.jointcommission.org/assets/1/6/ARoadmapforHospitalsfinalversion727.pdf.
21. *Advancing Effective Communication, Cultural Competence, and Patient- and Family-Centered Care: A Roadmap for Hospitals*. Retrieved from http://www.jointcommission.org/assets/1/6/ARoadmapforHospitalsfinalversion727.pdf.
22. Partnership for Clear Health Communication, National Patient Safety Foundation. *Ask Me 3: Program implementation guide for health care and information providers*. Retrieved from http://www.docstoc.com/docs/35459921/Program-Implementation-Guide-for-Health-Care-and-Information-Providers#.
23. American Medical Association. Criteria for informed consent. Retrieved from http://www.ama-assn.org/ama/pub/category/4608.html.
24. Pizzi, L. T., Goldfarb, N. I., & Nash, D. B. Procedures for obtaining informed consent. *Making health care safer: A critical analysis of patient safety practices*. Rockville, MD: Agency for Healthcare Research and Quality. Retrieved from http://ahrq.gov/clinic/ptsafety/chap48.htm.
25. American Medical Association. *Health Literacy Kit*. (2007). Retrieved from http://www.ama-assn.org/ama/pub/about-ama/ama-foundation/our-programs/public-health/health-literacy-program/health-literacy-kit.page.
26. Group Health Research Institute. *The PRISM Readability Toolkit*. Retrieved from http://www.grouphealthresearch.org/capabilities/readability/readability_home.html.
27. McLaughlin, G. H. SMOG: Simple Measure of Gobbledygook. Retrieved from www.harrymclaughlin.com/SMOG.htm.
28. MAXIMUS. (2005). *The health literacy style manual*. Retrieved from http://www.maximus.com/sites/default/files/filemanager/Health_Literacy_style_manual.pdf.
29. Harvard School of Public Health, Health Literacy Studies Department. Retrieved from http://www.hsph.harvard.edu/healthliteracy/.
30. Nowotny, M., & McCarthy, D. (2006). *Quality matters case study: Iowa's Health Literacy Collaborative is transforming patient–provider communication*. Retrieved from http://www.commonwealthfund.org/Newsletters/Quality-Matters/2006/November-December/Case-Study-Iowas-Health-Literacy-Collaborative-Is-Transforming-Patient-Provider-Communication.aspx.

16

The Leadership Role of the Chief Operating Officer in Aligning Strategy and Operations to Create Patient Safety

Julianne M. Morath, RN, MS

Patient safety will be a way of life for the chief operating officer (COO), given a more informed view of safety as a system, increased government regulation and oversight, specific accreditation standards through The Joint Commission and other organizations, payer requirements and incentives such as those proposed by the Leapfrog Group, and consumer demands for information and accountability. But most important, patient safety must be the fundamental aim or promise of the healthcare system to those who need and depend on us. As such, the COO role must be dedicated to unwavering and continuous attention, learning, and actions to design and operate systems that do no harm. This is what operations is all about. The other requirements in operations will follow when the design and operations for safety are done well.

Safety in health care is critical. Catastrophes can destroy an organization's reputation and profitability. The elements that form professional, national, and organizational cultures can come together to define and advance a safety culture or can create an unsafe operating environment.[1] A safety culture extends beyond a single organization's quest for world-class safety. Patient safety must become a value. Patient safety requires a joint belief in the importance of safety and a shared understanding of what it will take to create the culture of safety. The COO role is pivotal in initiating and continuing the dialogue and work strategies needed to accomplish this. The starting place is the operating environment, for which the COO has a direct responsibility.

The role of the COO in patient safety is to align and engage the energy of the organization to provide the highest quality of care and service, based on the most current professional knowledge and knowledge of patient and family needs and preferences. This includes the design and operation of systems in which this level of care and service delivery is not only possible but actively facilitated. The work of operations begins with building systems that do no harm. Although the focus of this chapter is patient safety, it is important to note that employee and environmental safety are inextricably linked to patient safety. In summary, the COO role is to engage others to

- Design and operate systems based on evidence in safety science
- Develop and support people who provide care and services to develop greater capacity in teamwork, risk awareness, risk mitigation, and resiliency
- Build a culture of safety and continuous learning in which care and services are delivered
- Focus and align resources to create greater safety
- Assure evidence-based, patient-centered, and system-centered work is being done

This chapter describes how this role can be operationalized.

Building systems that reduce the probability of accident and harm requires recognition and understanding of four basic concepts. These are as follows:[2]

1. Health care is a complex system, and complex systems are inherently risk prone, particularly operating rooms, intensive care units, and emergency rooms, where teamwork is essential and crises are common.
2. People, no matter how competent and vigilant, are fallible because they are human and hence physically and psychologically limited in memory capacity and the ability to deal with simultaneous multiple cognitive demands.
3. People create safety by defending against risk, intercepting error before it reaches the patient. They are also perpetrators of risk due to their being human, and are therefore subject to stressors such as fear, fatigue, and social factors that impair cognitive and motor function.
4. Safety is a system and can pose threats of failure from inadequate or clumsy equipment, fatigue-inducing schedules, flawed or incomplete procedures, excessive incentives for production, and risk-prone professional and organizational cultures often associated with faulty communications.

Accepting these concepts, the responsibility of the chief operating officer is to recognize the nature of emerging risks and operate a system of safety in the design and engineering of processes and in the management of processes to eliminate or mitigate risk. The foundation for this work is nurturing a culture, or people system, to see, live, and breathe safety. This is not about cautioning people to be more careful. It is rather about improving the systems in which people operate, and increasing their ability to perceive, identify, and close the gaps to eliminate or mitigate latent failures and vulnerabilities in those systems. Through an "alert field" in which people see and report risk, prediction and prevention of accidents can occur. A question that should be top of mind for the COO and actively pursued is: "Is this a safe place to give and receive care?"

A CALL TO ACTION

The work of patient safety is a challenge culturally, strategically, and technically. A starting place to examine these challenges is via a patient safety manifesto, or declaration of intent to act. Such a declaration was first organized by the Harvard Executive Session on Reducing Medical Error and Increasing Patient Safety.[3] The outline of the manifesto was an outcome of the sessions conducted semiannually over the course of three years, 1997 to 2000. The manifesto is a helpful organizing framework for the chief operating officer to examine, align, and mobilize the work to be done.

The elements of the patient safety manifesto are as follows:

1. Declare patient safety urgent and a priority.
2. Accept executive responsibility.
3. Import and apply new knowledge and skills.
4. Apply new tools and build infrastructure.
5. Assign accountability.

6. Establish blameless reporting.
7. Align external controls.

These elements will be described to explore the role of the COO.

DECLARE PATIENT SAFETY URGENT AND A PRIORITY

Declaring patient safety urgent and a priority must be done in a manner that is relevant, credible, and taps into attributes of the organization's culture that serve to inspire. The promise "we will do no harm" is a powerful change lever to engage the organization. However, despite the Institute of Medicine (IOM) report[4] and multiple studies of medical accident, most notably the Harvard Practice Study,[5] many healthcare leaders, clinicians, and consumers remain unaware of patient safety issues. They are also unaware that most adverse events and medical accidents that cause harm are recurrent, and therefore predictable and preventable. There are many reasons for this. Among the reasons are the belief that medical accidents and errors are an inevitable part of health care; gross underreporting; denial and fear of shame and punishment; or the belief that current performance is an acceptable standard of care. Communication of an urgent priority needs to reside in the belief that we can and must do better. This message needs to be coupled with an accurate understanding of the current reality of the safety experience within the organization.

From a practical perspective, arguments regarding the validity of research are futile. The question is: "What is your experience?" Bringing the stories of patient safety to life and relevance is part of the COO's role of knowing and defining current reality as the platform for change. This can be accomplished through multiple strategies. Following are two suggested strategies that not only bring forward local experience but also engage clinicians.

Patient Safety Dialogues

The first strategy is to convene thought-leaders or key influential people in the clinical environment. They are readily identifiable. They are the individuals who peers seek out to learn what is new, ask their opinions, and request consultations. Bringing them together to explore the questions "Is this a safe place to receive and give care?" "How do you know?" and "What is your experience?" invites and legitimizes conversations about events, near misses, barriers, and sources of safety. These stories are typically not shared, but rather individually experienced. In this dialogue, a collective consciousness regarding safety in the organization is raised. Such recognition of experience quickly leads to conversations regarding actions to prevent errors and accidents from occurring. It creates a safe place or architecture to expand such dialogue throughout the organization in pursuit of improvement.

Focus Groups

Another strategy is to conduct focus groups of key stakeholders by discipline, department, and patient and family consumer groups. A tool such as the one designed by Nancy Wilson at the VHA-Inc., a Texas-based healthcare alliance, can be adopted and used in all care environments to understand the culture of safety.[6] The strength of the focus group approach is that the data collection is in itself an intervention to build a safe, confidential, blameless environment in which to talk and learn about safety. Focus groups can provide specific information about perceived barriers to safety and processes that need to change.

These focus groups' data, rich in detail, create a portrait of the organization that can be reflected back and used to define its current state and serve as a baseline to measure change. Although the IOM report and studies reported in the literature are helpful to frame the issue and initiate a national conversation, it is the actual experience of the organization that provides traction for change.

Naming Safety as a Priority

Returning to the fundamental promise or pledge "do no harm" amplifies the characteristic of the healthcare culture that can be called upon to align its members to explicitly identify patient safety as a priority. This is not without risk. Explicitly and publicly addressing patient safety creates exposure for the organization and its members. It is therefore essential to engage the governing board, professional and medical staff, insurance carriers, and legal counsel in understanding the ethical imperative, issues, and strategy.

As risk perception and reporting are increased, historical methods of tracking safety, such as medication error rate, will dramatically increase. The need to understand what will occur and why is essential. Initially, such reporting can be experienced as a decline in safety or an increase in events. A more informed view will realize that risks and events are now becoming visible, and so may be addressed. Manipulating and chasing rates will not improve safety. At this time in the evolution of understanding safety in health care, the story of how the systems are operating is what is important. This assertion will be examined more closely in the section about establishing a blameless reporting system.

ACCEPT EXECUTIVE RESPONSIBILITY

The role of leadership requires personal commitment, strategy, and the use of tools. There are some critical "culture carriers," powerful messages usable to amplify aspects of the existing culture to build greater safety. The first such message is to publicly accept executive responsibility for patient safety. There can be no question of the priority of patient safety. The message must be clear, consistent, and concrete. The COO, as operations leader, provides a steady drumbeat of messages, measures, and feedback to the organization about patient safety. The COO also incorporates known practices to enhance safety in his or her work and requires the same of others. At the same time, the COO must incorporate strategies to remove barriers to safety as they are identified.

The COO role is to hardwire patient safety into the daily life and operations of the organization. Embracing and applying lessons learned from leaders in other industries, such as aviation, nuclear power, fire fighting, and manufacturing, can inform and accelerate action. Known safety principles from industry that can be incorporated into daily work include the following:[7]

- Train staff in effective teamwork, decision making, risk awareness, and error management as well as technical aspects of the job.
- Simplify and standardize work processes and products, such as the use of a consistent monitoring system.
- Design self-correcting systems or redundant systems that make it difficult to do the wrong thing, such as verifying messages about who will take what action when, or using technical monitors to complement judgment.
- Reduce reliance on human memory through protocols, checklists, and automated systems, and checking with colleagues.
- Use automation carefully through the meticulous design of manual processes that can be converted well to automation, such as the medication record documentation process.
- Learn how each function of the organization works by studying it as a flow process. This requires a comprehensive audit of each step in a sequence.
- Drive out fear of blame in error reporting and set up systems so that data can be collected to learn about error and near misses. The risk should be in failing to report, not in the act of bringing bad news.
- Find out what is going on by developing sources, asking questions, and walking

around. This is accomplished by being visible and actually reviewing in person the work activity.

- Do what obviously needs to be done one by one, step by step. When processes need correction, take action.
- Do not tolerate violation of standards or failure of staff to take available countermeasures against error (such as input from colleagues and use of checklists), and hold people accountable for their actions.

Another principle to incorporate into daily work is making implicit knowledge explicit.[8] Implicit knowledge is the information and know-how that individuals uniquely possess. In health care, a great deal of the work in developing care paths, clinical protocols, and best-of-practice models concerns making explicit each provider's knowledge about how a care process works. Working to define the knowledge that people have and don't know they have is a critical step in understanding workflow and seeing the whole picture. It also helps focus on these questions: Who in the system has knowledge and who gets to ask the questions?

The aviation industry would suggest that everyone has knowledge about different things and everyone can ask questions. The COO has a responsibility to both model and set the expectations for team-based communication, explicit sharing of information and knowledge, and tools to transfer knowledge and information such as those referenced earlier.

Leadership Exemplar: The Alcoa Story

An important example of leadership in safety is Paul O'Neill, former CEO of Alcoa. A Harvard case study describes O'Neill's leadership at Alcoa.[9]

> Paul O'Neill became CEO of Alcoa in June 1987 and was reported to have "immediately stunned corporate directors, industry analysts, and competitors when he announced his top priority: safety." He believed that the names of employees killed or injured should not be turned into numbers and rates. He didn't believe productivity necessitated increased risk or that accidents and injuries were the inevitable costs of doing business. He rather believed that to focus on safety required understanding of processes and systems in exquisite detail, and that understanding would lead to better and more productive operations. While Alcoa had an industry record for safety, O'Neill raised the bar and demanded management to zero defect. To eradicate accidents and injuries, he required recalibrating an operational approach from measuring what caused accidents to learning how to prevent them from occurring in the first place. For example, if a worker fell off a machine, he asked: "What was he doing on the machine anyway?" "Was the machine designed with control mechanisms that actually increased risk?"

The Alcoa story is an example of leadership's explicit focus on the basics of safety. O'Neill recognized that safety could be a rallying focus for the workforce. By focusing on safety and pursuing the root causes of accidents, the company prioritized improving process flow, which led to increased productivity and reduced the cost of accidents and errors. This is the boldness of approach required by the COO in operating a care delivery system of high reliability. The results at Alcoa are legendary. The same focus, discipline, and commitment can be executed in health care.

High Reliability

To fulfill the vision of creating a safety culture, one that consistently demonstrates the characteristics of high reliability, operational leadership tools must be learned and used. Before describing leadership tools, a brief reference to aspects of high reliability may be helpful. Martin Hatlie, president of the National Partnership for Patient Safety, summarizes these characteristics as being the following:[10]

- Trust and transparency
- Reporting
- Flexibility in hierarchy
- Perceived to be just and accountable
- Engaged and dedicated to continuous learning

An illustration of the characteristics of high reliability is provided in the article "When Failure Is Not an Option," by Robert Pool.[11] Berkeley researchers ask you to imagine the following:

> Shrink your airport to only one short runway and one ramp and gate. Make planes take off and land at the same time, at half the present time interval, rock the runway from side to side, and require everybody to leave in the morning and return the same day. Turn off the radar to avoid detection, impose strict controls on radios, fuel the aircraft in place with their engines running, wet the whole thing down with salt water and oil, and man it with 20-year-olds, half of whom have never seen a plane.

This is a depiction of the operating conditions of *Nimitz*-class naval aircraft carriers, an environment operated by an organization that is highly reliable in its ability to avoid error. There are lessons in this example for health care and the COO. The U.S. Navy requires command rules and manuals of operating procedures to govern the flight deck processes, making explicit lessons learned from years of experience. Navy training is designed so that these procedures are second nature to the individuals who serve.

The article also describes another dimension of this highly structured hierarchical organization. The organizational structure shifts as pressures and risk increase during the launch and recovery of planes. The crew interact as colleagues, not superiors and subordinates. Cooperation and continual communication is part of the operation. With planes taking off and landing once a minute, things happen too quickly for instruction, delegation, and authorization to occur. The crew works as a team by watching each other and by communicating constantly and repeatedly. Each member of the team understands his or her role and that of the other members of the team. The constant flow of observation and communication identifies mistakes, the latent errors, before they cause damage or an accident. Experienced personnel continually monitor the flow, listening for everything that doesn't fit and correcting mistakes before they cause error.

In an emergency, such as a deck fire, a third organizational structure emerges. If any emergency occurs, the crew reacts immediately and without direction. Each crew member assumes a preassigned role and fulfills the role according to carefully rehearsed procedures. The safety of the ship and crew is everyone's responsibility. Even the lowest-ranking crewmember has not only the authority but the obligation to halt operations immediately under proper circumstances. The researchers report, "Although his judgment may later be reviewed or even criticized, he will not be penalized for being wrong and will often be publicly congratulated if right."[12]

Apply this description to the operations of a healthcare organization, division, or department where the safety of patients, staff, and families is a paramount concern. This is the COO's challenge in orchestrating high reliability. High-reliability organizations are both centralized and decentralized, hierarchical and collegial, rule bound and learning centered.[13] They also emphasize constant communication directed toward avoiding mistakes. Constant watching and interacting are used to advise, detect, and act on any sign of trouble. In addition, high-reliability organizations look for ways to constantly improve and never take success or safety for granted.

IMPORT AND APPLY NEW KNOWLEDGE AND SKILLS

Researchers Carolyn B. Libuser and Karlene Roberts identified common factors in safety from studying high-reliability organizations.[14] These factors define skill sets and tools that the COO can import and apply from other industries. Among the most relevant tools that need to be applied in health care to create safety are the following.

Process Auditing

Process auditing involves establishing a system for ongoing checks and formal audits to spot unexpected safety problems. Questions for the COO include the following:

- Is there an objective process to inquire about, review, and measure critical areas of performance for the organization and its parts?
- Is there an internal audit function outside of defined workgroups, departments, or care units to conduct such audits and reporting?
- Are critical indicators systematically measured, reported, and reviewed with frequency and regularity?
- Is a formalized framework for safety self-assessment used, such as the ones now becoming available through the National Patient Safety Foundation and other professional organizations?
- Are accrediting and regulatory surveys used as an opportunity for rigorous self-assessment?

Reward Systems

Questions concerning incentives or rewards for the COO include the following:

- How are reward systems used to drive the attention and behavior of the organization?
- Are reward systems aligned consistently with promoting safe practices and behavior?
- Are shortcuts being made and rewarded to reduce costs?
- How are disclosures of risk- and failure-prone practices managed?

Pursual of Safety Standards

In studies of catastrophic accidents such as the *Exxon Valdez* oil spill, the Chernobyl nuclear power plant explosion, and the chemical gas spill in Bhophal, India, standards for safety and quality were found to be subordinated to cost. Industry standards of basic safety were not met. Questions concerning safety standards for the COO are as follows:

- Do clear standards exist that differentiate safe, high-quality practices from substandard practices?
- Are monitors of performance against relevant best-in-class standards in place and rigorously applied?
- Is performance improvement required and monitored to achieve best-in-class performance standards?

Perception of Risk

Perception of risk has two aspects: whether the organization or its members are aware of risks that exist and, if awareness of risk exists, what measures are being taken to minimize risk. This relates to what data are collected, monitored, and acted on. In high-reliability organizations, there are effective monitoring systems and the organization acknowledges and confronts existing reality. Questions for the COO include the following:

- Do you require and regularly use effective monitors?

- Are the measures used the right measures, and of sufficient sensitivity, to detect early signals of declining performance?
- Are actions to improve required, along with an ongoing follow-up to ensure improvement is sustained?

Command and Control

Formal rules and procedures are necessary. These are not meant to create bureaucratic complexity, but rather to ensure adherence to the standards and shared knowledge of best practices. This implies intelligent and thoughtful application of rules and procedures, not routinized compliance. The rules and procedures should foster knowledge-based decisions, in which experts can determine when a variation or innovation is required because of a unique condition. This factor is expanded by Roberts and Libuser, who outline the following command-and-control elements:[15]

- *Migrating decision making:* The person with the most expertise makes the decision.
- *Having redundancy:* Back-up systems are in place, whether consisting of people or technology support.
- *Seeing the big picture*: Senior managers see the big picture, and therefore do not micromanage, but attend to patterns and systems.
- *Establishing formal rules and procedures:* There is hierarchy, with procedure and protocol based on evidence.
- *Conducting ongoing training*: Investment is made in the knowledge and skills of workers at the front line. This includes training in teamwork, such as crew resource management technologies.

A self-assessment against these criteria or characteristics of high-reliability organizations is a helpful step in determining the status of an organization and provides a baseline for action. The COO must have ongoing rigorous assessment in place to continually understand the status of safety in the organization, starting with the highest-risk procedures or processes. This is a different process from that of investigating errors and failures after they occur. Partnering content experts with outside human factors and engineering expertise can proactively detect latent failure and system vulnerabilities, allowing preventive actions to close gaps in safety. Although health care is probably more complex than any other industry and has unique features, it has much to learn and apply from other industries and domains of science, such as the common factors that humans bring to all fields. The COO should seek these lessons out and calibrate the expectations of risk and quality professionals to increase their skill portfolios to include patient safety.

APPLY NEW TOOLS AND BUILD INFRASTRUCTURE

Because the domain of patient safety is vast, a considerable armamentarium of tools is required. Establishing clear expectations, policies, and mechanisms to engage the patient and family as partners in creating safety is a responsibility of the chief operating officer. The tools described in this chapter are instrumental for the COO role.

Knowledge Base

Numerous tools in education and training are required to build a knowledge base for patient safety. Three concepts are of particular utility. They are as follows:[16]

- *The Swiss cheese model.* This represents the nature of emerging risks in complex systems, with defenses and vulnerabilities.
- *The blunt and sharp end.* This illustrates how expertise is applied and error or accident is experienced at the point where provider and patient exist in exquisite vulnerability, at the sharp end. The table is set, however, for that encounter at the blunt end, or the governance and man-

agement end, where decisions regarding such things as policy, production, and resource allocation are made. The high influence of these two disparate but interrelated parts of health care is a powerful reminder of the need to close the distance between front office and front line to understand the complexity of technical work in health care.

- *Hindsight bias.*[17] This concept, from the field of human factors, illustrates that it is human nature for people in hindsight to simplify conditions and underestimate the complexity that people involved in an error or accident were dealing with at the time of the event. The most common result of hindsight bias is to attribute the cause of a medical accident to "human error." Having thus found a scapegoat, all learning stops and the conditions that were present lay in wait to realign to produce another accident in the future.

Rapid-Cycle Change

Rapid-change technologies, such as Plan-Do-Study-Act (PDSA) cycles[18] and rapid replication,[19] are proven best practices to accelerate change and improvement. The COO's urgency, focus, and skills in this area are critical in requiring and mentoring the changes needed to improve patient safety. For example, specific best practices to adopt and implement include the best medication practices identified by the Massachusetts Hospital Association and the National Patient Safety Partnership, the surgical site identification advanced by the professional association for orthopedic surgeons, and others reported in the literature.[20] Attention should be given to lessons from the aviation industry in applying crew resource management training for care teams in high-risk areas, such as operating rooms, labor and delivery suites, and intensive care suites. It is essential to build an arm of the organization to assist managers and front-line staff in acting on reported information of risk.

Language

Accepting that language shapes culture, thoughtful and deliberate use of a new vocabulary to reflect the new look of safety is required. Consider using the following replacement of terms and deliberately building new language into the COO and management vocabulary:[21]

- *System* versus *isolated event.* An accident results from latent failures or weaknesses in a system. These failures or weaknesses are cumulative and interactive. Research has revealed that at least four errors must align to produce an accident. A recent analysis of a catastrophic medical accident revealed 82 errors or system failures contributing to the event. An isolated single cause is rare.
- *Analysis* or *study* versus *investigation.* A process of analysis or study is used to learn how systems work and how the pieces fit together to create the whole. The learning from rigorous analysis can be applied to predict and inform interventions to prevent future failures. An investigation carries the connotation of a process to assign blame. It is typically a linear search to determine a single cause or "bad apple."
- *Accountable* versus *blame.* Healthcare professionals are accountable for their work. They have a responsibility to ensure they possess current knowledge and demonstrate competence in the work they perform, as well as the interdependence they have in that performance. In addition, they must appreciate how systems work and how people are the human components of systems that sometimes contribute to failure as well as create safety. Blame fixes on a scapegoat, rather than a pursuit of a deeper understanding of failure. Historical methods of blame, train, and punish have not worked to improve safety.
- *Blameless* versus *punitive* or *retaliatory.* A blameless environment is one where

healthcare personnel feel comfortable and compelled to report failures and near misses so they can be studied. Punitive or retaliatory environments create an atmosphere where healthcare staff are afraid to disclose failures and near misses, thus eliminating the opportunity to learn from mistakes.

- *Heedful procedure* versus *routine procedure.* Heedful procedures are designed so that they cannot be performed without thinking. Rather, they include steps that demand attention before action can take place. Routine procedures are those that are performed so many times they can become automatic, and as such introduce greater risk.
- *Hierarchy* versus *bureaucracy.* Hierarchy is a system of formal rules, procedures, training, and decision making based on evidence. Senior managers see the big picture and therefore do not micromanage, but attend to patterns and systems. Decisions are made by the person with the most expertise. Bureaucracy is a system of administration marked by adherence to fixed rules; authority by position, not expertise; red tape; specialized and isolated silos; and the politics of control.
- *What happened?* versus *Whose fault is it?* The question "What happened?" invites analysis of the conditions surrounding an error or accident. Asking "Whose fault is it?" immediately seeks to place blame and resorts to the social attribution of human error as cause.
- *Accident of failure* versus *human error as cause.* Accident describes a breakdown in a system, which is complex and needs analysis. Error suggests that only one factor, usually noted as human error, is the cause. If human error is assigned as the cause, all learning stops.
- *Multicausal* versus *root cause.* Studies of accidents reveal that at least four failures must occur and line up to create the conditions for an accident to occur. The Swiss cheese model illustrates the multicausal concept, suggesting that multiple failures or errors align to produce an accident versus a single source. Understanding this and pursuing the deeper story of an accident discloses the contributing conditions, latent vulnerabilities, or trajectories that lead to accidents. Analysis of the deeper story in turn allows for systemic actions to reduce the probability that a similar accident will occur in the future.
- *Learning* versus *judgment.* To build safer systems to prevent failures from happening again, an organization must be committed to learning from mistakes. A noted archeologist was quoted as saying, "Dig where you stumble, for that is where the treasure is." Such a mind-set directs a passionate curiosity to dig deeply into understanding sources of failure, where we stumbled, and also the sources of success, where error was averted. Judgment closes down inquiry.

Process Auditing Tools and Methods

This area was addressed under the section on high reliability. Process auditing tools and methods move safety into a proactive role.

Architecture for Learning

Minicourses with national experts, attended by interdisciplinary members of the organization; dialogues to invite informal exploration of safety; self-learning packets; orientation and training modules; and ongoing publications in the communication vehicles of the organization serve to teach, reinforce, and stimulate learning among all members of the healthcare delivery system.

Policies to Advance Partnerships with Patients and Their Families

- *"Nothing about me without me."* This policy embraces practices and tools to involve the patient and family in decision making and participation in the care process. It includes providing information to patient and family through multiple media such as print, Internet, video, courses, counseling, and conferencing, in a timely manner and in a way that can be understood. This includes ensuring translators and translated materials for the multicultural communities served. Informational content focused on what patient's families need to know, ask, and do to create safety with their providers is empowering and an essential part of care.

- *"If it looks wrong, it is wrong."* This is a policy that not only legitimizes but requires anyone who perceives a risk to safety to stop the process. This includes the patient and family. All participants in the care process have the responsibility to stop until the question of risk has been thoroughly examined and safety established. This policy, fashioned after the "Andon Cord" in industry, empowers all participants in the healthcare system to act to establish safety without regard to hierarchy.
- *Disclosure and truth telling.* This policy is one that provides guidance in working with patients and families in the face of an error or medical accident. It consists in establishing and guiding the practice of communication and is a powerful culture carrier. The National Patient Safety Foundation has published a statement of principle to talk to patients about healthcare accidents and adverse events. Elements of disclosure include a prompt and compassionate explanation of what is understood about what happened and the probable effects, what is being done to ensure safety, the assurance that a full analysis will take place to reduce the likelihood of a similar event happening to another patient, what changes are being made based on the findings of the analyses as they are known, and an acknowledgment of accountability.[22] Skills training in critical communication is needed, and the COO has the responsibility to ensure the necessary resources.

Response to Medical Accidents

It is the responsibility of the COO and other designated senior managers to be immediately notified and to respond to medical accidents, significant near misses, and sentinel events. Clear policies and operating procedures are required to set expectations and guide action. The response to medical accidents both defines and shapes a safety culture. The direct involvement of senior leadership with patient, family, and affected staff is an important statement of commitment and accountability.

Measures

An essential tool for the COO is measurement. Measures serve as the gauges to determine whether desired changes are taking place and desired effects are being achieved. Increasing the frequency of measures and providing feedback to front-line workers can accelerate and sustain change. Although measuring medical error is complicated, a starting point is to measure increased reporting. Measures also need to be built for public accountability as well as for internal and industry-specific learning and improvement.

ASSIGN ACCOUNTABILITY

A specific work plan with ambitious aims, goals, assigned accountabilities, and measures is an essential tool. Defined and focused resources to execute the plan are also needed. The work plan provides a road map to achieve the aims, as well as a method for the organization to align contributions and gauge effectiveness. Serious consideration should be given to the designation of a technical leader for patient safety to help execute the patient safety work plan. A patient safety leader or director is a role that complements the COO as content expert, consultative resource to managers and front line providers, and catalyst for the organization to develop greater capacity at the sharp end or front line of care.

Assigning accountability also carries with it the requirement to actively engage employees and professional staff in the design and execution of the safety agenda. Providing care that is free of defect is a shared interest among those who have committed their careers to health care. Actively engaging all stakeholders, however, starts with an inspiring aim, goals, and associated measures that are directly relevant to patient care. As mentioned throughout this chapter, the leadership strives to create a confidential and safe space, ask questions, and consistently follow through, eliminating the skepticism that patient safety is a fad, a buzzword, or shallow rhetoric. Such action emphasizes the work of patient safety as a long-term and never-ending disciplined pursuit.

Mentoring an Accountability System

The COO mentors the required accountability system by holding managers directly responsible for taking action to eliminate or mitigate known risks, urgently responding to near misses, and engaging in continual dialogue and learning about creating ever-increasing levels of safety. Every conversation becomes curriculum content of accountability in the management system of the organization.

Engaging the Organization

There are many examples of engagement strategies. A specific engagement strategy is to work with managers to establish a safety log in each unit for staff to enter safety information. Managers and medical leadership should meet regularly with an interdisciplinary team to review the content of the log, prioritize, and plan resolving actions to eliminate or mitigate risks identified.

A safety action team can be assembled at each local unit, populated by interdisciplinary and interdepartmental staff who are empowered to take the necessary actions to implement changes that increase safety and reduce the probability that accidents will occur. They can develop and use data sources, such as logs, safety reports, provider insights, and patient and family feedback. They can also scan relevant literature for ideas from the experience of others.

At a broad organizational level, a patient safety steering committee with membership from across the organization, including professional staff, clinical front-line staff, consumers, and board members, can be appointed to advise on strategy, formulate policy, and monitor results. They may also act as resources and emissaries of patient safety to the organization. The role of the COO in chartering and chairing such a forum is a powerful and visible message about the commitment to and priority of patient safety in the organization. It also provides a forum for practicing clinicians, clinical leaders, administrators, communication experts, consumers, and governing directors to engage in promoting safety and the changes that must be made to achieve ever-increasing levels of safety in care delivery.

Further areas of engagement include leveraging information technology and clinical staff expertise to design the necessary decision supports, alerts, documentation processes, information migration, and reports to enhance patient safety. Direct order entry, dose-range checking, bar coding, and alerts for incompatibilities and allergies in the medication use system are a starting point. The use of information technology is just beginning to be a fully realized domain of patient safety. Although not a technical expert, the COO's role involves gaining a working knowledge of what is possible, and engaging cross-functional experts to anticipate and build what is necessary.

ESTABLISH BLAMELESS REPORTING

Reporting for accountability, reporting for learning, and reporting for intervention are important COO considerations. The discussion of this facet of the patient safety manifesto will focus on reporting for learning and intervention, while noting that public accountability, by reporting medical accidents to the appropriate agencies and authorities, is an obligation and is addressed in the section "Align External Controls."

The reporting system is not only a tool, but a deep cultural intervention to nurture an "alert field" and empower front-line technical and clinical providers. Characteristics of the system include a blameless and confidential reporting system, robust analysis and pattern detection, feedback, and communication of lessons learned. The system should encourage and reward increased risk perception and reporting of near misses, vulnerabilities, and "accidents waiting to happen." A reporting format with limited fixed fields and greater room for text allows the story of existing conditions that contributed to error and accident to be identified, explored, and better understood. This requires greater analytical investment but yields richer intelligence about how systems and processes are actually operating. Transparency is a characteristic of the reporting process that enables everyone to learn from failures, accidents, and acts of prevention.

Reporting and tracking data for purposes of learning and improvement require an environment of confidentiality and privilege of protection. The healthcare workplace must be free of blame, punishment, and liability exposure so that full disclosure and learning can take place. This, however, does not apply to circumstances of gross negligence, intention to harm, unethical behavior, impairment due to drugs or alcohol, or failure to learn over time. These circumstances, although rare, pose a threat to patient safety and must be dealt with swiftly, fairly, and professionally from an administrative perspective.

Recognition and celebration of risk identification and reporting, through providing timely feedback, telegraphing lessons learned, taking action, and saying "thank you," reinforce a culture that is alert, critical, and heedful in its work. Rather than normalizing deviance through routine or through resignation and acceptance of the status quo as the standard, this environment critically examines everything it does and engages in learning and improvement. Changing the frame of reference from "incident reporting" to "safety reporting" removes historic connotations of performance judgment and expands reporting to a productive stance in identifying near misses and risks. Importing lessons from the aviation industry is one of the best practices for developing a reporting model for health care.

ALIGN EXTERNAL CONTROLS

Safety cultures are created through trust, knowledge, and well-designed interventions to produce desired effects. The role of the COO is to actively foster these characteristics inside the organization and in the societal context in which the organization operates.

The broad view of patient safety encompasses three domains: 1. how society understands and talks about safety, 2. how the legislative and legal system acts, and 3. what we do inside and across healthcare organizations and systems.

The emphasis of this chapter has been on what to do inside healthcare organizations and systems. However, the role of the COO must encompass influencing the public discourse on patient safety. The legal system and media are very challenging. The societal call for "heads to roll" when something goes wrong in medical care must be respected and met with accountability and open dialogue to appreciate the paradox of contemporary health care. This paradox is that with dramatic increases in the ability to cure and treat injury and disease and perform "miracles" of medicine comes the expectation of perfect outcomes and infallible providers. The very technology that introduces breakthroughs in science also introduces new and unprecedented risk that leads to medical accident. The COO role is one that must actively seek avenues to influence, interpret, and create forums to explore the complexities of patient safety. The exquisite tension between public accountability and the public's right to know versus provider confidentiality and privilege of protection in pursuit of improvement must be managed. These notions are not mutually exclusive, but require a balance-seeking dialogue.

The active involvement of the COO with regulatory and accrediting bodies is increasing. The need to align external controls to promote, rather than undermine, efforts to improve safety is critical. This involves mutually exploring messages and behaviors that create partnership, while also eliminating messages and conduct that create barriers. Working with professional organizations to promote patient safety through educational offerings, skills development, care competencies, and expanded research efforts is another leadership activity.

The COO role includes working with government and with professional organizations, especially those with purchasing power, to require pharmaceutical and device industries to submit products to human factors testing, engineer safety features into product design, and use labeling practices that elevate safety above marketing considerations. Engaging the media is increasingly important to encourage responsible reporting of the issues in medical accidents rather than sensationalizion of specific cases, which may cause internal safety reporting and analysis to go underground for fear of reprisals. Working toward tort reform is another COO consideration in preparing an environment for patient safety.

THE BUSINESS CASE

The COO is required to operate the organization cost-effectively in order to provide affordable care and services, allow for financial resources to reinvest in the growth and capability of the organization, and help ensure long-term viability. This chapter would be incomplete without explicitly addressing the business case for patient safety. Beyond the ethical imperative to improve safety, there is a compelling business case.

The business case for patient safety is reducing cost through improving care and eliminating the costs of poor quality. This serves as a more compelling rallying point for efficiency and productivity than the cost-cutting messages that plague the healthcare industry and may have had the effect of increasing risk and undermining safety. The original Harvard Practice Study concluded that 6.7% of all hospital admissions experience a medical error; of these, 3.4% result in an adverse event, and 14% of those events are fatal.[23] It was this study, extrapolated to national demographics, that created the compelling comparison that the number of annual hospital deaths is equivalent to the death toll that would result from the crash of two jumbo jet carriers each week. Studies are now suggesting that deaths from medical accident, currently reported as the number eight public health problem in the United States, are grossly underestimated. Applying these early findings allows an organization to model the predicted number of patients expected to experience an adverse event.

The studies further noted that each adverse event added $4,700 in costs of care.[24] A simple economic model can be constructed to estimate the increased cost to the burden of illness due to adverse events. Analyzing actual adverse events in an organization to determine the cost is a worthwhile initiative. Engaging the chief financial officer in this exercise is an important strategy to develop awareness and appreciation of the issue. It is important to note that few errors and adverse events are caused by unusual or rare circumstances.[25] Rather, these adverse events constitute a familiar list: wound infection, drug overdose, wrong drug, bleeding from anticoagulation, insulin reaction, missed diagnosis, and falls. Because these risks and events are known and predictable, they are also preventable. It is estimated that these preventable events represent over 72% of medical accidents and errors.[26]

Studies further found that the setting of care was not significant in preventability, thereby focusing attention systemwide to hospital, clinic, emergency department, free-standing ambulatory care, and diagnostic settings.[27] The work of patient safety is not isolated to the highest-risk clinical inpatient environments but is the work of the entire system of care, with particular attention to the handoffs and transitions between areas and functions.

The business case for patient safety involves reducing the costs of poor quality through the development of aligned and effective systems of care delivery in every part of the continuum from suppliers of products to care encounters. When patient safety, or the reduction of error and accident, becomes an explicit business strategy, then errors and accidents must be examined in enormous detail. The organization, not the individual, must be examined from a process flow perspective. Efficient and effective systems are safe systems.[28]

In most healthcare organizations, people have learned to work around unnecessary complexity, process failure, and other system issues. When people adapt their practices around faulty systems, waste is usually produced. Waste in processes adds additional cost burden and frustration to the work of patient care. This "normalization of deviance" is not only costly but adds risk of error and accident to the care system.

An engaged and stable workforce is a contribution to safety and reduces the cost of turnover and declining productivity. A safe organization builds confidence and a reputation that can translate to loyalty and market share. However, an investment is required. Designating an operating budget to support patient safety and sponsoring applied research funding are COO responsibilities. The business case, through economic modeling of preventable errors and adverse events, refocusing resources to the safety agenda, and integrating safety into the core expectations of all managers, allows providers to begin to identify sources of funding.

SUMMARY

The COO plays a pivotal role in defining, inspiring, and developing an aligned organization that consistently demonstrates the characteristics of high reliability. Ensuring effective human resources systems and management practices in recruitment, training, and ongoing ensurance of competence is essential. Setting and communicating clear expectations that risk perception, reporting, and error prevention are the responsibility of each individual and the collective obligation of everyone is essential. Dedicating the resources to educate about and advance patient safety underlies COO and organizational commitment. Hardwiring patient safety into the strategy, management and measurement system, and reward system of the organization integrates patient safety as part of the organization, not an initiative grafted onto it. Nurturing patient and family partnerships through policies, protocols, and practices is foundational. The willingness and enthusiasm to do the heavy lifting of the work in patient safety, and the courage to stay the course and model the way, is the COO's role in aligning operations to build systems that do no harm.

A final note: The more you know and do in patient safety, the more you will see to do. The stages in increasing patient safety create a clearer line of sight to the evolving knowledge of the topic and the greater depth of application and action that is called for. As our industry effectively tackles the known risks of today's environment, new knowledge, technology, pharmaceutical agents, and challenges, such as changes in workforce demographics, will be continually introduced, with new emerging risks. By aggressively learning the lessons of today, there will be greater intelligence and capacity to address the challenges of the future. This challenge is one of the worthy pursuits of the COO role that adds value to healthcare delivery.

References

1. Helmreich, R., and Merritt, A. *Culture at Work in Medicine and Aviation: National, Organizational and Professional Influences* (Aldershot, UK: Ashgate, 1998).
2. Helmreich, R. et al., "Applying Aviation Safety Initiatives to Medicine," *Focus on Patient Safety* 4, no. 1 (2001):1–2.
3. Weingart, S. "Patient Safety Manifesto," notes from the Executive Session on Medical Error and Patient Safety, Division of Health Policy Research and Education, Harvard University, Harvard Medical School, Malcolm Wiener Center for Social Policy, John F. Kennedy School of Government, January 29, 2000.
4. Institute of Medicine Committee of Healthcare in America, L. Kohn et al., eds., *To Err Is Human: Building a Safer Health System* (Washington, DC: National Academy Press, 1999).
5. Leape, L. L. et al., "The Nature of Adverse Events in Hospitalized Patients: Results from the Harvard Medical Practice Study II," *New England Journal of Medicine* 324 (1991):377–384.
6. Wilson, N., and Study Team, "Patient Safety: Listening to Healthcare Employees," Cooperative Study of Veterans Health Administration, Care Group, Kaiser Permanente, and National Patient Safety Foundation, sponsored by Department of Veterans Affairs, 1998.
7. Nance, J. D. "Managing Human Error in Aviation," *Scientific American* May (1997):62–70.
8. Norman, D. *The Psychology of Everyday Things* (New York: Basic Books, 1988).
9. Clark, K. B., and Margolis, J. D. "Workplace Safety at Alcoa," Case 9-692-042 (Boston: Harvard Business School Publishing, 1991), 1–2.
10. Hatlie, M. Patient Safety Collaborative Lecture Series, Voluntary Hospitals of American Regional Collaboratives, 2000.
11. Pool, R. "When Failure Is Not an Option," *Technology Review* 100 (1997):38–45.
12. Ibid.
13. Libuser, C. B., and Roberts, K. "Risk Mitigation Through Organizational Structure," paper to be submitted, 1998.
14. Ibid.
15. Ibid.
16. Reason, J. *Managing the Risks of Organizational Accidents* (Brookfield, NY: Ashgate, 1997).
17. Cook, R. for the Cognitive Technologies Laboratory, *How Systems Fail* (Chicago: Cognitive Technologies Laboratory, 2002).
18. Langley, G. J. et al., *The Improvement Guide: A Practical Approach to Enhancing Organizational Performance* (San Francisco: Jossey-Bass, 1996).
19. Cauldwell, C. *Mentoring Strategic Change in Health Care: An Action Guide* (Milwaukee, WI: ASQC Quality Press, 1995).
20. Joint Commission on Accreditation of Healthcare Organizations. *Sentinel Event Alert* 6 (Oakbrook Terrace, IL: JCAHO, 1998).
21. Minnesota Hospital and Healthcare Partnership and Minnesota Medical Association, "Redefining the Culture for Patient Safety [brochure]" (St. Paul, MN: Author, 2000).
22. National Patient Safety Foundation, "NPSF Statement Principle: Talk to Patients About Health Care Injury," *Focus on Patient Safety* 4, no. 1 (2000):3.
23. Brennan, T. A. et al., "Incidence of Adverse Events and Negligence in Hospitalized Patients: Results from the Harvard Medical Practice Study I," *New England Journal of Medicine* 324 (1991):370–376.
24. Leape et al., "The Nature of Adverse Events in Hospitalized Patients."
25. Johnson, J. A., and Bootman, J. L. "Drug-Related Morbidity and Mortality and the Economic Impact on Pharmaceutical Care," *American Journal of Hospital-System Pharmacy* 54 (1997).
26. Leape, L. L. et al., "Preventing Medical Injury," *Quality Review Bulletin* May (1993):144–149.
27. Ibid.
28. Massmann, J. as quoted in "Taking the Mistakes Out of Medicine," feature of the Children's Hospitals and Clinics of Minnesota, J. Shapiro, *U.S. News and World Report* July (2000):50–66.

17

The Role of the Risk Manager in Creating Patient Safety

Grena G. Porto, RN, MHA, ARM, CPHRM

The goal of healthcare risk management is to create and maintain a safe and effective healthcare environment for patients, visitors, and employees, thereby preventing or reducing loss to the organization.[1] This goal has remained constant since the birth of the profession 30 years ago, but the methods used to accomplish it have changed and evolved to accommodate evolution and innovation in the profession. The emergence of patient safety as a national priority following the release of the Institute of Medicine's report on medical error[2] has changed the way providers view risk and safety. Acceptance and complacency about the inevitability of patient injury is evaporating rapidly as providers confront increasing demands from patients, regulators, and payers for safer care.

There is some evidence that a safety culture is emerging in health care. High-reliability intensive care units have been identified by some authors.[3,4] However, more work is needed to make entire healthcare organizations high-reliability organizations. Risk managers can and must play a key role in this process if the transformation of health care into a high-reliability industry is to succeed. This chapter discusses the strategies and tactics that risk managers must employ to make health care safer in their organizations.

WHAT IS A HIGH-RELIABILITY ORGANIZATION?

Comparisons of error rates between health care and other industries have shown that the healthcare industry tolerates a rate of error that would be considered unacceptable by NASA, aviation, the nuclear power industry, and even the postal service.[5] In light of this, health care has begun to study these other industries to identify strategies that may be adapted to health care to help reduce error.

High-reliability organizations are highly complex and hazardous systems that are fraught with risk of error and injury, yet which operate over long periods of time without errors or injury. Examples of high-reliability organizations include aircraft carriers, NASA, and nuclear power. Studies of high-reliability organizations[6,7] have shown that they share common features:

- *Auditing of risk:* An ongoing system of checks designed to detect both expected and unexpected risk and safety problems.
- *Appropriate reward system:* A mechanism for rewarding both the organization and the people in it for safety-oriented behavior.
- *System quality standards:* An acknowledged system that is the "gold standard" in safety.
- *Acknowledgment of risk:* These organizations acknowledge that risk exists and address the risk by adopting strategies to mitigate it.
- *Command and control:* A management model that balances authority and teamwork and is characterized by migrating decision making, built-in redundancies in systems and people, senior managers with "big picture" orientation who do not micromanage, formal rules and procedures, and training.

Safety in high-reliability organizations is not left to chance; it is the result of careful planning and design. The challenge for healthcare risk managers is to find ways to design these features into their own organizations. Some parallels already exist; however, modification is needed to make these features more effective in creating safety. What follows is a discussion of each of the features of high-reliability organizations, the existing counterparts in health care, and the changes that are needed to enhance the features to create safety.

AUDITING OF RISK

Healthcare risk managers use a number of tools to audit risk, including incident reports, referrals from other departments such as quality improvement (QI), informal reports from staff, medical record reviews, and regular rounds of patient care units. Each of these methods of auditing risk has strengths and weaknesses. As cost pressures have escalated in healthcare organizations and resources have become scarce, there has been an increased reliance on voluntary reporting systems to identify risk, since they consume the least amount of resources. The information generated by these reports is analyzed, categorized, quantified, and often used to compare the organization's performance with respect to either its own past experience or the experience of other organizations.

There are several problems with this approach to auditing of risk. First, incident reporting systems are often burdensome, requiring the front-line worker, already pressed to attend to multiple competing priorities, to complete a written form. Second, the form itself tends to limit the information to that which can be described by a series of checkboxes. Narratives are discouraged, as is speculation about possible causes of events. Instead, emphasis is placed on aggregation of data; thus, much valuable information about the causes of events is lost. Third, incident reporting systems are punitive in nature because the reporter's identity is attached to the report and the information contained in the report often forms the basis for disciplinary action against the reporter or another party. This creates a disincentive for reporting. Finally, there are few incentives for reporting, because reporting is rarely rewarded and the reporter seldom receives feedback about the report or the outcome of the analysis.

One of the most successful risk auditing programs in existence is the Aviation Safety Reporting System (ASRS).[8] The system was implemented in 1975 with the goal of creating a safer aviation system by collecting information from the acknowledged safety experts in the field—front-line workers such as mechanics, pilots, and air traffic controllers. Today, it receives and processes approximately 35,000 reports annually. Some of the key characteristics that make ASRS successful are as follows:

- *Nonpunitive reporting structure.* The reporting system is operated by NASA rather than by the aviation industry or its regulators, thereby removing the threat of punitive or regulatory consequences for reporters. In addition, the name of the reporter is removed from the report after a brief evaluation period, ensuring that his or her identity will not be revealed. The ASRS has found that eliminating fear by safeguarding the identity of the reporter is key to encouraging reporting.

- *Emphasis on detailed narratives rather than on aggregate or frequency data.* The reporting system solicits detailed narratives from reporters, including their theories about what happened and why. The ASRS has learned that truly useful information about how accidents occur comes from the observations of those involved in the event, not from trending aggregate data.
- *Nonburdensome reporting.* The forms are simple and easy to use. Follow-up to the initial report occurs through telephone conversations with expert analysts who staff the reporting center. The reporter is not inconvenienced in any way by the reporting process; this also serves to encourage reporting.
- *Feedback to reporters.* Information about identified hazards is provided to front-line aviation workers in the form of alerts, newsletters, and other publications, which reinforces the importance of reporting. Currently, ASRS issues approximately 20 safety alerts per month.

Voluntary reporting systems currently in use in health care share few of the critical success factors of the ASRS model. However, healthcare risk managers, as custodians of voluntary reporting systems, can play a critical role in transforming these systems into successful risk auditing systems by emulating the ASRS model. This can be achieved by doing the following:

- Eliminate confusing and restrictive definitions about what is reportable, which creates barriers to reporting. Instead, encourage widespread and automatic reporting of all potential safety problems, including close calls, screening out information that is not useful after it is received.
- Eliminate duplicative reporting and standardize the reporting process to avoid confusion. Use the same system for reporting of all potential safety problems.
- Create multiple methods of accessing the reporting system, including oral, written, and electronic reporting options, to accommodate the needs and preferences of reporters.
- Offer anonymity in exchange for information when needed. Even in a nonpunitive reporting culture, some healthcare workers will feel threatened by reporting and will need the security of anonymity in order to participate in the reporting system.
- Press for a nonpunitive reporting policy that does not tie disciplinary action to reports. The risk manager must be prepared to educate the entire organization, including senior management, about the deleterious effects of tying discipline to voluntary reporting.
- Implement an amnesty policy that offers freedom from disciplinary action in exchange for timely good-faith reporting. Most errors are due to system defects rather than individual failure. An amnesty policy makes a convincing case for the organization's commitment to building a culture of safety while still allowing for disciplinary actions against those who intentionally harm patients.
- Encourage narratives that provide detail about how the event occurred and possible contributing factors. These narratives are the richest source of information about how accidents truly occur and therefore provide the best hope for designing system changes to prevent future accidents.
- Provide for a mechanism for immediate response to a serious hazard. This not only prevents recurrence of a problem, but also provides important feedback about the organization's commitment to the safety program and reinforces reporting.

- Discontinue counting, trending, and other quantitative analysis that provides little useful information. This activity consumes valuable resources that could be better devoted to analyzing narratives and disseminating important information about lessons learned.
- Create incentives for reporting, such as rewards for safety reports that lead to improvements. Adopt the strategies used by other industries, including commemorative plaques, small gifts, and other tokens to acknowledge the contribution of the "safety hero."
- Provide feedback about lessons learned from reporting to the front-line healthcare worker. This will reinforce the importance and utility of the reporting system. Feedback should take the form of stories about events reported, the causes identified, and actions taken to improve safety as a result. This type of feedback is more likely to be remembered and used by the healthcare worker than quantitative data on the frequency of events reported.
- Train staff on the importance and role of reporting in creating safety, and on their own role in patient safety.

APPROPRIATE REWARD SYSTEM

High-reliability organizations recognize that reward is more important than punishment in motivating and changing behavior. They know that in order for a specific behavior to take hold and become routine practice, it must be rewarded. At the same time, disincentives that might discourage the behavior must be removed. Healthcare organizations rarely reward employees for safety-related behavior, though this practice is commonplace in other settings, such as aerospace engineering and even the military. Experience from these industries has shown that even small rewards can have a profound effect on culture and morale.[9]

Healthcare risk managers are uniquely positioned to lead the development of a reward system that encourages safety-related behavior because of their access to a wide variety of identified problems and solutions. They can do this by:

- *Identifying the safety-related behaviors the organization wishes to encourage.* This can be done in consultation with other members of the management team as part of the development of an organization-wide safety plan. These behaviors might include timely reporting of actual or potential safety problems, questioning of decisions by others that seem to compromise patient safety, effective teamwork, and involvement in work process redesign to enhance safety.
- *Identifying and removing disincentives caused by undue burdens associated with the safety-related behaviors.* For example, if the organization wants to discourage a practice it deems unsafe, such as multiple-dose medication vials, but fails to provide a safe alternative that is convenient, such as timely delivery of unit doses, it has created a disincentive for the safety-related behavior it wishes to encourage. Until the disincentive is identified and removed, the safety-related behavior will not be widely adopted.
- *Identifying and removing disincentives caused by fear.* If a safety-related behavior, such as reporting actual or potential patient injury, is accompanied by a negative consequence for the reporter, such as reprimand from a superior or hostility from a coworker, the desired behavior will be avoided. Likewise, if the safety-related behavior is rewarded only when it is without negative consequences for the organization, a disincentive is created. For example, if employees are encouraged to halt a procedure when they have safety-related concerns, but are rewarded only when their concerns

are well founded and punished when they are not, a disincentive is created. It is important that all disincentives be removed and rewards applied consistently, even when safety-related behaviors prove unnecessary.

- *Identifying and removing disincentives caused by lack of knowledge or interest.* For a patient safety program to succeed, it must have the commitment and participation of all levels of the organization. Healthcare workers are not likely to support a program that is imposed on them with little opportunity for their input. By implementing training and outreach programs that enhance the knowledge of the healthcare worker and increase opportunities for involvement, the healthcare risk manager can promote the success of the safety program. As mentioned in the previous section, feedback and responsiveness are also important components that reinforce participation in the safety program and maintain commitment and interest.
- *Creating rewards for safety-related behaviors.* Rewards need not be costly or elaborate to have the desired effect. Even financially challenged organizations can implement a system of rewards that can greatly enhance employee commitment to and involvement in the safety program. For example, recognition at a meeting, perhaps accompanied by a plaque or other token, is a powerful reward that can greatly motivate not only the recipient but others in the organization to continue to support the safety program. This is especially true if the reward and recognition comes from a member of senior management, such as the CEO.
- *Publicizing rewards and success stories.* Rewards are most effective when they are well known and celebrated within the organization. Not every success story must be celebrated and not every safety-related behavior must be rewarded. But rewards, recognition, and celebrations should occur frequently enough to demonstrate the organization's commitment to the safety program. Newsletters can be an effective means of publicizing rewards and success stories.

SYSTEM QUALITY STANDARDS

In high-reliability industries, there is consensus regarding what constitutes safety, and standards exist against which organizations can measure themselves. Often there is an industry leader that is recognized as having achieved the highest standards of safety and that others try to emulate.

In health care, patient safety standards are still evolving. The Institute of Medicine (IOM) report[10] released in 1999 helped to accelerate this process and contained a number of recommendations that are becoming accepted as standards. The Joint Commission has also published standards on patient safety,[11] incorporating many components of the IOM's recommendations. In addition, the Leapfrog Group, a coalition of large national corporations representing their interests as purchasers of health care, has begun setting standards in patient safety.[12] They have identified three strategies—computerized physician order entry, evidence-based referrals, and intensive care unit (ICU) physician staffing—that have been shown to improve patient safety and have announced their intention to use these as selection criteria for the contracting of healthcare services on behalf of employees. Finally, the Institute for Safe Medication Practices (ISMP)[13] has been instrumental in developing and disseminating medication safety standards.

Patient safety leaders are beginning to emerge, and there have been well-recognized efforts by some organizations, such as Children's Hospital in Minneapolis, to create a high-reliability organization based on established principles.[14] The Veteran's Health

Administration has also demonstrated leadership in patient safety for its work in developing nonpunitive reporting systems.[15]

Although the healthcare risk manager is not in a position to propel the organization to a position of industry leadership, he or she can play an important role in helping the organization meet emerging standards in patients safety. This can be done by:

- Assisting in the development and implementation of an organization-wide patient safety plan that identifies patient safety as a top priority.
- Ensuring that there is a mechanism for prompt identification and analysis of patient safety problems, including identification of root causes and themes across events and root causes.
- Ensuring that corrective actions planned as a result of incident analysis incorporate principles of human factors engineering, cognitive bias, and adult learning so that risk of error can be minimized. This includes decreased reliance on memory and vigilance, use of constraints and forcing functions, and standardization and simplification of work processes when possible.
- Recognizing the importance of teamwork in error prevention and lobbying for organizational support and commitment of resources to teamwork training in high-risk areas, such as the emergency department, operating room, and ICU.
- Promoting a culture of safety in which all healthcare workers are empowered to make decisions that support patient safety without fear of retribution.
- Promoting inclusion of patients in the design of the systems and processes of care.
- Ensuring that patients who suffer a harm-causing adverse event are provided with all known information about what happened, why it happened, and what consequences they should expect as a result.
- Working to identify system failures prospectively, practicing failures, and designing for recovery from failure.
- Working to create a learning environment that encourages reporting of errors and close calls and focuses on learning from these rather than on blame and reprisal.
- Helping the organization to prepare for the installation of computerized order entry systems.
- Helping prepare the organization to meet evolving requirements in the area of evidence-based referrals and ICU physician staffing.
- Identifying and introducing emerging standards in the area of medication safety.
- Monitoring developments of technological solutions, such as bar coding, that help to prevent error.
- Monitoring and maintaining current knowledge about the development of other patient safety solutions that the organization may wish to consider adopting.

ACKNOWLEDGMENT OF RISK

High-reliability organizations acknowledge that risk exists rather than create unrealistic expectations about performance and outcomes. In addition to acknowledging risk, these organizations take steps to reduce or mitigate risk, designing a system focused on detection and recovery from error, rather than simply accepting that errors are inevitable.

To acknowledge risk, it is first necessary to talk openly about it. In healthcare organizations, discussion about risks or errors has been traditionally discouraged because of fears of liability and regulatory consequences. This tendency to avoid discussion of risk and error precludes mitigation of risk, because it is not possible to discuss potential solutions to a problem without discussing the problem.

However, healthcare providers' fears about discussing risk and errors are not well founded. Disclosure of medical errors, even to patients, does not lead to increased liability, and in fact has been shown to decrease the risk of a lawsuit. Further, discussion of errors with colleagues and patients has been shown to have benefits for both patients and providers, enabling patients to forgive, providers to be forgiven, and the organization to learn from the error and make plans to mitigate future risk of error.

Healthcare risk managers are in a unique position to lead an organization's journey to acknowledgment of risk. Because risk managers have traditionally been the guardians of information about errors and risk, they can begin to educate senior management and other levels of the organization about the benefits of information sharing as a means to acknowledge, demystify, and ultimately reduce risk of error. This can be done by:

- Developing a policy that permits and rewards reporting of errors and close calls, as outlined previously;
- Encouraging healthcare workers to share information about errors and close calls, permitting them to learn from one another's experiences;
- Promoting a shift toward a blame-free culture that recognizes that failure is a property of the system rather than the individual;
- Emphasizing the importance of error as an opportunity to learn how to prevent future errors;
- Focusing on rapid recognition and recovery from error; and
- Developing a program that addresses identified risk proactively, with system redesign and appropriate allocation of resources.

COMMAND AND CONTROL

In high-reliability organizations, command-and-control functions are management processes designed to balance authority and teamwork and enable rapid and easy transition between these two models as needed to create safety. Command-and-control functions in high-reliability organizations have five characteristics:

1. Migrating decision making that enables the person with the most expertise to make decisions, regardless of rank
2. Redundancy in people and equipment so that backups are always available when needed
3. Senior managers with strategic vision who don't micromanage, allowing experienced subordinates with more direct knowledge to make decisions as needed
4. Formal rules and procedures that provide true guidance and are followed
5. Training, so that expertise is planned for and developed, not left to chance

In health care, there exists a rigid hierarchy in which the physician is viewed as the "captain of the ship" to whom other members of the team must be subservient. This rigid management style does not change as circumstances change. Yet we know that this management model is not the best one for preventing error.

Making changes in the command-and-control model of a healthcare organization requires the commitment and leadership of senior management as well as a change in culture and thinking throughout the organization. However, as an organization evolves toward high reliability, the risk manager can assist in the transition to the new management model by:

- Encouraging front-line workers to become involved in problem solving and encouraging managers to involve them;
- Analyzing work processes and identifying gaps that require strategic redundancies to prevent errors, especially when the risk of error or the severity of the consequences is high;
- Developing policies, procedures, and guidance documents that are clear, easy

to use, and serve as useful resources for the front-line worker rather than as evidence of compliance for regulators and accreditation agencies; and

- Becoming a strong champion for training programs as a means to reduce risk of error, especially when budget pressures dictate otherwise.

CONCLUSION

Healthcare risk managers can play an important role in helping their organizations make a transition to high-reliability organizations. This involves not only changes in processes but also a shift in culture and thinking. The risk manager's own long-held views about the practice of risk management may be challenged by the changes necessary to achieve high reliability as an organization. Long-standing practices involving reporting of errors and sharing of information may have to be abandoned in favor of more progressive concepts that allow the organization and everyone in it to truly understand error, thereby learning how to prevent it. Although daunting, this shift provides the healthcare risk manager with a welcome opportunity to emerge as the organization's safety leader.

References

1. Carroll, R., ed. *Risk Management Handbook for Healthcare Organizations*, 3rd ed. San Francisco: Jossey-Bass, 2001.
2. Kohn, L. T., Corrigan, J. M., Donaldson, M. S., eds. *To Err Is Human: Building a Safer Health System*. Washington, DC: National Academy Press, 1999.
3. Roberts, K. H. Organizational change and a culture of safety. Paper presented at Enhancing Patient Safety and Reducing Errors in Health Care, Rancho Mirage, November 1998.
4. Knox, G. E., Simpson, K. R., Garite, T. J. High reliability perinatal units: an approach to the prevention of patient injury and medical malpractice claims. *Journal of Healthcare Risk Management*, Spring 1999:24–32.
5. Leape, L. L. Error in medicine. *JAMA*, 1994; 272:1851–1857.
6. Roberts, K. H. Some characteristics of high reliability organizations. *Organization Science*, 1990;1(2):160–177.
7. Roberts, 1998.
8. Reynard, W. D., Billings, C. E., Cheaney, E. S., et al. *The Development of the NASA Aviation Safety Reporting System*. NASA Reference Publication 1114. Washington, DC: NASA, 1986.
9. Roberts, 1998.
10. Kohn, 1999.
11. Available at www.jcaho.org.
12. Available at www.leapfroggroup.org/safety3.htm.
13. See www.ismp.org.
14. Shapiro, J. P. Taking the mistakes out of medicine. *US News & World Report*, 2000;129(3):50–66.
15. Adelson, R., Bieber, J., Blum, L., et al. *Patient Safety: Listening to Healthcare Employees*. Chicago: National Patient Safety Foundation, 1998.

18

Reducing Medical Errors: The Role of the Physician

Roy Magnusson, MD, MS, FACEP

THE CHANGING LANDSCAPE

The practice of medicine changed drastically over the past century. The discovery of hundreds of new medications, techniques, and technologies significantly expanded our ability to deliver care that improved the duration and quality of our lives. To support this tremendous expansion in knowledge and clinical practice, training programs grew longer and medical specialization became essential. Medical care was gradually transferred to an ever more complex health system environment. In today's hospital, a single patient may undergo several potentially dangerous procedures and treatments while interacting with dozens of people, including physicians, nurses, technologists, and other staff.

As care became more complex, the number of patients receiving medical services grew. Larger health systems now coordinate hundreds of thousands of patient visits, admissions, operations, or outpatient procedures each year. All of this occurs in a healthcare system in which the economic pressures are to provide medical services as rapidly and inexpensively as possible. Although health systems have spent large sums during the past decade developing information systems, the efforts were often focused on financial systems to either manage capitated contracts or bill efficiently and accurately to avoid being accused of fraud and abuse as the government changed payment guidelines.

Although the trends toward team management, aggressive therapeutic protocols, and large, efficient institutions were essential to progress, there was definitely a downside to these changes. The potential for a medical mishap or serious complication grew as well. Is it any wonder that there is growing concern about serious or even fatal mistakes being made?

The Institute of Medicine (IOM) report issued in late 1999 estimated that between 44,000 and 98,000 unnecessary deaths occur each year in the United States alone.[1] The IOM committee pointed out that although recent medical research and technological advances permit one set of ideal outcomes, the overall health system lags behind this standard in its ability to deliver an ideal level of care consistently to the population as a whole. The result is a frustrating gap between what we know to be the best care and what we provide on a daily basis.

In its follow-up report in March 2001 entitled *Crossing the Quality Chasm*, the Institute of Medicine outlined a strategy to close the gap between known best practice and the overall care delivered.[2] The committee called for a national commitment to improve the quality of care to new levels, with an emphasis on making medical services safe, effective, patient centered, timely, efficient, and equitable.

> To this end, the committee proposes the following agenda for redesigning the 21st century health care system . . . that purchasers, regulators, health professions, educational institutions, and the Department of Health and Human Services create an environment that fosters and rewards improvement by
>
> 1. Creating an infrastructure to support evidence-based medicine,
> 2. Facilitating the use of information technology to redesign safer and more efficient systems,
> 3. Aligning payment and financial incentives with clinical quality outcomes, and
> 4. Preparing the workforce to better service patients in a world of expanding knowledge and rapid change.[3]

If completely implemented, these recommendations will bring sweeping change once again to our health systems and the practice of medicine.

CENTRAL ROLE OF THE PHYSICIAN

In simpler times, physicians played the absolute leadership role in health care. As the expert and decision maker, the physician was the central figure in coordinating the care of patients by supervising small groups of support staff. In today's healthcare setting, physicians have less direct control over many of the decisions that affect their patients, often working in collaboration with scores of people in support of the clinical effort. Paradoxically, coordinating medical care under these complex circumstances requires even stronger physician leadership at all levels in the organization if consistently excellent clinical outcomes are to be achieved.

Physicians can assure quality in many concrete ways. Whether you are an active frontline clinician or the medical director of a large facility, your contributions toward the safe, effective delivery of care can be substantial. For any system, large or small, the delivery of excellent medical services really boils down to the ability of that system's providers to make the right clinical decisions and then execute the diagnostic and treatment plans without delay or mishap. Efforts to guarantee good care must therefore focus on the quality of the providers involved, the information available to them, the redesign of systems that support the effort, and the ability of the organization to evolve rapidly along with medical knowledge and technology.

SELECTING THE MEDICAL STAFF

The most important element in providing quality care is the caliber of the people making decisions and performing procedures. Traditional quality efforts recognized the central role of the physician; as a result, many of the early quality efforts focused on the selection and initial assessment of providers applying for medical staff privileges. Establishing training standards, verifying credentials, and carefully matching the physician's experience with the privileges given are all required practices in today's health systems. None of these activities can be done effectively without physician involvement. In recognition of this, these processes are a primary function of the medical staff organization.

Although the credentialing and privileging process is conducted routinely in all hospitals, the challenge of selecting good providers is far from routine. Many issues need careful consideration as reasonable new standards are set. How much additional training is required before a surgeon may independently perform a new technique such as laparoscopic surgery? How will allied health professionals such as nurse practitioners and physician's assistants be integrated into our healthcare system? Do we have the right mix of talent in our medical staff to meet the medical needs of our community? Physicians must be engaged in these medical staff discussions in order to avoid situations in which providers and level of care are not appropriately matched. Although some of these decisions may be controversial and therefore difficult, to ignore training standards is to invite serious potential for medical errors and a reduced overall quality of care.

THE VALUE OF PEER REVIEW AND ONGOING ASSESSMENT OF CLINICAL PERFORMANCE

Periodic review of the care provided is another basic building block of any quality effort. Quality committees, chart review, and morbidity and mortality conferences are all established methods of such review. Newer methods of collecting information electronically may reduce the time required to collect this information and help direct attention to serious issues. Peer review can only be done by physicians and must be done in a fair and confidential setting. For our residents and medical staff, honest review of cases is at times difficult but is always rewarding. These are the lessons we never forget. It is an essential part of our ongoing education.

It is essential that the medical staff leadership create a culture that discourages disparaging clinical anecdotes in the hallway and promotes honest, confidential, evidence-based dialogue among providers. Patients will benefit, physicians will benefit, and fewer medical errors will occur in the long run.

COLLECTING AND USING OUTCOMES DATA

More and more often the results of our work are measured at the program or institutional level. For example, transplant programs monitor the survival rates of transplant patients and the rejection rates of transplanted organs. This information is helpful in comparing institutional performance with that of other programs or evaluating the effect of newly implemented clinical practice changes.

As care becomes more complex and is performed by teams, this aggregate data can be used to direct discussion and problem solving within the team. This presents yet another leadership opportunity for physicians. Design of appropriate outcomes measures and collection methods will make the information credible. Regular review of outcome results, coupled with evidence-based medical decision making, is a very effective way to improve the outcomes of care over time. The strongest programs have in common one essential element: a physician leader who is committed to the program, works effectively with a team of providers, and uses information to continually improve clinical outcomes and reduce the potential for medical error.

IDENTIFYING AND ASSISTING THE IMPAIRED PHYSICIAN

The 1999 Institute of Medicine report, *To Err Is Human*, emphasized the importance of creating a "no blame" atmosphere in which systems issues can be identified and addressed. This approach is very important in the peer review, case review, and outcomes data approach outlined earlier. Still, on occasion we must turn our attention to the performance of an individual. We are human beings, with all the strengths and frailties that make us human. Alcohol use, drug dependence, depression, or physical changes can directly affect the performance of a physician and result in medical errors. It is the responsibility of the medical staff to encourage confidential reporting and evaluation of these delicate problems. A timely, complete assessment of the situation followed by treatment and monitoring recommendations can save the life of a patient and the career of an otherwise excellent physician.

Many medical staff organizations have a physician's committee that performs this function. Members of this committee must be both firm and compassionate in their approach. This is yet another opportunity for the medical community to assist in making health care safe and to gain credibility with the public at large. A further satisfaction is that of assisting a colleague by directing him or her to needed treatment.

DEALING WITH DISASTER

Regardless of the quality of the people involved, the unexpected occurs in medicine. The 1999 IOM report estimated that somewhere between 44,000 and 98,000 patients die unnecessarily in the United States each year as a result of less than optimal care. Anyone who has been in medicine for even a short time has been witness to a clinical event that has caused him or her to pause and ask some fairly disturbing questions. Should I have predicted this bad outcome? Would another approach have been better? Was this my fault?

Because physicians are on the front lines where clinical care takes place, they are often the first to realize that an unexpected outcome has occurred. Unfortunately, the physician is also likely to be seen as the individual most responsible by the patient or family. Emotions can run high at moments like this. The patient and family may experience pain, loss, fear, and anger. They often vent these emotions with aggressive questioning and even allegations of wrongdoing. Physicians and other healthcare staff also experience intense reactions of disappointment, fear, and anger. In the back of everyone's mind is the concern over possible litigation. Communication among the parties can become strained or may even be avoided altogether. This can result in further misunderstanding and inconsistent care. Errors can be perpetuated or compounded because routine clinical interactions are disrupted.

When things are not going well, it is human nature to look for someone or something to blame. Patients, families, and providers can jump to less than logical conclusions or superficial solutions, missing the opportunity to really study what happened, identify the root cause, and correct the circumstances that led to the incident. If we are to reduce the frequency of serious medical errors, physicians must be willing to participate and lead discussions about care not only in the peer review setting but also in the multidisciplinary setting of a team trying to find out what went wrong. Problems with quality are not isolated to decisions alone. Errors lurk in the handoffs between providers and in the assumptions we make about what happens in other parts of the hospital. The only way to sort out what really happened is to get all involved parties together and search for the root cause. This means opening up the discussion to pharmacists, nurses, technicians, managers, and other involved staff. This is the only way to fix systems issues.

Consider the following example. In order to provide a much more modern and comfortable facility, a hospital elects to build a new wing in the medical center to care specifically for children. Planning is extensive, and the process of building and moving into the facility is very smooth. One year later, surgery is being performed on a 2-year-old with a tumor in his liver. The anesthesiologist has 4 units of blood on hand since the tumor is known to be quite vascular. During the surgery, bleeding escalates. The surgeon cannot control the hemorrhage, and a call for more blood goes out. The blood bank, located some distance from this new wing, immediately begins routine cross matching, not knowing that this blood is needed emergently. A second call is made, upgrading this request to an emergency, and type-specific blood is matched and sent. The combined preparation and transport time, however, is too long. The child exsanguinates in the operating room despite all efforts of the surgical team to control the bleeding.

Very soon thereafter, the anger within the team becomes counterproductive. In their defensiveness, each group begins blaming the other. Positive working relations that took years to build are in jeopardy. To make matters worse, the team has no clear way to prevent what happened from recurring. Something needs to be done.

The team is called together 2 days after the incident, and a detailed root cause analysis is done. This has many positive effects. First, it gives each person a chance to express his or her feelings about the system that had let this happen. Second, care processes are diagrammed in step-by-step detail. As a result, several potential improvements are identified. Suggestions include having type O blood in the operating suite at all times, using the mass transfusion protocol that had been developed for trauma patients, and setting standards for clear communication between operating rooms and the blood bank. The case is also reviewed in the online journal *Mortality and Morbidity* to share the experience with other surgeons and residents and to discuss care options and alternatives that can be used in the future. Participants feel somewhat better knowing that some good came from the case, in that the system was improved. No similar episodes occurred in two additional years of operation.

Taking an emotionally charged disaster like this and creating something positive is not easy. Without strong physician leadership and the participation of all parties, it is impossible. Make sure that your facility has a process for reporting and investigating critical events. Encourage physicians to participate and work with nursing and administration to learn from these experiences and improve the systems supporting the clinical effort.

SYSTEMS REDESIGN

In the Institute of Medicine's follow-up report, *Crossing the Quality Chasm*, the importance of redesigning systems to compensate for the volume and complexity of today's health system was highlighted:

> The committee believes information technology must play a central role in the redesign of the health care system if a substantial improvement in quality is to be achieved over the coming decade. Automation of clinical, financial, and administrative transactions is essential to improving quality, preventing errors, enhancing consumer confidence in the health system and improving efficiency. . . .
>
> Sizable benefits can be derived in the near future from automating certain types of data, such as medication orders.[4]

The impact of computers on hospital workflow has been incredible. Sometimes helpful, sometimes frustrating, computers have become so plentiful in clinics that it is difficult to find enough counter space to write a simple note in the chart. This is not a trend that is likely to abate, as is evidenced by the IOM comments just quoted.

Over the next decade, physicians will see the automation and redesign of every aspect of their work. Office management systems, patient management systems, digital radiographs, electronic medical records, email communication with patients, Web-based software and physician access pages, physician order entry, and bar coding drugs are but a sampling of the information technology systems that administrators are considering right now. So many systems are being developed and piloted that the rate-limiting factor in this change is no longer technology—it is our ability to finance and deploy these new systems and then train people to use them.

I had the personal and painful experience of leading the implementation of a digital radiography system at a university health system that included both hospital and clinic use. This yearlong endeavor taught me several important lessons with respect to implementing new systems to be used by physicians. Here are just a few.

- Implementing systemwide change requires early involvement of key stakeholders, especially physicians who use that system extensively.
- There must be a clear and compelling advantage for physicians or they will not support the effort.
- Electronic systems are not necessarily an improvement, and issues of patient safety can develop as a result of the new technology.
- A clear understanding of how the physician uses the information and how the new system will affect the physician's workflow is required to plan a successful system.
- Training busy providers on new systems requires tremendous effort, creativity, and flexibility.

Assuming that the IOM report is correct and that these systems will be critical in our effort to become more efficient and error free, what is the role of the physician in system redesign? The answer is simple: early involvement of front-line practitioners in all major systems projects. This planning takes a considerable amount of time, but both the health system and the physicians have much to lose if it is done poorly. A willingness to work with information technologists and administrators to revise and redesign workflow has the potential for creating effective systems that make the practice of medicine easier and less error prone. Shortcuts in this initial planning stage prior to the selection of hardware and software options will result in a very expensive system that interferes with patient care and makes efficient practice impossible. If new systems are being planned at your institution, you must get in on the ground floor and have a clinician on the team.

Many larger organizations have taken this concept a step further by assigning one or two physicians with computer experience to the information technology (IT) planning team. The chief medical informatics officer can be very helpful in long-range strategic planning for clinical IT systems.

MATCHING RESOURCES TO NEEDS: PHYSICIANS AS SENIOR ADMINISTRATORS

Medical errors increase when the system designed to provide care is overwhelmed. In this era of managed care, many health systems are forced to make difficult resource allocation decisions that may affect the quality of patient care. Tighter and tighter control of costs must be balanced with outcomes and safety considerations. This can only be done if the providers who see the effects of administrative choices are actively involved in health system administration.

Physicians can contribute to this effort in many ways. Cooperating with reasonable cost containment efforts is a great first step. Set aside favorites and use less expensive implants, devices, or medications if the clinical results will be the same. Physicians can also set high expectations and quality standards while advocating for safe patient care in their own clinic or hospital.

Ideally, in your community, physicians are in leadership positions and participate regularly when both financial performance and clinical outcomes are measured and discussed. Make sure that physicians are actively participating in the highest levels of your organization.

ESTABLISHING STANDARDS AND POLICY

Certain aspects of care are high risk and therefore deserve focused discussion and guidelines. Examples of these include medication order writing, conscious sedation, and the restraint or seclusion of patients. Physicians can help reduce the potential for medical mishaps and prevent patient injury by authoring practical policies and then by enforcing safety guidelines.

We recently created an electronic medication administration record (MAR) at our institution in an effort to clean up the handwritten MAR and reduce the likelihood of error. In doing so, we discovered many nonspecific orders being used by medical staff. "Hold drug X" was one such common order. We became concerned when we realized that this order was interpreted differently depending on the nurse and the setting. Some nurses held a single dose, whereas others thought this order was equivalent to stopping the drug until a restart order was written.

The potential for error with vague orders like this is obvious, but let's face it, old habits are hard to break. The point here is a simple one. Physicians today are not working with a small group of people who "know what I mean when I say hold drug X." Physicians must be as clear as possible in their communication and order writing. Stricter guidelines will be required, and we must support that concept. The same is true of other policies directed at high-risk aspects of care. In the future, cooperation and understanding of the importance of making care safe will be expected of all healthcare professionals.

EVIDENCE-BASED MEDICINE

"In the current health care system, scientific knowledge about best practice is not applied systematically or expediently to clinical practice. An average of about 17 years is required for new knowledge generated by randomized controlled trials to be incorporated into practice, and even then application is highly uneven."[5]

Practice guidelines for the optimal care of many disease states have been created, but consistent application of these is still not a reality. According to the 2001 IOM report, "Patients should receive care that is based on the best available scientific knowledge. Care should not vary illogically from clinician to clinician or from place to place."[6]

This assessment prompted the IOM to recommend that the Department of Health and Human Services be given the responsibility and necessary resources to establish and maintain a comprehensive program aimed at making scientific evidence more useful and accessible to clinicians and patients.

Physician leadership in the development of these standards will be important. The acceptance and use of such guidelines will depend on the extent to which practicing physicians are involved and educated on the science behind the guidelines. Bringing best practices into an organization and implementing advances in medical science should be rapid and consistent. Physician leaders will be called upon to make it so.

CONCLUSION

All things considered, these are very exciting times to be a physician. The unbalanced emphasis on cost cutting and reduced reimbursement for medical care that defined the 1990s is being challenged by those interested in the results of what physicians do. Improved outcomes and preventing unnecessary complications are excellent goals that we can all support. The basic principles have been laid out in this chapter. They are easy to describe but difficult to implement. It will be well worth the effort, however, because each of these topics could contribute something positive to your patients if implemented well. Make sure your organization carefully selects and evaluates its providers. Offer your expertise in the development of more efficient systems of care. Set and meet standards that will make the hospital or clinic a safer place. Your patients will be better off, and it may even bring the joy back into the practice of medicine.

References

1. Kohn, L. T., Corrigan, J. M., Donaldson, M. S., eds. *To Err Is Human: Building a Safer Health System*. Washington, DC: National Academy Press, 1999.
2. Institute of Medicine. *Crossing the Quality Chasm*. Washington, DC: National Academy Press, 2001.
3. Ibid.
4. Ibid.
5. Ibid.
6. Ibid.

19

Engaging General Counsel in the Pursuit of Safety

Barbara J. Youngberg, BSN, MSW, JD

A critical stumbling block impeding many organizations from fully engaging in practices associated with the creation of high-reliability organizations may be the advice of counsel. Although it is easy to understand why counsel representing healthcare organizations are skittish, given the dramatic escalations in malpractice verdicts and settlements over the past few years,[1] perhaps in their zeal to protect the organization they are actually inhibiting the organization's ability to protect its patients. Healthcare professionals' concern over unwanted, at times nonmeritorious, and increasingly costly litigation is understandable, but they are often urged to consider these problems as a failure of the legal system. Although that may at times be the case, organizations and providers must recognize that it could also be related to failures of the healthcare system's peer review processes and quality improvement or risk management processes, which should be structured to identify and prevent adverse patient outcomes or medical complications and negligent care. Because the fear of litigation often discourages open discussion of error and methods of reducing those errors, it might be prudent for healthcare attorneys to assist their organizations in designing a more structured performance improvement system and peer review process so that care outcomes can be studied, rather than litigation outcomes. Because the escalating costs of malpractice frequently fuel discussions associated with the need for tort reform, healthcare organizations should also recognize that quality improvement opportunities hold the promise not only of significant improvement in patient outcomes, but also of significant reductions in healthcare costs.

In-house counsel often characterize their job as being the protection of the organization's assets—of course, meaning its financial assets. These costs are typically viewed as the costs traditionally associated with malpractice litigation (including indemnity payments made to injured patients and defense and legal expenses paid to those involved in developing and advancing a legal defense). Providing counsel with an understanding of the costs of poor quality might help them see their job more broadly and could allow them to focus on the importance of their role as it relates to assisting the organization to create an enhanced system for performing peer review that insulates the committee from antitrust claims when they actually invoke disciplinary actions and that holds all providers, leaders, and managers accountable. In addition, if patients (rather than money) were viewed as the primary asset of the organization, perhaps the role of in-house counsel could change its focus. Counsel could and should serve as an essential partner in the pursuit of a safe and error-free organization and should recognize their essential role in promoting and designing structures that identify practices, practitioners, and systems that are at the root of the cases they later must defend on behalf of their clients.

Equally important in this dialogue is the recognition that the damage component of our tort system is flawed and in need of reform, but that, more often than not, plaintiffs have sustained some type of injury at the hands of a healthcare provider or organization. It is the injury that generally fuels both the patient's need for information and the demand for retribution. Only by creating a structure that helps the organization understand and respond to the problems associated with error will the organization ever truly be able to get ahead of the problems inherent in the tort system.

The science surrounding the study of error and the factors contributing to it is advancing and can provide assistance to organizations seeking to get ahead of the problem, but it may require a different way of thinking for all of those who are part of the team. And for the first time, it might require that the organization's counsel see themselves as part of the team that not only contains errors but also proactively assists the organization in addressing the causes of them. This might include enhancing the nature of the peer review process and ensuring that all state requirements are met, thereby creating a process that ensures maximum likelihood of protection for all who participate.

What is clear from reading the literature about the safety practices of health care is that for many years very well-intentioned professionals have tried to make their environments safe, using a variety of new techniques and philosophies. What is equally clear is that in almost any organization, there are a number of individuals who know why errors occur, who is often involved, and what needs to be done to make the system more safe. It would seem, then, that having identified the problem, it would be relatively easy to fix it. But for many reasons, this has not been the case.

For years, the literature has been quick to blame many of the problems being faced by the healthcare system on a damaged legal system. The cost of defensive medicine, the rising costs of malpractice coverage, the plaintiff 's bar eager to make millions by wrongfully suing the competent provider—some of these problems and characterizations may be true, but what is equally true is that preventable errors continue to occur and they often result in injury to the very individuals our systems are supposed to protect. Only by truly reducing preventable medical errors can we hope to get in front of the malpractice problems.

You can't get ahead of the problem of medical error by hiding behind the law. The law of negligence, particularly medical malpractice, evolved in response to a need. It is equally compelling to note that you cannot change behavior if you design a system that continually looks the other way when it becomes aware of systemic and personal failures. A different system of learning and accountability must be established.

I have heard in-house attorneys and defense counsel advise against the sharing of error data for the purpose of learning, stating that they don't want to provide a road map for a plaintiff's attorney. My response has generally been, Better a road map than a client!

Many in health care today would state that the reason they cannot get their organizations behind the creation of an accountable system of quality is the fear of what might be discovered that will place the organization in an unfavorable light. Of equal concern is that many physicians fear legal retribution by their colleagues if indeed they institute actions that limit another physician's practice, and thus they are unwilling to truly assist in the disciplinary activities necessary to create an accountable healthcare system.

PROTECTION OF MEDICAL ERROR DATA

Three general rules of evidence could potentially protect medical error data in an online or paper-based reporting tool from disclosure: the remedial action privilege, attorney–client privilege, and the work product doctrine.[2] The IOM report says all three have major limitations. The remedial action privilege applies solely to information submitted to prove negligence or a product defect. Attorney–client privilege is limited to communication between an attorney and a client either seeking or providing advice or in anticipation of litigation: Disclosure of information to a third party under this protection destroys the privilege. Work product doctrine protects the thoughts and mental impressions of an attorney, data that are not typically found in paper or online medical error reports.

The remedial action privilege prevents admission of actions taken after an adverse event occurs to prove negligence or a defective product. The purpose of the privilege is to encourage defendants and potential defendants to take action to improve safety without the fear that the information will be used against them. It recognizes that remedial actions are not necessarily related to negligence. All states except Rhode Island have adopted this rule.[3] Some courts have extended this privilege to include self-evaluative reports or other postinjury analyses and reports. A California court ruled that hospital peer review activities were protected from discovery on the theory of remedial action privilege.[4] This privilege does not prevent admission of these reports to prove issues other than negligence or product defect.

In response to a poor benchmarking showing, plaintiffs would argue that a hospital's efforts to remediate the process or system that led to the poor performance are evidence that the prior system was defective. There is a strong public policy argument to be made that subsequent remedial measures, as in a product liability case, should not be admissible to prove negligence by the hospital for the medical error. For the same reason, a plaintiff suing a widget manufacturer cannot use evidence of a later design change as evidence the widget was previously defective or caused the injury.[5]

In Illinois, courts have made clear that the nature and content of the internal peer review process itself are privileged and confidential under the Medical Studies Act.[6] Because subsequent remediation is clearly part of the internal peer review process, it follows that such activities should be protected from disclosure in Illinois. Many states in addition to Illinois have created specific protections for healthcare facilities and providers in an effort to facilitate the creation of a process in healthcare settings or between peer providers that truly allows for the identification and correction of problems associated with providing healthcare. These statutes should be examined carefully and utilized fully to afford the organization the highest level of protection possible under each individual state's laws.

Attorney–client privilege protects communication between attorneys and clients, although a client may waive this privilege. In medical institutions, the client is usually limited to the "control group," or senior management, of the organization. The privilege will rarely protect data sent to an external entity and may not be useful in protecting reports that are prepared by those other than senior management. In *Chicago Trust Company v. Cook County Hospital*, the court found that incident reports submitted by a nurse and respiratory therapist were not protected under attorney–client privilege because the nurse and respiratory therapist were not part of the hospital control group;[7] that is, they were not clients of the attorney who received the reports. The reports were not addressed to an attorney or prepared by an attorney, they were not memoranda or communication to or advice from an attorney, and they contained only factual information. The court said that even if these documents were privileged, the privilege was waived when the documents were sent to the hospital quality committee.[8]

Attorney work product doctrine protects materials created by or on behalf of a lawyer in anticipation of litigation. It protects the thoughts and ideas of the attorney, and only the attorney can waive the privilege. Many states have found that this doctrine does not apply to incident reports because they are completed in the ordinary course of business and seldom contain the thoughts and ideas of attorneys. In addition, many current incident reporting systems are now designed to collect data on near miss events and data related to other types of situations in the organization that will never be the subject of legal action. In *Columbia/HCA Healthcare Corporation v. Eighth Judicial District Court*, the court found that incident reports are filled out in the ordinary course of business because Columbia requires hospital personnel to fill out preprinted forms when an unusual event occurs.[9] They are not completed in anticipation of litigation. Even if they were, if the plaintiffs can show that they have a substantial need for the information and cannot get the information in any other way, access to incident reports may be granted.

Peer Review Protection

The peer review privilege is one statutory protection that may provide legal protection for medical error data. It differs from state to state but is the most promising source of protection.[10] One common element of state peer review privileges is that they protect peer review or quality improvement committee activities if performed in a manner designed to ensure consistency and quality of purpose. Some states protect data collected at the direction of a quality improvement committee or the findings of quality improvement committees that are made in the interest of reducing morbidity and mortality and improving the quality of care. These privileges vary considerably in their reach and strength and typically do not protect documents that are prepared in the course of rendering services to patients or conducting business for an organization. Therefore, the peer review privilege does not typically protect medical records or accident reports that are a routine part of business, but will protect documents prepared as an organization identifies quality problems, discusses possible solutions, and modifies the environment to bring about desired change.

Most statutes require that all information collected remain confidential within the peer review or quality improvement committee and not be disclosed to others. Many statutes do not address interhospital collaboration, even when the hospitals are within an integrated delivery system.[11] In *Of the Estate of Stanley W. Howard*, the court found that the applicability of the medical peer review privilege relates to the way in which the document was created and the purpose for which it was used, not its content.[12] This case found that incident reports in the peer review system created by the Massachusetts legislature are a core component of peer review because they begin the process and are necessary to the committees' work product.[13] Many states only protect the case analysis by the quality improvement or peer review committee, not the information that was sent to the committee or the actions taken by the committee.

In a well-publicized case arising in the state of New York, *Zion v. New York Hospital*,[14] the plaintiffs sought production of documents from The Joint Commission (formerly JCAHO) that they believed would support their claims of negligence against the hospital. The hospital denied the release of these documents, citing the New York education law that allows for protection of privileged information. The hospital prevailed in its argument in a strong opinion of the court, which wrote: "Affording such a privilege to the records of the JCAHO furthers the goal of improving the quality of hospital care, a goal which both the statute (see, *Matter of Albany Medical Center Hospital v. Denis*, 161 AD 2d 1030: *Lilly v. Turecki*, 112 AD 2d 788) and JCAHO seek to achieve."

Confidentiality of these records encourages the surveyed hospital to engage in open and candid discussion of hospital conditions, thereby enabling the hospital to learn from mistakes. Stripping the records of the confidentiality the Joint Commission guarantees to the hospitals that seek its services would frustrate this purpose. Although "the exemption from disclosure for the JCAHO records, may, on occasion, hamper a malpractice plaintiff 's ability to ascertain relevant information, the legislature has made a determination that, on balance, this consideration is outweighed by the benefit the privilege confers on the general public."[15]

Plaintiffs' attorneys have tried to get access to peer review–protected materials when bringing suits against a hospital for corporate negligence in credentialing physicians. They have argued that the data must be available in these cases because it is the only way to judge if the hospital is fulfilling its responsibility to assess the competence of providers. In California, Colorado, and New York, the courts have held that peer review activity is protected from discovery and is not available even when the issue is the adequacy of the hospital in carrying out its role of assessing the competence of its medical staff.[16] In Texas, however, the court found that there was no legislative intent in the peer review statute to protect hospitals from negligent credentialing claims.[17]

The Health Care Quality Improvement Act[18] provides federal protection for peer review activities and those who participate in the process in good faith. The act protects the participants from antitrust or libel allegations, but it was not crafted to protect the information reviewed by the quality improvement or peer review committees. It is unclear whether this act would be useful in protecting online reporting activity or information shared to facilitate discussions about improving quality or promoting safety from discovery, so legislation at the federal level would be helpful to protect these data. Legislation has been enacted by Congress to protect some medical quality assurance records, but it limited the scope to federally operated healthcare facilities. These examples demonstrate that Congress is at least aware of the need for federal protection of peer review information.

With the focus now on patient safety, multiple bills have been advanced in the House and the Senate to protect information gathered to study and improve patient safety. Bills by Nancy Johnson (D-CT),[19] Jim Jeffords (D-VT),[20] and Ted Kennedy (D-MA)[21] provide definitions of the term *patient safety data* and create protections for organizations that share such data to study error reduction. Each bill also creates a role for the Department of Health and Human Services as its relates to furthering the study and science of error.

Web-based error collection tools are relatively new to health care, and protection of these data is untested in most states. There are several reasons, however, why sending medical error data to a Web-based error collection system may not waive the hospital's peer review privilege. As the recipient of medical error data from a hospital, any collecting or aggregating agency could be deemed to be acting as an agent or designee of that hospital's peer review committee; those activities, therefore, including the data collected, could be protected. The Illinois Medical Studies Act (MSA) specifically provides protection for the peer review activities of "Patient Care Audit Committees, Medical Care Evaluation Committees, Utilization Review Committees, Credential Committees and Executive Committees, or their designees."[22] Current protection afforded under the Health Insurance Portability and Accountability Act for business associates may also serve to provide protection for these types of data.

THE VALUE OF ERROR DATA TO PLAINTIFF ATTORNEYS

There are three types of data that may be of interest to plaintiff attorneys: (1) patient-identifiable data about the specific event, (2) aggregate data about the involved institution's performance in similar events, and (3) similar-occurrence data that relate to a specific aspect of the case where the plaintiff's attorney is attempting to prove negligence.[23]

The last two categories of data are available to plaintiff attorneys without a medical error report, online reporting tool, or collaborative data project. Hospital-identifiable aggregate data regarding complications and mortalities are publicly available and can easily be used to infer negligence or to support or impute an organization's mismanagement of specific diseases or diagnoses. Examples of aggregate data are the coronary artery bypass graft mortality rates and total joint replacement complication rates available through Internet sites such as www.healthgrades.com. Plaintiff attorneys have not used these data frequently, but they could use the data to show that the organization had prior notice of an issue that it had not addressed. Similarly, many states (Pennsylvania and New York among them) have mandatory reporting requirements for specific groups of patients or specific types of adverse events and periodically make this data public to show practice variations (and possibly quality variations) among organizations or providers. Participation in data-sharing projects, coupled with a strong safety or performance improvement program, could be used to offset data that may one day present an organization unfavorably in a public format; participation also may be used to argue that the organization has a strong commitment to quality improvement and the prevention of harm to patients.

In a Florida medical malpractice case, similar-occurrence data were used when an obese plaintiff alleged that the defendant obstetrician injured her child by delivering her on a standard bed versus a drop-down bed.[24] The court held that the records of other obese women who the obstetrician had delivered were relevant and discoverable to show whether other infants of obese women sustained injuries when delivered on a standard bed. The defendant had to provide the records of obese patients, with their names redacted.[25] An internal or external reporting system coupled with a safety management program would have alerted the organization and provider if there were newborn complications when obese women delivered on standard beds or would have provided the organization with data to refute the allegation.

The first category of data of interest to plaintiff attorneys, patient-identifiable data about the specific event, is mainly of interest to fortify one or more elements in a malpractice action against an individual or healthcare facility. The elements of a negligence suit include duty owed by the provider to the plaintiff, a breach of that duty, the breach of duty being the proximate cause of injury to the plaintiff, and damages suffered related to the injury. Incident reports are highly sought after by plaintiff attorneys because they are viewed as the "real story" behind the event. Whereas the medical record contains (mostly) objective information and data, the incident report fills out the story with details that may definitively show provider error or negligence.

Each organization must determine if the risk of possible discovery outweighs the benefits of collecting and analyzing information from an incident report. The major benefit of having knowledge of a medical error is that the mishap can be fully investigated, with a root cause or criticality analysis performed as necessary. Early claims processing can begin also, if warranted. The benefits of tracking and trending all reported errors include the ability to identify systems issues, detect individual practitioner or practice issues, and focus on clinical risk areas in need of support and education. Instructing staff on the importance of objective nonretaliatory reporting of incidents can go a long way toward reducing the value of these reports for plaintiff's counsel, and a policy of open disclosure to patients when errors do occur could certainly alleviate the need for a plaintiff's attorney to find value in these reports.

A DEFENSE ATTORNEY'S STRATEGY

As more sophisticated error data collection becomes prevalent and hospitals look to enhance their reporting structures, defense attorneys are increasingly being asked whether this information is legally protected from disclosure in litigation. The answer is a qualified "yes," with the following caveats: Data can be protected from disclosure if they are limited, there is limited distribution of the data collected, there is a limited purpose for collecting the data, and the structure of the committees and processes designed by the organization comports with the requirements of the law.

Every state has enacted legislation protecting peer review activities in hospitals, to some extent. Certain states have very strong protections for data generated by those activities, whereas other states have weaker protections that might allow for disclosure.

The Joint Commission states that "performance monitoring and improvements are data driven. Every organization must choose which processes and outcomes (and thus which types of data) are important to monitor based on its mission and the scope of care and services it provides."[26]

The challenge to hospitals is to comply with this Joint Commission standard while protecting the collected data under state peer review legislation, such as the Illinois MSA.[27] Like many state peer review statutes, the MSA outlines what data and peer review activities are protected, whose data and activities are protected, and when they are protected. On its face, the MSA protects computer-based medical error data as "reports . . . or other data." The MSA protects "All information, interviews, reports, statements, memoranda, recommendations . . . or other data . . . of accredited hospitals or their medical staffs . . . used in the course of internal quality control or . . . for improving patient care."[28]

The court in *Chicago Trust v. Cook County Hospital*[29] ("Cook County") said that the Illinois MSA does not protect the following:

- Material created in the ordinary course of business
- Material created for the purpose of rendering a legal opinion
- Material created to weigh potential liability risk
- Material created for later corrective action by the hospital staff
- Pre-committee material used by a peer review committee

The Cook County case instructs Illinois hospitals that they must establish how, when, and why certain material is privileged before it is collected.

Various ways to protect data before they are collected are as follows:

- *Refer to medical error data collection in your hospital's peer review policy:* All hospital peer review committee policies and procedures should specifically incorporate medical error data collection as part of the information gathering, tracking, trending, monitoring, and deliberation process that is used in medical staff peer review.
- *Encourage anonymous reporting:* The MSA is premised on the belief that without statutory peer review privilege, the medical staff would hesitate to frankly evaluate their colleagues.[30] Allowing anonymous medical error reporting advances this policy of encouraging an open flow of information through the peer review process.
- *Stress performance improvement rather than peer review:* The Joint Commission's new patient safety initiative speaks primarily of performance improvement and patient safety activities. Since successful performance improvement will reduce the need for peer review activities, because of fewer errors, review committee policies with an eye toward tying performance

improvement, patient safety, and peer review together more closely.

Although Illinois law obviously is not controlling outside of Illinois, some of the logic behind it might be helpful for all healthcare organizations to consider. The best approach for hospitals still concerned about discoverability is to consider error data collection as a minimalist incident report, which simply serves as a trigger for further detailed peer review. Unfortunately, many paper-based incident reporting systems allow for healthcare providers to enter an unlimited amount of subjective information, often pointing fingers of blame at specific parties.

Another consideration: The data in a medical error reporting system or paper tool do not provide plaintiff attorneys with any information that is not available through other discoverable tools such as the medical record, personnel files, or depositions. At a deposition, a plaintiff 's attorney will gather far more, and more detailed, information from the involved healthcare professionals than he or she will get from the medical error report. Therefore, data protection through peer review statutes is only temporary until the litigation discovery process begins.

Another area of concern is what effect benchmarking of data has on legal protection of the information collected. The Joint Commission states that "Certain types of data and information need to be accumulated over time to support the hospital's clinical and management functions . . . [including] analysis of trends over time . . . [and] performance comparisons over time within the hospital and with other hospitals."[31] Accordingly, The Joint Commission clearly supports an organization that benchmarks or shares medical error data "to effect behavioral changes in itself and other health care organizations to improve patient safety."[32]

What a hospital does when faced with the bad news that it has scored poorly when benchmarked against other hospitals for a given indicator is critically important. This is true whether the benchmarking project is related to reported medical errors or complication rates developed from public information. If hospital leadership dismisses the poor benchmarking performance, forbids future benchmark study participation, builds obstacles to error improvement efforts, or otherwise does nothing, consider the ramifications:

- A plaintiff 's attorney could argue that the hospital does not place a high priority on patient safety and high-quality medical care—a public relations problem.
- Quitting a benchmarking program after poor performance results, if even a possibility, will not be well received by any jury—a legal problem.
- Increased claims arise from medical errors—an economic problem.
- Ignoring benchmarking data allows a known, documented potential danger to patients to continue—a moral and ethical problem that could become a serious legal problem in those states allowing punitive damages against hospitals and healthcare providers.

The appropriate response is for the hospital risk or quality manager to launch an investigation and assessment of the root causes of that poor performance, determine whether it is a true systemic problem or a data problem, then implement an action plan to improve performance, and monitor progress to ensure the effectiveness of the solution. This response will reduce future claims. In the event of a claim, such preventive and remedial activity may be useful to mitigate damages by showing that the hospital had instituted an aggressive program to identify and correct systemic problems and had acted reasonably to prevent the occurrence.

If hospitals share benchmarking data with other organizations that are outside the scope of the peer review process, will that action waive the privilege? If The Joint Commission mandates hospitals to conduct ongoing monitoring of patient safety, the public policy behind state peer review statutes should protect data generated by that monitoring. To encourage frank and open information gathering during this "monitoring process," all data gathered by these systems should be protected.

The Joint Commission has effectively expanded the scope of the performance improvement or peer review process outside the hospital by expressly encouraging the ongoing proactive reduction of medical errors. In fact, the Intent section of Standard PI.2 specifically states that performance review processes, when they are designed well, draw on a variety of information sources, including sources external to the hospital: Such a process "incorporates available information from within the organization and from other organizations, about potential risks to patients."[33]

Similarly, The Joint Commission contemplates that a hospital will "link with external databases and information networks."[34] The cited Joint Commission language demonstrates the intent to expand the current idea of performance review to include data from external databases and information from other hospitals. Therefore, protections for such data must likewise expand. Hospitals are well advised to carefully limit their data to the dictates of the relevant state peer review statute. The biggest patient safety problem is not bad people but good people working in bad systems. Fostering open communication and disclosure of errors and encouraging systemic fixes throughout the healthcare industry are parts of an important new public policy that has yet to be adopted by state courts or incorporated into state or federal data and peer review protection legislation. In the meantime, hospitals are advised to limit the data reported, limit who has access to those data, and limit the use of those data to ensure greatest protection for those data.

In-house attorneys, external defense counsel, and any lawyers working with healthcare organizations and providers have many opportunities to use their knowledge and skills to assist in creating high-reliability organizations. Providing excuses related to the ineffectiveness of current laws, the lack of predictability of the current tort system, or the current antagonism felt by the public toward the healthcare system may not be the most effective way for their value to be realized.

References

1. *Addressing the New Health Care Crisis: Reforming the Medical Litigation System to Improve the Quality of Health Care.* U.S. Department of Health and Human Services, Office of the Assistant Secretary for Planning and Evaluation, Washington, DC, March 3, 2003.
2. Kohn, L. T., Corrigan, J. M., Donaldson, M. S., eds. *To Err Is Human: Building a Safer Health System.* Washington, DC: National Academy Press, 2000, 117.
3. Ibid.
4. *Fox v Kramer*, 22 Cal. 4th 531, 994 P2d 343, 2000 Cal LEXIS 1566, 93 Cal Rptr 2d 497, 2000 Cal Daily Op Service 2082, 2000 DAR 2805 (2000).
5. Restatement of Torts.
6. *Zajac v St. Mary of Nazareth Hospital*, 212 Ill App 3d 779, 571 NE2d 840 (1st District 1991).
7. *Chicago Trust Company v Cook County Hospital*, 298 Ill App 3d 396, 698 NE2d 641 (1st Dist 1998).
8. Ibid.
9. *Columbia/HCA Healthcare Corporation v Eighth Judicial District Court*, 113 Nev 521, 1997, 5–6.
10. Kohn, Corrigan, Donaldson, eds. *To Err Is Human*, 119.
11. Ibid., 120.
12. *Carr v Howard, administratrix of the Estate of Stanley W. Howard*, 426 Mass 514, 689 NE2d 1304, 1998 Mass Lexis 24.
13. Ibid.
14. *Sidney E. Zion, as administrator of the Estate of Libby Zion, Deceased v New York Hospital, et al.*, 183 AD2d 386, 590 NYS2d 188, 1992 NY App Div.
15. Ibid.

16. *Posey v Supreme Court of Colorado*, 196 Colo 396, 1978; *West Covian Hospital v Superior Court of Los Angeles County*, 153 Cal App3d 134, 1984; *Parker v St. Clare's Hospital et al.*, 159 AD2d 919.
17. *AGBOR v St. Luke's Episcopal Hospital*, 912 SW2d 354; 1995 Tex App LEXIS 3007.
18. Health Care Quality Improvement Act of 1986, 38 USC 5705; 38 CFR 17.501; 10 USC 1102.
19. Patient Safety Improvement Act of 2002 (HR 4889). House Ways and Means Committee, September 10, 2002.
20. Patient Safety and Quality Improvement Act (SR 2590), June 5, 2002.
21. Patient Safety Improvement and Medical Injury Reduction Act (SR 3029), September 24, 2002.
22. Illinois Medical Studies Act, 735 ILCS 5/8-2101 (1997).
23. Kohn, Corrigan, Donaldson, eds. *To Err Is Human*, 114–115.
24. *Amente v Newman*, 653 So2d 1030, 20 FLW S172 (1995, Fla).
25. Ibid.
26. *Comprehensive Accreditation Manual for Hospitals: The Official Handbook*. Oakbrook Terrace, IL: Joint Commission on Accreditation of Healthcare Organizations, 2002, Intent of Standard PI.3.1.
27. Illinois Medical Studies Act.
28. Ibid.
29. *Chicago Trust Company v Cook County Hospital*.
30. *Stricklin v Becan*, 293 Ill App 3d 866, 689 NE2d 328 (4th Dist 1997).
31. *Comprehensive Accreditation Manual*, Intent of Standard IM.8.
32. *Comprehensive Accreditation Manual*, LD.39.
33. Ibid.
34. *Comprehensive Accreditation Manual*, Intent of Standard IM.1.

20

Growing Nursing Leadership in the Field of Patient Safety

Mary L. Salisbury, RN, MSN and Robert Simon, EdD, CPE

We have had the privilege and the opportunity of traveling to healthcare organizations across the country. Maintaining a practice that spans the continent broadens the spectrum of professional input beyond that of the institution-based provider. In our travels, we find that professionals easily discuss and eagerly entertain the considered perspective of others. Beyond engaging discussion, our responsibility as researchers is to listen and log conditions, observe, and postulate solutions. We find that whenever we visit a healthcare organization, we are confronted by caregivers characterizing the condition of patient safety with an identical exclamation and inquiry:

- "It is awful out there; we are working in the worst of times and the best of times."
- "Beyond the issue of staffing, why is the voice of nursing seemingly silent regarding patient safety and the development of comprehensive solutions?"

The exclamation is intensely expressed and appears omnipresent. Caregivers state that a gulf exists between the standards of healthcare delivery and actual outcomes. Our investigation, direct observations, and patient interviews serve to confirm their perspective. The specific aim of this chapter, therefore, is to sort this out and do the following:

1. Describe what is happening relative to health care, nursing, and patient safety, and summarize the history, duty, and current perspective of nursing
2. Establish the key characteristics of a comprehensive solution to the problem of patient safety
3. Explicate the form and function of patient safety (form as it exists in the concept of *vision*; function as it exists in the concept of *teamwork*)
4. Present a comprehensive patient safety solution that can move health care from the worst of times toward the best of times

THE WORST OF TIMES

The healthcare arena is a battlefield rife with the cratered remains of the repeated and haphazard bombs of change. Within a period of 4 years, two-thirds of the nation's healthcare organizations merged (Danzon, 1994). Of these conglomerations, undeterminable numbers have disaffiliated and remerged, giving rise to tidal crashes of cultures. So ravaged, the healthcare geography little resembles the healing arenas where once we received and delivered the fruits of our education.

Displaced from healthcare homelands by the ongoing maneuvers of organizational mergers, joint ventures, and managed care affiliations, nurses and physicians alike are separated from the work they once knew and understood. Stunned caregivers tell stories regarding their professional alienation and that of their equally stunned leaders, who stagger about like mapless captains on rudderless ships. One of our client hospitals characterized changes in the healthcare arena this way, "First we downsized; then we right sized; now we capsize." To further the alienation, jargons du jour constantly emerge to create a new and unrecognizable language of health care. Unable to interpret the landscape or the language of these newly merged worlds, caregivers fail to anticipate the lurking patient care dangers and for these reasons fail to establish safe arenas of care. Isolated, caregivers believe that they are left to respond, or react, alone.

THE BEST OF TIMES

Professionals are seeking solutions. We care. The vehicle that will carry many of these solutions is this simple yet profound handbook. This particular handbook's topic is patient safety, and the book carries with it the acknowledgment that any solution addressing patient safety would be incomplete without the perspective of nursing. This fact and opportunity provide a segue to the interrogative regarding the absent voice of nursing and the subsequent perception that nursing problem solves in isolation, along the lines of the discipline. Perhaps the two most compelling perspectives are summarized by the following:

- With nursing absent from the table, no patient safety solution can be considered comprehensive. The term *comprehensive* prescribes a solution that is inclusive and therefore mandates an outcome-based solution that includes all disciplines and aspects of care that affect patient experience. The issue of proper and appropriate staffing, although central to the concept, does not provide the single link to safety. Staffing is a necessary condition, but proper staffing alone is not sufficient to prevent the occurrence of error.
- With nursing absent from the table, any solution developed along a discipline's line fails to recognize the agenda for national patient safety and a central tenet of the National Patient Safety Foundation (1998), namely, that safety does not reside in an individual. Rather, patient safety is a condition that emerges from the collective interactivities of caregivers working in systems designed to produce desired outcomes.

BACKGROUND: HISTORY AND DUTY OF NURSING IN COMPREHENSIVE PATIENT SAFETY

Patient safety, for nursing, is encapsulated in the term *advocacy*. Advocacy is the intent of the profession. Despite that fact, the concept grows vague as organizations fail to respond to the wisdom of its providers and as the term disappears into the riptides and undertow caused by the breaking waves of new language. Corporate mergers, cultural collisions, changing professional perspectives, and emerging patient safety collaboratives all serve as sweeping reasons why the language of advocacy has been pulled into the sea of patient safety rhetoric. Although nursing is rooted in patient safety under the term advocacy, the changes have been too many and caregivers have grown weary. Unable to make sense of these changes, many caregivers have shut down (Clemmer, 1992). Still, the historic and current vision of the discipline embodies the concept of patient advocacy. Nurses believe that they are advocates and are quick to attest the same. An emergency department (ED) nurse of greater than 30 years' experience contributes the following exemplar that illustrates this point:

> As a nurse of many years, I speak to a time when my colleagues and I were educated to commit our lives and organize our care around a simple philosophy: "to do for the patient the things that they could not do for themselves." We were the conscience for the unconscious, the voice for the voiceless, the mobility for the immobile, the courage for the disheartened, and the anticipator of danger for those rendered unable to anticipate. This philosophy was core to each provider and created a vertical snap to our ranks that resulted in the delivery of care through and towards a common ideal. This philosophy of advocacy was integrated deep into the culture of caring; a fact that served to further buffer us against the frailty of our humanness, that of the potential to err. Despite its brevity, the statement was comprehensive, easily assimilated, and continues to organize my care yet today.

To respond to this philosophy fully is to fully advocate, and to plead in favor of the patient's best interest necessitates comprehensive patient safety. The two concepts are inextricably linked, and for nursing the concept of patient advocacy is integrated deep into the action of caring.

When informally surveyed, nurses do not see patient safety as some new and late-breaking insight; rather, it is their belief that it has always been and continues to be a part of what they do. Line-level nurses are clear that they are not absent from the patient safety movement; rather, their impact has been limited. They believe that their voices are not heard within their organizations, and that this perspective is further reinforced by the constant presence of consultants du jour. Caregivers are clear that although the rhetoric of organizations spins along the line of patient safety, corporate decisions follow the line of economics.

CHARACTERISTICS OF A COMPREHENSIVE PATIENT SAFETY SOLUTION

The first set of characteristics of a comprehensive patient safety solution must be as follows: one vision, one language, but all disciplines.

Awareness, always the first characteristic to arrive, is not enough. Despite growing efforts and approaches to patient safety education, knowledgeable caregivers with excellent clinical skills do not ensure the success of a safety program. Millensen (1997) unequivocally stated that knowledge does not equal action. The question remains, "If everyone agrees that patient safety is desired and is a worthy aim of providers, why then don't all healthcare professionals provide safe care?" The answer is complex, but considerable observations indicate the following:

- *Leaders are lost to their staff.* Daily, leaders are reassigned, cross-assigned, or overassigned and are, therefore, rarely present to observe the nature of staff work or to mentor actions of safety.
- *Staff are lost to their leaders.* Visionless, staff work without a corporate meaning; they determine and decide for themselves what needs to be done and then defer performance to the skills installed by their primary discipline.
- *Vision is meaningless.* The healthcare merger experiences have created foreign corporate entities with unknown climates. Unsettled and alienated from the organizations they once knew, caregivers

are suspicious of the overnight appearance and disappearance of visions. As the universe of patient safety becomes further stratified within a national agenda, there is neither universal vision nor understanding among disciplines regarding the language and the symbols of comprehensive safety. We have not been able to agree on what it should look like and what it should do.

A call to duty is one means to reduce the disconnect between knowledge and action and to ensure outcomes. The judicial perspective regarding the standards of clinical duty is well defined (American Nurses Association [ANA], 1995), but less delineated are the standards and the language necessary to assess patient safety solutions. Although the disciplines are seeking support from the professional organizations, in lieu of forthcoming standards and language, patient safety advocates preliminarily state that comprehensive patient safety solutions must provide three core outcomes:

1. *Unity.* One vision ensures safety by demonstrating an understanding that safety is a condition that emerges from the collective interactivities of caregivers working in systems designed to prevent inadvertent outcomes (National Patient Safety Foundation [NPSF], 1998). Therefore, a comprehensive patient safety solution must be unifying, establishing a common work with a common language and providing the initiative that organizes multilevel caregivers around a common goal. That goal is to ensure patients' access to safe, cost-effective, high-quality care that is composed of repeatable processes with predictable and positive outcomes.
2. *Error reduction.* High-reliability theories support the conclusions that errors are reduced in systems with repeatable processes producing predictable and positive outcomes (Sagan, 1993). These processes assume stable and appropriate staffing patterns at the unit of delivery.
3. *Patient and staff satisfaction.* Satisfaction is one outcome of fulfilling expectations, and patient and provider safety are often linked (Institute of Medicine [IOM], 2000). Moreover, when healthcare systems are designed to ensure that caregivers are safe and can deliver safe care, patients benefit.

The second set of characteristics of a comprehensive patient safety solution must therefore be as follows: unity of vision, error management and reduction, and patient and staff satisfaction.

If the original premise is true and nursing is absent from the discussion table, how then does nursing leverage its collective knowledge and considerable lessons learned to ensure its presence in the face of the emerging body of patient safety literature and findings and ensuing actions (IOM, 2000)? When examined,

- *The solution in form is vision.* Staff are caught in the aftermath of the daily healthcare eruptions; blinded, they roam alone. A meaningful vision from leaders is essential to restore their sight. Although a thorough examination of vision exceeds the scope of this chapter, a short discussion is provided.
- *The solution in function is teamwork.* Teamwork offers the practical skills required to assist caregivers in understanding their work by establishing clear roles, a common and meaningful language, and unity through shared vision, goals, and outcomes. A case study later in this chapter provides an example for exploring teamwork as a solution to ensure the three core outcomes of unity of vision, error management and reduction, and patient and staff satisfaction.

THE FORM OF PATIENT SAFETY IS EMBODIED IN VISION

Vision is important to the actions of creating meaning and providing a clear sense of direction to the work that individuals do; organizations cannot survive without vision. The literature indicates that individuals delivering care within an organization that has a clearly established vision and leadership skilled in the translation of that vision have a higher level of commitment, productivity, and job satisfaction than individuals who do not (Senge, 1990; Pritchett and Pound, 1991). Both the vision and the language must be shared within an organization. The language used within an organization and the staff 's recognition and understanding of that language are vitally important to the leader's ability to translate statements of vision into something meaningful. Caregivers, connected and engaged in meaningful work, translate statements of vision into outcomes for patients (Westrope, Vaughn, Bott, and Taunton, 1995). Absent a clear organizational vision and outspoken, decisive leaders, caregivers and their patients will be troubled.

THE FUNCTION OF COMPREHENSIVE PATIENT SAFETY IS EMBODIED IN TEAMWORK

Teamwork provides a concrete set of practical skills that everyone can learn and use. Teamwork organizes caregivers around a common operational language that is used to articulate patient safety. Individuals organized around a specific goal influence the behaviors of others to work and achieve together (Cannon-Bowers, Oser, and Flannagan, 1992). In health care, individuals are challenged to work within and across department lines; at times they form teams (e.g., code teams), but in general they are trained, evaluated, and socialized to succeed as individuals (Morey et al., 2001; Risser, Simon, Rice, and Salisbury, 1999; Swezey and Salas, 1992). So, how does teamwork achieve the effect of comprehensive patient safety? Our experience has shown that teamwork helps to ensure the three core outcomes of patient safety: unity, reduction in errors, and improved patient and staff satisfaction.

Caregivers organized into healthcare teams deliver improved outcomes (Morey et al., 2001). Teamwork is multidimensional: Individuals bring to bear their individual skill sets, exercise those skills while functioning within their team role, and coordinate activities with their teammates to achieve the expected work outcomes (Swezey and Salas, 1992, p. 13). Additionally, teamwork mitigates three key issues that undermine patient safety: unclear roles, lack of accountability, and humans providing care in poorly designed and organized complex systems.

Error, the type of error (whether active or latent), and the subsequent development of safeguards against that type of error are really at the heart of what safety is all about. A large factor in active and latent medical error is that humans traditionally function as individuals working in poorly organized groups to deliver care in poorly designed and organized, complex healthcare systems. These systems provide little support regarding stable climates and established structure, and often fail to provide the necessary resources to caregivers. In this context caregivers must make complex decisions that are tightly coupled to emerging and unstable conditions of high-acuity care delivery (Cook and Woods, 1994; IOM, 2000). To support this discourse, and develop a common understanding, three terms must be defined: coupling, active error, and latent error.

- *Coupling*, a mechanical term, refers to the degree to which an environment is forgiving or unforgiving of certain actions. The provision of health care is often in the context of time-compressed multidimensional events wherein decisions must be made in an environment that is not tolerant of errors (IOM, 2000). The tightly coupled nature of health care defines an added dimension of urgency; lives are at stake.
- *Active errors* are inadvertent events that occur during the delivery of care and whose effects are immediate (IOM, 2000).
- *Latent errors* are embedded into the environment, are a part of operations, and may be termed "precursors or preconditions" to error (IOM, 2000).

Unrecognized and therefore unaddressed latent errors lead to provider errors (Reason, 1990). Latent errors may plague caregivers repeatedly but become normalized into a climate of deviance and lie dormant in the environment until a tightly coupled event emerges, catalyzing the latent system error into an active error. Examples are chronic understaffing; similar names or packaging of medications; breach of standards, such as improper monitoring during conscious sedation procedures; and improper use of equipment. The following is an example of the improper use of equipment: In many places it has become a standard practice to use one monitor to serve two cubicles. The monitor viewed in cubicle A is connected to the patient in cubicle B. A tightly coupled event results and catalyzes the latent error into an emerging event when an overloaded attending physician views the worrisome vitals and EKG and, not recognizing that the vital signs belong to the patient in the adjacent cubicle, prescribes an intervention on the wrong patient's chart.

Principle 3 of the Institute of Medicine's principles for the design of safety systems in healthcare organizations (IOM, 2000) recommends the following: "Train in teams those who are expected to work in teams." The danger of a latent error manifesting itself is reduced when the precursors and preconditions of care are optimized, that is, when the structure and climate for teamwork are secured: Processes and procedures are standardized, resources are optimal, and individuals know and understand their roles. The chances for active error are reduced when information is maximized by sharing situation awareness factors; plans and decisions are made, communicated, and updated as necessary; a common mental model of the expected outcomes is established; caregivers cross-monitor the activities of others; workload is balanced; and timely individual and team feedback is provided constantly and consistently, thereby informing the team processes (IOM, 2000).

TEAMWORK CASE STUDY: MEDTEAMS

When designing comprehensive patient safety solutions, teamwork provides a compelling multidisciplinary model of healthcare delivery. The following is a case study of the MedTeams research project and provides a concrete demonstration of teamwork's power to unify staff and improve performance; reduce error by trapping, managing, and mitigating the outcome of active and latent errors embedded in the reality of our humanity and in healthcare systems; and provide patient and staff satisfaction.

History

Aviation has been examining safety issues and actively seeking and engaging solutions for decades. Safety in aviation is something that all the stakeholders (i.e., government officials, management, pilots, and passengers) want. Previous research performed for U.S. army aviation showed that aircrew coordination training developed by Dynamics Research Corporation (DRC) improved mission performance by at least 20%, reduced safety-related task errors by over 40%, and resulted in estimated annual savings (from accident avoidance) in excess of $30 million. Based on these results, DRC and government researchers began to look for other high-stress, high-stakes environments that would benefit from team training.

Strong parallels were observed between the fields of tactical aviation and emergency health care (Simon et al., 1997; Weiner et al., 1993; Westrope, Vaughn, Bott, and Taunton, 1993). It was noted that the delivery of emergency care, like aviation, is composed of events where individuals undertake time-compressed, critical decisions and actions often based on incomplete information; demand effective coordination of interdisciplinary professionals; and understand that poor decision making and performance can lead to costly or deadly results.

Although teamwork is not a substitute for an excellent operational or clinical skill set, the initial advantages of teamwork are intuitive to participants. When applied to the domains of aviation and emergency care, those benefits became apparent to all stakeholders. Safety is something that aviators and caregivers want, passengers and patients need, and that managers and leaders can support by creating climates that actively promote teamwork behaviors (Clemmer, 1992; IOM, 2000; Morey et al., 2001; Risser et al., 1999; Simon et al., 1997).

Despite the strong parallels, it was important that the teamwork principles and the lessons learned in aviation undergo review, adaptation, and adoption by the caregivers who deliver emergency care (IOM, 2000). To execute the MedTeams project, a national panel was formed, composed of emergency care physicians and nurses from around the country, a cadre of knowledgeable consultants, emergency care professional societies, and clinical and behavioral experts from DRC. This MedTeams Project Subject Matter Expert Panel worked to adapt aviation-oriented teamwork training to the field of emergency care delivery, evaluate the effectiveness of MedTeams in operational settings, and ensure that the final MedTeams system could be sustained after the research dollars had been spent.

Needs Assessment: Teamwork in Emergency Health Care

To determine need, the initial MedTeams work focused on a closed-case review. Using a Teamwork Failure tool, closed cases were reviewed and assessed for teamwork failures (Risser et al., 1999). Physician and nurse pairs systematically reviewed 68 medical malpractice claims that arose through 4.7 million patient visits from eight emergency departments (EDs) across the country. A total of 476 teamwork failures were identified within the closed cases, for an average of about seven failures per case. These findings led to the conclusion that in each case effective teamwork could have prevented patient harm or injury, avoided over half the documented deaths, and avoided expensive litigation. Using actual costs and applying a national index, researchers calculated the cost of the teamwork failures as $350,000 in malpractice costs (indemnity and expenses) per 100,000 ED patient visits. Translated into practical terms, this means that the conservative amount added to each ED patient's visit to cover the litigated cost of teamwork failures is $3.50.

The behaviors that frequently led to teamwork failures were documented and subsequently integrated into a core curriculum. Central to that curriculum development was a fourfold premise:

1. Teamwork behaviors that improve caregiver coordination and prevent errors are a learnable set of skills (Morey et al., 2001).
2. Individuals trained and skilled in the behaviors of teamwork are equipped to work together to deliver more reliable, high-quality patient-focused care with improved outcomes as well as enhanced patient and staff satisfaction (Morey et al., 2001).
3. Each member of the team remains responsible and accountable to maintain an awareness of the patient's assessment and plan of care and to advocate and assert a position on behalf of the patient. This action of asserting a position and advocating on behalf of the patient is key to breaking the chain of errors (Cook and Woods, 1994, pp. 273–277; Morey et al., 2001; Risser et al., 1999).
4. Most errors unfold over an extended period of time and are observable and recognizable; therefore, they are interruptible (Cook and Woods, 1994, p. 274).

The MedTeams Teamwork Training System

MedTeams is an outcome-based patient safety solution initially delivered to the department as a teamwork training course. MedTeams is a behaviorally-oriented, theory-grounded, scientifically-based, comprehensive solution to the problem of patient safety.

MedTeams delivers the adapted aviation-based teamwork training to ED staffs, with specific attention paid to team operating rules and the use of a set of standardized teamwork behaviors. The start-up training course, entitled Emergency Team Coordination Course (ETCC), addresses how teams form, the principles of teamwork, the essential operational issues, and the reinforcements required to promote the effective delivery of emergency care. The MedTeams behaviors and course are organized around the five dimensions of teamwork principles common to highly effective teams: (1) maintaining team structure and climate, (2) planning and problem solving, (3) communication, (4) workload management, and (5) improving teamwork skills.

The MedTeams teamwork training system equips clinically expert caregivers to work as a team organized around the goal of the right care delivered in the right way. MedTeams training equips team members with the skills to identify, capture, and manage or mitigate the active or latent errors that unfold or lie dormant within their system. The details of each MedTeams teamwork dimension are discussed next.

Team Dimension 1: Team Structure and Climate

The care delivery unit of a MedTeams organization is its team. As an organizational model, MedTeams divides an ED into functional units called *core teams*. These core teams are composed of 4 to 10 staff members, including physicians, nurses, technical caregivers, and administrative assistants. Each team member clearly knows which team he or she belongs to and which patients are assigned to the team. An ED maintains from one to four core teams during any given shift, depending on the expected patient volume and the actual staffing level. During the course of emerging events, such as incoming trauma or medical resuscitations, team members peel off from the core team and join with others to form an ad hoc team that delivers care until patients are handed off or members are relieved to return to their core team function and role. Leadership is trained to become skilled in the duties and responsibilities relative to creating and maintaining the climate and structuring the supports that are required to implement and sustain teamwork behaviors.

Team dimension 1 safeguards against latent error by ensuring that the proper climate and system structures for the delivery of care are in place, that team members are knowledgeable of their roles, and that upon arrival each new team meets to discuss resource and patient flow issues and takes the necessary actions to correct any existing issues.

Team Dimension 2: Plan and Problem Solve

Failure to advocate and assert a position on behalf of the patient was recognized in the needs assessment by the MedTeams physician–nurse pairs as core to teamwork failures that too often resulted in patient harm or injury. Team dimension 2 is designed specifically to safeguard against that failure. The action of advocating and asserting a position on behalf of the patient is key to interrupting active and unfolding errors. In traditional care, individuals assess their patients and develop and hold a mental model of the patient's problems, needs, and expected outcomes. A working diagnosis is developed, plans are designed, and all actions prescribed proceed along nursing and along medical discipline lines. In MedTeams, the essential act of communicating across the disciplines moves information from the mental model of an individual to a shared mental model within a team. The patient's plan is shared and agreement held by all members, who in return effectively cross-monitor the actions of each other against the established plan.

When the actions of a provider differ from the expected actions, any team member recognizing that difference is responsible for advocating and asserting a position on behalf of the patient. This expectation is not a license to mutiny. Rather, the asserting individual assumes a difference in information between caregivers. That is, the unstated assumption is "I have information that you do not. If you had the additional information that I have it would alter the patient's plan of care." Therefore, this action effectively traps the active error and manages or mitigates its outcome.

Team Dimension 3: Communicate with the Team

Effective communication is essential to timely and accurate information exchange, ensuring proper plans of care, and creating the team's shared mental model for each patient. Team dimension 3 establishes the common language necessary for understanding the actions of team members. The practical skills of communication and conflict resolution are taught and practiced. Effective communication ensures that caregivers maintain a shared mental model for each patient; moves information forward to the key decision maker, who in return acts on the patient's plan of care; and maintains situation awareness across the team.

Team Dimension 4: Manage Workload

MedTeams is not a substitute for appropriate staffing; without the proper staffing level, no patient safety solution is effective. Research indicates that caregivers are at risk when workload is too high (Serig, 1994). Team dimension 4 equips caregivers with the skills necessary to monitor and balance workload within and across teams.

Team Dimension 5: Improve Team Skills

Team dimension 5 establishes the formal and informal means for teams to share their information, improve processes, and enhance the safe delivery of care.

Improving the Delivery of Emergency Care: MedTeams Validation

The statistics representing validation of MedTeams are pending publication (Morey et al., 2001). The data demonstrate the effectiveness of MedTeams in improving patient outcomes, caregiver effectiveness, patient and staff satisfaction, and patient safety. Additionally, an analysis of the savings attributed to reduced litigation costs and improved outcomes has been completed and demonstrates a savings that substantially exceeds the $3.50 per patient figure initially estimated in the project needs assessment.

The MedTeams Research Project results show conclusively that when staff are trained and MedTeams is implemented, the quality of care delivery improves, as evidenced by the following:

- *Error rates drop significantly.* Additionally, patients admitted to the hospital are "packaged" more completely (i.e., patients and their families know why they are being admitted, patients have their ID bands on, and intravenous and intravenous medications are run or given as prescribed).
- *Performance improves.* Data indicated that despite increases in acuity and volume, the length of stay remained steady and several specific quality indices improved.
- *Patients' perception of care is more positive.* The number of patients reporting a high level of satisfaction and an improvement in their sense of well-being is greater for the sites with MedTeams implementation.

A MedTeams organization with individuals properly engaged and exercising their MedTeams teamwork training skill set can ensure the reliable delivery of high-quality care to the communities it serves. The leaders of a MedTeams organization can measure the impact: Staff can reduce errors and improve the effectiveness of their performance, and patients can sense and communicate the difference.

Leadership Considerations

Leaders must establish the infrastructure that ensures principle 3 of the Institute of Medicine's principles for the design of safety systems in healthcare organizations: "training in teams those who are expected to work in teams" (IOM, 2000). Latent, embedded error is reduced when the optimal precursors and preconditions to the successful delivery of care are in place, the structure and climate for teamwork are secured, processes and procedures are standardized, resources are optimal, and individuals who recognize and understand their roles are free to focus on the delivery of care. However, leading a human behavior change process requires education and support, careful planning and preparation, concrete and decisive actions, and great consideration afforded to the details of department operations and care delivery (Locke, 2000). Although these essential leadership actions begin to cull the latent errors embedded within systems, they take time to learn.

MedTeams addresses this issue and is designed to move departments from the single dimension of quality initiatives to the multiple dimensionality of true culture change by providing training and support over time (Clemmer, 1992; Locke, 2000). The following describes each delivery phase of the MedTeams System:

- Delivery phase I engages leadership in preparing the climate and structuring the environment for the transition to a team-based care delivery system, including planning the details of the change initiative (Locke, 2000).
- Delivery phase II provides training to physician and nurse pairs and their leadership in the practical steps for undertaking a cultural change and installing MedTeams in their department (Locke, 2000).
- Delivery phase III provides a forward focus on obtaining a change in culture. If unattended, the good effects of MedTeams will disappear. Fostering MedTeams behaviors within and across departments through sustainment and integration methods is essential. Leadership receives education specific to coaching and mentoring these skills. Our ongoing research in sustainment indicates that the active involvement of leadership is essential to optimal MedTeams implementation.

For the purpose of this discourse, *leaders* are those who have the power to formally influence caregivers. The following discussion contains the seeds of action that are relevant and applicable for both formal and informal leaders. MedTeams establishes a structure and climate of care delivery through concrete actions and environmental improvements to install and sustain teamwork behaviors. Leaders engage in the following actions:

1. *Assess the organization's readiness to change.* Leaders are assisted in performing a readiness-to-change assessment. The department assesses its operations or resources for positive and negative resources. Leadership reviews the department against specific criteria (e.g., whether there be a change of leadership in the next 12 months, whether leadership is willing to organize staff as small teams, whether leadership is willing to incorporate MedTeams standard procedures and techniques into routine or daily activities). Additionally, leaders assess for stability relative to organizational structure, leadership, and staffing. These actions further identify and mitigate some of the preconditions to errors.
2. *Establish the vision.* Leaders must establish and communicate the vision and the purpose for change. They train to develop and communicate the strategic implementation plan; determine and communicate the expected performance accountabilities; and develop and communicate which outcomes are important. When these determinations are made, the staff can be engaged to unify around common goals.
3. *Plan for MedTeams success and prepare the climate.* During this aspect of implementation, leaders clarify the purpose of change and gain the commitment of key stakeholders. Leaders enlist the on-

going commitment and support of the organization by establishing MedTeams as an infrastructure that adds a vertical snap to operations and ensures the strategic plan. Additionally, this commitment ensures the necessary resources of money, staff replacement, classroom and audiovisual support, training time, and sustainment activities. Leaders and their staff must determine the necessary team structure for their department and then coordinate and communicate the structure to all staff. Planning and coordinating the decision-making process is essential.

4. *Implement behaviors.* Leaders and certified ETCC instructors train the staff and provide ongoing coaching and mentoring. Leaders continue to monitor the growth of their staff into MedTeams behaviors. A multidisciplinary MedTeams patient safety committee is established and provides the methodology for reviewing active errors and identifying and resolving the preconditions for latent error.
5. *Sustain behaviors.* This is a critical component. It is an area where management initiatives traditionally have stumbled. Leaders and their staff evaluate and formalize structures and processes essential to MedTeams performance. Leaders continue their focus on teams by coaching and role modeling, and the instructors continue to teach new staff and refresh current staff on the behaviors and updates of MedTeams.
6. *Integrate the behaviors into a comprehensive cultural change.* Individuals serving on the MedTeams patient safety committee add to their problem-solving methodology by creating methods for fostering MedTeams behaviors into staff performance over time. A new culture of patient safety is obtained when vision moves from an external existence displayed in the form of slogans and initiatives to an internal initiative that emerges as an outcome of professionals engaged in the collective process of purposeful and cooperative care delivery.
7. *Evaluate outcomes.* The processes of leadership are informed by a data-driven evaluation system. Leadership determines and defines the state of excellence at their organization and is supported in their ongoing processes with a suite of measures that enhances their current process improvement efforts and that is sensitive to teamwork.

Teamwork Summary

Teamwork is a powerful tool. It provides the medium for leaders and staff to communicate with each other and to provide information to their patients. Teamwork ensures (1) the hearing and understanding of patient safety in multidisciplinary multidirectional ways, (2) the creation of outcome-based solutions, and (3) leadership and caregiver accountability.

Teamwork cannot solve everything. The profession must be educated about the national patient safety agenda. It is undeniable that staffing shortages threaten to undercut patient care initiatives, but nursing cannot abdicate its obligation to patient safety. It is clear that patient safety in the form of advocacy is deeply rooted in the profession of nursing, but this fact is of little use in responding to the national agenda of patient safety unless nursing leverages its extensive knowledge of this advocacy. To achieve comprehensive change, a concerted effort by providers is required to research, adapt, and adopt solutions that are multifaceted and multidisciplinary. Synergy will develop between the disciplines and, over time, outcomes will result that bring us full cycle, from the worst to the best of times.

The MedTeams teamwork training system achieves and ensures lasting comprehensive patient safety. It establishes the characteristics of a comprehensive patient safety solution:

- *Unity.* Safety emerges from the collective interactivities of caregivers working in a system designed to prevent inadvertent outcomes. MedTeams establishes the proper and appropriate climate and structure for care provision; clear vision and roles that organize multiple levels of caregivers around the common goal of safe, efficient, and effective patient care; and a common language for providers. In so doing, patients are ensured access to safe and effective care that is composed of repeatable processes with predictable and positive outcomes.

- *Error reduction.* Individuals trained in the MedTeams behaviors develop responses and repeatable processes to deliver predictable outcomes that in return ensure high-reliability health care promulgated at the unit of delivery.
- *Patient and staff satisfaction.* The high-reliability outcomes achieved by MedTeams-trained caregivers are evidenced by improved delivery of effective care and reduced active and latent errors. As a result, patients and staff are more satisfied. MedTeams is designed to ensure that caregivers are safe and can safely deliver care. Patients and staff both benefit.

MedTeams responds to and ensures the IOM recommendation in principle 3. Caregivers trained in MedTeams teamwork behaviors:

- Work to manage and mitigate active and latent errors.
- Ensure that team climate, structures, and processes are in place that identify and address the precursors and preconditions of error and in return ensure proper outcomes.
- Ensure against normalizing system deviance.
- Ensure maximal flow of information to decision makers. That information translates into the right patient receiving the right plan accompanied by the right prescriptives and procedures to result in the right outcome.
- Ensure clear roles, standardize terms and processes, and simplify procedures.

CONCLUSION

Health care is spinning out of control. It is time to sort things out. As it relates to patient safety, control and meaning are established through a common language and lexicon of error. To move from the static condition of control into the dynamics of progress, patient safety research must build on its emerging knowledge base to provide unity of vision, reduction of error, and patient and staff satisfaction. To ensure the construction of this research framework, the disciplines must hold a common vision, speak a common language of patient safety, and research aspects of comprehensive patient safety. Research development must proceed to theory that will give rise to form and function. Form is embedded in vision, and function manifests in teamwork. Without that vision and a language that is understood and accepted by all disciplines, knowledge will not equal action, and patient safety will not happen.

Teamwork brings us full circle. Teamwork provides form and function for comprehensive patient safety, teamwork assesses for and ensures the presence of nursing, and teamwork is a multidisciplinary vehicle to move us from the worst to the best of times.

References

1. American Nurses Association. (1995). *Scope and Standards for Nurse Administrators*. Washington, DC: American Nurses Publishing.
2. Cannon-Bowers, J. A., Oser, F., and Flanagan, D. L. (1992). "Work Teams in Industry: A Selected Review and Proposed Framework."

In R. Swezy and E. Salas (Eds.), *Teams: Their Training and Performance* (pp. 355–377). Norwood, NJ: Ablex.

3. Clemmer, J. (1992). *Firing on all Cylinders: The Service/Quality System for High-Powered Corporate Performance*. Homewood, IL: Business One Irwin.
4. Cook, R. I., and Woods, D. D. (1994). "Operating at the Sharp End: The Complexity of Human Error." In M. S. Bogner (Ed.), *Human Error in Medicine* (pp. 255–310). Hinsdale, NJ: Lawrence Erlbaum.
5. Danzon, P. M. (1994). "Merger Mania: An Analysis." *Health Systems Rev* 27 (6), 18–28.
6. Institute for Healthcare Improvement. (1997). "The Quest for Error-Proof Medicine." *Drug Benefit Trends* 9 (6), 27–29.
7. Institute of Medicine. Kohn, L. T., Corrigan, J. M., and Donaldson, M. S. (Eds.). (2000). *To Err Is Human: Building a Safer Health System*. Washington, DC: National Academy Press.
8. Leape, L. (1994). "Error in Medicine." *JAMA* 272 (23), 4.
9. Locke, A. (2000). *MedTeams Teamwork System Implementation Guide*. (Training materials: Available from Dynamics Research Corporation, 60 Frontage Road, Andover, MA 01810.)
10. Millensen, M. (1997). *Demanding Medical Excellence: Doctors and Accountability in the Information Age*. Chicago: University of Chicago Press.
11. Morey, J., Simon, R., Jay, G., Wears, R., Salisbury, M., Dukes, K., and Berns, S. (2002). "Error Reduction and Performance Improvement in the Emergency Department through Formal Teamwork Training: Evaluation Results of the MedTeams Project." *Health Science Research*, December 2002, 1553–1581.
12. National Patient Safety Foundation. (1998). *A Tale of Two Stories: Contrasting Views of Patient Safety*. Chicago: NPSF, p. 1. Available: http://www.npsf.org/exec.front.html.
13. Pritchett, P. L., and Pound, R. (1991). *Business as Usual: The Handbook for Managing and Supervising Organizational Change*. Dallas: Pritchett Publishing.
14. Reason, J. (1990). *Human Error*. New York: Cambridge University Press.
15. Risser, D., Simon, R., Rice, M., and Salisbury, M. (1999). "The Potential for Improved Teamwork to Reduce Medical Errors in the Emergency Department." *Annals of Emergency Medicine* 34, 373–383.
16. Sagan, S. (1993). *The Limits of Safety*. Princeton, NJ: Princeton University Press.
17. Senge, P. (1990). *The Fifth Discipline*. New York: Doubleday-Currency.
18. Serig, D. I. (1994). "Radiopharmaceutical Misadministrations: What's Wrong." In M. S. Bogner (Ed.). *Human Error in Medicine* (pp. 179–195). Hinsdale, NJ: Lawrence Erlbaum.
19. Simon, R., Morey, J., and Locke, A. (1997). *Full Scale Development of the Emergency Team Coordination Course and Evaluation Measures*. (Available from Dynamics Research Corporation, 60 Frontage Road, Andover, MA 01810.)
20. Swezey, R. W., and Salas, E. (Eds.). (1992). *Teams: Their Training and Performance*. Norwood, NJ: Ablex.
21. Weiner, E. L., Kanki, B. G., and Helmreich, R. L. (Eds.). (1993). *Cockpit Resource Management*. San Diego: Academic Press.
22. Westrope, R. A., Vaughn, L., Bott, M., and Taunton, R. L. (1995). "Shared Governance: From Vision to Reality." *JONA* 25 (12), 45–54.

21

TEAMWORK COMMUNICATIONS AND TRAINING

Richard Lauve, MD

There is no limit to what one man can achieve so long as he does not require getting credit for it all.

—Henry Grady

It's easy gettin' good players. The hard part is gettin' them to play with each other.

—Casey Stengel

DEFINITIONS AND INITIAL THOUGHTS

Teamwork is by definition the work done by groups of individuals greater than one. While this may seem obvious, what is not so obvious is what is required for groups of individuals to work together. Many of us have not been trained in the intricacies of working together with other individuals. Indeed, a great many of us have been trained in organizations or professions where individual work is highly valued and rewarded, and the only communication required is giving orders to others. The central command-and-control management style may be highly effective for organizations such as an army, where rote obedience and an established hierarchical chain of command best maintain order and safety, but is inadequate for organizations that deal with constant variation and rapid change and must rely on individuals, each with a particular set of knowledge, skills, or perspectives.

If individuals are to come together and collaborate (i.e., work as a team in intellectual endeavors for a common purpose), attention must be given to training these individuals in the expected collaborative behaviors and the communication styles necessary for collaboration to succeed.

REDUCING THE BARRIERS TO COLLABORATION

The Need for a Team

The more complex the system to be improved, the more complex the team that must be brought together and the more difficult will be true collaboration. Having a clear vision and common goal for the group certainly provides motivation, but even the highly motivated group runs the risk of achieving little, if attention is not paid to the barriers to collaboration. Therefore, the first task for you, as the leader, is to instill in each individual on the newly formed team an awareness that the group has a purpose. This involves more than simply establishing a mission and a vision; instead, the need for the team itself must be established. I am referring now to the realization that no individual can achieve what the team is required to achieve.

This concept will be foreign to the culture of many healthcare organizations, because individualistic work and organization have been the historical standards and ideals of health care. This reality is probably best demonstrated by the mandate from The Joint Commission in recent years that performance improvement initiatives in its accredited organizations should involve "cross silo" efforts by several components of the organization. This revealing requirement demonstrates years of Joint Commission observation of the fragmented nature of quality improvement in hospitals, where quality departments rarely coordinated with medical staffs or other operational areas within the hospital. This often resulted in simultaneous but disjointed efforts to address similar opportunities by the quality department, operating room nursing leadership, materials management, the medical staff, and others, without significant collaboration or communication between the silos. The Joint Commission observed not only inefficient duplicative efforts within the organization, but also movements by the various parties at cross-purposes to the other components of the organization.

With a mission as significant and complex as improving the environment of safety that our patients experience, it becomes difficult to imagine how any single individual or, for that matter, any focused silo could possibly achieve improvement without involvement of other components of the hospital. If we are to seize the full potential of possible gains in reducing medication errors, as a specific example, not only will product acquisition/materials management departments and pharmacies need to be involved, but nurses, physicians, group purchasing organizations, and ultimately product manufacturers will need to be components of the improvement effort.

If your organization is having difficulty understanding why performance improvement or quality can't handle patient safety alone, try emphasizing the benefits of collaboration. The concept is relatively simple, yet escapes those not familiar with it. Collaboration allows for the possibility of *synthesis*, a product by definition not possible without the input of at least two individuals. Many will be confused by this concept, and believe that *collaboration* is a euphemism for *compromise*. Synthesis is far from compromise. Synthesis is the product of two or more distinct perspectives, separate and apart before coming together, combining to make something not possible without the joining of the two (or more). The process of synthesis produces something new, never before realized or imagined prior to the joining. Compromise is more akin to a reduction or an overlap, usually involving areas of commonality and agreement.

Try this example to stimulate the proper vision of collaborative synthesis: children. Who can view a child as a compromise between the genetic materials of their parents? The bringing together of two separate influences has the potential for creating something totally new, never before imagined, and not possible without the joining of the two.

One more hint on breaking through the barrier of understanding the need for a team: I find that many times one party to the potential collaboration (a new team member, for example) will believe that his or her perspective is the correct one and will not value the richness of potential possible through synthesis with others. The following exercise can be done with two people, or mini-teams of two formed solely for the exercise. Show one person, or one half of the teams, a square with an X through it. Show the other person, or other half of the teams, a right triangle. The two views look something like Figure 21.1. Now

FIGURE 21.1 Two Views of the Same Object

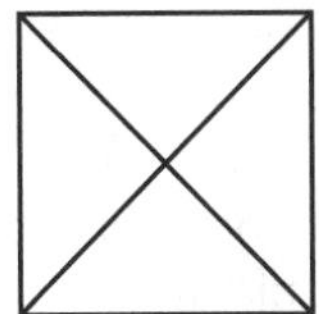
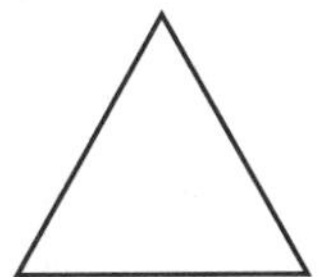

tell the two individuals, or both members of the mini-teams, that they have seen two views of the same thing. What is it?

The dynamics that emerge are phenomenal. Some groups won't show each other what they have seen. Some will converse and conclude that you are lying to them, that it can't possibly be the same thing. But eventually, two people will think, using full input from both groups, and realize that these simple figures can only represent two views of a pyramid—one from close up at ground level, and the other from directly above. It is nearly impossible for anyone to conclude with accuracy the true nature of the object from a single view. Combining the information from both observations almost always leads to the correct conclusion. After this exercise, I once had the CEO of a 750-bed hospital, a retired general and decidedly a central command-and-control authoritarian manager, approach me. "You know," he said, "its never bothered me before that other people have different points of view than mine. They have every right to be wrong. But that pyramid thing, that really got to me."

Individual Domination

Very commonly, when groups are formed from a pool of individuals who have not previously collaborated, certain persons or a person within the group tends to dominate over others. This is particularly true when the group members come from an organization that fosters and supports individualism, and whenever people of disparate rank come together on a team. The challenge for the group leader is then to give the more shy, docile, subordinate, or quiet individuals a structured environment that promotes their participation.

The solution to the dominating individual, in most cases, lies with the team leader's knowledge and execution of the nominal group technique combined occasionally with a small dose of parliamentary procedure. In the nominal group technique, the team is posed a question, problem, idea, challenge, or opportunity followed by the request that each member of the group work silently for a few moments to record his or her own ideas. For example, the group might be considering the high incidence of drug administration error during code blue or resuscitation efforts. The group might be told, after some discussion of the facts known about the problem, "Take a few moments to write down what you feel should be done about this problem. Writing just one idea is acceptable, but if you have several, please record them all." Asked openly, this is the ideal invitation for the dominating individual to climb aboard the soapbox and espouse his or her views, solutions, and implementation plans to secure a 100% cure. The input of the group might easily be lost. With each member working silently alone, the individuals gain the opportunity to think without contamination of others' ideas.

Next, the leader asks each individual to report to the group one idea from his or her list. One member of the group is asked to record the reported ideas on a flip chart. This job is ideally given to the dominating member. Not only does it give that individual an important job that distracts him from feeling the need to dominate the conversation, but it materially takes him out of immediate participation mode and forces him to listen in order to record correctly. After each person has reported one idea, the leader goes around the room again, and again if necessary, until all ideas have been recorded. Only then is a discussion allowed about the ideas. Grouping and splitting ideas is allowed and will promote the discussion.

After all the ideas are grouped, related, split out, and discussed, the group votes on prioritization. Sequential multivote ballots have the greatest probability of building consensus.

For example, if the group has identified eleven possible actions, force each member to vote for three. After tallying the votes—notice that your group's previously dominating individual is being kept very busy—make a cut where the votes fall off abruptly. If five ideas each got more than seven votes, but the next-highest vote getter only got four votes, consider the five ideas your "top five." More discussion is often needed at this point, but if no consensus emerges, vote again. This time each member gets two votes. If two or three ideas are separated from the others, then vote again, eventually getting to one vote per member and identifying a single top-priority action item. With a little practice, this technique can be used very rapidly to focus even a medium-sized group of seven to nine individuals.

Another way to deal with dominating individuals, particularly when they are repeating the same speech about their preferences, is to "call the question." This parliamentary maneuver of calling for a vote is best performed by a member of the group, and not the leader; however, the group's leader can promote the maneuver with questions such as "Can I take that as a motion?" or "Would you like to make that in the form of a motion?" This is very powerful when immediately following the dominating individual's speech. Either the dominator's idea will be adopted, or the group can move on to other ideas. Whichever course the group takes, progress will be made, and the group will avoid a paralysis of analysis and the domination of a single member.

Resources

I often hear complaints about not having enough resources to carry out actions, and sometimes even enough resources to have meetings. People not being able to give their time to sit and think about a new approach, a new set of ideas, or a new problem is often the greatest barrier to a new team. There is no doubt that time is our greatest resource, and few healthcare organizations have slack time when it comes to the skilled problem solvers you will want on your team.

Conflicting agendas of team members and frank turf protection frequently manifest as inadequate time to attend meetings. It is possible that individuals have been asked to do more than humanly possible. If so, top management must resolve this situation, as will be discussed in a moment. On the other hand, the individual that "simply does not have the time for another meeting" may be engaged in turf-protecting behavior. The team leader's job is to search for the possibility that a team member may be threatened by the formation of the new team. Candidates for this behavior include all of the members important to the function of the new team and for whom a similar function was previously under their purview. For a patient safety initiative, this could be the head of pharmacy, materials management, quality, performance improvement, risk management, corporate compliance, or any other silo of the hospital that previously dealt with safety issues.

The team leader's job is to reduce turf as a barrier to progress for the new team. Recall Henry Grady's quote from the beginning of this chapter. The truly inspired and safety-motivated leader will have no difficulty approaching a turf protector. The withdrawn individual needs reassurance that her participation is critical and that by definition she is under no particular threat from the new group. In fact, the participation of the corporate compliance officer (substitute whatever title is appropriate) is so critical that the individual's job is in jeopardy only if she does not participate. Appeal to her ego: "We need your perspective on this issue," or "We cannot get this done without you." Emphasize that the job is bigger than any single department, and that this effort is an attempt to work across departments, not replace any one. It's a team effort. The job requires more than a corporate compliance perspective (to continue with the previous example), but that perspective is a critical part that the team cannot be without.

Inadequate prioritization from top management can kill any endeavor, but especially one that requires bridging previously recognized silos. Only the CEO and board can make it clear to recalcitrant participants that their position's involvement is critical and that their involvement is an important part of their job description.

It is the job of any given individual's superior to require his or her participation in the organization and to assist with prioritizing the many issues before that individual. Above the supervisor lies the workings of the board's strategy process. Ultimately, the board must make it clear that the proper resources are to be made available to succeed in a patient safety initiative. Conversely, confusion over which task or unprioritized items on your full plate to tackle first is the difficult but primary task of the midlevel manager to sort out. Few CEOs will long tolerate the middle manager who constantly complains about "too much to do." Resolving this conundrum is a daunting task for many middle managers. I suggest always approaching your superior with a suggested course of action to resolve these issues. "I can do that. Will it be acceptable for Project B to take a back seat to this?" is always preferable to "I just have too much to do."

For any manager who is "on board" with patient safety as a high-priority item but is having trouble securing resources from the CEO or others above, I suggest the following strategies. First, find ways to communicate that patient safety is an investment, not an expense. For medication error interventions, this is already done for you. Get and distribute the following: *Pharmacotherapy* vol. 16, no. 6 (1996), which shows a 16.7 to 1 return on investment in certain pharmacy error reduction efforts, and *JAMA* vol. 280, no. 15 (October 21, 1998), which demonstrates a 5 to 1 return on computer-assisted programs for drug selection.

Second, show how you can quickly measure and report the results of your intervention. For example, measure the difference between the pharmacy time needed to clarify orders using preprinted order forms and handwritten forms for a focused intervention—say, chemotherapy orders. Give the feedback the following month (e.g., 123 minutes of pharmacy and nursing time for handwritten orders versus 27 minutes for preprinted orders over a one-month period).

Third, realize that the top leadership is not your enemy in this. They—your board, CEO, and CFO—have distinct and valid obligations to the financial well-being of the organization. Nothing will secure the support of the top leadership faster than showing them the aligned incentives of what's best for the patient and what's best for the bottom line. Remind them that "best performers" all over the country are doing this, with decidedly positive effects on their public relations image, and positive financial results.

Training

The team leader is the only individual who needs team dynamics training. Such training is ideal for all members, but not necessary, and impractical in our budget-constrained environment. One aspect of training, however, is very difficult to do without everyone at least having a taste, and that is systems thinking. If your team has never thought in an interdisciplinary manner before, you will have difficulty accomplishing collaborative synthesis. Ideally, your team should attend a team collaboration workshop. This experience not only teaches the fundamentals but also, if properly done, provides the opportunity for the team to practice under the guidance of experts in team systems thinking as applied to evidence-based medicine.

If the budget allows for additional training, seek out an experienced trainer in chaos theory as it applies to groups and management of organizations. (Of course, if you are lucky enough to find a collaborative-team workshop that includes chaos theory concepts, grab it.) Chaos, or emergent control as it is sometimes called, is (among many other things) a dynamic way of viewing what happens in a group of people. It uses organic models that are inherently meaningful to healthcare workers. Metaphors such as the immune system understood as a hive of bees or a forest are very easy for most healthcare professionals to relate to. The further elucidation of these concepts is far beyond the scope of this chapter, but one of the underlying constructs encourages a team to celebrate its self-determined direction. This is particularly useful for the team leader. Your ideas about how to begin addressing patient safety may be very different from the risk manager's ideas. If the team identifies with his or her ideas, celebrate that direction for the team. Remember that part of the "getting credit for it" thing that Henry Grady referred to includes not having to always "do it your way." Be happy that you have a team that wants to do something, whatever it is!

Allowing the team to determine its own direction is intimately connected to the modern concepts of power, or authority, within an organization. When we think of authority in an organization, we often think of the *formal authority*. This is also referred to as the legitimate, official, or titled authority. As a team leader or committee chair, such authority rests in you. It also rests in the CEO of your organization. By virtue of title, job description, designation by a higher authority, or sometimes just history, these figures have responsibility. They may or may not actually have authority to act, not act, choose a course of action, secure resources, allocate those resources, prioritize, and so forth. These are the classic measures of "real" authority. The individual with formal authority is, however, always the one held responsible or rewarded for action, lack of actions, and so forth. Unfortunately, we have all seen the designation of formal authority with responsibility, but without the true ability to take action.

The ability to take action always lies with what is referred to as the *informal authority*. Sometimes, this informal authority resides with a superior, who has the real power to allow or not allow action. For a discussion of the need to manage a superior who constrains results by restricting resources, refer to the Resources section earlier in this chapter. If you are lucky, you have both, and this is certainly possible. For now, consider the ability to take action as residing within the group itself, as it ultimately does—always.

Just as commonly as informal authority resides with a superior, so too the real control of results actually lies with the members of the team. Remember that we started this whole discussion with the premise that "it takes a team." One person can't get the job done. So without the cooperation, at a minimum, of the team members, no action will be taken. Even with all the resources in the world, a leader will accomplish nothing without followers. It is their "ownership" of the plan of action that is critical to accomplishments. Therefore, it is the realization by the team leader that the team has the true authority to act or not act that frees him or her to celebrate the emergent control seen within a well-functioning group.

To paraphrase Harlan Cleveland in *The Knowledge Executive*, authority is always delegated upward within any educated group. The instant the group ceases to delegate authority to the leadership (whether it be the formal or informal authority figure), that individual loses all power to accomplish anything. Remember Casey Stengel. You could in theory be the best team leader in the world, with great ideas, but you will accomplish nothing if you can't get the team to "play together."

Communications

The most important aspect of communications in a group, indeed the sine qua non, is to value input from every member. The lowest-ranking participant can provide the group with a unique insight that inspires breakthrough change in your organization. This is diametrically opposed to the central command-and-control mind-set. As the team leader, you must truly believe and have as a contagious attitude that it is the line troops who really know what the problem is and have the unique perspective on how to fix it.

In the culture of the Ritz Carlton organization, whomever the guest approaches is the right person. If that individual can't help the guest, he or she won't leave the guest until someone who can has been found. Once I was participating in a group effort to cut the time from call to answer when a patient rings the call button. A night housekeeping employee on the team listened attentively to the discussion and finally said, "I don't know why they think I can't help with this. They don't want me talking to patients. I can tell if they need a spill cleaned up or something else. I can't help with chest pain, but if they really need a nurse I'll bet I can make that clearer than any call button!" The comment hit most of us like a ton of bricks, and initiated a culture change in the organization. Everyone responded to calls for help. What a novel idea in a hospital. Clerks and housekeeping staff were trained in the recognition of medical emergencies, and patient satisfaction scores skyrocketed.

As a team leader, you will have to be sensitive to the group's dynamics. If conflict or simple inattention to a member emerges, try Rogers' Rule. Carl Rogers, in *On Becoming A Person*, recommends this simple tool: Every speaker must repeat the message of the previous speaker, to the satisfaction of the previous speaker, before being allowed to voice his or her own opinion or ideas. You don't have to actually announce this rule. I find if you simply begin using it, others will follow. Everyone will listen more attentively. Emotional reaction will dissipate. "Positions" will be replaced by concepts, ideas, clarified understandings, and synthesis of ideas. Leaders will hear themselves and others saying, "So if I understand you correctly . . ." and "Did you mean this or that?" We cannot synthesize new ideas from the input of others if we cannot listen to them and understand their meaning. Real listening and clearly presented ideas are the basis of true communication and are required for collaborative synthesis to take place.

SOME FINAL ADVICE

You're changing the culture of your organization, not your shorts. Don't be discouraged with slow progress and the persistence of the smell of dirty laundry. Team collaboration, synthesis of new ideas, and investment in performance improvement that has demonstrated financial returns are all new ideas for many healthcare organizations.

Celebrate your victories. You don't need the entire medical staff to adopt the new standard order set for sliding-scale insulin. Just one physician will do. With one, you have the opportunity to measure the difference between his or her performance and the others. Now measure the right thing and demonstrate the differences. Physicians are highly competitive individuals. Show them a better way and they will follow. And now, your one physician will become your champion to get the word out to his or her peers. In the words of a Native American proverb, "You don't have to turn the whole herd, just the buffalo in front."

22

Teamwork: The Fundamental Building Block of High-Reliability Organizations and Patient Safety

G. Eric Knox, MD and Kathleen Rice Simpson, PhD, RNC, FAAN

In today's healthcare environment, *teams*, *teamwork*, and *team building* are words often said, seldom heard, and only rarely considered an operational reality.[1] This is true in spite of the relentless cost, production, and efficiency pressures operating to diminish patient safety in all contemporary healthcare organizations. Understanding how multiple diverse professionals can most efficiently and effectively work together on clinical units (the "sharp end") remains a clear organizational imperative.[2]

Unfortunately, most clinical units responsible for delivering safe patient care continue to function as discrete and separate collections of nurses, physicians, and other patient care professionals rather than as a single team with mutually agreed-upon goals, tactics, and incentives. In extreme examples, the critical relationship between nurses and physicians (which heavily influences the professional relationships of all other team members) has been described as "strained or barely tolerable."[3] The result is a demanding, complex, and fragmented system in which both patients and clinicians must heroically—often unsuccessfully—struggle to reach the elusive goal of providing safe patient care.[4]

By contrast, successful organizations in a wide variety of other professional and technical industries facing similar or more difficult challenges have come to recognize multidisciplinary teams as the unifying principle for creating operational excellence and success.[5] Recently, similar thoughts applied to health care have begun to be reported. Morey and colleagues have suggested that increased patient safety and operational efficiency in emergency departments can result from formalized team-based training and operational structure.[6] Team simulation in the domain of anesthesia or surgery is being proposed as a means to increase human performance.[7]

In addition, characteristics of safe obstetrical units with a decreased likelihood of system error or medical accident occurring have been described.[8] These clinical units function in a manner similar to what has been defined as *high-reliability organizations*.[9] High-reliability organizations are those that operate highly complex and hazardous technological systems essentially without mistakes over long periods of time.[10] Examples of this type of organization are nuclear power plants, airline inflight and traffic control operations, and the technical side of the banking industry.[11]

In high-reliability organizations, safety is the hallmark of organizational culture and professional behavior. In addition, teamwork is the key operating principle, with both production and safety thought to be created by teams (rather than individuals). Safety is spoken and thought about and has at least as high a priority as does production in all operational decisions. Team interaction is collegial rather than hierarchical, and each team member has an obligation to speak up if a question of safety arises.[12] Communication (including reporting of accidents and near misses) is highly valued and rewarded. It is understood that when team members fail to engage in respectful interactions, errors can occur.[13] Emergencies are rehearsed, and the unexpected is practiced. Successful operations are viewed as potentially dangerous because success leads to system simplification and shortcuts.[14] Preparation, practice, and evaluation of team decision making and the resulting consequences are a constant feature of day-to-day operations.

It is hypothesized that increased patient safety would result if the principles of teamwork and high reliability could be more widely introduced and applied in sharp-end clinical units.[15] This chapter explores three questions regarding why wider adoption of teamwork has not occurred in the healthcare domain:

1. What are the factors that prevent key clinical leaders (i.e., nurses and physicians) from realizing what other service groups assume to be self-evident?
2. What needs to be done by health system and organizational leadership to create teamwork and high reliability at the clinical sharp-end point of care?
3. What behaviors and attributes distinguish a team-based model of delivering safe care from the current silo-based model of coexisting individual professionals?

THE WHY, WHAT, AND WHY NOT OF TEAMWORK

Why Teams Are Superior

In virtually every performance domain studied, teams perform better than collections of individuals operating within confined job roles and responsibilities.[16] Whether it is customer service, innovation, product development, healthcare quality, safety in high-risk technically complex domains, healthcare resource utilization, or decision-making competence, the conclusion is invariably the same.[17–21] In any situation requiring a real-time combination of multiple skills, experiences, and judgment, teams—as opposed to individuals—create superior performance.

Katzenbach and Smith[22] have summarized the factors that explain the superior performance inherent in teams:

- No single individual can possess the complementary skills and experience required to respond efficiently to operational challenges such as innovation, quality, customer service, or patient care emergencies.
- Communication established between professionals during team formation creates the basis for efficient real-time problem solving.
- Teams build trust and confidence in each member's information, intellectual challenges, and differing adaptability to change.
- Importantly, working in teams that achieve significant performance goals provides personal satisfaction and fun. Given the inherent external stress existing in health care, maintaining a pleasant, nonhostile work environment is a key component in every organization's attempt to survive.

What Is a Team?

One of the most difficult tasks in creating an effective team is understanding what it is and, importantly, what it is not.[23] Although the chemistry of personalities, "getting along," and team building are important components in the creation of teams, they do not, individually or collectively, define or describe a team in a functional or operational sense. Rather, a team is a *discrete unit of performance*, not a positive set of values. True teams (as opposed to simple work groups or social interaction) can be identified by the following operational principles:

- *Consensus (agreeing to agree):* The primary purpose of any clinical unit can be defined very differently from different professional vantages. Physicians, nurses, and other professionals simply see the world differently. To be successful, each clinical management team needs to articulate and reach consensus on mission, vision, goals, and objectives.[24] Although different professionals are indeed different, it is necessary to acknowledge and respect the unique contributions that each can make toward reaching team goals and objectives. Ultimately, if increased and increasing patient safety is the stated and desired goal, it will be necessary to develop a common methodology for creating that reality.

  It is important to note that it may not be possible or desirable to gain complete consensus for each decision.[25] The concept of consensus is sometimes used by those who refuse to agree to anything, as a barrier to stop the group from moving forward. They suggest that consensus means each and every team member must agree to all points of any initiative. Consensus in that model actually means minority rule and can effectively halt any progress toward articulating and reaching common goals. As an alternative, the use of consensus to indicate that the majority of the team *agrees to agree* and to acknowledge that complete consensus may not always be possible and therefore not necessary for the group to go forward is a critical first step toward successful teamwork.
- *Mutual accountability:* Each member of a team-based operational unit must be willing to hold the team rather than himself, herself, or other individuals accountable for success or failure.
- *Organizational discipline:* Teams will only succeed in an organization that recognizes the team rather than the individual as the operating unit, has strong overall performance standards, pushes for ever larger achievement goals, and has sufficient discipline to adhere to these principles.
- *Task:* The more demanding the performance challenge, the better the resulting team. Creating "the safest hospital" works much better as a catalyst for teamwork than simply "doing pathways" in an effort to "enhance collaboration."
- *Time:* A specific time limit within which ultimate or temporary goals must be achieved keeps teams on task and focused.

Behaviors and Attributes of Effective Teams

Effective teams exhibit the following behaviors and attributes:[26]

- *Clear purpose:* The vision, mission, goal, or task of the team has been defined and is now accepted by everyone. There is an action plan that supports and gives definition to the stated organizational purpose.
- *Informality:* The climate tends to be informal, comfortable, and relaxed. There are no obvious tensions or signs of boredom.
- *Participation:* There is much discussion, and everyone is encouraged to participate.
- *Listening:* The members use effective listening techniques such as questioning, paraphrasing, and summarizing to get multiple ideas and perspectives into all discussions.

- *Civilized disagreements:* There is disagreement, but the team is comfortable with this and shows no signs of avoiding, smoothing over, or suppressing conflict.
- *Consensus decisions:* For important decisions, the goal is substantial, but not necessarily unanimous, agreement through open discussion of everyone's ideas, and avoidance of voting or easy compromises.
- *Open communication:* Team members feel free to express their feelings on the tasks as well as on the group's operation. There are few hidden agendas. Ongoing communication takes place outside of meetings.
- *Clear roles and work assignments:* There are clear expectations about the roles played by each team member. When action is taken, clear assignments are made, accepted, and carried out. Work is fairly distributed among team members.
- *Shared leadership:* Although the team has a formal leader, leadership functions shift from time to time depending on the circumstances and the needs of the group and the skills of the members. The formal leader models the appropriate behavior and helps establish norms.
- *External relations:* The team spends time developing key outside relationships, mobilizing resources, and building credibility with important players in other parts of the organization.
- *Style diversity:* The team has a broad spectrum of team-player types, including members who emphasize attention to task, goal setting, focus on process, and questions about how the team is functioning.
- *Self-assessment:* Periodically, the team stops to examine how well it is functioning and what may be interfering with its effectiveness.

Why Not Teams? Existing Barriers to Teamwork in the Healthcare Environment

Given what appears to be a universal and irrefutable organizational truism, why haven't teams become the predominant unit of performance in the delivery of health care at the sharp end? The answer to this question is complex and involves many interrelated factors:[27]

- Historical roles of women in society
- Traditional roles of physicians and nurses
- Institutional territory and politics
- Licensure and professional accountability
- Type and quantity of education
- Different styles of learning and information exchange
- Socialization of each group
- Methods and amounts of compensation
- Power of social and professional position
- Collaboration—an impediment because it assumes separation of groups
- Unresolved conflict, setting the stage for the expectation of future discord
- Inability to get common incentives
- Healthcare organizations operating under extreme stress and pressure

Some of these factors may be easily changed or overcome, whereas others represent challenges deeply embedded in the structure of our current healthcare system and therefore represent particularly difficult issues that stand in the way of effective team performance.

Historical Roles of Men and Women: The Gender Issue

Although women have made significant political, social, and economic progress in the last century, the historical role of women in society remains a factor in how nurses and physicians communicate, interact, and ultimately work together in the clinical setting. Ninety-five percent of nurses in the United States are women.[28] This ratio of male to female professionals in the healthcare workplace perpetuates the traditional male physician (dominant)–female nurse (submissive) model of interaction, rather than the equality needed for true team behavior.[29] How this form of interaction affects other potential team members remains to be elucidated.

Although the increasing numbers of female physicians might be expected to alter the historical way nurses and doctors relate to each other, current observations suggest that the current socialization of female physicians during medical education perpetuates the traditional male–female roles rather than creating behavior based more on female–female interaction.[30] The resulting interactional dichotomy between what might be expected based on gender and the reality created by professional training is confusing and disappointing to many nurses. For example, informal conversations between female physicians and nurses about common challenges faced by working women (e.g., childcare difficulties and long hours away from families) that could invite camaraderie and collaboration can be quickly followed by unilateral and authoritarian "physician orders" with no input invited or desired from the nurses providing direct care. What could have been the basis for establishing the trust required for effective team performance quickly disappears under the differential socialization of the involved professionals.

Understanding the powerful effect of socialization and how resulting roles influence behavior may be helpful in explaining how gender differences have an impact on nurse–physician relationships. Kearny and White examined behaviors associated with work and categorized people as "warriors" or "villagers" based on the way they interacted with each other and approached the tasks to be completed.[31] Warriors are aggressive, competitive, and distrustful of others, viewing life as a struggle or contest to be won on the battlefield of living.[32] Warriors are not inclined to ask other warriors for help, fearing that would imply weakness or incompetence. However, warriors make excellent leaders because they have a firm resolve to meet their objectives and their confident attitude inspires others to follow their directions.[33] Warriors make decisions on data they see as black or white, rarely letting emotion influence the decisions they make.

By contrast, villagers are cooperative and eager to please, even if that means giving in to the needs of others.[34] The goals of the village outweigh individual objectives or desires. Villagers reach decisions by consensus and are generous in giving praise to other team members, irrespective of whether those praised are pulling their own weight on the team.[35] Villagers excel at working together, recognizing the value of cooperation and fostering relationships. They are generally sensitive and caring and use these feelings to guide decision making over more objective data.[36]

Importantly, these behaviors are *not* determined by genetics, but rather are learned as an integral by-product of the socialization that defines the unique culture of each society. Historically (and stereotypically) in this society (the United States), men have been taught the characteristics and behaviors of warriors, whereas women have been assigned the villager role. Traditional training of both nurses and physicians has reinforced these generalized societal expectations. While the place and status of women in society and in health care has been altered toward more equality in recent years, the male–female/physician–nurse hierarchy and the personality types attracted to these roles remain a strong barrier to the establishment of effective service teams.

Traditional Roles of Physicians and Nurses: Who Is in Charge and How Do We Talk to Each Other?

Interaction and communication among physicians, nurses, and other professionals occurs in a hierarchical model (based on tradition and training) in which physicians give orders and nurses (and everyone else) are expected to follow those orders without question.[37] Communication of this type does not always create optimal patient care and is potentially dangerous. Examples include rapidly changing patient status, where the nurse at the bedside has more information than the physician at home or in the office; training situations, where the nurse has more experience than the physician in training; situations where the nurse has more up-to-date knowledge than the attending physician; or situations where the nurse has learned important information from the patient or family that the family has chosen not to communicate with the physician. In circumstances such as these, experienced nurses have developed strategies designed to overcome the fact that many physicians are not comfortable with nurses making overt diagnoses or clinical suggestions concerning how their patients should be cared for (i.e., violating the expected hierarchal model of communication).

Instead of mutually desirable direct communication leading to a plan of care developed through the wisdom and experience of two knowledgeable professionals, nurses are forced to revert to the "doctor–nurse" game to achieve what they believe is in the patient's best interest. Although this technique was first described in the literature over 30 years ago,[38] it was used for many years before Dr. Stein's classic article was published and is still alive and well today. Tips on how to play this game are given by experienced nurses to new graduates as part of socialization to the role of the professional registered nurse.[39] For example, one of the most common techniques taught is how to get physicians to think it was their idea to order an intervention, medication, or laboratory test rather than that of the nurse. The doctor–nurse game avoids open disagreement and conflict and allows the nurse to give recommendations and the physician to request recommendations without appearing to do so.[40] Nurses are expected to learn how to phrase suggestions (different for each physician) in such a way that the physician will reach the same clinical decision or course of management that the nurse thinks is correct.

This situation can be dangerous for patients and lead to adverse outcomes or decreased patient safety in multiple ways: first, when nurses are unable to find the right "story" or words that convey the emergent nature of an evolving clinical situation;[41] second, when the nurse is wrong in her assessment because of a clinical fact known to the physician but not the nurse; and finally, when the assessment is correct but the description is misunderstood by the physician. In these as well as other easily imagined clinical scenarios, patient safety suffers because of delays and clinical miscues inherent in the dysfunctional communication adopted as part of the doctor–nurse game. A recent study described common strategies used by intrapartum nurses in dealing with obstetricians. These strategies included letting them feel in control; avoiding making them feel threatened; not lying for them, but not contradicting them; being tactful and subservient; and doing whatever would keep them happy.[42] Routinely using these strategies serves as a powerful barrier to real communication and collaboration. The doctor–nurse game is a real problem because it does not foster the open dialogue needed to provide safe patient care.[43]

By contrast, one hallmark of team behavior is clear language agreed to and understood by all members. Patient care would be much better if telephone communication with the physician were direct and to the point. For example, "Patient status is deteriorating quickly and I need you here now." Instead, many nurses find themselves searching for the "right words or story" designed primarily to not offend the attending physician while at the same time attempting to obtain the required clinical action. The result is indirect, inefficient, and often inaccurate communication.

Physicians may not understand the real sense of clinical urgency when nurses are reluctant to communicate directly. In cases resulting in medical accident or patient injury, physicians are often quoted as saying, "If she had only told me this was a real emergency, I would have come right in, but I didn't know things were that bad." This can be a valid concern and legitimate statement if the nurse did not communicate effectively. Urgent time is lost playing the doctor–nurse game, and miscommunications are common with this approach to physician–nurse interactions.

An important by-product of this dysfunctional communication is an underlying attempt to shift blame away from oneself and onto other professionals. Mutual accountability, the hallmark of successful teams, does not develop or is easily destroyed in the resulting "culture of blame."[44] Ultimately, an escalating cycle of mistrust between healthcare providers is created, accentuated, and perpetuated, with resulting deterioration in patient care.

This is more than a theoretical possibility. In a classic study of how the quality of nurse–physician interactions in an intensive care setting affects patient outcomes, Knaus and colleagues demonstrated that the most powerful determinant of severity-adjusted patient death rates was how well nurses and physicians worked together in the planning and subsequent delivery of patient care.[45] They concluded that a high degree of involvement and interaction between nurses and physicians directly influences patient outcomes. Another study found that for each severity level of medical condition studied, patients were at greater risk of dying or being readmitted when nurses and resident physicians failed to communicate and effectively work together.[46] The current system of nurse–physician and other team professional interaction could benefit from a significant reevaluation and fundamental change to minimize the chances of system error or medical accident.[47]

Institutional Politics and Organizational Structure

In addition to the factors previously discussed, institutional politics and organizational structure contribute to difficulties in physician–nurse interactions and, by implication, entire healthcare team interactions. Physicians traditionally have been viewed as customers who bring patients and revenue to the healthcare system or institution. As a result, physicians are treated with a level of organizational deference and respect not afforded the registered nurse or other professionals employed by the healthcare organization (who, after all, are a cost on the balance sheet). An institution can more easily replace a nurse or pharmacist than a revenue-generating physician. Historically and in the extreme, a physician could demand that a particular nurse be terminated (for good reasons or bad) and expect that the institution would cause it to happen. By contrast, physician behavior that is inappropriate and disruptive will often be tolerated by those same institutions.[48] Nurses or other professionals behaving similarly would be terminated. In addition to these behavioral and operational observations, the differential status of nurses and physicians may be seen in hospital organizational charts, where nursing services are placed on a lower level than that of the medical departments.

Methods and Amount of Compensation

Differences in methods and amount of compensation for physicians, nurses, and other team members further divide the professions. Nurses are compensated for hours worked, and unless they are in a managerial role, responsibility and accountability for patient care end when a nursing shift is completed. Physician compensation is commensurate with years of education and 24-hour ultimate responsibility for patients under their care. This results in physicians earning 5 to 10 times more than staff nurses who provide most of the direct hands-on care. The disparity in compensation creates not only a professional barrier but a social barrier as well. There are distinct differences in lifestyles between those who are middle class and those who are upper class, and these discrepancies carry over into professional attitudes and interaction as well.[49]

Wide Disparity in Level of Educational Preparation

The disparity in educational preparation between physicians and nurses affects professional working relationships in multiple ways. Differential levels of education influence clinical interactions, contribute to inequity in compensation and professional respect, and result in real or perceived differences in social status. One of the most serious challenges facing nurses today is the issue of educational criteria and entry level into professional practice. According to the latest data, 59% of registered professional nurses in the United States do not hold a four-year college degree.[50] This inequity in education when compared with other healthcare disciplines is not only a significant barrier for advancing the professional practice of nursing, but also a significant barrier to team work. Consider that laboratory and radiation technicians are required to hold a baccalaureate degree; social workers and speech, occupational, and physical therapists require a master's degree; and pharmacists require a doctorate in pharmacology. There is no other profession that nurses must collaborate with professionally that does not require at least a four-year college degree.

For reasons not entirely clear, nurses do not insist that they cease to be the poorest prepared of all healthcare professionals.[51] Because nurses are the least educated, they are also the lowest-earning and least respected of the healthcare professionals.[52] Given the wide disparity in education between nurses and other members of the healthcare team, clinical discussions that involve research, outcomes, and clinical judgment can be challenging at best. Without at least a baccalaureate education, nurses have a hard time evaluating evidence and deciding how to provide care that is based on science rather than tradition.[53] All members of the healthcare team need a solid background in science and the scientific method in order to effectively collaborate with the medical profession. Access to the latest scientific information and use of the most appropriate technology to gather information and provide care are critical.[54] This knowledge is critical for nurses when planning with physicians and other team members the pros and cons, risks and benefits, and expected outcomes based on what is known about interventions for specific clinical conditions.[55] An equal voice in clinical discussions must be the voice of one who has been educated in an institution of higher learning in a manner similar to the other members of the healthcare team. The discrepancy in educational preparation between physicians and nurses plays an important role in less than optimal professional communication and clinical interactions and thus ultimately adversely affects patient outcomes.

Interestingly, physicians have a paradoxical view regarding nurses increasing their level of education. When asked to list weaknesses of nurses in a recent survey, some physicians noted that nurses had too many credentials and spent too much time in the classroom, whereas others believed that nurses had low initiative and suffered from a failure to seek advanced education.[56] By contrast, in a July 1999 Harris poll, 76% of Americans indicated they expected nurses to have four or more years of education to be successful clinicians. Perhaps the time has come for the nursing profession to stop arguing about the entry level into practice issue and set a date by which nurses would be required to hold a baccalaureate degree in nursing. Movement toward higher and more uniform educational requirements could significantly increase the potential of the nursing profession as well as teamwork in the clinical arena.

Licensure and Professional Accountability

Licensure and professional accountability are generally not thought of when factors that inhibit collaboration and teamwork between physicians, nurses, and other professionals are considered. However, their effect may be as powerful as any of the previously mentioned factors. Physician licensure gives the physician authority and demands accountability for admission, discharge, treatment (including all procedures and medications), and general oversight of all patient care. In short, physicians have the ultimate responsibility for patient care. Nurses, by contrast, provide the majority of direct patient care ordered by physicians, with other professionals contributing on a more fragmented or limited basis. However, nurses and other professionals have an independent responsibility for ensuring that orders received and followed are reasonable and appropriate. This differential responsibility is highlighted when litigation ensues as a result of patient injury. For example, nurses are responsible for their own clinical judgments and interventions. It is unacceptable to "delegate up" (a process whereby nurses avoid responsibility for their decisions for implementing care by invoking the authority of physicians as the basis for their decision making) when there is a question about appropriateness of orders.[57] However, it is not uncommon for some nurses to claim in retrospect that "the doctor made me do it," even when they were aware that the ordered course of treatment was not in the best interests of the patient. If patient well-being is at risk, nurses or other professionals have the moral responsibility to refuse to carry out that order and should be given institutional protection from potential physician-initiated repercussions.[58] This clearly defined principle of high-reliability organizations ("anyone can stop it") is not widely known or adhered to in contemporary healthcare organizations.

From the regulatory and legal perspective, a nurse is expected to know which orders given by a physician (who has many more years of education, training, and experience) are unreasonable or inappropriate; that is, which should be questioned either directly with the physician or, alternatively, result in a request for additional assistance (going up the chain of command) in the event of physician nonresponsiveness to a question asked by a nurse. This nursing accountability specified by licensure is in conflict with the hierarchical roles of physicians giving orders and nurses following those orders without question; in addition, it reinforces the factors previously cited that led to the historical role definition in the first place. Licensing requirements place a nurse in the difficult theoretical position of needing to know more than the physician giving the order. Nurses are compelled to take steps to directly go against physician orders, with serious institutional and professional ramifications if they are found to be wrong in retrospect. Clinical conflicts not able to be resolved by direct communication that result in chain-of-command initiatives not only inhibit physician–nurse trust and collaboration, but also are a strong indicator that teamwork is nonexistent in the first place.

Health Care Under Pressure: Resulting Stress Makes Teamwork Difficult

Teamwork, although logical and intuitive, is not the organizational norm found in health care today. In large part, this is because of the antiteam forces previously discussed, but in addition and importantly, it is because of the extreme challenges produced by the rapid, constant change facing all healthcare organizations. Under stress, the natural reaction of any professional is to revert to previous individual history, socialization, and teaching, all of which conflict with the fundamental operational descriptors and characteristics of teamwork.[59]

Effective teams operate in an informal, comfortable, and relaxed atmosphere,[60] the very antithesis of the professional climate found in health care today. Cost pressure, staff reductions, legal and regulatory concerns, and marketplace competition all combine to create time pressure, nonaligned incentives, and potential mistrust among the professionals who must cooperate for a team to succeed. In addition, these same environmental forces serve to confuse teams in selecting and maintaining effective necessary partnerships. Cooperating and competing simultaneously with stakeholders who, at the same time, may likewise be competing and cooperating with each other can occupy inordinate amounts of energy that could otherwise be devoted to productive team activity. Finally, the characteristics of participation, listening, civilized disagreement, consensus decisions, open communication, and shared leadership are often difficult to achieve because of the socialization and psychology of physician participants.[61]

Highly individualistic, trained to be self-reliant, competitively aggressive under stress, and imbedded with a historical mistrust of hospital administration, physicians do not easily adapt to team dynamics and participation. In fact, the key ingredient necessary for effective clinical team development is physician leadership that understands the importance and operating principle of the team as the functional unit of production. Absent physician leadership, nurses and other professionals are forced to develop secondary, much less effective, often dysfunctional coping mechanisms for the delivery of clinical care.[62]

Within the clinical team, physicians have ultimate legal and regulatory responsibility and accountability for patient assessment and diagnosis, as well as for ordering treatments, interventions, surgeries, and medications. However, these responsibilities can be, and in fact are, best met through the coordinated and supportive efforts of the entire clinical team. Some believe that the historical paradigm of the physician as the "captain of the ship" precludes true teamwork because in a real team all members are mutually accountable as they work toward a common goal. Even some leaders in the nursing profession have contributed to this perception by describing nursing as an "inherently subservient role." To defeat these traditional but outdated views, physicians must learn to appreciate, value, and invite each member of the healthcare team to contribute the diverse opinions and perspectives that create superior decision making and performance. Although every team requires a leader, and in health care this role typically is assumed by a physician, it is necessary for physicians to remember that different roles or contributions do not necessarily mean unequal or no value.

Fortunately, nurse and physician perceptions of each other have improved significantly over the last few years. A 1998 study of physician–nurse relationships revealed that in general, nurses and physicians have positive perceptions about each other.[63] Nurses and physicians were asked to describe the role of the other's profession and to list respective strengths and weaknesses. In this study, nurses described physicians as leaders and the most important member of the healthcare team, collaborative, involved, and caring.[64] Physicians described nurses as patient and physician advocates, emotionally supportive and comforting to patients, the ones who provide minute-to-minute care, and as partners with physicians.[65] Thus, mutual respect and admiration between professionals appears to be increasing and needs to be nurtured so that teamwork becomes the model for delivering clinical care.

It should be noted however, that the social and organizational reality previously described is powerful and not easily ignored or dismissed. Therefore, it should be apparent that transforming these disparate professional groups into a team-based model of clinical care will not be accomplished easily. Nor will the transformation occur quickly or without a significant commitment of organizational resources. Nonetheless, it is our belief that if the commitment is understood, planned, and budgeted appropriately, the result will be well worth the dollars and effort expended. After all, despite many historical, professional, and cultural differences, nurses, physicians, and other members of the healthcare team share a powerful common goal around which effective teamwork can be developed: the safest care possible for patients who have placed their trust in us.

ALIGNING OPERATIONS TO BUILD TEAM-BASED HIGH-RELIABILITY ORGANIZATIONS: WHERE TO START AND HOW TO SUCCEED

The Blunt End: Organizational Leadership Shapes the Clinical Environment

The Role of Organizational Leaders

Although all healthcare professionals have the potential to substantially contribute to the development of effective team development, two participants hold significant enabling influence: physicians (see the previous discussion) and healthcare administrators. Healthcare administrators have the basic responsibility for ensuring that adequate financial, personnel, and other organizational resources (i.e., training and equipment) are available to provide safe and effective care. Without continued commitment of these resources, the clinical team faces significant and at times insurmountable challenges and frustration.

In addition, all clinical teams reflect explicit organizational culture and values; thus, an assessment of executive organizational group process and work environment is the first step in evaluating the potential for successful clinical teamwork. Unfortunately, in many healthcare organizations, senior management currently use group processes that resemble ineffective or nonfunctioning teams[66] and therefore create conditions under which clinical teamwork cannot emerge or flourish.

Safety is a fundamental patient right. Establishing an organizational culture that can deliver on that promise falls squarely on the shoulders of senior leadership. Moving to establish an organizational culture that creates teamwork and maximizes patient safety requires that four principles be focused on and visibly displayed at all times:

1. Commit and accept responsibility for safety.
2. Invite communication and dialogue.
3. Encourage risk taking and thinking and reward behaving courageously.
4. Foster creative thinking and seek innovative solutions and systems.

Leadership's Commitment to and Acceptance of Responsibility for Safety

The importance of patient safety relative to production is a fundamental clue to all employees and medical staff of how serious the organizational commitment is. When production and safety come into conflict, it is important that the choices made are explicit and the consequences clear to everyone throughout the organization.[67,68]

Without executive leadership continuously championing patient safety, the fundamental shifts necessary in an organization's behavior, in the work, in the systems, and in the relationships necessary for high reliability will be minimal. Becoming informed and knowledgeable about the principles of safety science is fundamental. A commitment to educate staff in these principles must follow. Using the language of safety in day-to-day conversation is a must; a demonstration to staff that leadership understands the basic concepts of "sharp end/blunt end," "Swiss cheese" thinking, and the pitfalls of "hindsight bias" (to use Reason's terminology) is paramount. With a grounded perspective in the principles of safety science, adopting a nonpunitive policy in reporting accidents becomes second nature. Essentially, these principles must be on public display at all times (especially in those difficult times following the accidents that inevitably will occur).

Armed with the language and informed of safety science literature, the next step is to "walk the talk" and lead by example. Strategies to demonstrate leadership commitment to patient safety include the following:

- Establish patient safety goals in department and unit work plans.
- Integrate patient safety into management and staff incentive programs.
- Acknowledge patient safety and medical accident reduction as a foundation for quality.
- Conduct walking rounds and eliminate weak links in the systems as they become known.
- Make sure that zero tolerance for procedural violations through intent or negligence is fundamental to organizational operations.
- Celebrate increased reporting of hazard identification and unnecessary system complexities and weaknesses. Eliminate those discovered.
- Create blameless reporting loops so all can stay informed about patient safety issues.
- Foster ongoing real-time dialogue about patient safety and the lessons learned from medical accidents.

Inviting Communication and Dialogue

The second leadership principle necessary in advancing a patient safety agenda is to consistently model inviting communication and dialogue. By listening more and using "inviting" questions, leaders can gain greater understanding of the culture and more in-depth analysis of the patient safety issues. Using simple and standard language and "inviting" communication techniques sets the stage for blameless reporting. Senior leadership must constantly model the approach. Examples of inviting questions include the following:

- What happened? (rather than, Who did it?)
- What is getting in the way of your ability to do your job effectively?
- Tell me about a significant accident waiting to happen.

Leadership must create opportunities for staff to develop communication skills, to understand the principles of effective communication, and to practice discussing bad outcomes with colleagues. Intentionally improving all communication processes is a significant patient safety success strategy. The message of safety is contained in the series of stories waiting to be told and retold throughout every organization.

Risk Taking and Thinking and Behaving Courageously

The third principle essential for advancing a patient safety agenda is to encourage risk taking and reward acting courageously. The traditional hierarchical culture of health care and silence will not easily be eliminated. Without effective teamwork, reporting lines continue to be rigidly defined and are not often crossed, even in the name of safety. Nurses often report using extreme caution in approaching certain physicians or not mentioning a concern at all because of the risk of a punitive or even abusive response. This fearful, blame-ridden, individual-driven hierarchy is detrimental to patient safety. Instead, leaders should demand a culture driven by respectful professional, patient, and family partnerships. Everyone must hear the message from those in leadership positions that it's a necessity and a fundamental responsibility to speak up, identify risks, avert risks, and always act thoughtfully to ensure patient safety. A leader can readily interview key personnel, posing the question, "Have you ever held back and hesitated to intervene or speak up when a patient's safety was in jeopardy?" The "inviting" interviewer needs to ensure the ground rules of honesty and nonpunitive reporting. The resulting leadership strategy is to further encourage risk taking and courageous behavior and not reward risk aversion. Leaders must deliver the following key message: The voice of safety belongs to us all, and all of us have a duty to speak directly and clearly.

Creative Thinking and Innovative Solutions and Systems

The fourth principle of leadership essential in solidifying a culture of patient safety is fostering creative thinking and seeking innovative solutions and systems. Simultaneous production and safety goals cannot be met by continuing to work in the manner to which we have currently become accustomed. Changes in the way our highly complex system works are necessary. Rigorous, increasing demands on the systems, the staff, and the infrastructure are created by 24-7-365 needs. Additionally, much has changed over the last decade, with a spiraling evolution of technology, excessive drug manufacturing, shrinking workforce, and dwindling reimbursement dollars. Yet the care delivery systems and the work of the patient care team remain essentially unchanged. Attempts to simplify and reduce the inherent complexity in the systems and the infrastructure have been largely unsuccessful. Healthcare providers have been placed in reactionary positions to all the forces of change coming to a confluence at the sharp end. Leaders, by being open to ideas and thinking more creatively, can encourage an infusion of lessons from highly reliable industries. The work of leadership is to design and operate systems. Increased patient safety is an outcome of reliable systems based on teamwork. Leaders must dispel the myths of traditional thinking and infuse energy, enthusiasm, and innovative approaches to the work, systems, and relationships currently existing in the organizations they lead.

The Sharp End: A Reflection of Blunt-End Organizational Priorities

Self-Assessment

After reviewing the operational principles and characteristics of successful teams, it should be possible to decide if a given clinical unit is functioning as an effective highly reliable team with safety as its primary mission. For example, it should be evident whether patient safety is a clearly stated organizational goal. From that starting point, it should then be possible using the following tools to determine whether the behaviors of the clinical professionals working together exhibit any or all of the attributes of a well-functioning team.

The Teamwork Continuum

Based on established work patterns and observed professional communication, a point along the continuum of teamwork (Figure 22.1) can be assigned to any clinical work group. Most clinical units fall midway between peaceful coexistence and collaboration. Much has been written about moving clinical professionals toward teamwork, and many suggestions for creating fully operational teams have been offered. However, for any of these techniques to be effective, it is first up to the sharp-end clinicians to decide that teamwork is a desirable goal. Simply put, they *must agree to agree*. This is much easier said than done because of long-standing barriers (previously discussed) as well as current cynicism rooted in the beliefs of many that true teamwork is an impossible goal in the current healthcare environment.

Hostile Competing Forces This is the most dysfunctional and potentially dangerous work environment for both patients and healthcare workers. When healthcare professionals are openly abusive or distrustful of each other and in effect are working against each other, it is self-evident that patient care will suffer. Absent effective clinical leadership and mutually agreed-upon goals to achieve patient well-being, healthcare professionals tend to compete for resources, favor, and rewards from both administrators and patients. If this natural form of competition is not held in check (or worse, is openly encouraged) by senior management or decision-making processes, open hostility at the sharp end will be the result. Decisions are then made on the basis of power, politics, or the squeaky wheel rather than data or common sense based on what is in the patient's best interest. Fortunately, this extreme of the continuum is rare in the current healthcare environment, but where it exists, it is often driven by long-standing personal and professional animosity and often requires expert outside consultation to eliminate it.

Peaceful Coexistence In this predominately unit practice structure, physicians, nurses, and other allied healthcare workers meet separately to discuss clinical issues or processes that have implications or consequences for all team members and patients. Goals defined by each professional group remain part of the agenda in attempting to set and achieve larger work group objectives. Representatives from each group typically meet to "let each other know" what their group has decided. These parallel committee processes and resulting need to check back create inefficient duplication and excessive use of time and energy.

FIGURE 22.1 The Continuum of Teamwork

Hostile (Open or Covert) Competing Forces —> Peaceful Coexistence —> Collaboration —> Teamwork

Because no clinical issue or process definition can be decided or implemented without simultaneous input from all representatives of the healthcare team, peaceful coexistence is ultimately not sustainable. Eventually, more and more meetings must be scheduled to reach consensus among representatives of each discipline to determine plans for implementing anything, with the process ultimately sinking under its own weight. However, an interesting paradox exists in peaceful coexistence because the absence of overt hostility leads clinicians to believe they are truly functioning as a team rather than at the low end of the teamwork continuum. While seeing themselves as cooperating and doing their best in trying to improve existing clinical processes or patient care outcomes, clinicians often become frustrated by the lack of observable progress that is part and parcel of peaceful coexistence. A peaceful retreat of all parties to the "land of nothing getting done" ultimately occurs.

Collaboration Collaboration implies members of at least two different professional groups agreeing to simultaneously work together toward defined clinical unit goals. Often, goals are brought forward or are championed from one member group rather than being first agreed on collectively. Working simultaneously together, with collaborative decisions taking precedence over those of member interests (in theory, if not often in practice), distinguishes this organizational form from peaceful coexistence. Importantly however, collaboration differs from true teamwork in that different interests or priorities of collaborating groups are *not subsumed* to those of the larger group. Patient care goals can be achieved only if the interests of each participating group represented in the collaborative process are also achieved (which does not occur very often). Often, the result is a compromise that is not entirely satisfactory to anyone. Although collaboration is preferable to peaceful coexistence because some operational and clinical decisions actually occur, collaboration is an inefficient and fragile means of working together.

Teamwork A team implies professionals working collectively and in nonhierarchical fashion toward mutually agreed-upon common goals, with each member contributing and being valued for his or her unique talents, education, experience, background, and perspective. Individual member contributions are evaluated based on merit without regard for that member's status in the traditional healthcare hierarchy. For example, the ideas of a staff nurse have as much value as those of an attending physician, and the input from a resident physician is just as important as that of an advanced practice nurse. The value of contributions is defined by existing data or merit rather than presumed organizational position. Further, the needs of individual members are subsumed to those of the group. Importantly, team members hold each other mutually accountable for achieving the agreed-upon goals. Team members may offer views of the implications of operational and clinical initiatives on their respective disciplines, but they are not acting as "representatives" of these disciplines. The focus of any potential change in practice remains on patient outcomes rather than provider convenience. Forming, maintaining, and effectively working as a clinical team is very hard personal work and requires immense organizational support; thus, it does not occur very often in contemporary health care.

How close to teamwork is any clinical group operating? The position on the teamwork continuum may be defined by observing the following behaviors and characteristics.

Characteristics of Clinical Groups Operating Without Teamwork or High Reliability (Those at High Risk for Medical Accidents)

- The mission, vision, or goals of the clinical team are not uniformly agreed to or able to be described by all participants. Several subagendas, often in conflict with each other, are readily apparent.
- Safety is not explicitly stated as a primary and important goal or value.

- Reporting of accidents and near misses is not done or valued.
- Errors are blamed on people rather than prompting an evaluation of system processes and unit operations.
- Accidents are often attributed to an "act of God" or "circumstances beyond our control."
- Meetings are formal, tense, and uncomfortable when multidisciplinary professionals are present.
- Trust among members is low or nonexistent.
- Hierarchical professional relationships are emphasized.
- Physician–nurse conflict is ongoing (may be open or underlying).
- Dysfunctional or disruptive team members are not held accountable for their behavior or lack of action.
- Conflict is downplayed or avoided rather than used as an opportunity for learning.
- Professional communication often requires deception (i.e., the "doctor–nurse" game) in a misguided attempt at patient advocacy.
- A formal chain of command is frequently used instead of informal group norms to regulate behavior.
- The ratio of output to discussion in meetings is low. Similar agenda items appear over and over again.
- Little accountability for work assignments or follow-up exists.
- Disagreements and discussion continue outside of team meetings.
- Parallel group processes are in place, duplicating work efforts and creating boundaries, ownership of issues, and lack of effective coordination.
- Decisions are made unilaterally after "input" was sought, rather than by consensus.
- There are wide variations in clinical practice for which clear national standards and guidelines exist.
- Practices are based on what is most convenient for providers rather than what is best for patients.
- Practices are based on "the way we've always done it" instead of evidence and standards.
- Consistent external or internal assessment of teams as a discrete unit of production is not done.

Strategies for Implementing Effective Teamwork at the Sharp End

Successful clinical services in which teamwork is an operational reality are found selectively throughout health care. In our experience, there are key characteristics and strategies that set them apart from units functioning at the opposite end of the teamwork continuum. A review of these behavioral and organizational characteristics and how clinical teams can implement them may be helpful in further evaluating the status of teamwork in any clinical setting as well as in moving forward on the teamwork continuum.

At the outset, it should be noted that high-reliability clinical environments that support teamwork and patient safety do not occur randomly or by luck. They are the result of strong interdisciplinary leadership that instills and frequently communicates safety as its main value and operational principle. Teamwork requires more time and more professional energy than traditional models of care and traditional methods of communication and workplace behavior. It is possible, however, for an organization to learn and refocus on the principles of high reliability, teamwork, and the clinical practices that are needed to ensure patient safety. In our experience, effective teamwork within a high-reliability organization will result in fewer preventable adverse events as well as a more pleasant and energized work environment.

Characteristics of and Strategies to Create High-Reliability Clinical Units and Teamwork

- Safety is the hallmark of the organizational clinical culture and individual behavior, actions, and decision making.

Safety is understood to be the shared responsibility and individual duty of every team member. It is explicitly stated repeatedly that "we will not knowingly compromise safety." Patient safety is the number one consideration when care practices that may cost more, generate controversy among team members, or are deemed inconvenient to providers are under consideration. When the philosophy of safe care is challenged, it is up to all team members to keep everyone focused on the ultimate goal. For example, if controversial clinical practices or new technologies are being considered for introduction to a clinical unit, care providers promoting the new practice will sometimes insist that professionals who are opposed produce rigorous data to prove the practice is unsafe (and therefore should not be used or introduced). However, the elementary principle underlying consideration of risks and benefits of all clinical interventions is "first do no harm." Clearly, it would be much better for our patients if the alternative argument were needed (i.e., "prove" the practice is safe) before a specific clinical practice was implemented.

Because many patient injuries and adverse outcomes are not reported in the literature, it is difficult to quantify the risks of questionable practices with any degree of certainty. In the absence of a mature and robust reporting system, patient injuries are many times discovered only as a result of accident or litigation. Although all healthcare providers have been educated to rely on the best evidence from rigorously designed research studies to guide clinical practice, prospective randomized controlled trials do not exist to provide definitive "proof " that a questionable practice is unsafe. These types of trials cannot be done because it is difficult to prove a negative, plus there are medico-legal implications and ethical issues regarding what is commonly known (but not formally reported in the literature) about the adverse risks of certain practices. Lack of data to prove it's *not* safe does not mean it *is* safe. Redefining risk based on what has not happened as opposed to what may occur will not create safety. This lesson in safety was learned (unfortunately too late) by the members of the team at NASA who made the decision to launch the *Challenger* space shuttle.[69] Sometimes anecdotal data, common sense, and a gut feeling about doing the right thing will be the best and only guides to determining the best approach to handling controversy about questionable clinical or organizational (e.g., staffing) practices. An open, interdisciplinary approach to reaching consensus in the face of clinical or administrative controversy based on "safety first" creates an optimal process for managing organizational risk. Erring on the side of patient safety is always preferable to using a technique that could potentially cause patient injuries.

- Operation of the system is considered to be a team rather than individual function.

In a high-reliability organization, whatever hierarchical organizational relationships otherwise exist, at the point of service or care they are replaced with teamwork and cohesiveness. Because this is a concept generally foreign to health care, introduction of this important concept usually requires education and training based on simulation or example taken from other high-risk industries. Following a systematic validation of individual credentials, training, and skill sets, all team members are considered competent and therefore have an obligation to speak up ("call it off") if a question of safety arises. Leadership backing and congratulations to those who "stop the line" is absolutely essential. Teams, rather than individuals, are defined as the unit of production and safety creation. This concept needs to be introduced at employee orientation and periodically reinforced. Systems are designed to prevent, detect, and minimize the likelihood of a medical accident, rather than attributing blame or error to individuals. The process of effective teamwork is subject to ongoing examination and improvement. Individuals are evaluated and are provided incentives through their contribution to team performance.

- Communication is highly valued and rewarded.

All professionals use open and extensive communication to orient, plan, update, adjust to the unexpected, test assumptions, and debrief regarding unusual or unexpected events. Introducing debriefings in the normal course of doing business instead of just when things go wrong is a good way to create team communication and organizational learning. It is understood that when professionals fail to engage in respectful interactions, effective communication is hindered and patient safety is threatened. To avoid preventable adverse outcomes, an environment where healthcare professionals respect each other and value input into clinical decision making is developed and nurtured. Different perspectives are valued and contribute to successful outcomes. Each team member has the opportunity, indeed the obligation, to add a viewpoint that others may have overlooked or not previously considered. In many instances, the otherwise overlooked information may prove to be the essential missing component necessary to make a good decision. Simulations based on role playing are useful practice in this regard.

- Clinical standards and unit practices are developed by an interdisciplinary committee.

Important aspects of creating effective teamwork and a safe environment for patients and healthcare workers include creating a unified picture of what needs to be accomplished (shared vision) as well as agreed-upon operational goals, standards, and tactics of each clinical unit. Fostering teamwork through the creation and adoption of "the way we do business" is best accomplished within the structure of an interdisciplinary unit practice committee.

An interdisciplinary practice committee has two purposes: first, to establish the basis for and to define current clinical practice; second, to redefine practice accordingly as knowledge, professional guidelines, or regulatory requirements change.[70] Clinical teamwork within a practice committee enhances the quality of the decision-making processes for practice issues. There should be frequent and established meetings, with the expectation that all team members will make every attempt to attend. The committee should be empowered to make decisions about practice changes based on review of appropriate literature and standards.

A systematic team process for evaluating clinical practice, products, and services in terms of their respective contribution to patient outcomes has been described.[71] Through the use of quantitative data, evidence from the "safety scientists," and a measure of common sense, practices without an apparent or adverse effect on patient safety can be reevaluated, while practices thought to be beneficial can be enhanced and supported. It is possible to offset some of the costs of the additional resources necessary to provide safe care by eliminating routine practices not proven clinically effective or valued by patients.

Joint nurse–physician leadership of the clinical practice committee is essential for success.[72] Selection of these leaders should be based on peer respect, clinical expertise, and ability to influence and manage change. This latter attribute may need formal development or training for the individuals involved. Skilled clinicians are not necessarily skilled at effective group processes. In some cases, the leaders may be the physician chairperson of the clinical department and the nurse manager. However, today many of those in administrative roles are not clinical experts. In this situation, a clinical nurse specialist, nurse educator, charge nurse, or nurse expert in an informal leadership position and a designated expert physician may be better choices. The key requirements for co-chairmanship of the practice committee are recognized clinical expertise, peer respect and support, and enough influence to implement committee decisions (simple positional power will not succeed).

Committee membership should include physicians from specialties represented by the unit patient population, advanced practice nurses, and staff nurses. Members should be selected based on their ability to be articulate and assertive and their willingness to share their perspectives with professional colleagues. A physician or nurse researcher with experience in critiquing evidence would be a valuable member of the committee. Providers from other disciplines and departments such as pharmacy, social services, occupational and physical therapy, grief support, and risk management are also important committee members and should be encouraged to attend and participate.

Based on our experience working with institutions that have implemented this type of committee successfully, the following ground rules work well:

1. Professionals requesting practice or product/technical change are responsible for developing a proposal that includes a review of appropriate standards and guidelines for care (if available); review of available literature; the potential impact on the unit resources, such as staffing or clinical operations; cost data; and potential benefits to patients, as well as any foreseeable safety issues or concerns.
2. The proposal should be distributed well in advance of the committee meeting when it will be discussed so members have the opportunity to gather additional data if desired.
3. There should be an agreement that no practice change will be approved that is inconsistent with available research or established standards and guidelines from professional organizations. Likewise, no change will occur until all potential patient safety concerns have been addressed.

After team consensus is obtained, these best practices can be outlined in the form of protocols or routine order sets and presented to the entire group of healthcare providers. Administrative support and influential committee members are key factors in implementing practice changes using this type of process.

Commitment to practice based on evidence, standards, and concern for patient safety is an ongoing process and may require substantial changes from the usual methods of implementing and evaluating changes in patient care. Discussions about clinical practice that are based on evidence and standards of care rather than hierarchical relationships, personal preferences, and old routines can be helpful in setting the stage for real teamwork.

For some, the process of agreeing to establish this type of committee and select committee members may require months of negotiation. It may be foreign to some unit cultures for nurses to have an equal voice in clinical practice development and to be viewed as credible members of an interdisciplinary clinical practice committee. The "way we've always done it" may include physicians telling nurses about the latest research and standards of care and nurses "complying" without discussion or reviewing these data themselves. Ability to critically review literature and evaluate published standards as the basis for clinical practice changes is not inherently dependent on professional group membership. It is a skill that can be learned by both nurses and physicians who are committed to the process and open to changes that can enhance patient care.

Significant changes in unit culture will not occur overnight. Professional relationships between nurses and physicians that include trust and mutual respect evolve progressively and are based on many interactions. Developing and nurturing an environment that supports real teamwork may take years. It may be helpful for the committee members to participate in team-building exercises to enhance the likelihood of success. Initial success may be measured in small steps and implementation of simple practice changes that do not involve controversy or conflict. Once members are more comfortable with the process and with working together, more complex clinical practice issues can be addressed.

Based on our experiences, it is not unusual for there to be periods of time when it seems that nothing can be accomplished and that group consensus is impossible or—even more frustrating—when members revert to the old ways of interacting and decision making. A firm resolve to focus on the mutual goal of providing the safest possible patient care can help get through these periods. Addition of new members or rotation of membership may help energize the committee. One key to success is to expect these frustrations at times and acknowledge that the process is ongoing and dynamic. Although a team approach to clinical decision making may not evolve as quickly as desired and may involve significant professional energy, the initial investment of time to get oriented to this process is worth the effort. The main advantages of care based on the latest evidence, standards, and guidelines from professional associations and regulatory agencies are as follows: care practices that can be defended as internal budgets become more restricted (almost guaranteed to happen); establishment of true teamwork between nurse and physician colleagues that will have a positive spillover effect on clinical operations and therefore patient safety; and the assurance to the public and purchasers that practices are clinically sound, consistent with scientific data and existing professional standards of care.

- Professionals learn through interdisciplinary education.

Physicians, nurses, and other healthcare professionals work together to provide patient care; thus, education about patient care practices should occur in sessions with all members in attendance. Everyone can learn the same lessons, and there is opportunity to discuss methods of implementation and communication about clinical practices. Issues with the potential to cause controversy in the middle of the night can be openly discussed in the light of day, and strategies to avoid clinical disagreements that can adversely affect patient care can be developed.

- Professional competence is a necessity.

Healthcare providers who are responsible for patient care must be competent in both clinical assessment skills and intervention strategies. Various methods to validate competence have been used over the years, and there are pros and cons to each of these methods. One method that avoids the inherent observer bias of skills checklists and the limitations of written examinations is periodic evaluation of clinical practice via medical record audits. Audit tools can be developed using guidelines and standards from professional associations and regulatory agencies. Consistency with published guidelines and standards can help to avoid preventable adverse outcomes and decrease liability should the institution be involved in litigation related to patient care.

- Technology and interventions are used appropriately and only when indicated.

Use of technology and interventions should be appropriate for the clinical situation, rather than based on provider convenience and cost issues. Overuse of technology and unnecessary interventions can result in iatrogenic patient injuries as well as drain financial and human resources that could be better used in more effective methods of providing patient care.

- Emergencies are rehearsed and the unexpected practiced.

In each practice specialty, clinical situations occur with the potential to result in great harm, or even death, to a patient. These clinical situations should be identified and emergency procedures developed and rehearsed. For example, every team member should be competent in cardiopulmonary resuscitation, know how to make preparations for emergency surgery, and know what to do when there are adverse reactions to blood products and medications. Rehearsing the unexpected but possible clinical emergency promotes patient safety. Clinical appropriateness and timeliness during rehearsed emergencies can be evaluated by the interdisciplinary team retrospectively in a systematic manner. Opportunities for improvement can be identified and incorporated into future emergent clinical situations.

- Successful operations are viewed as potentially dangerous.

Routine, repetitive, successful operations naturally lead to process shortcuts and simplification, or what Vaughan in her analysis of the *Challenger* space shuttle disaster termed "normalization of deviance."[73] She concluded that all work groups continuously redefine risk in the context of accidents that do not occur. Unknowingly, professional, technical, and behavioral standards degrade as time goes on. Incrementally, all group cultures become unsafe over time because "they get away with it." Because accidents are rare, there are no immediate or apparent consequences for not strictly adhering to defenses created to prevent their occurrence. When the inevitable disaster occurs (and it always does), the negative impact is magnified because risk is then redefined in terms of impact on the individual(s), rather than the number of times the accident did not previously happen.

At times operational systems and clinical practices that are known to be risky may continue because the unit is short-staffed or because some team members feel powerless to challenge other team members. Ongoing limited financial and human resources contribute to a stressful, error-prone clinical environment. Physicians react to the pressures of demands for efficiency by third-party payers and hospital administrators. For example, they are sometimes tempted to speed things up and may override clinical protocols in the interest of time. Nurses may initially go along unwillingly but develop mistrust and hostility toward physicians in the process. Physicians in turn, often play "I told you so," thereby perpetuating the developing deviance until disaster strikes. As an alternative, nurses may use deceptive countermeasures in a misguided attempt to advocate for their patients; however, at times, lacking knowledge of the complete clinical situation, these techniques may actually result in patient harm.

To combat this natural tendency toward normalizing deviance, high-reliability clinical units actively and continuously question assumptions. They promote orderly challenge of operating systems and practices so that the successful lessons of the past do not become routine to the point of safety degradation. The "outside" view is actively solicited or created through interdisciplinary review of the routine and debriefing of the unusual. Clinical units are especially vulnerable to normalizing deviance. Because an outcome is "good" (no harm, no foul in legal terms), near misses are frequently not viewed as opportunities to learn about or improve system behaviors. Once the concepts are understood, however, it is very easy for a clinical unit to identify specific deviances it has normalized over time. Professionals new to a unit are frequently amazed at potentially unsafe conditions or clinical practices attributed to "the way we've always done it." Six months later these same professionals are just as amazed by newcomers questioning the same practices with which they themselves have now grown comfortable. Newcomers present an ideal opportunity for an "outsider view" of clinical practices. Their perspectives and suggestions for improvement should be given serious consideration.

- Clear language is routinely used to describe clinical conditions and patient well-being in all professional communication and medical record documentation.

Members of the unit team should establish clear language to describe common clinical situations and deviations, and that language should be used in all professional communication and medical record documentation.[74] A common language enhances communication and avoids misconceptions about patient status. This is especially important when communicating over the telephone. Much of the communication about patient conditions occurs over the telephone between the nurse at the bedside and the physician at home or in the office. Each team member must be able to accurately convey the patient's clinical status and clearly understand the substance, implications, and urgency of what is being communicated.

- Clearly defined policies and practices exist that everyone knows and agrees to follow.

Policies and practices promulgated by the unit practice committee should be clearly written and widely disseminated. There should be a process in place to ensure that every team member is made aware of practice changes and updates. An expectation that all professionals agree to follow established unit policies and practices is critical to safe care. A system of accountability and zero tolerance for violations (or repeated violations) of these policies and practices should be developed and followed.

- Organizational resources and systems are in place to support clinically timely interventions in the event of unexpected patient deterioration.

Sufficient nurse-to-patient ratios are critical to identifying deterioration in a patient's condition in a timely manner. There is ample evidence to support the idea that patient outcomes improve and adverse events are less frequent as the number of nurses per patient is increased.[75-81] A higher number of registered nurses per patient is consistently related to lower adverse outcome rates, shorter lengths of stay, and lower patient morbidity. The nurse manager can use these data to argue that any plans for downsizing, reengineering, or restructuring of the clinical workforce should be evaluated in the context of the potential impact on patient safety. Although decreasing the number of registered nurses may appear to be a cost-saving measure initially, over time patient morbidity and adverse incidents will increase and patient and nursing satisfaction decrease. Thus, there may be significant unplanned negative financial implications in addition to lower-quality care.

Accurate identification of deteriorating or significant changes in patient condition should be followed with clinically timely interventions. Twenty-four-hour availability of a medical emergency or surgical team (including an anesthesia provider, scrub nurse, circulating nurse, surgical first assistant, and surgeon) is essential. Institutional financial constraints that do not permit intensive care, anesthesia, or surgical standby for potential emergencies or for calling the surgical team in before the attending physician has arrived when there is clear evidence of patient deterioration are inconsistent with safe care.

- Interdisciplinary debriefings are held for near misses and medical accidents.

When clinical situations result in an adverse outcome, an interdisciplinary process that allows all parties to review the events in a blame-free environment works well as a strategy to potentially prevent future occurrences. The key issue is to focus on the process and systems that contributed to the adverse outcome rather than assigning fault to individual professionals.

WHEN A PREVENTABLE ADVERSE OUTCOME OCCURS IN A HIGH-RELIABILITY CLINICAL UNIT

It is important to realize that medical accidents, mistakes, and patient injuries cannot be avoided with absolute certainty.[82] The best clinical teams on occasion experience adverse patient outcomes. When these unfortunate incidents do occur, a lawsuit is not inevitable, and therefore organizational response should not use the medicolegal system as the primary basis for determining communication policy for providers and patients. Data suggest that six patient injuries occur for every one that results in legal action.[83] The key variable that separates these outcomes is effective patient communication.[84] The ability to communicate effectively in times of crisis is a skill that can be learned and must be practiced.[85] Clinical units with few lawsuits are succeeding at setting realistic patient expectations as well as communicating effectively when those expectations are not met. Self-appraisal and the practice of an effective communication style are taken seriously by every team member involved.

In addition to communicating with patients and families following adverse outcomes, healthcare professionals on effective clinical units communicate with and support each other. Besides debriefing following patient injuries in an effort to learn and improve system performance, there is recognition that an adverse event has high potential for personal and professional costs as well. Most professionals are perfectionists, and failure creates extreme vulnerability that can result in personal disruption and suboptimal future performance, and therefore the potential for further errors.[86,87] The ultimate success of a high-reliability clinical unit is its ability to avoid casting personal blame while creating an environment that is mutually supportive at the time of high stress secondary to catastrophic outcome. A supportive environment that maintains psychological well-being protects future individual performance and diminishes the chances of recurrent patient injury.

CONCLUSION

Ultimately, the creation and maintenance of teamwork, high reliability, and an environment safe for both patients and healthcare providers come down to a series of decisions. Organizations are composed of professionals who have the ability to decide what the conditions of where they work and how they work will be. Safety is an active choice that can be embraced or rejected. Although the principles and benefits of teamwork are easily summarized, the choice to move forward has proved to be more difficult. The answer to this paradox is as important as any question facing health care today. The work required in "first doing no harm" will only occur when people make up their minds to embrace it seriously.

References

1. Simpson, K. R., and Knox, G. E. (2001). Perinatal teamwork: Turning rhetoric into reality. In K. R. Simpson and P. A. Creehan (Eds.). *AWHONN's Perinatal Nursing* (2nd ed., pp. 53–67). Philadelphia: Lippincott.
2. Knox, G. E., Kelley, M., Simpson, K. R., Carrier, L., and Berry, D. (1999). Downsizing, reengineering and patient safety: Numbers, newness and resultant risk. *Journal of Healthcare Risk Management, 19*(4), 18–25.
3. Pavlovich-Davis, S., Forman, H., and Simek, P. F. (1998). The nurse-physician relationship: Can it be saved? *Journal of Nursing Administration, 28*(7), 17–20.
4. Harvard Risk Management Foundation, personal communication (2000).
5. Katzenbach, J. R., and Smith, D. K. (1993). *The Wisdom of Teams*. Boston: Harvard Business School Press.
6. Morey, J. C., Simon, R., Jay, G. D., Wears, R. L., Salisbury, M., Dukes, K. A., and Berns, S. D. (2002). Error reduction and performance improvement in the emergency department through formal teamwork training: Evaluation results of the Med-Teams project. *Health Services Research, 37*(6), 1553–1581.
7. Gaba, D. M., Howard, S. K., Flanagan, B., Smith, B. E., Fish, K. J., and Botney, R. (1998). Assessment of clinical performance during simulated crises using both technical and behavioral ratings. *Anesthesiology, 89*, 8–18.
8. Knox, G. E., Simpson, K. R., and Garite, T. J. (1999). High reliability perinatal units: An approach to the prevention of patient injury and medical malpractice claims. *Journal of Healthcare Risk Management, 19*(2), 27–35.
9. Roberts, K. H. (1990). Some characteristics of high reliability organizations. *Organization Science, 1*(2), 160–177.
10. Ibid.
11. Knox et al. (1999). Downsizing, reengineering and patient safety.

12. Ibid.
13. Ibid.
14. Roberts (1990). Some characteristics of high reliability organizations.
15. Simpson, K. R. (2000). Creating a culture of safety: A shared responsibility. *MCN American Journal of Maternal Child Nursing, 25*(2), 61.
16. Katzenbach and Smith (1993). *The Wisdom of Teams.*
17. Briscoe, G., and Authur, G. (1998). CQI teamwork: Reevaluate, restructure, renew. *Nursing Management, 29*(10), 73–80.
18. Klein, G. (1998). *Sources of Power: How People Make Decisions*. Cambridge, MA: MIT Press.
19. Roberts (1990). Some characteristics of high reliability organizations.
20. Mannarelli, T., Roberts, K. H., and Bea, R. G. (1996). Learning how organizations mitigate risk. *Journal of Contingencies and Crisis Management, 4*, 83–92.
21. Smith, P. G., and Reinhart, D. G. (1991). *Developing Products in Half the Time*. New York: Van Nostrand Reinhold.
22. Katzenbach and Smith (1993). *The Wisdom of Teams.*
23. Ibid.
24. Knox et al. (1999). Downsizing, reengineering and patient safety.
25. Simpson and Knox (2001). Perinatal teamwork.
26. Parker, G. A. (1996). *Team Players and Teamwork: The New Competitive Business Strategy*. San Francisco: Jossey-Bass.
27. Simpson and Knox (2001). Perinatal teamwork.
28. Department of Health and Human Services (2001). Sample survey of registered nurses. Washington, DC: Author.
29. Bickel, J. (1997). Gender stereotypes and misconceptions: Unresolved issues in physician's professional development. *Journal of the American Medical Association, 277*(17), 1405–1407.
30. Pasko, T., and Seidman, B. (1999). *Physician Characteristics and Distribution in the Workplace*. Chicago: American Medical Association.
31. Kearny, K. G., and White, T. I. (Eds.). (1994). *Men and Women at Work: Warriors and Villagers on the Job*. Hawthorne, NJ: Cancer Press.
32. Ibid.
33. Ibid.
34. Ibid.
35. Ibid.
36. Ibid.
37. Keenan, G. M., Cooke, R., and Hillis, S. L. (1998). Norms and nurse management of conflicts: Keys to understanding nurse-physician collaboration. *Research in Nursing and Health, 21*, 59–72.
38. Stein, L. I. (1967). The doctor-nurse game. *Archives in General Psychiatry, 16*, 699–703.
39. Willis, E., and Parish, K. (1997). Managing the doctor-nurse game: A nursing and social science analysis. *Contemporary Nurse, 6*(3), 136–144.
40. Peter, E. (2000). Ethical conflicts or political problems in intrapartum nursing care. *Birth: Issues in Perinatal Care, 27*(1), 46–48.
41. Knaus, W. A., Draper, E. A., and Wagner, D. P. (1986). An evaluation of outcome from intensive care units in major medical centers. *Annals of Internal Medicine, 104*, 410–418.
42. Sleutel, M. R. (2000). Intrapartum nursing care: A case study of supportive interventions and ethical conflicts. *Birth: Issues in Perinatal Care, 27*(1), 38–45.
43. Peter (2000). Ethical conflicts or political problems.
44. Leape, L. L. (1994). Error in medicine. *Journal of the American Medical Association, 272*, 1851–1857.
45. Knaus, Draper, and Wagner (1986). An evaluation of outcome.
46. Baggs, J. G., Ryan, S. A., and Phelps, C. E. (1992). The association between interdisciplinary collaboration and patient outcomes in a medical intensive care unit. *Heart and Lung, 21*, 18–24.
47. Katzman, E. M., and Roberts, J. I. (1988). Nurse-physician conflicts as barriers to enactment of nursing roles. *Western Journal of Nursing Research, 10*, 576–590.
48. Knox, G. E. (1999). Doctors behaving badly and the people who let them. *Trustees, 52*(4), 18–19.
49. Roberts, S. J. (1983). Oppressed group behavior: Implications for nurses. *Advances in Nursing Science, 5*(4), 21–30.
50. Department of Health and Human Services (2001). Sample survey of registered nurses. Washington, DC: Author.
51. Christman, L. (1998). Who is a nurse? *Image: The Journal of Nursing Scholarship, 30*, 211–214.

52. Gennaro, S., and Lewis, J. (2000)..Is the goal of a BSN as the criteria for entry into professional nursing practice still worthwhile and realistic? *MCN American Journal of Maternal Child Nursing, 25*(2), 62–63.
53. Ibid.
54. Ibid.
55. Simpson, K. R., and Knox, G. E. (1999). Strategies for developing an evidence-based approach to perinatal care. *MCN American Journal of Maternal Child Nursing, 24*(3), 122–132.
56. Pavlovich-Davis, Forman, and Simek (1998). The nurse-physician relationship.
57. Rubin, J. (1996). Impediments to the development of clinical knowledge and ethical judgment in critical care nursing. In P. Benner, C. A. Tanner, and C. Chelsa (Eds.). *Expertise in Nursing Practice: Caring Clinical Judgment and Ethics* (pp. 170–192). New York: Springer Publishing.
58. Peter (2000). Ethical conflicts or political problems.
59. Simpson and Knox (2001). Perinatal teamwork.
60. Parker (1996). *Team Players and Teamwork.*
61. Kassebaum, D., and Culter, E. (1998). On the culture of student abuse in medical school. *Academic Medicine, 73*(11), 1149–1158.
62. Simpson and Knox (2001). Perinatal teamwork.
63. Pavlovich-Davis, Forman, and Simek (1998). The nurse-physician relationship.
64. Ibid.
65. Ibid.
66. Parker (1996). *Team Players and Teamwork.*
67. Reason, J. T. (1997). *Managing the Risks of Organizational Accidents.* Aldershot, UK: Ashgate Publishing.
68. Reason, J. T. (2001). Understanding adverse events: The human factor. In C. Vincent (Ed.). *Clinical Risk Management* (2nd ed.). London: BMJ Books.
69. Vaughn, D. (1996). *The Challenger Launch Decision: Risky Technology, Culture and Deviance at NASA.* Chicago: University of Chicago Press.
70. Simpson and Knox (1999). Strategies for developing an evidence-based approach to perinatal care.
71. Ibid.
72. Ibid.
73. Vaughn (1996). *Challenger launch decision.*
74. Simpson, K. R., and Knox, G. E. (2003). Communication of fetal heart monitoring information. In N. Feinstein, K. L. Torgersen, and J. Atterbury (Eds.). *Fetal Heart Monitoring Principles and Practices.* Washington, DC: Association of Women's Health, Obstetric and Neonatal Nurses.
75. Aiken, L. H., Clarke, S. P., Sloane, D. M., Sochalski, J., and Siber, J. H. (2002). Hospital nurse staffing and patient mortality, nurse burnout, and job satisfaction. *Journal of the American Medical Association, 288*(16), 1987–1993.
76. Blegen, M. A., Goode, C. J., and Reed, L. (1998). Nurse staffing and patient outcomes. *Nursing Research, 47*(1), 43–50.
77. Bond, C. A., Raehl, C. L., Pitterle, M. E., and Franke, T. (1999). Health care professional staffing, hospital characteristics, and hospital mortality rates. *Pharmacotherapy, 19*(2), 130–138.
78. Callaghan, L. A., Cartwright, D. W., O'Rourke, P., and Davies, M. W. (2003). Infant to staff ratios and risk of mortality in very low birthweight infants. *Archives of Disease in Childhood: Fetal and Neonatal Edition, 88*(2), F94–F97.
79. Kovner, C., and Gergen, P. J. (1998). Nurse staffing levels and adverse events following surgery in U. S. hospitals. *Image: Journal of Nursing Scholarship, 30*(4), 315–321.
80. Lichtig, L. K., Knauf, R. A., and Milholland, D. K. (1999). Some impacts of nursing on acute care hospital outcomes. *Journal of Nursing Administration, 29*(2), 25–33.
81. Needleman, J., Buerhaus, P., Mattke, S., Stewart, M., and Zelevinsky, K. (2002). Nurse-staffing levels and the quality of care in hospitals. *New England Journal of Medicine, 346*(22), 1715–1722.
82. Kohn, L. T., Corrigan, J., and Donaldson, M. S. (Eds.). (1999). *To Err Is Human: Building a Safe Health System.* Washington, DC: National Academy of Sciences Press.
83. Localio, A. R., Lawthers, A. G., Brennan, T. A., Laird, N. M., Hebert, L. E., Peterson, L. M., Newhouse, J. P., Weiler, P. C., and Hiatt, H. H. (1991). Relation between malpractice claims and adverse events due to negligence: Results of the Harvard Medical Practice Study III. *New England Journal of Medicine, 325*(4), 245–251.

84. Hickson, G. B., Clayton, E. W., Githens, P. B., and Sloan, F. A. (1992). Factors that prompted families to file malpractice claims following perinatal injury. *Journal of the American Medical Association, 287*(10), 1359–1363.
85. Markakis, K. M., Beckman, H. B., Suchman, A. L., and Frankel, R. M. (2000). The path to professionalism: Cultivating humanistic values and attitudes in residency training. *Academic Medicine, 75*(2), 141–150.
86. Charles, S. C. (1986). Malpractice litigation and its impact on physicians. *Current Psychiatric Therapies, 23*, 173–180.
87. Charles, S. C. (1991). The psychological trauma of a medical malpractice suit: A practical guide. *Bulletin of the American College of Surgeons, 76*(11), 22–26.

23

Health Information Technology and Patient Safety

Laura B. Morgan

INTRODUCTION

Health information technology (HIT) has been lauded by many for its potential to enhance the safety and quality of the U.S. healthcare system. Despite this widespread belief, only about 17% of U.S. doctors and 10% of U.S. hospitals currently have even basic HIT systems.[1,2] This percentage will increase dramatically in the coming years, however, because the Health Information Technology for Economic and Clinical Health (HITECH) Act of the American Recovery and Reinvestment Act of 2009 (ARRA) promises billions of dollars in extra Medicare and Medicaid payments to providers who implement and achieve *meaningful use* of HIT systems. *Meaningful use* is defined as using a certified EHR system (1) in a meaningful way, such as e-prescribing; (2) to exchange health information in order to advance quality of care; and (3) to submit clinical measures, such as quality.[12,13]

However, many healthcare providers who have already implemented HIT have discovered that this new technology often produces unintended consequences that undermine—not enhance—patient safety.[3] As providers rush to implement HIT systems to receive HITECH Act incentive payments beginning in 2011 and avoid penalties beginning in 2015,[1] caution must be exercised to ensure that the use of this new technology facilitates rather than impedes the provision of safe and high-quality health care in the United States. With this context in mind, in this chapter, I will analyze the potential of various HIT systems to enhance patient safety and the actual outcomes of these systems in practice and I will analyze the actual outcomes. Then, I will propose various ways by which HIT can be harnessed to support a culture of safety in the healthcare industry.

THE POTENTIAL OF HIT TO IMPROVE PATIENT SAFETY

In theory, HIT—which includes electronic health records, computerized physician order entry, and decision support systems[1]—has innumerable benefits that could greatly increase the provision of safe health care. Electronic health records (EHRs), also known as electronic medical records (EMRs), are the most well-known and widely used form of HIT, and, for this reason, the terms HIT and EHR are often used interchangeably. An EHR is an electronic repository of information about an individual's health care and health status. An EHR system has electronic tools—such as a display of the patient's medications, allergies, laboratory results, diagnoses, and providers' notes—which can greatly assist clinicians in managing a patient's health information.[2] EHRs could be particularly helpful to providers of emergent care, who could view a patient's medical history, allergies, and medications even if the patient had never received care at that facility, thus preventing potential adverse drug events and unnecessary diagnostic tests.[4]

Another significant benefit of EHR systems is the personal health record (PHR), through which individuals can electronically access, manage, and share the information contained in their EHRs. Ideally, a PHR integrates the provider-maintained EHR information with the patient's own notes about his or her health status. In this way, the PHR can enable a patient to take a more active role in managing his or her health and can facilitate shared decision making with the physician about the most appropriate course of treatment for acute conditions or management of chronic conditions.[5]

Next, computerized physician order entry (CPOE), or e-prescribing, has been praised by the Institute of Medicine (IOM) for its potential to improve patient safety by reducing medication errors.[6] According to an IOM report, more than 1.5 million preventable medication errors occur each year.[7] Most of these errors occur during the ordering step,[6] for reasons such as illegible handwriting, calculation and transcription errors, lack of specificity in the order, and physicians having insufficient information about the drug or the patient.[8] A CPOE system addresses many of these issues because it compels the physician to make complete and legible orders and provides access to a patient's full medical history.[9] It can also include *forcing functions* that limit a clinician's choice of drugs to prescribe, which according to Bates and Gawande is a primary way in which CPOE can reduce medication errors.[8] Further, CPOE could improve patient outcomes by providing more efficient treatment. In a study by Stone et al. of CPOE implementation in an inpatient hospital setting, the electronic ordering process was found to be 38 minutes faster than its paper counterpart.[10]

Finally, a decision support system (DSS) is a computer application designed to assist a clinician in his or her decision-making process about the most appropriate course of treatment for a patient.[2] A DSS can be a part of a CPOE system, assisting the clinician at the time of ordering medication, or a separate system.[6] A DSS can include alerts about drug allergies and interactions and abnormal laboratory results, and provide recommendations for tests and treatment modalities.[2] DSS can support the provision of safe and high-quality health care by encouraging adherence to evidence-based medicine and reducing errors of omission.[11]

Significantly, the *meaningful use* requirement to receive funding through the HITECH Act may encourage the provision of safe and effective HIT systems. The ability of EHR systems to submit clinical measures would enable data mining of medical records for the purpose of researching diseases and could assist with the reporting of adverse events.[11] Also, the ability of EHR systems to exchange information, known as *interoperability*, is the essential feature that would allow physicians to access a patient's medical records from other facilities and thus make optimally informed decisions about the patient's care.[2]

UNINTENDED CONSEQUENCES OF HIT ON PATIENT SAFETY

For the reasons discussed above, HIT does have many potential advantages over traditional paper record keeping and medication ordering. However, this new technology also has considerable downsides, which have been underemphasized by the medical informatics industry.[12,13] Although HIT can strengthen many areas of health care, it can also introduce new sources of potential error that can nullify its beneficial potential.[14,15] In the enthusiasm to implement HIT in the wake of the HITECH Act, it is crucial to not overlook the negative aspects of this new technology.

For example, although DSS can support the provision of safe health care, many researchers have found that decision support tools are frequently disregarded. Physicians may ignore suggestions from the DSS because they may be too busy to fully consider them, may take offense to a computer telling them what to do, or may distrust the suggested course of action.[2] Several studies have also shown that DSS can cause *alert fatigue:* up to 85% of suggestions from a DSS are ignored because they are disruptive and unwanted.[13] This pattern of ignoring DSS suggestions can lead a clinician to disregard the DSS when it notifies him or her of an important alert about allergies or drug interactions, thus undermining the intention of the DSS to support the provision of safer patient care.

Similarly, CPOE systems have been found to negligibly impact patient safety in many contexts and have negatively impacted patient safety in others. In the above-referenced study by Stone et al. of CPOE implementation in an inpatient hospital setting, a slight improvement was recorded in the medication error rate after the system was in place.[10] However, in that study and others like it, the rate of adverse drug events (ADEs)—medication errors or adverse drug reactions resulting in patient harm[6]—actually increased after the CPOE system was in place.[6,10] This is because, although the CPOE may eliminate some sources of error, it also introduces new sources of potential error.[6,10] For example, the CPOE system creates an *illusion of communication*—the belief that once an order is entered, other clinicians will see and act upon it, without verifying that this actually took place—and also takes away redundant checks by multiple clinicians, which can catch errors.[3]

Another example of a new source of potential error is the time that HIT takes away from a clinician's interaction with the patient. When clinicians have less time to examine and talk with their patients, they may provide poorer quality care.[2] In the study by Stone et al., for instance, although overall efficiency was gained after the CPOE was in place, doctors actually spent more time processing orders and thus spent less time with patients.[10]

EHR systems have also been found to impose greater demands on a physician's time. One study found that EHR documentation increased the time a physician spent away from a patient during a consultation by as much as 28%, and this figure did not change when the physician became more proficient with the EHR system.[4] This is because the templates in EHR systems require a physician to document much more information than he or she was accustomed to documenting in paper records. And according to some commentators, not all of the information required in the EHR template is necessary to provide quality patient care.[2]

Moreover, the large amount of information required by the EHR template may sacrifice efficacy for what appears to be *completeness*. For example, many clinicians simply copy and paste a patient's record from a previous encounter into the new EHR entry. Thus, the record may appear complete, but the next clinician who views it will not be able to tell whether it represents thoughtful analysis or is merely a repeat of previous data.[14]

Copying and pasting is just one of the workarounds that clinicians have discovered to bypass HIT system barriers. Such workarounds are understandable because, especially in an emergent or intensive-care setting, the need to immediately help the patient outweighs the need to comply with HIT protocols.[3] However, workarounds can complicate the job of other clinicians down the road and can negatively affect patients. For instance, if a hospital patient is in urgent need of an I.V., a clinician may grab a prepared I.V. bag from another patient's supply. But if this bag was barcoded for the other patient through the CPOE and EHR system, this may wreak havoc in both the record keeping and ordering for that patient. Likewise, if a patient needs a laboratory test and the HIT system requires input of a diagnostic code to order the test, a busy clinician may make up a code, which then erroneously becomes part of the patient's EHR history.[13]

These examples show how HIT systems are often incompatible with the high-stress nature of many healthcare settings. It is very difficult for clinicians to accurately enter data into the EHR while they are caring for patients and dealing with interruptions from other clinicians and from DSS alerts. In this highly interruptive context, *juxtaposition errors*—when the wrong option on the screen is clicked because it appears close to the correct option—and other input errors can easily occur.[14] Additionally, information is frequently entered into the wrong patient's EHR, which can lead to confusion and misdiagnosis for those who consult the record in the future.[2] In one such instance, a patient with AIDS was mistakenly told that he had skin cancer because a clinician entered a lab result for a different patient in his EHR. Clearly, such input errors can endanger patient safety, often to a greater degree than illegible handwriting. Using barcodes for EHR and CPOE systems may help to protect against inputting information in the wrong patient record but also produces new sources of potential error.[13]

In addition to input errors, overdependence on information technology in the healthcare industry may also have grave implications for patient safety efforts. Physicians who become accustomed to relying on HIT for decision support and error prevention may have difficulty transitioning to work in an area that does not provide such technology and may forget basic information about standard dosages or drug interactions.[3] Of even greater concern is the possibility of software defects or failure. As physicians and entire hospital systems fully implement HITs, these systems will become essential to the delivery of care, and computer crashes and software problems could have dire consequences for patients.[2,4] For example, the U.S. Department of Veterans Affairs (VA) Health Administration has the largest EHR system in the country.[4] Despite the size of the system and the praise it has received from many sources, a recent software glitch caused the erroneous administration of life-threatening dosages of heparin, a blood thinner, to VA patients across the country.[2,16]

A final concern with the current state of HIT is a lack of interoperability within and across HIT systems. Even within a single hospital, not all floors will use the same EHR system, and some floors may not have access to the system at all. In the case discussed above in which the skin cancer diagnosis was reported to the wrong patient, this error might have been prevented if the hospital had installed the EHR in the lab so the laboratory technicians could have noted that the patient did not have any skin lesions.[13] Further, the benefits of EHRs cannot be fully realized if physicians and hospitals cannot share EHR information with other provider institutions. For this reason, as discussed above, the HITECH Act encourages interoperability of EHR systems so that HIT can be exchanged electronically among providers.[2]

However, the interoperability of HIT systems across provider institutions may introduce new sources of error. As more HIT systems become interoperable, a single data input error, technical problem, or computer crash can have widespread implications for a large number of patients across many healthcare institutions.[4] And with access to a patient's medical data from previous providers, coupled with pressure to keep costs down, physicians may rely on other clinicians' findings rather than ordering new tests, even when the patient could benefit from a second opinion.[2]

Another concern with interoperability is that clinicians may be overwhelmed by the amount of information from previous providers that they need to sift through when treating their patients.[2] Physicians may have access to medical information from other providers, but if the display formats and features of the different systems are not well integrated, it may be difficult to find necessary information, leading to confusion rather than clinical insight.[13] The practice of copying and pasting, described above, also exacerbates data overload.[14] Although clinicians may have immediate access to essential patient information when making a diagnosis or processing an order, such access may not assist in the provision of quality patient care if it requires searching through seemingly endless amounts of information and clicking through multiple screens that may contain irrelevant and repetitive data.[13]

HARNESSING HIT'S POTENTIAL TO IMPROVE PATIENT SAFETY AND MANAGING HIT'S UNINTENDED CONSEQUENCES

Despite these significant concerns about the effect of HIT on patient safety, with the provision of incentive payments through the HITECH Act, widespread promulgation will certainly occur in the coming years. In HIT design, implementation, and use, it is crucial for healthcare providers to be vigilantly aware of how to harness this new technology to support rather than undermine the development of a culture of safety within their institutions. Providers should keep the following steps in mind to use HIT implementation as a tool to improve overall patient safety efforts: (1) purchase the safest possible HIT products, (2) develop HIT systems that are customized to the unique workflow processes of their institutions, (3) optimize patient safety in the implementation stage, and (4) engage in constant improvement of HIT practices. Each of these steps will be addressed in turn below.

Purchase the Safest Possible HIT Products

HIT systems must be developed and maintained with the highest quality software engineering to prevent technical errors from happening in the future. These errors, such as the erroneous heparin administration to VA patients due to a software glitch, can be life threatening. As more systems implement HIT and increasingly rely on their DSS and CPOE functions, they will assume an even larger role in diagnosis and treatment of disease, and the dependability of these systems will be essential to proper patient care.[4]

Thus, HIT products should be regulated to ensure they are as dependable as possible. The HITECH Act takes an important step in the right direction in this regard. For providers to receive Medicare and Medicaid incentive payments, they must use certified EHR programs, according to standards set by the Department of Health and Human Services (HHS).[17] Within HHS, the Office of the National Coordinator for Health Information Technology (ONCHIT)[1] tests and certifies HIT products through authorized testing and certification bodies (ATCBs).[17] Products that have passed such certification are listed on the ONCHIT Web site for other providers to view.[18] Hopefully, the regulation and certification of HIT through ONCHIT will facilitate the promulgation and purchase of the safest possible products.

Develop HIT Systems That Align with the Provider's Sociotechnical Context

The mere act of purchasing safe and dependable HIT products does not guarantee that the HIT system supports the provision of safe healthcare practices. Providers often assume that HIT will provide the results promised by vendors, but they may not consider how the new technology will interact with their existing workflow practices.[3] It is important to note that some of the first healthcare providers to successfully implement safe and effective EHR systems spent decades working closely with software designers to customize a program that fits the work processes of their institutions. Because most other provider institutions will not use such highly customized

EHR systems, they may not realize the same positive effect on patient safety.[19]

To minimize the impact of HIT's new potential sources of error, however, it is essential for providers to customize their HIT systems as much as possible. This is because the new sources of error inherent in HIT do not necessarily flow from the technology itself or from its users. Rather, they come from the interplay of HIT with the already existing workflow, culture, and social interactions of the provider institution.[3] This *sociotechnical* approach recognizes that new technology must be tested where it is actually used (*ergonomically*) to determine what unintended consequences it may produce and to verify that it can improve patient safety rather than cause harm.[15] At the same time, it is important to balance customization with the need to standardize HIT platforms so that the information can be interoperable with HIT systems of other institutions.[3]

To facilitate optimal customization, clinicians at the provider institution must be involved as early as possible in designing the HIT system, long before it is actually implemented. Having clinicians involved at this stage will encourage greater acceptance of the technology in the future.[20] More important, these clinicians can provide vital information about the *clinical workflow* of the institution—the patterns of actions clinicians use to perform routine tasks such as scheduling appointments, performing examinations, ordering medications, and following up with patients.[11] With this input, HIT can be designed to support clinicians' cognitive processes and the workflow among clinicians within the organization.[21] Thus, HIT software will fit the ecology of the practice and will provide as little interruption as possible in the clinical workflow necessary to ensure patient safety.[14] However, rather than modeling existing clinical practices that may not provide the safest possible care, HIT development can be used, where necessary, to improve care practices and redesign outdated or error-prone processes.[11,19,20]

Optimize Patient Safety During the HIT Implementation Phase

If the development process outlined above is followed, providers will be able to anticipate how the implementation of HIT will change their clinical and administrative work processes.[21] They will also need to anticipate further changes that will likely be necessary for safe implementation, including new organization policies and job descriptions, and training of clinicians on the new technology.[19] Ideally, clinicians will be able to use the new technology, especially DSS and CPOE systems, in a training context before using it with patients.[20]

Furthermore, studies have shown that the appointment of a *HIT champion* within the institution can greatly assist with this transition phase. In a hospital setting, this individual could work closely with the quality and risk management staff. He or she would be responsible for promoting the benefits of the HIT system for patient safety, assisting with training efforts, and addressing any issues or concerns from clinical staff. The champion could help assure that productivity remains high and patient safety is not compromised during the transition to the HIT system.[11]

Engage in Constant Improvement of HIT Practices

The work of assuring safety of HIT systems does not end once implementation is complete.[13,14] Even with clinician involvement in the development stage and a HIT champion during the implementation stage, it is impossible to anticipate all of the sociotechnical implications of HIT. Thus, it is essential to evaluate the actual uses of the new technology once it is in place rather than the uses that were envisioned. This includes evaluating how HIT affects clinical workflow and how clinicians have reinterpreted the technology, such as by finding workarounds.[3]

Clinicians, HIT designers, and managers at the provider institutions must continually interact with one another about the sociotechnical implications of the HIT system and resolve any unanticipated consequences of the system before they harm patients. If necessary, these parties should change the pace of HIT implementation or redesign software components to ensure that the system supports the provision of high-quality heath care.[3] This process should be viewed as an opportunity to continually improve all aspects of care at the institution. In this way, HIT can live up to its potential to enhance the safety and quality of health care.

CONCLUSION

HIT—in the form of EHRs, CPOE, and DSS—certainly has many promising features. However, it is crucial that healthcare providers are aware of the unintended consequences of this technology, which can undermine patient safety efforts. In the enthusiasm about implementing HIT to receive HITECH Act incentive payments, providers must be continually vigilant to ensure that their efforts do not compromise quality care. HIT must be implemented with caution and with mindfulness of its sociotechnical implications to successfully harness it to support a culture of safety in the healthcare industry.

References

1. Blumenthal, D. (2009). Stimulating the adoption of health information technology. *New England Journal of Medicine, 360*, 1477–1479.
2. Hoffman, S., & Podgurski, A. (2009). E-health hazards: Provider liability and electronic health record systems. *Berkeley Technology Law Journal, 24*, 1523–1581.
3. Harrison, M. I., Koppel, R., & Bar-Lev, S. (2007). Unintended consequences of information technologies in health care—An interactive sociotechnical analysis. *Journal of the American Medical Informatics Association, 14*, 542–549.
4. Hoffman, S., & Podgurski, A. (2008). Finding a cure: The case for regulation and oversight of electronic health record systems. *Harvard Journal of Law & Technology, 22*, 103–165. [hereinafter Hoffman & Podgurski, Finding a Cure].
5. Goldstein, M. M. (2010). Health information technology and the idea of informed consent. *The Journal of Law, Medicine & Ethics, 38*, 27–35.
6. Eslami, S., de Keizer, N. F., & Abu-Hanna, A. (2007). The impact of computerized physician medication order entry in hospitalized patients—A systematic review. *International Journal of Medical Informatics, 77*, 365–376.
7. Committee on Identifying and Preventing Medication Errors, Aspden, P., Wolcott, J., Bootman, J. L., & Cronenwett, L. R. (Eds.). (2006). *Preventing medication errors*. Quality Chasm Series. Washington, DC: National Academies Press.
8. Bates, D. W., & Gawande, A. A. (2003). Improving safety with information technology. *New England Journal of Medicine, 348*, 2526–2534.
9. Lundy, S. H. et al. (2009). Just what the doctor ordered? CMS and DEA introduce new measures to facilitate e-prescribing. *Journal of Health & Life Sciences Law, 2*, 79, 81–114.
10. Stone, W. M, Smith B. E., Shaft, J. D., Nelson, R. D, & Money, S. R. (2009). Impact of computerized physician order-entry system. *Journal of the American College of Surgeons, 208*, 960–967.
11. Kilbridge, P. M., & Classen, D. C. (2008). The informatics opportunities at the intersection of patient safety and clinical informatics. *Journal of the American Medical Informatics Association, 15*, 397–407.
12. Pallin, D. J., Sullivan, A. F., Kaushal, R., & Camargo, C. A. (2010). Health information technology in US emergency departments. *International Journal of Emergency Medicine, 3*, 181–185.
13. Koppel, R. (2009). *EMR entry error: Not so benign*. AHRQ Morbidity & Mortality Rounds. Retrieved from http://www.webmm.ahrq.gov/case.aspx?caseID= 199.

14. Ash, J. S., Berg, M., & Coiera, E. (2004). Some unintended consequences of information technology in health care: The nature of patient care information system-related errors. *Journal of the American Medical Informatics Association 11*, 104–112.
15. Balka, E., Doyle-Waters, M., Lecznarowicz, D., & FitzGerald, J. M. (2006). Technology, governance and patient safety: systems issues in technology and patient safety. *International Journal of Medical Informatics, 76*, S35–S47.
16. Yen, H. (2009, January 14). Veterans exposed to incorrect drug doses. Retrieved from http://www.bcbs.com/news/national/veterans-exposed-to-incorrect-drug-doses.html.
17. Centers for Medicare & Medicaid Services. *EHR Incentive Program—Certified EHR Technology*. Retrieved from https://www.cms.gov/Regulations-and-Guidance/Legislation/EHRIncentivePrograms/Certification.html.
18. U.S. Department of Health and Human Services, Office of the National Coordinator for Health Information Technology. *Certified Health IT Product List*. (2010). Retrieved from http://onc-chpl.force.com/ehrcert.
19. Walker, J. M., Carayon, P., Leveson, N., Paulus, R. A., Tooker, J., Chin, H., & Bothe, A. Jr., & Stewart, W. F. (2008). EHR safety: the way forward to safe and effective systems. *Journal of the American Medical Informatics Association, 15*, 272–277.
20. Brokel, J. M., & Harrison, M. I. (2009). Redesigning care processes using an electronic health record: A system's experience. *Joint Commission Journal on Quality and Patient Safety, 35*, 82–92.
21. U.S. Department of Health and Human Services, Agency for Healthcare Research and Quality. (2010). *Incorporating health it into workflow redesign: Request for information summary report*. Retrieved from http://archive.ahrq.gov/downloads/pub/contract/rfp0810036a.htm.

24

Sleep Deprivation in Healthcare Professionals: The Effect on Patient Safety

Mahendr S. Kochar, MD, MS, MBA, JD and Barbara A. Connelly, RN, MJ

Sleep is a restful state during which body and mind functions are restored. Most people require seven to eight hours of sleep daily. Prolonged or chronic sleep loss leads to sleep deprivation and fatigue, which result in decreased cognitive functioning and performance deficits. Although there are strict government rules regulating daily work hours for airline pilots and truck drivers, no such restrictions exist for physicians, nurses, and other healthcare providers in the United States.

Research has demonstrated an increase in the number of medical errors made by residents and nurses working extended hours who are sleep deprived. Sometimes these errors are serious and result in permanent injury or death. Occasionally, the media focuses on such injuries; sometimes they are sensationalized. The medical and nursing professions should work to eliminate sleep deprivation and related medical errors by redesigning work schedules and educating their members on communication techniques and other patient safety measures to avoid errors. They should also educate their members on sleep deprivation so that the culture, which currently accepts sleep deprivation as a *necessary evil* is changed.

INTRODUCTION

The catch phrases *I am too tired to think straight* and *I am dead on my feet*, when uttered by healthcare providers, should not be dismissed out of hand given what is known about sleep deprivation and related medical errors. To provide high-quality health care around the clock, physicians and nurses are required to work extended hours and night shifts and take overnight calls. Such scheduling requirements result in incredibly long hours, which may impair their cognitive skills and ability to provide safe medical care. A growing body of research demonstrates that sleep deprivation results in decreased performance by physicians in training (residents) and nurses, which in turn leads to greater numbers of medical errors and increased risk to patients.[1–4]

The training of physicians is largely based on experiential learning set within a system balanced by supervision and graduated responsibility. Graduate medical education (GME) has a dual purpose. The first is to provide medical care to patients, especially in urban medical centers, and the second is to acquire knowledge and skills through clinical experience and study. For the purpose of this chapter, intern, resident, senior resident, and fellow will be referred to as resident. Historically, residents worked up to 100 to 120 hours per week, and it was common for them to work 36 consecutive hours. In response to growing concerns about patient safety and the threat of government regulation, the Accreditation Council of Graduate Medical Education (ACGME), the organization that accredits GME programs, adopted maximum duty-hour requirements in 2003.[5] The ACGME accredits more than 8,500 residency and fellowship programs at more than 1,000 institutions. ACGME accreditation is required by the Centers for Medicare and Medicaid Services (CMS) for hospitals to receive reimbursement for GME services.

Currently, the ACGME duty-hour requirements permit residents to work 80 hours each week and to be on call every third night averaged over a four-week period. On-call duty generally entails a 24-hour shift with up to six additional hours for clinical care responsibilities and educational purposes. Other duty-hour restrictions require that no new patients may be accepted by the resident after 24 hours of continuous duty and there must be a 10-hour period between duty. Home call must not be so frequent as to preclude rest and personal time. When a resident is called into the hospital from home call, that time must be counted in the 80-hour limit, and there must be one day in seven free from all educational and clinical responsibilities when averaged over a four-week period.[2] Although these duty-hour restrictions have reduced the total number of work hours, residents still work extremely long hours.

Similarly, nurses also work extended shifts. This is due in part to a shortage of nurses and an increase in complex and ill hospitalized patients. In 2004 the Institute of Medicine (IOM) published a report, *Keeping Patients Safe: Transforming the Work Environment for Nurses and Patient Safety*, in which the IOM recognized the critical role nurses play in the safety of patients and recommended that state regulatory bodies prohibit nurses from providing patient care in excess of 12 hours in a 24-hour period and in excess of 60 hours in a seven-day period to reduce error-producing fatigue.[3] A 2004 study of American Nurses Association (ANA) members identified the extent of nurses working long work hours by reporting that 39% of all nurses worked shifts of 12.5 hours long or longer. In addition, 14% of the nurses in the study responded that they had worked shifts 16 hours or longer during the preceding four weeks and mandatory overtime was required in many hospitals.[4] Just as the IOM has recommended shorter work hours for nurses, so too has the American Nurses Association;[5] but no organization or agency enforces these recommendations. Currently, only a few states prohibit mandatory overtime and none prohibit voluntary overtime.[6] A reduction in nursing work hours occurring without regulatory or accreditation enforcement is unlikely.

Extended work hours, especially over time, lead to decrements in physical and psychological performance and an increase in serious medical errors.[3] This chapter focuses on the effects of extended work hours of both residents and nurses. We review the current scientific understanding of sleep, sleep deprivation, and research regarding the effect of sleep deprivation and fatigue on the safety of patients. We discuss how the healthcare industry in the United States does not implement work-hour restrictions for healthcare providers and why many in the medical community object to such restrictions. Last, we consider potential solutions to prevent or minimize sleep deprivation and discuss patient safety practices that can be utilized to reduce the potential for medical errors.

UNDERSTANDING SLEEP, SLEEP DEPRIVATION, AND FATIGUE

Sleep is a restful state occurring naturally and regularly during which consciousness is suspended and power of body and mind are restored. It is an essential need of all humans and animals, similar to the need for food and water. Most people require seven to eight hours of sleep every 24 hours. Sleep deprivation causes fatigue, a feeling of tiredness, reduced energy, and decreased cognitive ability.[7] A fatigued individual requires increased effort to perform tasks effectively and to avoid errors. Going 24 hours without sleep is comparable to having a blood alcohol level of 0.1%, which is considered legally drunk in every state in the country.[8] Adequate sleep is necessary for healthcare professionals to perform their duties safely.

Circadian Rhythm and Sleep

Sleep and wakefulness have independent controls and functions. The endogenous circadian pacemaker, often referred to as the biological clock, is located in the suprachiastmatic nuclei of the hypothalamus. It controls all physiological and psychological functions of the body including temperature, the secretions of hormones, and the rhythms of sleep and wakefulness.[9,10] The circadian cycle is 24 hours long and has periods of peak and low activity. In the early morning hours, the body is at its nadir, or lowest period, of activity; thus residents and nurses working at night must struggle to function while at their lowest level of physiological and psychological activity, alertness, and behavioral response.[12]

Sleep studies utilize electroencephalography (EEG) and other modalities. The exact physiology of sleep is not known; however, sleep is required for proper physical and mental functioning. Sleep is divided into two independent states: nonrapid eye movement (NREM) and rapid eye movement (REM) sleep. NREM and REM sleep alternate, each cycle lasting about 90 to 100 minutes. The first third of a normal sleep period is primarily NREM sleep and the last third is REM sleep. REM sleep is essential to a restful sleep. During sleep, the somatic (voluntary) nervous system shuts down and the autonomic (involuntary) nervous system slows down. Most hormonal secretions except testosterone are also reduced at night; however, melatonin, a brain hormone, increases between 3 am and 5 am. The neurohormone serotonin rises during sleep and nonepinephrine rises during wakefulness in the brain. Body temperature begins to fall at the onset of sleep and reaches its lowest point at about 2 am. The human circadian rhythm is set to induce sleep at night; therefore, daytime sleep is not as restful as nocturnal sleep.[11]

Sleep Deprivation

Three distinct types of sleep loss or impairment lead to sleep deprivation. The first is acute sleep loss. Acute sleep loss begins when an individual stays awake beyond 16 to 18 hours especially during the habitual nocturnal period for sleep.[12] Neuroimaging studies have shown that a night without sleep results in changes in brain function that are associated with unstable and inaccurate performance on a wide range of cognitive tasks such as attention, memory, problem solving, and decision making.[1] Residents and nurses working extended hours, as described above, frequently experience acute sleep loss. It is common for residents to report for work at 7 am and work straight through for the next 30 hours. Akerstedt reported that workers are often awake 20 to 22 hours their first night of duty.[13] Because of the difficulty of daytime sleep, it is unlikely that nurses sleep much prior to the start of their first night shift.

The second type of impairment is chronic partial sleep loss. It is the cumulative result of not getting enough sleep over a period of time. Young adults normally need 8.5 hours of sleep at night. A loss of two hours per night is sufficient to lead to chronic partial sleep loss.[12] Loss of sleep also occurs when transitioning from night shift back to day shift. The scientific literature indicates that recovery from night-shift work requires more days off due to the repeated challenges it poses to the circadian rhythm and the sleep restriction, which occur during the typical four to five nights' work by healthcare providers. Recovery from the cumulative sleep loss and circadian disturbance of consecutive night shifts requires at least two nocturnal sleep periods of uninterrupted extended sleep to allow recovery,[12] but as many as three to four days may be necessary due to the disturbance of normal circadian rhythms.[13]

The third is sleep inertia. Sleep inertia is the term used to describe the waking recovery period when someone is suddenly awakened from sleep. Although not sleep deprivation per se, sleep inertia can result in the inability to function safely. It is less likely that a person is able to be alert and perform well during the first 15 to 30 minutes after being awakened. Lockley discussed how performance during times of sleep inertia can be far more impaired than performance during prolonged periods of wakefulness.[12] Being suddenly awakened from sleep while on call and having to make patient care decisions is a common experience for residents whether they are taking calls from home or they are physically present in the hospital. Making medical decisions while experiencing sleep inertia can lead to or cause serious patient safety risks.

Fatigue

As noted earlier, fatigue is a feeling of tiredness or exhaustion that most of us experience from time to time. It can range from sluggishness to an inability to respond. Acute and chronic sleep deprivation has a profound effect on fatigue, but other factors such as continuous physical or mental activity, workload, shift start time, total hours worked in a week, rotation of work shifts between day and night work, caregiving outside of work, illness, and substance abuse can lead to or contribute to fatigue as well.[10] Even without loss of sleep, night-shift work in and of itself can create fatigue because of the disassociation of awake time to the circadian rhythm.[13]

THE EFFECTS OF HEALTHCARE PROVIDER SLEEP DEPRIVATION AND FATIGUE ON PATIENT SAFETY

The effect of sleep deprivation and fatigue on humans is well documented. Sleep deprivation leads to a greater drive to sleep and increased periods of poor, inefficient, and variable performance. As cognitive and neurobehavioral functioning declines, response times are delayed and it takes longer to process information. Short-term memory is affected and it takes more time to perform tasks. The ability to be vigilant decreases.[1,9] Sleep deprivation and fatigue also exact an emotional toll on individuals. Cavallo et al. studied residents on night float rotations and reported a significant correlation between fatigue and mood measures such as tension, anxiety, anger, hostility, and depression.[16] After having worked for four contiguous nights, a person should break 48 hours to allow catch-up sleep.[16]

Over the past 20 to 30 years, a body of research identifying the negative impact of sleep deprivation and fatigue on performance has been emerging; however, some studies, cited by many in the medical community, reported that sleep deprivation has no effect. Philibert conducted a meta-analysis of 60 studies on the effects of sleep deprivation in physician and nonphysicians reported since 1971.[4] Her analysis confirmed that sleep loss has a negative effect on cognitive and clinical performance. One finding was that a sleep loss of 30 hours or less reduced a physician's overall performance.[4]

Until recently, little information was available on the actual correlation of sleep loss with medical errors. In 2004, Landrigan et al. published a report on serious medical errors made by residents rotating in an intensive care unit. The study compared errors made by interns working a traditional resident work schedule to errors made by interns working fewer hours per week with no 24-hour shifts. The conclusion was that residents working 24 hours or more made substantially more-serious medical errors.[3] The group working the traditional hours made 36% more-serious errors, were five times as likely to make serious diagnostic errors, and made twice as many attention-related errors at night.[3] Similarly, Rogers et al. found that nurses are also more likely to make errors or have near misses when they worked more than 12 hours, worked overtime, or worked more than 40 hours per week.[7]

A professional workforce that is sleep deprived increases the risk of harm to patients, but it is often hard to fully grasp the devastating effect that serious medical errors have on individual patients. Recounting true events can help. We give an account of two patients. Each case was widely publicized; one event had a significant effect on resident work hours whereas the other did not lead to any change in nursing work hours. Like all serious errors, these events involved multiple causal factors; however, sleep deprivation played a significant role in both cases.

In 1984, Libby Zion, an 18-year-old woman, died at a New York hospital within a few hours of admission.[14] The Zion family refused to accept that Libby's death was simply a bad outcome. As they sought answers, they learned of multiple missteps and errors. One of the most shocking factors they discovered was that their daughter was being cared for by residents who had worked 36-hour shifts.[17] Libby's father was an attorney and a columnist for the *New York Daily News*. Through his column, he brought national attention to the long hours that residents work. As a result, in 1989 the state of New York regulated resident work hours.[17] Fifteen years later, the ACGME instituted similar duty-hour regulations for training programs across the country.[5]

On July 4, 2006, Julie Thao, RN, worked two back-to-back eight-hour shifts in a hospital in Madison, Wisconsin. She slept at the hospital and started her next shift at 7 the following morning. Jasimine Grant was a 16-year-old patient admitted on July 5th for the delivery of her baby, and Ms. Thao was the nurse assigned to care for her. During the day, Ms. Thao anticipated that the patient would need an epidural, so she brought an I.V. bag prepared for epidural anesthesia to the room. She laid the bag on the counter. The physician ordered an infusion of antibiotics to treat a streptococcal infection, and another nurse brought an I.V. bag mixed with the prescribed antibiotics to the room and laid it on the same counter. Despite clear labeling, Ms. Thao mistakenly picked up the I.V. epidural infusion bag and piggybacked it onto the I.V. line being used for venous infusion. Within minutes Jasimine Grant was in distress. She died several hours later.[15] As with all serious adverse events, there were multiple performance errors and contributing factors, but little attention was paid to the potential for cognitive impairment due to sleep deprivation and fatigue. Ms. Thao was criminally charged by the Wisconsin Attorney General with neglect of a patient causing great bodily harm. The healthcare community in Wisconsin and across the country was shocked that a nurse was charged with criminal negligence for an error due to inattention. Ultimately, Ms. Thao entered into a plea agreement of no contest to two misdemeanors for obtaining and dispensing a prescription drug without a prescription. In return, prosecutors dropped the felony count of neglect of causing a patient great bodily harm, and Ms. Thao was placed on probation for three years. While on probation, she was prohibited from practicing critical care nursing in obstetrics, emergency room, and recovery room nursing.[18] The Wisconsin Board of Nursing suspended Ms. Thao's license for nine months after which her nursing practice was limited for two years. One of the limitations on her practice was that for two years she could not work more than 12 hours in any 24 consecutive hours and could work no more than 60 hours in any seven consecutive days.[16]

Although it is impossible to conclude that these two deaths could have been avoided if the healthcare professionals had been well rested, it seems likely that fatigue was a contributing factor. In the United States, the nuclear power, transportation, and many other industries that provide 24-hour-per-day service have restricted extended work hours because of accidents related to sleep deprivation. Airline pilots and truck drivers have had their work hours restricted by the Occupational Safety and Health Agency (OSHA) for a long time. Airline pilots are not permitted to work for more than eight hours. There are two crews on international flights lasting more than eight hours. The second crew takes over in midair after the first crew has completed its shift. Truck drivers have to take an eight-hour break after a 12-hour shift.[1] The European Union developed the European Working Time Directive in 1993 as a result of sleep deprivation studies. Now, all European countries, including the United Kingdom, have restricted the maximum number of work hours to 48 to 56 hours per week for all workers including those in health care. Denmark limits the work hours of doctors in training to 37 hours per week. New Zealand has had work restrictions for physicians in training for more than 20 years. Their hours are limited to 72 hours per week and 16 hours of consecutive work.[17]

CURRENT STATUS OF WORK-HOUR RESTRICTIONS AND THE POTENTIAL FOR CHANGE

As more is written and more serious harmful events in health care occur where fatigue and extended scheduling are identified as a root cause, patient safety experts, clinicians, and hospital administrators are recognizing the need to address fatigue as a legitimate patient safety concern. Many approaches are being implemented to both raise awareness about the impact of fatigue on clinicians so that they will speak up if they are concerned about their own ability to provide safe care and to design safer systems that limit fatigue in caregivers.

Residents

At present, no restrictions in the United States limit physician work hours other than those for residents as described earlier in this chapter. See the middle column on Table 24.1 for the 2003 ACGME-mandated duty restrictions.

Although critics generally agree that resident sleep deprivation and fatigue is an issue, many in the medical community openly voice their objections to the 2003 ACGME-mandated duty-hour restrictions because of other competing and compelling needs. These objections include:

- Residents do not work enough hours to gain adequate experience and education. As a result they are not prepared to practice independently upon graduation.[18] In the United States, physicians must be competent to work independently upon completion of their graduate medical education. This is dissimilar from physicians who train in Europe where they continue to be mentored for years following training until they function at an expert level.[19]
- Limited duty hours do not prepare residents for the rigors of medical practice. Today, many residents work fewer hours than attending physicians. Residents must experience long hours so they are trained to endure difficult circumstances when providing medical services.[21]
- Duty hour restrictions foster a shift mentality rather than professionalism because residents are required to leave once they have reached the maximum duty-hour limit, even if it is at a critical moment in their patients' care.[22,23]
- Residents falsify documentation of the hours they work because they are highly motivated to avoid accreditation citations related to noncompliance of duty-hour restrictions for their programs, which would place their training at risk.[20] This is true even when they stay to complete their work, remain with a patient, or want to gain additional hands-on experience.
- Duty-hour restrictions have increased the number of handovers of patients among the residents, thus increasing discontinuity of care and increasing the risks of communication failures.[21]

2008 Recommendations of the Institute of Medicine on Duty Hours

The Institute of Medicine (IOM) serves as adviser to the nation to improve health. Established in 1970 under the charter of the National Academy of Sciences, the IOM provides independent, objective, evidence-based advice to

TABLE 24.1. Comparison of the 2003 ACGME Duty Hour Limits with the Current Requirements

Variables	2003 Acgme Duty Hour Limits	2011 Acgme Duty Hour Limits
Maximum hours of work per week	80 hours, averaged over 4 weeks	The same including moonlighting.
Maximum shift length	30 hours (admitting patients up to 24 hours then 6 additional hours for transitional and educational activities)	• Duty period of PGY-1 residents must not exceed 16 hours in duration. • Duty residents of PGY-2 residents and above may be scheduled to a maximum of 24 hours of continuing duty in the hospital. Strategic napping, especially after 16 hours of continuous duty, and between the hours of 10pm and 8am is strongly suggested. • Residents may remain on site for an additional 4 hours for patient safety and education under exceptional circumstances.
Maximum in-hospital on-call frequency	Every third night, on average	Every third night on average for PGY-2 and above residents.
Minimum time off between scheduled shifts	10 hours after shift length	• PGY-1 residents should have 10 hours and must have 8 hours, free of duty between scheduled duty periods. • Intermediate-level residents should have 10 hours free of duty, and must have 8 hours between scheduled duty periods. They must have at least 14 hours free of duty after 24 hours of in-house duty. • Residents in the final years of education may care for patients over irregular or extended periods.
Maximum frequency of in-hospital night float	Not addressed	• Residents must not be scheduled for more than 6 consecutive nights of night float.
Mandatory time off duty	4 days off per month 1 day (24 hours) off per week, averaged over 4 weeks	• The same. • At-home calls cannot be assigned on the free days.

(*continues*)

TABLE 24.1. Comparison of the 2003 ACGME Duty Hour Limits with the Current Requirements (*Continued*)

Variables	2003 Acgme Duty Hour Limits	2011 Acgme Duty Hour Limits
Moonlighting	Internal moonlighting is counted against 80-hour weekly limit	Internal and external moonlighting is counted against 80-hour weekly limit. All other duty hour limits apply to moonlighting in combination with scheduled work. PGY-1 residents are not allowed to moonlight.
Limit on hours for exceptions	88 hours for select programs with a sound educational rationale	No change.
Emergency room limits	12-hour shift limit, at least an equivalent period of time off between shifts; 60-hour work week with additional 12 hours for education	No change.
At-home call	No limit	Time spent in the hospital must count towards the 80-hour maximum weekly hour limit. It must not be so frequent or taxing as to preclude rest or reasonable personal time.

policy makers, health professionals, the private sector, and the public. At the request of Congress and under a contract with the Agency for Health Care Research and Quality (AHRQ), IOM formed a committee to:

1. synthesize current evidence on medical residents' schedules and healthcare safety, and
2. develop strategies to enable optimization of work schedules to improve safety in the healthcare work environment.[22]

The Committee was formed in 2007 and released its report a year later. The Committee was called Committee on Optimizing Graduate Medical Training (Resident) Hours and Work Schedules to Improve Patient Safety. The report is titled "Resident Duty Hours: Enhancing Sleep, Supervision, and Safety." The Committee examined whether residents' duty hours and schedules could be improved to reduce sleep deprivation, performance degradation, and the risk of error. It had 17 members and was chaired by Michael M. E. Jonce, MD, Chancellor of Emory University, Atlanta, Georgia. It performed extensive literature reviews and conducted hearings in which testimony was received from multiple stakeholders.[25]

The report calls for reduction in resident duty hours currently permitted by the ACGME. Table 24.1 shows a comparison of IOM Committee recommendations to current ACGME duty-hour limits.

A study conducted for the IOM estimates that adopting their recommendations will cost the healthcare system at least $1.7 billion per year. Although this is a large sum of money, it is less than 0.1 % of what is currently spent on health care in the United States. Although uncertain at this time, if implementation of the IOM recommendations improves patient safety and reduces medical errors in the nation's teaching hospitals, it may prove cost effective.[23]

ACGME Response to the 2008 IOM Report on Duty Hours

In an open letter to the GME community, dated October 28, 2009, Thomas Nasca, MD, chief executive officer of the ACGME, discussed the work of the ACGME Resident Duty Hour Task Force (Task Force), chaired by Susan Day, MD, chair of the ACGME board of directors, and E. Stephen Amis, MD, chair of the Council of Review Committees of the ACGME. The Task Force is charged with responding to the IOM's recommendations on duty hours. In December 2008, upon receipt of the IOM report, the Task Force began its review of literature, data regarding the duty-hour restrictions, and the testimony of many stakeholders. The work of the Task Force also coincides with the ACGME's commitment to review the effectiveness of 2003 duty-hour restrictions five years after their implementation. In his letter, Dr. Nasca thoughtfully discussed duty-hour restrictions, along with other complex issues involved in resident education and training. These issues include patient safety, supervision, the need to prepare residents for independent practice, the traditional model of resident assignments, and the need to understand a multitude of factors that contribute to fatigue in addition to loss of sleep.[22] The ACGME will consider all of these issues as it moves forward with its revised standards on duty hours. The Task Force is expected to complete its recommendations by September 2010. Any new or revised standards are to be implemented in July 2011.[22]

Nursing Profession's Response to the 2004 IOM Report on Nursing and Patient Safety

Longer shifts and the use of overtime have increased as hospitals face a shortage of nurses.[7] Despite evidence that shift work and sleep deprivation result in nursing errors, and the explicit recommendations of the IOM on nurses' work hours, little has been done. As of March 2010, only 15 states had restricted mandatory overtime. Of these 16 states, only California, Illinois, Maine, and West Virginia limit the length of work hours or require prescribed time off between shifts.[24]

No state precludes voluntary overtime. The practice of having nurses volunteer to work overtime after a very long shift is especially concerning because self-assessment of one's alertness and performance is unreliable when deprived of sleep. Such self-assessment often reflects a perception of being in control of a situation rather than an accurate assessment of the risk of making an error.[1,7] Disappointingly, the ANA shifted sole responsibility to the individual nurse in its position statement in 2006, *Assuring Patient Safety: Registered Nurses' Responsibility in All Roles and Settings to Guard Against Working When Fatigued.* It states that it is the ethical duty of each nurse to self-determine whether she or he will accept longer hours.[25] Self-regulation in light of compelling economic needs or employer demands is a weak and unreliable method of addressing safety concerns related to sleep deprivation and fatigue.

Solutions and Alternatives

Solutions that are dependent on an increase in full-time equivalent positions are not possible because there is a lack of resources and a fixed supply, or shortage, of qualified individuals. This is especially true given the economic difficulties facing health care in the United States today; therefore, we need to look at other creative approaches to ensure that residents and nurses are rested and able to perform safely.

Increasing Sleep Through Alternative Schedules

The best way to overcome sleep deprivation is to sleep an adequate number of hours in sync with one's circadian rhythm. Although the care and treatment of patients at night will always be needed, resident training programs and the nursing profession should research new and varying approaches to shift work to find better alternatives to extended work hours. Many residency programs have successfully utilized *night float* physician coverage, which allows for 12-hour shifts rather than the current 24- to 30-hour shifts. The night float resident comes in at 8 pm and leaves at 8 am.

Several program directors reported at the annual ACGME Annual Educational Conference in March 2010 that they have eliminated 30-hour on-call shifts because they found the 2003 duty-hour restrictions were not meeting the intended goal for patient safety and resident well-being. For example, Mautone and Cennimo reported that since July 2004 they have successfully eliminated on-call duty in their respective pediatric and internal medicine programs by implementing day and night shift rotations incorporating a team approach. Because of a sufficient number of residents and converting from an every fourth night call schedule, the number of hours residents worked per week has remained consistent with the 2003 ACGME duty-hour model. They found instituting day and night shifts increased continuity of patient care because residents were on two week block schedules caring for their own team's patients.[26]

Many sleep studies have found that naps and longer sleep periods of four to five hours can help mitigate some of the effects of fatigue during night shifts and extended duty periods. A 15-minute nap benefits fatigue and performance for a few hours whereas a four-hour sleep period benefits performance for up to 10 hours.[27] The longer the sleep, the greater are the benefits on performance and the longer the benefits last. However, if naps are used to combat the effects of sleep deprivation while on call, sleep inertia should be taken into consideration when a resident needs to be suddenly awakened. All residents and nurses should be educated on the strategic use of naps and sleep inertia.

Improve Communication Techniques

Utilizing effective communication techniques at all times when discussing patient information is important, but it is especially critical when one is tired. It is essential that all physicians and nurses receive education and training on effectively communicating patient information. All healthcare institutions should require effective communication and monitor it for quality. The process of communicating when transitioning responsibility for patient care is commonly called *handovers*. Handovers in patient care have always been a part of providing care to patients, yet breakdowns in communication remain a substantial source of errors and risks to patients. Handovers are also referred to as hand-offs, transfers, or sign out. It is handing over a responsibility from one healthcare provider to another. Information transferred during handovers includes the patient's name, bed location, vital signs, diagnosis, medications, treatment, psychosocial background, and other critical data. Because healthcare services must be available 24 hours daily, transferring information and responsibility from one team member to another is necessary, sometimes several times a day. In a hospital setting, where teams of attending physicians, residents, and nurses are responsible for a single patient's continuity of care, comprehensive handover of patient information from one to another is a necessity. Because the number of hours that residents work decreased with the ACGME 2003 duty-hour restrictions, the frequency of handovers between residents increased. Many believe that the increased need to transfer patient information has negated any benefit gained from the duty-hour restrictions.[24]

Handovers take place at multiple levels. They occur between individual providers from one shift to the next, as well as among teams of nurses, teams of physicians, and teams of residents. They also occur between the primary provider and consulting physicians and occur when the patient is transferred between care units and different clinical departments. For example, multiple handovers occur among various teams within hours when a patient is seen in the emergency department and then sent to surgery, postoperative care, and to the floor for care. Handovers also occur between different hospitals and between hospitals and nursing homes or home care settings.

With each handover, there is the possibility for the dilution, or omission, of information that can lead to inaccuracies that affect patient care and outcomes.[24] The Joint Commission, which accredits hospitals, has required a standardized approach to handovers since 2006. Handovers should incorporate the following elements:

- Face-to-face interactions
- A set location and time for handovers to occur
- Minimal interruptions
- Structured content to ensure that all relevant information is transmitted
- Uniform language or terminology
- Sufficient time to interact and clarify questions or concerns with overlapping shifts
- Presence of a supervisor to oversee the process and answer additional questions[31]

In addition to the above elements, handovers must be tailored to meet the needs of specific specialties and units. For example, the critical details in a handover for obstetrical patients differ significantly from those for a cardiac patient.

With the increasing use of electronic health records in hospitals, patient information should be more readily accessible around the clock to all healthcare providers, thus reducing medical errors and improving patient safety.

Good communication is required every time information is exchanged. Many healthcare systems are adopting situational briefing techniques such as situation, background, assessment, and recommendation (SBAR). Such techniques provide a standardized framework that facilitates communication of critical information.[32] Other techniques or processes that integrate an opportunity to confirm information and ask questions, such as multidisciplinary rounds, read-backs, and face-to-face conversations should be used to improve communication.

Education and Research

Education on patient safety is fundamental in establishing a culture of safety in medicine and nursing. All healthcare providers and administrators should be educated on sleep deprivation and fatigue, and their associated effects on medical and nursing errors, to create a greater understanding among those who control the scheduling of residents and nurses. Additionally, education regarding communication techniques for handovers and the exchange of information is critical so that those working on the same patient care team have a common framework and understand the organizational expectation.

As mentioned earlier, one of the core purposes of resident training is education. If resident training hours are redesigned to utilize night shift work, graduate medical education must establish educational opportunities during those shifts. This can be accomplished by employing multiple approaches to night time education by utilizing electronic and online resources. Similarly, nursing must ensure that nursing education is equally available for those who work night shifts as it is for those who work day shifts.

Although a great deal of research is already available, more is needed on managing sleep deprivation and fatigue in healthcare settings. This will be particularly true as extended work hours are eliminated and alternate scheduling is attempted. Before major changes are made, pilot testing and research should be conducted to determine whether various staffing patterns increase the quantity or quality of sleep and reduce the number and severity of medical errors. As noted earlier, there are empirical reports from many within the medical community that it is imperative to train residents to endure long work hours so that they can function under stressful circumstances. It is important to objectively measure this. Last, to address concerns within the medical community as to whether graduating residents are ready for unsupervised practice, research should be conducted to determine whether residents' fund of medical knowledge and skills are diminished with reduced hours.

CONCLUSION

Generations of physicians have accepted that sleep deprivation is a necessary part of resident training. More recently, nurses have been required to work longer hours. Research clearly demonstrates that residents and nurses who are sleep deprived are more likely to make serious medical errors because of decreased cognitive functioning and performance. Graduate medical education and the nursing profession should address sleep deprivation and fatigue by implementing scheduling designs that are supported by research. They must also use known communication techniques and other patient safety measures that support healthcare providers in delivering safe patient care. Failure to do so will lead to avoidable medical errors and may ultimately result in governmental and regulatory oversight at the expense of professional self-governance.

References

1. Dinges, D. F. An overview of sleepiness and accidents. (1995). *Journal of Sleep Research, 4*(Suppl 2), 4–14.
2. Friedman, R. C., Bigger, J. T., & Kornfield, D. S. (1971). The intern and sleep loss. *New England Journal of Medicine, 285*, 201–203.
3. Landrigan, C. P., Rothschild, J. M., Croniu, J. W., Kauschal, R., Burdick, E., Katz, J. T., . . . Czeisler, C. A. (2004). Effect of reducing interns' work hours on serious medical errors in intensive care units. *New England Journal of Medicine, 351*(18), 1838–1848.
4. Philibert, I. (2005). Sleep loss and performance in residents and nonphysicians: A meta-analytic examination. *Sleep, 28*(11), 1392–1402.
5. Accreditation Council for Graduate Medical Education. *Common requirements for one-year fellowships*. Retrieved from http://www.acgme.org/acWebsite/home/One_Year_Common_Program_Requirements.pdf.
6. Page, A. (ed.). (2004). *Keeping patients safe: Transforming the work environment of nurses*. Washington, DC: National Academies Press.
7. Rogers, A. E., Wei-Ting, H., Scott, L.D., Aiken, L. H., & Dinges, D. F. (2004). The working hours of hospital staff nurses and patient safety. *Health Affairs, 24*(4), 202–212.
8. American Nurses Association. (2006). *Assuring patient safety: The employers' role in promoting healthy nursing work hours for registered nurses in all roles and settings*. Retrieved from http://gm6.nursingworld.org/MainMenuCategories/Policy-Advocacy/Positions-and-Resolutions/ANAPositionStatements/Position-Statements-Alphabetically/AssuringPatientSafety.pdf.
9. Rogers, A. E. (2002). Sleep deprivation and the ED night shift. *Journal of Emergency Nursing, 28*, 469–470.
10. Joint Commission Resources. (2008). *Strategies for addressing health care worker fatigue*. Oakbrook Terrace, IL: Joint Commission on Accreditation of Healthcare Organizations.
11. Williamson, A. M., & Feyer, A. (2000). Moderate sleep deprivation produces impairments in cognitive and motor performance equivalent to legally proscribed levels of alcohol intoxication. *Occupational and Environmental Medicine, 57*, 649–655.
12. Lockley, S. W., Barger, L. K., Ayas, N. T., Rothschild, J. M., Czeisler, C. A., Landrigan, C. P., & Harvard Work Hours, Health and Safety Group. (2007). Effects of health care provider work hours and sleep deprivation on safety and performance. *Joint Commission Journal on Quality and Patient Safety, 33*(11 Supp), 7–18.
13. Akerstedt, T. (2003). Shift work and disturbed sleep/wakefulness. *Occupational Medicine, 53*(2), 89–94.

14. Chokroverty, S. (2006). Sleep disorders. *ACP Medicine Eds*. Dale, David et al. WebMD and American College of Physicians, Philadelphia; 2360–2362. Retrieved from http://www.acpmedicine.com/bcdecker/pdfs/acp/1176.pdf.
15. Jay, S. M., Lemond, N., Ferguson, S. A., Dorrian, J., Jones, C. B., & Dawson, D. (2007). The characteristics of recovery sleep when recovery opportunity is restricted. *Sleep, 30*(3), 353–360.
16. Cavallo, A., Ris, M. D., & Succop, P. (2003). The night float paradigm to decrease sleep deprivation: Good solution or a new problem? *Ergonomics, 46*(7), 653–663.
17. Lerner, B. H. (2011, August 14). A life-changing case for doctors in training. *The New York Times*. Retrieved from http://www.nytimes.com/2009/03/03/health/03zion.html?_r = 1.
18. Cady, R. F. (2009). Criminal prosecution for nursing errors. *JONA's Healthcare Law, Ethics and Regulation, 11*(1), 10–6.
19. State of Wisconsin before the Board of Nursing. (2006, December 14). Final Decision and Order LS0612145NUR. Retrieved from https://online.drl.wi.gov/decisions/2006/ls0612145nur-00075545.pdf.
20. Landrigan, C. P., Czeisler, C. A., Barger, L. K., Ayow, N. T., Rothschild, J. M., & Lockley, S. W. (2007). Effective implementation of work hour limits and systemic improvements. *Joint Commission Journal on Quality and Patient Safety, 33*(11 Suppl), 19–29.
21. Millard, W. B. (2009). For whom the bell tolls: Unintended effects of limiting residents' hours. *Annals of Emergency Medicine, 54*(4), 25A–29A.
22. Nasca, T. J. (2009, October 27). *Open letter to the GME Community*. Retrieved from http://www.acgme.org/acWebsite/home/NascaLetterCommunity10_27_09.pdf.
23. American Medical Association. *Can the profession effectively self-regulate residents' duty hours?* Retrieved from http://www.ama-assn.org/ama/pub/education-careers/graduate-medical-education/question-of-month/can-profession-self-regulate.page.
24. Arora, V. M., Johnson, J. K., Meltzer, D. O., & Humphrey, H. J. (2008). A theoretical framework and competency-based approach to improving handoffs. *Quality & Safety in Health Care, 17*, 11–14.
25. Institute of Medicine. (2008). *Resident duty hours: Enhancing sleep, supervision, and safety*. Washington, DC: National Academies Press. Retrieved from http://www.iom.edu/~/media/Files/Report%20Files/2008/Resident-Duty-Hours/residency%20hours%20revised%20for%20web.pdf.
26. Nuckols, T. K., Bhattacharya, J., Wolman, D. M., Ulmer, C., & Escarca, J. J. (2009). Cost implications of reduced work hours and workloads for resident physicians. *New England Journal of Medicine, 360*, 2202–2215.
27. American Nurses Association. *Mandatory overtime*. Available at: http://indiananurses.org/documents/Mandatory-ovettime-article.pdf.
28. American Nurses Association. (2006, December 8). *Assuring patient safety: Registered nurses' responsibility in all roles and settings to guard against working when fatigued*. Retrieved from http://www.nursingworld.org/MainMenuCategories/WorkplaceSafety/Work-Environment/NurseFatigue/AssuringPatientSafety_1.pdf.
29. Mautone, S., & Cennimo, D. (2010, March 6). *Surviving and thriving without 24-hour call: The art and science of schedule re-engineering*. Presentation at the 2010 ACGME Annual Educational Conference in Nashville, Tennessee. Retrieved from http://www.hourswatch.org/storage/PPT-%20Surviving%20and%20Thriving.pdf.
30. Driskell, J. E., & Mullen, B. (2005). The efficacy of naps as a fatigue countermeasure: A meta-analytic integration. *Human Factors, 47*(2), 360–377.
31. Arora, V. M., & Farnan, J. M. (2008). Care transitions for hospitalized patients. *Medical Clinics of North America, 92*(2), 315–324.
32. Joint Commission on Accreditation of Healthcare Organizations. *Facts about 2006 National Patient Safety Goals*. Retrieved from http://www.teacherweb.com/NY/StBarnabas/Law-PublicPolicy/JCAHO-JCAHO-NPSG-2006~.pdf.
33. World Health Organization Collaborating Centre for Patient Safety Solutions. (2007). *Communication during patient hand-overs*. Geneva, Switzerland: World Health Organization. Retrieved from http://www.ccforpatientsafety.org/common/pdfs/fpdf/presskit/PS-Solution3.pdf.

25

Supporting Healthcare Providers Impacted by Adverse Medical Events

Allison Caravana Lilly, MSW, LICSW, CEAP

Although our healthcare systems have begun to focus on patient safety and disclosure and apology for unanticipated outcomes in the past decade, less emphasis has been placed on the impact of adverse medical events on the healthcare provider. Dr. Robert Wears in his article, *Human Error in Medicine: Promise and Pitfalls*, eloquently outlines how our healthcare systems are lacking in providing support to both patients and providers when injury is caused to a patient. "There are two sets of victims after a system failure of human error has led to injury, and we have not done a good job helping either. The first group of victims is patients and their families; the second is the healthcare workers involved in the incident."[1] The purpose of this chapter is to look at the impact of adverse medical events on healthcare providers and to outline a program at Brigham and Women's Hospital in Boston, Massachusetts that offers support to clinicians involved in adverse medical events.

Healthcare providers often feel isolated and alone when adverse medical events occur, and in many healthcare environments talking about the event is taboo. However, if we expect our caregivers to disclose their errors to patients and family members, we need to provide a supportive environment that enables them to recover from the event, and in turn, effectively communicate regarding the error or adverse event to both patients and their family members. The term "second victim"[2] is now commonly used to identify the care provider impacted by an adverse medical event.

When clinicians make errors that impact the health and well-being of their patients, it is contrary to the reasons they have gone into medicine: to help alleviate suffering and to cure patients. One study looks at the impact of mistakes on the care provider. Mistakes can cause a "cognitive dissonance between the self-attribution of hard-working, altruistic caregiver and the self-attribution of having harmed the patient."[3] In this small study of 11 physicians, the "mistake" was defined by the physician. Some of the mistakes reported were missed diagnosis and medication errors, and some of the results included death, admission to an intensive care unit, and surgery. The study looked at problem-focused and emotion-focused coping strategies and found that in many cases the emphasis was problem focused versus emotion focused. Study participants perceived that their peers avoided communicating regarding the emotional aspects of their experiences, instead preferring to address the facts of the event.

Medical errors impact physicians on many levels. In a 2007 study by Waterman et al., "The Emotional Impact of Medical Errors on Practicing Physicians in the United States and Canada," 3,171 U.S. and Canadian physicians from internal medicine, surgery, family medicine, and pediatrics were surveyed. Waterman and colleagues looked at five work and life domains of physicians: how medical errors impacted the physicians' job satisfaction, confidence in their ability as physicians, professional reputations, anxiety about future errors, and ability to sleep. The study indicated that 61 % of the physicians reported anxiety about future errors, 44 % reported loss of confidence, 42 % sleep difficulties, and 42 % reduced job satisfaction.[4]

In terms of perceived supports offered by the hospitals in which they worked, 90 % of physicians surveyed in the Waterman et al. study reported that their hospitals did not offer adequate support. Eighty-two percent of those surveyed expressed an interest in counseling but gave the following reasons not to seek help: they believed counseling would not be helpful, they had concerns about confidentiality if sued, and they were concerned that counseling would go on their permanent records.

It is important to examine the support systems of physicians who have been affected by an adverse medical event. In a 2002 study of internal medicine residents, the residents identified "two personal coping strategies most often rated as 'significant' or 'essential for managing stress.'" These strategies involved talking with either family or significant others and talking with other residents.[5]

It is clearly evident that adverse medical events impact caregivers in both their work and personal lives. Healthcare providers report an interest in seeking support and most often find it through peers and family. Yet few healthcare institutions offer formal support mechanisms for clinicians involved in an adverse medical event. An adverse medical event can be career ending for some physicians. Hospital administrative staff and physician leadership must consider what formal supports can be put into place to support clinicians following an adverse medical event.

During the 1980s, Dr. Jeffrey Mitchell coined the phrase "critical incident stress debriefing" (CISD), which was embraced by the world of emergency service personnel. He went on to develop the International Critical Incident Stress Foundation (ICISF), which trains and supports teams of first responders to provide psychological debriefing to those having experienced a critical incident. CISDs were expanded to include a multifaceted response to personnel faced with critical incidents. Some of the components include management support, peer support, workplace interventions, and chaplain support. This multifaceted support system is referred to as "critical incident stress management," or CISM.

However, the group intervention outlined in the literature as a critical incident stress debriefing has been hotly contested and researched in the past decade, and the findings have been controversial. Much of the controversy relates to the lack of evidence that debriefings prevent posttraumatic stress disorder. Some literature presents findings that debriefings can create more harm than good. In Devilly, Gist, and Cotton's 2006 article, *Ready! Fire! Aim!*, they review literature related to this controversy and look closely at each component of a CISD and the potential concerns.[6]

One of the major concerns presented by the healthcare system in which I work is described in Devilly et al.'s article regarding reconstruction of a critical event: "Reconstruction may serve to . . . intensify already disturbing reactions by reconnecting the individual with the sources of discomfort well before sufficient distancing has been achieved."[6] We also know that "the vast majority of individuals recover from a traumatic experience without experiencing significant psychopathology."[7,8,9]

In 2002, 58 experts in the field of disaster mental health got together to discuss evidence-based early intervention for victims and survivors of mass violence. Some of their recommendations were to offer psychological first aid, to provide a needs assessment of the individual and groups, to monitor the environment and those affected, and to provide information on resources. Psychological first aid includes protecting survivors from further harm, reducing physiological arousal, mobilizing support for those who are most distressed, keeping families together and facilitating reunions, providing information, and fostering communication and education.[10]

How does a healthcare setting support healthcare providers impacted by an adverse medical event? First one needs to define an adverse medical event. The Harvard Hospitals Concensus Statement defines it as "An injury that was caused by medical management rather than the patient's underlying disease; also sometimes called 'harm', 'injury', or 'complication'. . . . 'Medical management' refers to all aspects of health care, not just the actions or decisions of physicians or nurses."[11] An adverse event may or may not result from an error. An example of an adverse medical event that is not an error is a reaction to a medication or radiology dye. A complication is an amniotic embolism during labor and delivery.

After years of working in the field of health care, I believe that much of what is experienced by healthcare providers has great effect and can be a critical event in their lives and careers. However, the effect of an adverse medical event is different from exposure to a traditional critical incident often defined as a mass casualty or an incident involving violence. An adapted definition of critical incident used by ICISF is any event or series of events which may cause an individual or group to experience unusually strong emotional, cognitive, physical and/or behavioral reactions and have the potential to interfere with the ability to function effectively at work or at home. It is for these events that Partners Healthcare employee assistance program (Partners EAP) has worked to develop an institutional response to supporting healthcare providers. The model used by Partners EAP is adapted from ICISF in consideration of related research and studies.

In any adverse medical event or critical incident that impacts healthcare providers, we consider the Hippocratic Oath, "Do no harm," whenever any form of support or intervention is offered following an adverse medical event. This is why before any service is offered an assessment of the event is conducted.

CONDUCTING AN ASSESSMENT

When a call comes in reporting an adverse medical event or critical incident in one of our healthcare settings, it is important to note the name and position of the caller, time of the call, and a call back number. The caller will naturally tell you the event about which he or she is contacting you. However, one needs to confirm that all those involved have been identified, which shifts have been affected, and how others who were not present at the time of the event may be impacted. For example, there may have been a particularly long resuscitation during a night shift on a unit that led to a patient's death, but the day shift may have been connected to the patient or the patient's family. In assault situations the assessment of the current safety of the staff and/or the unit needs to be determined; until safety is addressed, staff members will be unable to process the impact the event had on them. The demographics of the staff are also important information to gather. Are the nurses on the unit fairly new? Is this their first patient death? What has been the history on this unit related to critical incidents or adverse medical events? Have there been others and what was the response to them? Are there any administrative issues impacting this work group that may be seen as impacting this event (e.g., staffing)?

Although at times it may be obvious why a situation is perceived as a critical incident, at times it may not be so clear. In such situations, the following questions need to be asked: What makes this a critical incident for this work group? Was it a patient who was in such ill health that the outcome was inevitable and the need for treatment in question? Was it that the family was watching the code, or was it that the code should have been called much sooner? By understanding this, responders can best help the caregivers affected by such an event.

PARTNERS EAP'S MODEL FOR RESPONSE: BRIGHAM AND WOMEN'S HOSPITAL PEER SUPPORT TEAM

Partners Healthcare System is made up of multiple Massachusetts hospitals with varying needs and differing opinions on ways to respond to these needs. I have had the privilege to work with Partners hospitals in a variety of ways to respond to caregivers affected by both adverse medical events and critical incidents. The most comprehensive model is at Brigham and Women's Hospital (BWH) in Boston, Massachusetts. As with many new and innovative programs, it took a crisis and a champion to initiate this service. Dr. Frederick van Pelt, while an anesthesiologist at BWH, had a career-altering adverse medical event that led him to champion getting a program off the ground to support caregivers affected by events. In his article, *Peer Support: Healthcare Professionals Supporting Each Other After Adverse Medical Events*,[12] he shares his personal story that led him to gain the support of BWH Chief Medical Officer Dr. Anthony Whittemore and BWH Executive Director of Clinical Compliance and Risk Management Janet Barnes, RN, JD, in 2004 to develop a task force to implement a service to support caregivers like himself affected by adverse medical events. In addition to adverse medical events, the peer support team responds to critical incidents. Critical incidents in a healthcare setting are events that may include but are not limited to sudden death of a coworker, patient death (not involving an adverse event), verbal/physical assault by a patient, and multiple patient deaths.

I had the privilege of working with Dr. van Pelt and EAP Quality Manager Henrietta Menco, LICSW, CEAP, with the support of Partners EAP Director Andrea Stidsen, LICSW, CEAP, in developing a program at BWH.

The BWH model for support for clinicians involved in an adverse medical event includes both individual peer and group support. Individual support is offered to clinicians, ideally by a trained peer provider in the same profession (physicians, nursing, and social work). Group support is offered when a team is involved in an adverse event. All team members are invited to the staff support session, and trained peers assist in facilitation. The group interventions are always led by a mental health clinician. At Partners hospitals, the trained mental health clinicians are from Partners EAP.

In 2004, the first round of training for individual peer and group interventions and team development took place; a large group of hospital staff from multiple disciplines and departments was trained using the ICISF trainers. In 2006–2007, I developed this training by adapting the ICISF model, taking into consideration some of the research concerns outlined earlier in this chapter. Based on my experiences with this model and implementation at other hospitals, I have outlined some recommended steps in developing a team to respond to adverse medical events or critical incidents in a healthcare setting.

GETTING BUY IN

In an ideal situation, a program supporting hospital staff impacted by adverse medical events and critical incidents should be backed by hospital leadership. Besides medicine and nursing, departments with a vested interest in such a program would be the risk management and quality/safety departments. Although Partners EAP has taken the lead with physicians and nurses in the efforts at Partners hospitals, in other systems it may be other departments that take the lead. The model set up at a hospital may vary depending on the role of various departments at the hospital developing such a program. During a time in which many hospitals are working on patient disclosure and apology programs, programs supporting the clinician are a natural extension.

One of the most significant concerns that each team needs to consider is whether the confidentiality of information shared during peer support is protected under state law from discovery in legal proceedings. The peer support process is not covered by peer review protection statutes in Massachusetts. This fact was considered at the early inception of the team and is brought up at team training. Thus, in the worst case scenario, a peer can be subpoenaed to testify in a legal case related to the medical event. At BWH, the decision was made that the value of the support provided to the care providers outweighed the possible legal ramifications, and the team development was supported. At BWH, it was important for team members to hear that hospital leadership supported the benefit of the team over the legal risk related to the medical malpractice case.

ICISF has a training program on team development, much of what has guided me over the years in developing many of the teams I have been involved with. This program is recommended for anyone considering a team at his or her healthcare institution.

CHOOSING TEAM MEMBERS

Team members should be chosen carefully and should represent the multiple disciplines within the hospital. Representation from a variety of disciplines is ideal. In a teaching hospital such as BWH, surgeons, anesthesiologists, primary care, and larger specialty practices should have physician representation. Nursing should have representation from surgical areas, intensive care nursing, and general nursing. The most important aspect of choosing team members is finding people who are respected and compassionate. The people who clinicians reach out to naturally are the ideal people to become members of a team to support peers facing an adverse event. In presenting to managers the need to identify appropriate team members, managers are asked to consider staff members who best fit the criteria: compassionate, interested in helping others impacted by adverse medical events, flexible with their schedules, and respected by their peers.

Part of choosing team members can involve an application and/or an interview of potential candidates, which allows for screening team members. Application information should include applicants' experience with adverse medical events, how they manage their stress, and whether they have had any training in critical incident and stress management. One danger is that if a clinician is still struggling with an adverse event, he or she may be unable to support someone else in a similar situation without his or her own unresolved issues impacting the process. Providing references is another option to consider in choosing team members but can be time consuming depending on the size of the team.

PEER SUPPORT TEAM TRAINING

Partners EAP has developed two-day long trainings for staff interested in participating in a peer support team. The first day is focused on one-to-one support, and the second on group support. These trainings are modeled after the ICISF program.

ONE-TO-ONE PEER SUPPORT TRAINING

One-to-one peer support training begins with defining critical incidents and adverse medical events. Peer support means providing a listening ear in a nonjudgmental way. Peer support is not a critique of medical care because there are other venues for that. Peer support is always voluntary, and some staff, for reasons outlined earlier, may find it harmful rather than helpful. Some stress theory is introduced using the work of Dr. Patricia Watson and Dr. Arieh Y. Shalev[13] and focuses on indicators of successful coping, initial response to trauma, and adaptive and less adaptive responses to stress/trauma. Communication techniques involving listening and meta-messages are discussed.

Next is a group exercise in which participants break out into their disciplines to discuss how to best approach a peer to offer one-on-one peer support. Partners EAP's model for intervention is then outlined. A one-to-one peer support begins with discussing what peer support is, that team members will maintain confidentiality of what is shared within the team, and that the process is voluntary. The second stage of the one-on-one support is listening to peers share their experiences using active listening as outlined earlier. Some time is then spent asking peers who they have for support and how they plan to spend the next few days. Resource information is given about the EAP and psychiatry, and follow-up contact with the peer is coordinated. Throughout the day, team-building exercises are done so group members representing multiple disciplines and departments get a chance to know each other. Role-plays are done to practice listening techniques, one-on-one interventions modeled by the facilitators, and newly learned skill sets.

After the training, all participants are given a card to attach to their hospital badges. One side of the card has the outline for a peer intervention so it can be carried with the peer supporter at all times. On the opposite side of the card is a listing of departments and contact numbers that a peer supporter may need: peer support team leader, EAP, psychiatry, social work, patient relations, and chaplaincy.

GROUP PEER SUPPORT TRAINING

In the group training, the general concepts of critical incidents and adverse medical events are reviewed, along with what one-on-one support involves. After the review, assessment of when a critical incident request comes to the EAP is discussed, emphasizing the importance of gathering information before providing any type of service. Assessment is made to reinforce that it may not be appropriate to provide a group intervention to any or all groups requesting and that enough information should be gathered to make this decision. It is made clear throughout the training that all group interventions are led by a trained mental health clinician. At Partners hospitals, group interventions are led by licensed mental health EAP clinicians who have had training in critical incident stress intervention. After being trained, EAP clinicians are initially paired with experienced EAP clinicians for several interventions prior to facilitating on their own.

Recent research and literature on group interventions is then reviewed at the training. The ICISF model for CISD is discussed and the intervention outlined. Based on the research, the Partners EAP model and its adaptations are presented. The Partners EAP group intervention outlined during the training is a similar process to the one-on-one peer support. However, because the intervention involves a group of people, not just an individual, confidentiality takes a different shape. In the introduction, group members are asked to respect the privacy of each other in terms of what is shared with others during the group session. The second phase of the group is open for members to share their experiences related to the critical incident or adverse medical event. As a means of transition, group facilitators may choose to note some of the themes brought up during the discussion. The third phase of the group process is education on reactions when one is exposed to adverse events. Ideally a facilitator would incorporate some of the information shared during the group process. Potential reactions are normalized and a general time frame for when they should subside is discussed. The final phase in a group support intervention is informing the group about resources, and follow up is offered. During the support session, group members may mention something for which they would like hospital leadership to be made aware. Prior to ending, group facilitators should confirm that the group would like the issue brought to management. Similar to one-on-one support, group training involves team-building exercises and didactic with role-plays to help practice skills being taught.

TEAM DEVELOPMENT

Now that team members have been chosen and have participated in training, the team needs to come together to meet on a regular basis and decide the best way to be activated. The decision regarding this is often done based on the size of the team, the number of possible interventions a team may experience, and the best means for contacting team members at a given institution. At a large hospital that may have several critical incident stress interventions in a month, a monthly team meeting may make sense. At a smaller hospital with an intervention requested every few months, a quarterly meeting may be all that is needed.

In terms of activation, a call to the employee assistance program (EAP) starts the process. The EAP clinician who takes the initial call should complete the assessment. Consideration is made for which team members are most appropriate; an email is then sent to the team. A page is sent to the peer nurse/physician team members in the case of an adverse medical event; a page is sent to a chaplain in the case of a sudden employee death. At BWH, in addition to a call to the EAP, a team pager is held by one of the team leaders. Team leaders are nurses, physicians, and the EAP. The team leaders are responsible for activating the peer clinician supporters and the EAP works to activate the supporting departments: chaplaincy, social work, psychiatry, ethics, and others.

The purpose for regular team meetings is for the team to review any interventions that have occurred since the last team meeting. This serves as a means for the team members to debrief their experiences. Any upcoming training, recent articles, or related information that needs to be shared is done at the meeting. Finally, the team meeting is the place where ongoing training and practice for both individual and group interventions can take place. Maintaining team meetings can be challenging in a healthcare setting where staff members work 24/7.

MARKETING THE SERVICES

After the team has been trained, some of the initial team meetings can be spent working on a marketing plan for how to educate the hospital or healthcare entity about the service. At Partners EAP, we have developed a few educational slides that define adverse medical events/critical incidents, peer and group support services, and how to activate the service. At the team meeting, it is discussed which departments the team feels most would benefit from the service. Managers from those areas are contacted to offer an orientation at a standing staff meeting. Often these departments are represented on the team, and the team member will present to the department the services offered and coordinate with the department manager. Ideally, a few team members from different disciplines will attend orientations.

LESSONS LEARNED

One size does not fit all. Each healthcare institution/entity has different cultures and different needs. One has to develop a response to adverse medical events and critical incidents being fully aware of the culture. BWH has embraced peer support, both one-on-one support and the group model.

The peer support model previously described at BWH is not the same model that is used at Massachusetts General Hospital (MGH). MGH has the number one psychiatry department in the country; while group support is offered by the EAP and peers, the individual interventions are done only by mental health professionals.

One must always be aware of the current treatment trends and research in the area of adverse events and critical incidents. Critical incident stress interventions have been a standard intervention in EAPs for the past 30-plus years, but we must continually assess the efficacy of these interventions. EAPs need to be aware of the risks associated with secondary trauma, must make all their services related to adverse events voluntary, and not offer services if there is any risk of potential further harm for participants.

It has been my honor to have been able to bear witness to the incredible healthcare offered at Partners Healthcare hospitals and to support the caregivers impacted by adverse medical events. Every intervention illustrates the level of commitment and care that Partners physicians and nurses give to every patient. The struggle that staff members feel when things do not go as planned or patient outcome is not as expected exhibits the degree of commitment, compassion, and dedication they have to providing the best patient care possible.

References

1. Wears, R. L., Janiak, B., Moorhead, J. C., Kellermann, A. L., Yeh, C. S., Rice, M. M., Jay, G., . . . Woolard, R. (2000). Human error in medicine: Promise and pitfalls, part 1. *Annals of Emergency Medicine, 36*, 58–60.
2. Wu, A. W. (2000). Medical error: The second victim. The doctor who makes the mistake needs help too. *BMJ, 320*, 726–727.
3. Christensen, J. F., Levinson, W., & Dunn, P. M. (1992). The heart of darkness: The impact of perceived mistakes on physicians. *Journal of General Internal Medicine, 7*, 424–431.
4. Waterman, A. D., Garbutt, J., Hazel, E., Dunagan, W. C., Levinson, W., Fraser, V. J., & Gallagher, T. H. (2007). The emotional impact of medical errors on practicing physicians in the United States and Canada. *Joint Commission Journal on Quality and Patient Safety, 33*(8), 467–576.
5. Shanafelt, T. D., Bradley, K. A., Wipf, J. E., & Back, A. L. (2002). Burnout and self-reported patient care in an internal medicine residency program. *Annals of Internal Medicine, 136*(5), 358–367.
6. Devilly, G. J., Gist, R., & Cotton, P. (2006). Ready! Fire! Aim! The status of psychological debriefing and therapeutic interventions: In the work place and after disasters. *Review of General Psychology, 10*(4), 318–345.
7. Cook, J. D., & Bickman, L. (1990). Social support and psychological symptomatology following a natural disaster. *Journal of Traumatic Stress, 3*, 541–556.
8. Rubonis, A., & Bickman, L. (1991). Psychological impairment in the wake of disaster: The disaster-psychopathology relationship. *Psychological Bulletin, 109*, 384–399.
9. Salzer, M., & Bickman, L. (1999). The short and long term psychological impact of disasters: Implications for mental health interventions and policy. In *Response to Disaster: Psychosocial, Community, and Ecological Approaches*, ed. R. Gist and B. Lubin, pp. 63–82. Philadelphia: Brunner/Maze.
10. National Institute of Mental Health. (2002). *Mental health and mass violence: Evidence-based early psychological intervention for victims/survivors of mass violence. A workshop to reach consensus on best practices.* NIH Publication No. 02-5138. Washington, DC: U.S. Government Printing Office. Retrieved from http://www.nimh.nih.gov/health/publications/massviolence.pdf.
11. Massachusetts Coalition for the Prevention of Medical Errors. (2006). *When things go wrong: Responding to adverse events. A consensus statement of the Harvard hospitals.* Retrieved from http://www.macoalition.org/documents/respondingToAdverseEvents.pdf.

12. van Peelt, F. (2008). Peer Support: Healthcare Professionals Supporting Each Other After Adverse Medical Events. *Qual Saf Health Care, 17*(4), 249–252.

13. Watson, P. J., & Shalev, A. Y. (2005). Assessment and treatment of adult acute responses to traumatic stress following mass traumatic events. *CNS Spectrums, 10*(2), 123–131.

Acknowledgments

The work outlined in this chapter was a joint effort by a multitude of individuals. Thanks to the BWH task force, made up of leaders from various departments in the hospital who spent months conceptualizing the peer support program. Dr. Frederick van Pelt and his relationship with his patient, Linda Kenney, was a catalyst for this program. Countless hours were spent with Dr. van Pelt and Henri Menco, MSW, in developing the ideas and program outlined in this chapter and making them happen. Nursing support was added by Barbara DiTullio, RN, and Carole Kubiak, RN. After Dr. van Pelt left his position at BWH, Dr. Jo Shapiro stepped into the leadership role and further developed the education and resources for physicians. Last, but not least, are the hours spent by the team supporting each other in the face of adverse events.

On a personal level, I would like to thank my colleague and editor Lisa Staffiere, MSW, for her continued support and red pen.

26

Patient Handoffs—Perils and Opportunities

George R. Cybulski, MD, FACS

INTRODUCTION

Few situations illustrate more significantly the degree of fragmentation and disjointedness of healthcare delivery and its contribution to potential perils for patient safety than the transition of responsibility between various caregiver groups or areas of a healthcare organization and the communication of vital clinical information during this transition that occurs with patient handoffs. Patient handoffs as a transfer of responsibility between caregivers and a transition with potential for gaps in continuity of care require pointed and specific conveyance of a patient's clinical and social information from one caregiver to another. As such, essential information about the identity and the medical condition of the patient including present health statistics (vital signs), diagnosis, ongoing treatment, prior history of response to treatment, and a potential plethora of additional relevant clinical and social information must be communicated in a comprehensive and meaningful way between the groups or individuals exchanging responsibility for the patient. Examples of handoffs include nursing shift changes, on-call overnight residents signing out to day-shift residents, patient transfers from medicine service to surgery service, patients leaving a nursing unit to go to diagnostic testing, and patients entering the operating room for surgery or leaving the operating room for the recovery room.

Patient handoffs in the healthcare setting differ substantially from handoffs in other arenas, such as sports, and in industries such as air traffic control. In sports, for example, the handoff involving a football entails mechanical performance of transferring an object from one player to another. These steps are typically outlined, choreographed, and rehearsed repeatedly. Similarly, air traffic control handoffs of aircraft follow a tightly scripted algorithm with standardized communication formats that air traffic controllers and flight crews have been trained to follow repeatedly, with emphasis on teamwork that is instrumental in developing consistency and trust in the instructions provided by air traffic controllers and air crews.

In contrast, patient handoffs historically have not been standardized, analyzed for effective communication technique, nor practiced to improve efficiency and decrease error.[1] In addition, the sheer volume of data, including laboratory results and radiology and pathology reports available for patient handoffs, is daunting not only from the aspect of collating and presentation but also from the clinically more significant aspect of discriminating the importance of data. Consequently, the patient handoff often becomes a rote recitation of laboratory values for each patient, which numbs the senses with its monotony and, as in the sports analogy, results in dropping the ball or failing to recognize the significance of a change in the trend of the laboratory values or a radiology finding.

The essential nature of the communication process, which is a key component of handoffs, and its link to patient care and safety is a serious problem in the United States healthcare delivery system. The Joint Commission's Sentinel Event Database indicates that breakdown in communication was the root cause of error in more than 65% of 3,811 sentinel events, of which 75% of the communication breakdowns were linked to fatal events. Patient handoffs themselves were associated with more than half of the sentinel events analyzed by The Joint Commission.[2] The significance of these findings, along with indications that during an average five-day hospitalization a patient is passed between doctors an average of 15 times and that on average a first-year internal medical resident will sign over as many as 300 patients in a single month, points to the frequency of exposure of patients to handoffs and their accompanying risks.[3]

To identify the source of these communication lapses involved in handoffs the "moving parts" of a healthcare organization, including the nature of the patient care groups, must be analyzed. Analysis involves looking at the makeup of the provider groups and their unique training, motivation, culture, and philosophical perspectives and how these factors influence communication.

The healthcare delivery system in which these groups operate must also be understood in terms of the effect that systems thinking has on communication processes during patient handoffs. With this information, the strategies to improve patient handoffs currently in practice can be assessed, and paradigms from other critical responsibility industries such as aviation and nuclear power, along with opportunities for innovation and improvement in patient handoffs, can be considered.

ROOT CAUSE ANALYSIS OF HANDOFF ERRORS: PROCESS OF HANDOFFS

The essence of handoffs is communication. Communication, whether by person to person or by person to machine (audio recordings) is usually a two-way process.[4] Communication can either be written or oral and therefore the process and the content form the most important components of communication. The communication process itself is affected by many variables or characteristics of the sender and receiver and the environment in which the exchange of information takes place. The person providing the handoff has significant discretionary control over the information provided. Such subjectivity can influence the quality and quantity of information provided. For example, the person providing the handoff may be influenced by factors such as fatigue and outside social commitments. Similarly, the person receiving the handoff may be experiencing sensory overload in attempting to assimilate new information involving several patients. The level of experience of the person providing the handoff weighs heavily on the emphasis placed on the various bits of clinical data, as well as their inclusion or exclusion. Pasteur said, "the eye sees what the mind knows." Horwitz et al. showed that the omission of key information, such as the patient's clinical condition, results of recent events, tasks to complete, and specific action plan, occurred routinely resulting in significant patient consequences.[5] Furthermore, medical training is heavily concentrated on assimilation of medical knowledge, but the history taking—physical examination process that stresses physician-to-patient communication, physician-to-physician communication, and physician communication with other clinical staff—is not emphasized nor practiced.[1] Analysis of communication failures in patient handoffs in a university teaching hospital medical service that led to adverse events or near misses indicated mainly content omissions (e.g., medications, treatments, test results, consult recommendations, active medical problems, etc.) or lack of face-to-face communication. Other studies of the taxonomy of communication failures in handoffs identified lack of supervision and anticipatory guidance (instructions for possible contingencies) and rationale for the plan of action. As a consequence, other types of inefficiencies also arise due to delays in the implementation of the care plan.[5] A recommendation to address this issue is the implementation of standardized handoff communication as identified in The Joint Commission's 2006 National Patient Safety Goals.[6]

In addition, Moorman points out that, although in reality the process of patient care involves many interdependent processes (e.g., nursing, clinical laboratory, radiology, medicine, surgery), historically in medical care there has been a reliance on silos of individual performance in which the potential for flawed communication often leads to adverse patient outcomes.[7]

In a typical handoff scenario, the solitary overnight on-call resident hands off to the oncoming day-shift resident on a number of overnight newly admitted patients amid the hustle and bustle of the hospital awakening for another day. I have participated in this process many times as a resident and I have observed the process as an attending physician supervising residents in training. I can attest that there is a consistently inconsistent aspect of the process of handing off the service.

This situation has become a more frequent and harried scenario since 2003, when the Accreditation Council for Graduate Medical Education (ACGME) mandated the Standards on Resident Duty Hours for resident training programs in the United States in which resident physician duty-hours were limited to 80 hours per week and 24 hours per shift. Formerly on-call residents continued to work well into the next day after being on call and while this effect of fatigue on patient safety led to the restriction of duty hours by the ACGME sign-outs or handoffs were fewer previously than today.[8] Although better-rested resident physicians may arguably lead to improvements in certain aspects of quality of patient care (e.g., better performance of manual tasks), fragmentation of care is exacerbated by more handoffs taking place.

The present restriction of duty hours also creates a type of shift-worker mentality among residents who are basically fighting a holding action on patient care issues during the night on call and offload their responsibilities to the oncoming call resident the next day.

In addition to the stresses placed on the communication process in this context, most resident handoff processes occur in an ad hoc informal, unstructured, and idiosyncratic manner.[9] Further analysis of resident handoffs indicated that the accompanying environment in more than half the cases was compromised by noise and in a third of the cases frequent interruption.[10]

These findings contrast with nursing handoffs, which occur at shift change, where for the most part there are no tolerated interruptions. In addition, the processes of handoffs for physicians/residents and nurses mostly occur in parallel with no formal interchange between the two groups of professionals. This fact leads to consideration of another major component of root cause analysis of handoff errors: the culture of health care.

As with many other endeavors (e.g., law, police work, firefighters, soldiers), impartation of culture is an integral component of professional training with strong roots in the historical development of the particular profession. Health care is no exception.

ROOT CAUSE ANALYSIS OF HANDOFF ERRORS: "TRIBES"

In addition to problems with communication of vital patient information during handoffs between members of the same group, such as illustrated with handoffs between resident physicians, the fragmented structure of healthcare organizations creates silos of caregivers with disparate training, motivation, philosophies, and cultures. These groups or tribes as part of their culture develop their own loyalties and jargon that also affect the communication process involved with handoffs.

The culture of health care is composed of a number of groups in some degree as Winston Churchill once said of the British and Americans separated by the English language. The various subcultures or tribes of healthcare providers, while sharing a common goal of patient care, have identified strongly with the philosophies of their own unique training. The two biggest tribes of health care are physicians and nurses ("lions and lambs"). Nurses, in general spend more of their time with hands-on care of patients and are charged with implementing physician orders. Accordingly, nurses often develop strong bonds, attachments, and protective postures for the patients under their care. On the other hand, physicians spend less time with patients performing physical diagnosis as the increased use of technology and procedures positions physicians more and more as proceduralists rather than bedside healers. Physicians themselves are further sub-divided into the camps of internal medicine and surgery with their own philosophies, practice patterns, and esprit de corps, which creates additional barriers to communication across specialties.

Furthermore, the organizational structure of hospitals as the predominant healthcare provider (38% of all U.S. healthcare expenditures in 2004 as reported by the Center for Medical Services) has historically solidified the power of resource allocation and care decisions to physicians operating autonomously.[11] As such, the interactions between nurses and physicians, the principal caregiver groups, separated by distinct cultural backgrounds and inequities of power, are ripe for dispute, conflict, and miscommunication, which create barriers to safe and effective patient care. Asymmetry of power, in particular, inhibits a free flow of communication.

The authors of a 2004 survey reported that less than 15% of nurses and physicians had an "excellent" relationship and less than 25% characterized their professional relationship as "very good" (Bartholomew and Bujack, personal communication). Consequently, the Institute of Healthcare Improvement has cited culture as the greatest impediment to patient safety.[2]

WAYS TO IMPROVE HANDOFFS

To improve patient handoffs and accordingly patient safety, modalities to improve the process of communication have been developed, including methods used by other industries. The problem with patient handoffs is in developing a standardized format. Vidyarthi et al. proposed the Who, What, Where, When, and How checklist: *Who* should participate in the handoff process? *What* content needs to be verbally communicated? *Where* should the handoff occur? *When* is the optimal time for handing off? *How* should verbal communication be performed?[9]

Another method is the Top 10 List for a safe and effective handoff for surgical patients.[12] The Top 10 List of guidelines for surgical resident handoffs include:

1. Time (ensure enough time for adequate handoff on every patient).
2. Active (make handing off an interactive process as opposed to a passive send–receive recitation of patient lab values.
3. Sick (emphasize sick patients).
4. Senior (know who the senior resident is).
5. One list (use one standardized list).
6. Details (list every key surgical and medical condition for each patient).

7. Outstanding tasks, labs/studies (hand off all pending lab tests, studies, and consults).
8. Outstanding labs/studies (sign-out or hand off all pending laboratory tests, studies, consults).
9. Admissions (detail expected patient admissions and their plan, for example, OR tomorrow).
10. Morning update (answer or dispose of all pending questions from prior shift).

Regardless of the handoff system employed, training on the system is critical. In addition, breaking down the silos that isolate groups of caregivers has been emphasized, along with larger systemic initiatives that aim to create an overarching culture of safety for a healthcare organization.

Standardizing Handoffs Using Techniques and Tools

Different forms of handoffs have included audiotapes, which have been used for nursing handoffs for years. Checklists and forms have also been utilized for handoffs and allow for a record that can be viewed and referred to by the receiving team.

Sentara Health Care, in Norfolk, Virginia, developed a format called the Five-Ps to organize handoffs.[13] The Sentara model uses the following categories:

- Patient: name, identifiers, age, sex, location
- Plan: diagnosis, treatment plan, next steps
- Purpose: rationale for the care plan
- Problems: explanation about what's different or unusual about this patient
- Precautions: explain what's different or unusual about this specific patient

The Department of Defense's Patient Safety Program uses the mnemonic phrase I PASS the BATON for improving communication in both simple and complex handoffs.[14] The phrase stands for the following: **I**ntroduction, **P**atient, **A**ssessment, **S**ituation, **S**afety concerns (IPASS) the **Ba**ckground, **A**ctions, **T**iming, **O**wnership, **N**ext (BATON).

The SBAR (**S**ituation, **B**ackground, **A**ssessment, **R**ecommendation) is adapted from a communication technique used on nuclear submarines and is used for improving communication exchanges among clinicians.[15]

Studies purporting to identify the use of any specific content for handoffs fail to provide data supporting this premise.[9,16] Due to this lack of supporting data, recommendations for handoffs are based on opinion or personal experience.[16] Another potentially confounding issue with the use of handoff data is the subjectivity of decision making due to anchoring bias, that is the pressure of preformed ideas about clinical data that inhibits processing of new hypotheses based on changing clinical signs and symptoms.[16] Along with the dispersion of responsibility that occurs with multiple handoffs, the opportunity for enlarging gaps due to failure to synthesize data and execute a plan will not be solved by handoff schematics.

Other Lessons from Industry

Continuous process tasks occur in industries such as chemical manufacturing, oil refining, and nuclear material reprocessing. Due to the significant consequences of breakdown of these processes, their study reinforces the focus on communication. Components of communication failure that figured prominently in accidents in these industries were ambiguity of language, failure to consider the different levels of information comprehension (analogous to the difference in clinical acumen and experiences between junior and senior residents), and overreliance on one means of communication, namely one-way, written communication (analogous to handoff lists).

SURGEON INFORMATION TRANSFER AND COMMUNICATION (ITC)

The Information Transfer and Communication Practices (ITCP) project (2007) was a multi-institutional attempt to understand and improve the role of communication in surgical patient care. Among other areas, it was recommended that handoffs or briefings be designed to assure reception, comprehension, action plan, and understanding of barriers to the action plan.[17] Face-to-face communication with interactive communication was the optimal method for clarifying information about complex clinical situations.

More important, the ITCP project emphasized the study and delineation of other unique identifiers that impact resident communication involving patient handoffs for the surgical service. Principally, surgical residents and surgeons are uniquely fluid in their activities in the hospital, going for example from the operating room to the emergency department to see a consult and then "flying" back to the operating room. This common type of encounter involves interaction with a number of different patients and healthcare workers. Opportunities for failure of handoff of care plans are plentiful during these "drive-by" encounters. In such a situation, the ITCP project recommends including in all patient care handoffs all patients seen by the respective surgical team irrespective of their locale (emergency department, medicine floor, etc.) and their disposition plan. A "flash" message would be electronically sent to the respective unit involved in outing the care plan (see below).

INFORMATION TECHNOLOGY

Linking electronic medical records with a handoff tool incorporating automatic real-time downloading of laboratory tests and radiologic procedure results would help to provide critical data to all members of the respective caregiver teams. However, these data still do not supply the rationale for safe decision making, which depends on knowledgeable interpretation that is experiential and discriminatory and is based on familiarity with factors beyond mere data access.

The greater use of asynchronous channels of communication (e.g., PDAs), tightly linked to alerts for significant clinical data (e.g., panic laboratory values, positive chest x-rays, abnormal ECGs), would create a boundaryless modem for communication but must be informed by other process components and cannot replace face-to-face communication.

However, two-way communication, including instant messaging, is still not de riguer even in hospitals that consider themselves savvy in information technology. In one such hospital, for example, I still carry a pager similar to one I carried as an intern in 1980.

Cross Talk Instead of Groupthink

Because health care is delivered by a team of individuals the need to gain the perspective from all members of the team as to how information is best communicated is paramount. Differences in communication style by these team members necessitates discussion between all parties as to how to most effectively communicate essential information.

Cultural Transformation

Standardization of handoff communication and using techniques and tools from other organizations serve as a guide to improving the handoff process. However, the barriers formed by culture among groups require a separate dedicated approach.

One such approach at cultural transformation that breaks down the isolation of groups involved in patient care is the Transforming Care at the Bedside (TCAB) technique. This technique consists of three major components: "moving the location of the shift change report to the bedside, implementing the safety huddle, and establishing nurse-physician rounds at the bedside." The initiative creates a system of interdisciplinary engagement of nurses, physicians, and patients at the bedside.[15]

Additional initiatives for dealing with the multiplicity of cultures and their contributions to the fragmentation of healthcare delivery and its contribution to patient harm is the creation of an overarching culture of safety.

Creating such a culture, which spreads into all of the hospital subcultures of nursing, medicine, and support staff, requires a commitment from senior management. The Singapore-based National Healthcare Group (NHG) describes implementation of such a system in which NHG senior leaders demonstrate their commitment to safety by participating in daily safety walkrounds.[18] In addition, patient safety officers and departmental safety champions are trained to conduct patient safety workshops, perform patient safety surveys, and implement open incident reporting policies.[18]

The involvement of NHG senior hospital management committed to grassroots clinical safety issues offers a unique and contrasting management style from most management styles employed in U.S. companies, especially in healthcare organizations in which a great divide exists between the domain knowledge workers (e.g., nurses and physicians in health care) and the upper-level hospital management (financial engineers).

Teamwork

Inculcation of a team-based culture through interdisciplinary workflow practice is essential to improve communication, break down the silos, and help to develop the innovative systems to improve handoff safety and other processes that cause harm to patients.[7]

A Battle Between Reductionism (Checklists) and Systems Thinking

Newtonian reductionism searches for a single-factor explanation for the complexity of providing health care and the oftentimes unaccountable results of patient reactions to disease processes and treatment.[19] The seduction of searching for a single "broken part" and fixing it explains why as Dekker puts it "Newton has been on retainer for more than three centuries."[19] Are checklists really the answer for increasing healthcare safety, or are we confusing quality for safety?[19]

"The Checklist Manifesto"

The allure of applying checklists to patient handoffs has developed principally from the aviation industry. Parallels do exist. For example crew resource management (CRM), developed by United Airlines in 1980, recognized that, although pilots were technically proficient, their communication or people skills were deficient, a situation not unlike the position of physicians in health care. In the aviation industry, emphasis on communication, prioritizing tasks, delegating authority, and monitoring automated equipment was implemented.[20]

Similar emphasis on checklists has been applied to medicine and surgical handoffs,[9,12] but the efficacy of checklists for surgical handoffs has received mixed reviews. Surgical checklists take handoffs to a point, but the major component of the actual operation lies in the surgeon's head. Unlike an airplane's route, which is strictly outlined point to point, the major component of the actual operation may not be effectively communicated to the rest of the operating room personnel, who therefore may not be able to effectively intervene in the case of an error. In other words, integrated surgical procedures may not be effectively reduced to simple components. Nemeth et al. notes that "operators" do this job so well that observation of the act is not apparent to outsiders or in fact close observers.[21] More comprehensive system thinking required to perform an operation is not easily translatable beyond the marking of the correct side or site of the surgical procedure with surgical checklists. As such, poor surgical results occur with perfect presurgical checklists and time-outs.

CONCLUSION

Handoffs are a significant source of miscommunication and peril for patients. Conversely, handoffs also offer the opportunity for a time of recovery and detection of error. With this emphasis, the stimulus for renewed focus, analysis, and creation of systems for effecting safe patient handoffs is essential. Significant lasting changes that enhance patient safety will be with system change built on the foundation of improving communication and breaking down cultural barriers. Checklists are presently rudimentary at best in achieving these goals.

Therefore, borrowing of systems from other industries to improve patient handoffs is a limited solution. The special nature and culture of patient care requires creation of unique systems developed by healthcare providers with the vested interest and aptitude for improving patient safety.

References

1. Solet, D., Norvell, J., Rutan, G., & Frankel, R. (2005). Lost in translation: Challenges and opportunities in physician-to-physician communication during patient handoffs. *Academic Medicine, 80*(12), 1094–099.
2. Bartholomew, K., & Bujak, J. (2010, March). *Of lions and lambs: Transforming physician-nurse communication*. Presentation at the meeting of the American College of Healthcare Executives, Chicago, Illinois. Retrieved from http://www.youtube.com/watch?v=SyFArqgenzU accessed May 10, 2012.
3. Chen, P. W. (2009, September 3). When patient handoffs go terribly wrong. *The New York Times*. Retrieved from www.nytimes.com/2009/09/03/health/03chen.html.
4. Arora, V., Manjarrez, E., Dressler, D., Basaviah, P., Halasyamani, L., & Kripalani, S. (2009). Hospitalist handoffs: A systematic review and task force recommendations. *Journal of Hospital Medicine, 4*(7), 433–440.
5. Horwitz, L., Moin, J., Krumholz, H., Wang, L., & Bradley, E. (2008). Consequences of inadequate sign-out for patient care. *Archives of Internal Medicine, 168*(16), 1755–1768.
6. Joint Commission on Accreditation of Healthcare Organizations. *National patient safety goals for 2006*. Retrieved from www.jointcommission.org/patientsafety/nationalpatientsafetygoals.
7. Moorman, D. (2007). Communication, teams, and medical mistakes. *Annals of Surgery, 245*(2), 173–175.
8. Grady, M., Batjer, H., & Dacey, R. (2009). Resident duty hour regulation and patient safety: Establishing a balance between concerns about resident fatigue and adequate training in neurosurgery. *Journal of Neurosurgery, 110*(5), 828–836.
9. Vidyarthi, A., Arora, V., Schnipper, J., Wall, S., & Wachter, R. (2006). Managing discontinuity in academic medical centers: Strategies for a safe and effective resident sign-out. *Journal of Hospital Medicine, 1*(4), 257–266.
10. Kitch, B., Cooper, J., Zapol, W., Marder, J., Karson, A., Hutter, M., & Campbell, E. (2008). Handoffs causing patient harm: A survey of medical and surgical house staff. *The Joint Commission Journal on Quality and Patient Safety, 34*(10), 563–570.
11. Cebul, R., Rebitzer, J., Taylor, L., & Votruba, M. (2008). Organizational fragmentation and care quality in the U.S. healthcare system. *Journal of Economic Perspectives, 22*(4), 93–113.
12. Kemp, C., Bath, J., Berger, J., Bergsman, A., Ellison, T., Emery, K., Garonzik-Wang, J., . . . Freischlag, J. (2008). The Top 10 List for a safe and effective sign-out. *Archives of Surgery, 143*(10), 1008–1010.
13. Sentara Health Care (2008). *Quality & patient safety*. Retrieved from www.sentara.com/quality.
14. Department of Defense. (2008). *Patient safety program: Healthcare communications toolkit to improve transitions in care*. Retrieved from http://www.oumedicine.com/docs/ad-obgyn-workfiles/handofftoolkit.pdf?sfvrsn=2.
15. Chapman, K. Improving communication among nurses, patients, and physicians. *American Journal of Nursing, 109*(11), 21–25.

16. Enfield, K., & Hoke, G. (2007). Discontinuity of care: Further thoughts on standardized processes. *Journal of Hospital Medicine, 2*(2), 115–116.
17. Williams, R., Silverman, R., Schwind, C., Fortune, J., Sutyak, J., Horvath, K., Van Eaton, E., . . . Dunnington, G. Surgeon information transfer and communication. Factors affecting quality and efficiency of inpatient care. *Annals of Surgery, 245*(7), 159–169.
18. National Healthcare Group. (2008). Create a culture of safety: A case study from the field. *Joint Commission International eZine, 3*(3), 1–12.
19. Dekker, S. W. (2010). We have Newton on a retainer: Reductionism when we need systems thinking. *Joint Commission Journal on Quality and Patient Safety, 36*(4), 147–149.
20. Baron, R. (2002). *CRM: From the instructor viewpoint.* Retrieved from http://airlinesafety.com/editorials/CRM-InstructorsView.htm.
21. Nemeth, C., Cook, R., & Woods, D. (2004). The messy details: Insights from the study of technical work in healthcare. *IEEE Transactions of Systems and Manual Cybernetics, 34,* 689–691.

27

When Employees Are Safe, Patients Are Safer

Kathy Gerwig

INTRODUCTION

When employees are safe, patients are safer. Healthcare workers are at high risk for workplace injuries. Serious injuries result in lost work days and potentially decreased staffing levels; staffing levels directly correlate to patient safety. Injuries can cause discomfort or pain, which makes it more difficult to provide superior care. Organizational culture and policies impact employees and patients and system performance. Improving the organizational climate of hospitals is likely to improve the safety of the employees and the profitability of hospitals through improved system outcomes (such as lower turnover of employees), as well as improved quality of patient care delivered.[1] In this chapter, I will describe what has been written about the hazards inherent in the delivery of health care and the steps that Kaiser Permanente (KP) has taken to improve patient safety by focusing on worker safety.

HEALTH CARE IS A HAZARDOUS OCCUPATION

Health care has one of the highest incidents of occupational injury and illness of any industry in the country. Of the 14 industries with the highest numbers of occupational injuries/illnesses, three are in health care. Hospitals have the greatest number of occupational injuries/illnesses in the private sector according to the Bureau of Labor Statistics (BLS).[2]

Healthcare workers face a wide range of hazards in the workplace according to the National Institute for Occupational Safety and Health (NIOSH). Musculoskeletal disorders and ergonomic issues challenge those who move patients. Lifting, pushing, pulling, carrying, and working in awkward postures can cause injuries, especially to the backs and shoulders of workers. Slips, trips, and falls are significant problems that affect both healthcare workers and patients. And sometimes, one may lead to another—that is, a nurse trying to stop a patient's fall becomes injured or a patient is injured while a nurse slips or trips. Trends indicate that patients are getting older, sicker, and heavier while healthcare workers are also getting older.[3]

The most common injuries among healthcare workers are back injuries and back pain. Healthcare workers experience significantly higher rates of low back disorders than the general population, and nurses are among the professionals with the highest rates. More than 40% of nursing injuries that result in lost workdays are strains and sprains—mostly of the back—and 10.5% of all occupational back injuries in the United States are caused by moving and assisting patients.[4]

Scientific evidence exists that healthcare worker injuries, particularly among nurses, negatively affect patient safety. According to Charney and Schirmer, nursing injuries yield negative patient outcomes because nursing injuries influence staffing ratios, which in turn influence patient safety.[5] Richer nurse staffing is associated with lower failure to rescue rates, lower inpatient mortality rates, and shorter hospital stays.[6] Since the Institute of Medicine released *Crossing the Quality Chasm* in 2001, there has been a growing recognition that improving patient safety must include improving healthcare worker occupational safety.[7]

Injuries can cause discomfort or pain that makes it more difficult to provide superior care. For example, we know from the science of human factors that fatigue, lack of sleep, interruptions and distractions, noise, and stress can adversely impact human performance. It is not unreasonable to assume that the pain associated with serious workplace injuries, and where applicable, medication-based pain management, is another factor that may contribute to human error.

When patient care staff members are involved in medical errors, they experience a tremendous emotional toll. There is also an

FIGURE 27.1 Number of Cases and Incidence Rates of Nonfatal Occupational Injuries/Illnesses for Industries with 100,000 or more Cases, 2010 (numbers are in thousands)

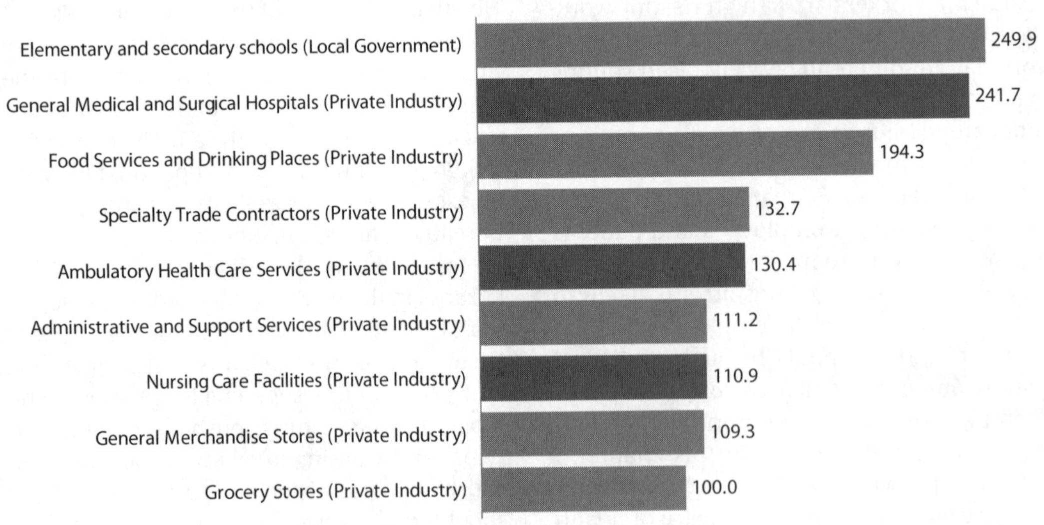
Elementary and secondary schools (Local Government)
249.9
General Medical and Surgical Hospitals (Private Industry)
241.7
Food Services and Drinking Places (Private Industry)
194.3
Specialty Trade Contractors (Private Industry)
132.7
Ambulatory Health Care Services (Private Industry)
130.4
Administrative and Support Services (Private Industry)
111.2
Nursing Care Facilities (Private Industry)
110.9
General Merchandise Stores (Private Industry)
109.3
Grocery Stores (Private Industry)
100.0

Adapted from Bureau of Labor Statistics.[16] Economic News Release: Table 4. Number of cases and incidence rate of nonfatal occupational injuries and illnesses for industries with 100,000 or more cases, 2010. http://www.bls.gov/news.release/osh.t04.htm Last Modified October 20, 2011. Accessed March 21, 2012.

emotional effect when healthcare workers suffer debilitating injuries and can't continue to practice the job they love. Occupational injuries can also result in the loss of income that creates financial hardship for entire families. Coworkers are affected due to staff shortages and staff turnover. Understanding the full consequences of workplace injuries—which go far beyond physical pain—allows leaders from labor unions and KP managers to appreciate the need for comprehensive solutions.

CASE STUDY: CREATING SAFE ENVIRONMENTS AT KAISER PERMANENTE

Kaiser Permanente enjoys excellent relations with its labor unions, and its workplace safety programs have benefited from the involvement of frontline workers who are deeply engaged in program design, implementation, and continuous improvement. In addition to tapping into representative frontline staff to work directly on programs, safety leaders at KP want everyone to understand their role in ensuring safety. Accountability is framed as follows: It is the responsibility of management to create and maintain a safe environment by having the right policies, procedures, systems, tools, equipment, and training in place, and by addressing unsafe conditions in a timely manner. It is everyone's responsibility to work safely and to report any unsafe conditions immediately.

Experience at Kaiser Permanente has taught safety leaders at KP that many of the root causes of adverse patient outcomes are common to root causes of worker injuries. These include:

- Lack of consistent, timely, and positive feedback for performance improvement
- Lack of employee engagement and empowerment
- Unresponsive systems (hazards go uncorrected)
- Miscommunication
- Information deficits
- Conflict between immediate and long-term goals (e.g., performance standards such as operating room turnover may conflict with adequate time to perform the tasks safely)
- Misaligned or conflicting goals among departments
- Lack of contingency planning and response
- Unclear allocation of responsibility
- Breakdown in coordination
- Lack of teamwork
- Inadequate training
- Poor supervision
- Inflexible policies
- Poor labor relations
- Cumbersome technology
- Undue time pressure
- Understaffing/overtasking
- Interruptions/distractions
- Inadequate policies and procedures
- "Drift" or noncompliance with policies and procedures
- Difficulty in speaking up when another staff member is doing something that is unsafe
- Lack of leadership engagement and sponsorship

Addressing these common problems with common solutions can improve both worker and patient safety. Table 27.1 shows some of the concepts, tools, and processes that are applicable to both.

Figure 27.2 shows the 14 drivers of workplace safety, which Kaiser Permanente developed as part of its work with DuPont Sustainable Solutions. All 14 elements need to be in place to achieve the leadership, accountabilities, and actions needed to create a culture of safety. The glue that holds workplace safety and patient safety together is culture—a value of first do no harm to anyone, coupled with measurable attitudes and observable behaviors of safety excellence.

TABLE 27.1 Concepts, tools, and processes for identifying patient and worker safety hazards

Concepts, Tools, and Processes	Patient Safety	Worker Safety
Common causes and contributing factors to adverse events (e.g., excess workload/inadequate staff, fatigue, interruptions or distractions, ergonomics)	X	X
Organizational and system factors are common causes to adverse events	X	X
Human factors analysis	X	X
Hierarchy of controls	X	X
Safety rules, policies, and procedures	X	X
Incident investigation and root-cause analysis	X	X
Performance management and use of metrics and dashboards	X	X
Safety observations and conversations	X	X
Risk prioritization and risk mapping	X	X
Hazard identification	X	X
Walk-arounds	X	X
Time-outs called by staff when significant hazard is present	X	X
Never events reporting and response	X	X
Effective practice sharing improves safety for patients and workers	X	X
Individual accountability and unit-based ownership	X	X
Build safe systems and structures rather than focus on individual staff members	X	X
Requires a culture of safety for success	X	X

FIGURE 27.2 The 14 Drivers of Workplace Safety

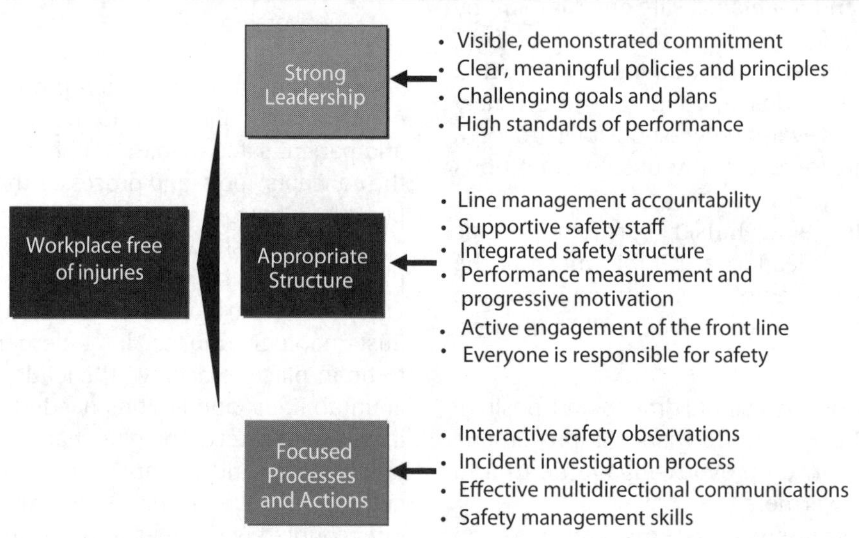
Strong Leadership
• Visible, demonstrated commitment
• Clear, meaningful policies and principles
• Challenging goals and plans
• High standards of performance
Workplace free of injuries
Appropriate Structure
• Line management accountability
• Supportive safety staff
• Integrated safety structure
• Performance measurement and progressive motivation
• Active engagement of the front line
• Everyone is responsible for safety
Focused Processes and Actions
• Interactive safety observations
• Incident investigation process
• Effective multidirectional communications
• Safety management skills

Source:

WORKPLACE SAFETY PROGRAMS AT KAISER PERMANENTE

Kaiser Permanente has committed to pursuing an injury-free workplace. Achievement of safety goals requires a culture of safety, one where employee safety is incorporated into every task, every day. These elements of a culture of workplace safety were created by labor and management representatives at Kaiser Permanente who work in partnership on workplace safety:

- At Kaiser Permanente, safety is a core business and personal value.
- All injuries and all safety incidents are preventable: the goal is zero.
- Line managers are accountable for the safety performance of their employees.
- All employees are accountable for working safely.
- Prevention is more effective and sustainable than postinjury management.
- Safety feedback and observation are everyone's responsibility.
- Employee involvement is critical.
- Employees must receive appropriate training.
- Managers are responsible for ensuring that the systems, equipment, training, and support allow employees to work safely.

These same tenets permeate Kaiser Permanente's patient safety program which recognizes the primacy of frontline engagement, looks to eliminate so-called never events, and strives to create a just culture where staff is accountable for making safe choices and management is accountable for creating and sustaining safe systems.

The following programs at Kaiser Permanente will be detailed in the following sections of this text: comprehensive safety management program, safe patient handling, walkarounds, and systems of safety (SOS), including the hierarchy of controls.

Comprehensive Safety Management Program

The comprehensive safety management program refers to an integrated approach to safety at the medical center and department levels that creates safety through strong leadership, clear accountability structures, and five processes that support safety (safety conversations, incident analysis, multidirectional communication, policies and procedures, and performance management). The program was adapted from an approach developed by DuPont Safety Resources, Inc., who was engaged by Kaiser Permanente from 2004 to 2006 to support implementation of the program at selected Kaiser Permanente medical centers in California. Where all of the program elements are fully effective, the program significantly improves worker safety. Kaiser Permanente is continuing to expand the program to all of its medical centers.

Workplace Safety Program Elements that Support Patient Safety

- Safety conversations (sometimes called safety observations) are in-the-moment, brief communications between staff who engage each other in a positive, proactive discussion about conditions and behaviors. This type of communication does not come naturally to everyone and Kaiser Permanente has training programs to support these conversations. Infusing staff members with freedom to discuss safe behaviors and conditions is consistent with open communication among caregivers about patient safety.
- Incident analysis and root-cause identification prevent recurrence of both worker and patient incidents. Leaders from labor and management create systems to address contributing factors and ensure appropriate improvements.
- Multidirectional communication channels ensure that frontline workers can

easily make their ideas and concerns known to those who can act on them. The channels also facilitate dissemination of effective practices, communication about emergent issues, and improved policies and protocols.

- Incorporating worker and patient safety considerations into all policies and procedures ensures that safety is not an afterthought but a key value that is codified.
- Understanding leading indicators, having systems to track and trend emergent issues, and having feedback mechanisms to see whether performance improvement activities resulted in positive outcomes are all part of worker and patient safety performance management.
- Positive reinforcement is fundamental to securing and sustaining worker involvement in building a culture of safety.
- Clarity of accountabilities enables follow up and follow through, which in turn builds trust—a necessary ingredient to effective and open communication about safety hazards.
- Frontline engagement taps into the experts who are best positioned to determine how to perform work safely.

Safe Patient Handling

Safe patient handling at Kaiser Permanente includes providing lift equipment and devices that reduce hazards associated with transferring, moving, and lifting patients. The program includes training in lift equipment and proper body mechanics. Although they are designed to reduce the incidence, severity, and cost of nursing injuries associated with patient handling, safe patient-handling programs also improve patient care as measured by (1) physical functioning, (2) activity level, (3) ability to maintain activities of daily living, (4) fall prevention, and (5) more wakefulness in the morning.[8] The equipment also minimizes the risk of patient injury caused by poor handling techniques.

Workplace Safety Leadership Walkarounds

Walkarounds are conducted by leaders from labor and management. They include nonthreatening conversations demonstrating that safety is a high priority by listening to frontline workers and asking them to share their workplace safety thoughts and observations. These interactions allow learning opportunities regarding risks, hazards, and root causes. They help improve reporting systems and enhance knowledge about how to ensure a safe workplace. When given the opportunity, with barriers of shame and punishment removed, staff members will effectively voice their thoughts around safety hazards and develop and implement best practices.

Walkarounds create a safer workplace by:

- Visibly showing leadership's support
- Listening to the worker
- Paving a way for improvement
- Tracking it all to measure success

Walkarounds *are*:

- A place for frontline staff to contribute
- Friendly and conversational
- Announced and informal
- Focused on glitches and barriers, not people
- Ideally conducted by a leader from management and labor

Walkarounds *are not*:

- Punitive
- Compliance or regulatory audits
- Demonstrations of authority
- Targeted to only problem departments

Sample Questions to Ask Frontline Staff on a Walkaround

The leader introduces herself or himself to the staff member and says, "Think about your day-to-day work life, and answer the questions based on what causes or could cause injury."

- Can you think of any events in the past few days that have resulted in an employee injury?
- Can you think of any close calls that almost caused an injury?
- In your view, what are three things that contribute to workplace injuries on your unit?
- Where do you think the next injury will happen? Why?
- What do you think this unit/area could do regularly to improve safety?
- How are you involved in workplace safety?
- How are the past workplace safety solutions working out for you? Why?
- Have there been changes to work practices?
- Are behaviors changing to sustain your efforts?
- If you had $5,000 to fix any one thing that would most likely reduce injury here, where would you spend it?
- How do you think workplace injuries and safety affect our members' experience?
- Are there issues with simple, quick solutions that have been overlooked?
- Have you ever reported anything that never got fixed? What do you think prevented us from fixing it?
- If you make or report an injury or close call, are you concerned about personal consequences?
- Do you know what happens with information that you report?
- Do you feel your efforts are getting to the root causes of your injuries?

Ideas and concerns are noted in a "glitch book," and at the conclusion of a walkaround, the leader assigns follow up for each glitch noted. Thank you notes are sent to all employees and physicians who provided input during the walkaround and includes a statement of the planned follow up.

In addition to the benefits of a safer work environment that derive from workplace safety walkarounds, they can be performed in conjunction with patient safety or service rounding, or other priority areas being addressed by leaders. Most of the sample questions can be adjusted to be patient safety related.

Systems of Safety

Systems of Safety (SOS) is an action-planning program developed by Kaiser Permanente and the University of California at Berkeley Labor Occupational Health Program. It is positioned within the comprehensive safety management program, at the unit level, and offers a hands-on way for frontline workers to understand the hazards within their immediate work environments and then create a plan to resolve them. The training consists of four modules:

- Identify underlying causes of accidents and injuries
- Identify job hazards in the work area
- Identify ways hazards can be controlled and injuries prevented
- Create a plan to eliminate job hazards

Figure 27.3 shows one of the key concepts applicable to patient and worker safety—the hierarchy of controls—which is taught in Kaiser Permanente's SOS program and through patient safety training. The preferred option (at the bottom of the pyramid) is to eliminate the safety hazard altogether. If that is not possible, then establish systems to facilitate safety by making the safe choice the easy choice (e.g., patient lift equipment is readily accessible). If that is not possible, then mitigate the hazard through training, using personal protective equipment, reinforcement mechanisms, and so on. There is increased reliance on human choice, and therefore risk of human error, as one moves toward the top of the pyramid.

Routine tasks are the enemy of safety. It is human nature to become complacent and even begin to drift away from known safe

FIGURE 27.3 Hierarchy of controls taught in Kaiser Permanente's SOS program

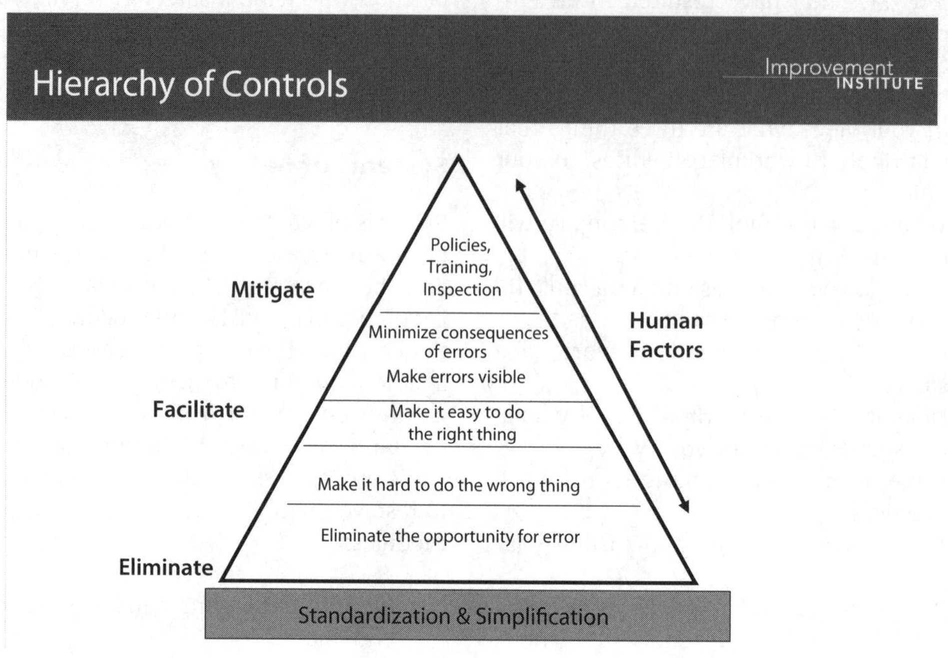

Courtesy of Kaiser Permanente

practices into riskier ones without realizing that the new "normal" is unsafe. One way that Kaiser Permanente has attempted to address the need for paying attention at all times, especially when doing the most routine activities, is a campaign called the "Ten Foot Circle of Safety," developed by the team at Kaiser Sunnyside Medical Center, in Portland, Oregon. With posters and other communications tailored to different care environments, workers are encouraged to think about the potential hazards around them, within a 10-foot circle, at all times. As they move, new hazards appear. Hazards may be sharps, chemicals, or doorways and even other workers. By training staff to be alert at all times for the hazards around them, management is encouraging constant mindfulness.

Top 10 Evidence-Based Practices for Improving Injury Reduction Performance

One of the core values of medicine is an ongoing review of the evidence, coupled with a strong ethic, to reliably deliver the best evidence-based medicine to every patient, every time. Workplace safety has benefited from this attention with its own growing focus on evidence-based workplace safety practices. To accelerate improvement in workplace safety, Kaiser Permanente requires that the following proven practices be in place across all their hospitals.[9–14]

1. Minimize manual lifting of patients by properly using mechanical lift

equipment, slide sheets, slide boards, and devices such as shower chairs and height adjustable electric beds.

2. Evaluate the lift and provide sufficient staff to handle the lift (i.e., get help). Use proper patient lifting techniques and good body mechanics. Bend knees, use arm and leg muscles, keep back straight, use smooth and steady lifting motions, avoid lifting or working above shoulder height, avoid awkward postures such as twisting while lifting, and lift patient close to the body.
3. Adjust computer work station. Arrange materials and supplies in front of the body so they can be easily reached with the elbows in close to the torso. Provide adjustable, supportive padded chairs that support the forearms, legs, and low back. Arm rests should allow the elbows to hang normally at the side of the body. Arrange monitor so that the most commonly viewed area is slightly below (about 20 degrees) horizontal eye level and can be seen without looking up or leaning forward. Provide engineering controls to limit awkward positions (e.g., provide headsets for employees to use when answering phones). Use a keyboard, which includes an adjustable mouse support that can be easily reached from a keying position. Keep wrists straight while typing and use wrist pads to rest on when not typing. Promote regular stretch breaks.
4. Wear proper footwear to reduce slips and falls by as much as 40 to 50%. Wear footwear that is appropriate for the conditions inside and outside. On smooth or wet surfaces, wear slip-resistant soles. Avoid wearing high heels. On snowy, icy, and rainy days, wear boots to work and change after arriving. Clean footwear of mud, snow, and so on when entering a building. Promote awareness of surroundings; everyone pays attention to where they are walking.
5. Keep floors clean and dry. Ensure spills are reported and cleaned up immediately. Provide warning signs for wet floor areas. Where wet processes are used, maintain drainage and provide false floors, platforms, mats, or other dry standing places where practicable or provide appropriate waterproof footgear. Use prudent housekeeping procedures such as cleaning only one side of a passageway at a time. Use no-skid waxes and surfaces coated with grit to create nonslip surfaces in slippery areas such as toilet and shower areas.
6. Eliminate clutter and obstructed areas. Keep aisles and passageways clear and in good repair, with no obstruction across or in aisles that could create a hazard. Provide plugs for equipment so power cords need not run across pathways. Keep exits free from obstruction. Re-lay or stretch carpets that bulge or have become bunched to prevent tripping hazards. Temporary electrical cords that cross aisles should be taped or anchored to the floor. Instruct workers to use the handrail on stairs, to avoid undue speed, and to maintain an unobstructed view of the stairs ahead of them even if that means requesting help to manage a bulky load.
7. Avoid manually lifting or lowering materials to or from the floor. Store materials and/or products off the floor. Arrange materials to arrive on pallets, and keep materials on pallets during storage. Use mechanical devices or equipment to lift the load or lower the entire pallet of material rather than lifting or lowering the material individually. Arrange to have material off loaded directly onto storage shelves. Store only lightweight or infrequently lifted items on the floor. Avoid designing jobs that require workers to lift or lower materials to or from floor level. Minimize the distances loads are lifted and lowered. Position pallet loads

of materials at a height that allows workers to lift and lower within their power zone (i.e., above the knees, below the shoulders, and close to the body).

8. Eliminate reaching and pushing hazards when moving heavy carts by keeping carts, hampers, gurneys, or other carts well maintained to minimize the amount of force exerted while using these items. Use carts with large, low rolling resistance wheels that can roll easily over mixed flooring, as well as gaps between elevators and hallways. Keep handles of devices to be pushed at waist to chest height. Use handles to move carts rather than the side of the cart to prevent the accidental smashing of hands and fingers. Keep floors clean and well maintained. Push rather than pull whenever possible. Remove from use all malfunctioning carts. Get help with heavy or bulky loads.
9. Eliminate reaching or lifting hazards when handling trash or laundry bags. Use handling bags for laundry, garbage, and housekeeping that have side openings to allow for easy disposal without reaching into and pulling bags up and out. The bags should be able to slide off the cart without lifting. Limit the size and weight of these bags and provide handles to further decrease lifting hazards. Use garbage cans that have a frame versus a solid can to prevent plastic bags from sticking to the inside of the can. Limit the size of the container to restrict the weight of the load the employee must lift and dump. Place receptacles in unobstructed and easy-to-reach places. Use spring-loaded platforms to help lift items such as laundry, keeping work at a comfortable uniform level.
10. Use safe housekeeping practices. Alternate leading hand, avoid tight and static grip, and use padded nonslip handles. Clean objects at waist level if possible rather than bending over them. Use knee pads when kneeling, tools with extended handles, or step stools or ladders to avoid or limit overhead reaching. When sweeping or dusting, use flat head dusters and push with the leading edge; sweep all areas into one pile and pick up with a vacuum. Use light head mops, such as fiber mops, frequently change mopping styles when mopping (e.g., push/pull, figure 8, and rocking side to side) to alternate stress on muscles. Be sure buckets, vacuums, and other cleaning tools have wheels or are on wheeled containers with functional brakes. Use carts to transport supplies rather than carrying. Alternate tasks or rotate employees through stressful tasks. Use buffers and vacuums that have lightweight construction and adjustable handle heights. Use spray bottles that have trigger arms rather than single-finger triggers.[15]

In addition to the benefits to patients that derive from improved worker safety, several of the above effective practices can directly improve patient safety, including proper patient handling/lifting, keeping floors clean and dry, and eliminating clutter and obstructed areas.

WORKPLACE SAFETY PERFORMANCE MEASUREMENT AT KAISER PERMANENTE

In order to ascertain whether the safety improvements are having the desired impact, feedback is obtained from employees and correlated to injury rates. This enables adjustments to the employee safety program.

Employee Perceptions

Kaiser Permanente's employee survey, called People Pulse, shows that locations with the most favorable safety perceptions by staff have lower worker injury rates and locations with the least favorable safety perceptions had higher injury rates (based on responses to the statement: "Necessary steps are taken in my department to ensure employee and physician safety.").

Lagging Indicators: Accepted Claims Injury Rate

For a systemwide measure of workplace safety performance, Kaiser Permanente uses an injury rate based on accepted workers' compensation claims, and applies a standard formula used by the Bureau of Labor Statistics, which converts the injury rate to a measure of injuries per 100 full-time equivalents (FTEs):

Injury rate = (N/EH) × 200,000
where:

- N is the number of workers' compensation claims accepted,
- EH is employee hours worked, and
- 200,000 represents 100 employees working 40 hours per week, 50 weeks per year.

Many hospitals use the Occupational Safety & Health Administration's (OSHA) 300 injury logs to track performance. Most Kaiser Permanente facilities are medical office buildings that are not required to complete OSHA logs, making that measure unsuitable for systemwide performance tracking. By using a measure of accepted claims, we can aggressively encourage reporting of all incidents, knowing that only those judged by workers' compensation claims staff to be compensable will be counted in the metric. This overcomes the problem with inadvertently underreporting, and it gives managers assurances that all claims counted are legitimate. The data are highly reliable because they go through a legal vetting process.

Leading Indicators or Outcome Drivers

Activities that drive injury reductions are referred to as outcome drivers. The following measures are tracked regularly for all Kaiser Permanente facilities:

1. Quantified outcome driver measures
   - Incident investigation driver: Percentage of injury reports that are fully investigated
   - Safety conversations driver: Percentage of people who are achieving 100% of their safety conversation goals
   - Ergonomic driver: Percentage of employees receiving ergonomics assessments
2. Subjective outcome driver measures
   - Leadership and sponsorship
   - Accountability structures at the facility level
   - Performance management (leading indicators, aligned plans)
   - Policies and procedures that promote safety
   - Safe patient handling
   - Frontline engagement, multidirectional communication

These measures are reported quarterly using the following categories:

- Effective in at least 85% of facilities in the region
- Effective in more than 50% of facilities in the region
- Effective in less than 50% of facilities in the region
- Not effective in most facilities in the region
- In pilot stage

Establishing Benchmarks

To compare performance to the healthcare sector as a whole, Kaiser Permanente established benchmarks, which were then used to set hospital-specific goals. As described previously, Kaiser Permanente's injury rate metric is based on accepted workers' compensation claims, which are a subset of the injury data available through the BLS and OSHA. To derive a comparable industry benchmark, we make two adjustments to the BLS/OSHA data:

- Adjust BLS data to be comparable to Kaiser Permanente's operations. For

example, we exclude the injuries and productive hours from the Social Assistance sector because we do not provide those services.
- Adjust BLS data to reflect the subset we use for benchmarking (i.e., accepted workers' compensation claims).

We utilized 2006 BLS data to establish the benchmarks in 2007:

- The calculated industry benchmark for Kaiser Permanente's hospital-based regions is 3.3 injuries per 100 full-time equivalent workers.
- The benchmark for Kaiser Permanente's regions that don't operate hospitals is 1.5 injuries per 100 full-time equivalent workers.

Refer to Table 27.2 for a breakdown of methods for deriving these benchmarks.

Never Events

Borrowing from patient safety nomenclature, Kaiser Permanente created *never events* for workplace injuries. The following workplace safety incidents are treated similarly to patient safety never events that require prompt action and escalated reporting. Kaiser Permanente requires internal (and where required external) reporting of any work-related incidents involving:

- Fatality
- Hospitalization
- More than one person requiring medical treatment injured in the same incident

TABLE 27.2 Method for Deriving Benchmarks

Injury Rate (2007 Data)	Method for Deriving Benchmarks
5.8	This is the 2006 BLS injury rate for the total "Health Care and Social Assistance" industry. This rate includes activities that do not take place at Kaiser Permanente, such as day care services and community food and housing; thus, this rate is not comparable to Kaiser Permanente's operations.
8.1	This is the 2006 BLS injury rate for hospitals only. This rate is also not directly comparable to Kaiser Permanente's operations because it does not reflect outpatient or other services provided by their regions.
6.2	This is the adjusted BLS rate that is comparable to Kaiser Permanente's operations. This calculation is performed as follows: Start with the total "Health Care and Social Assistance" industry rate of 5.8, then subtract the injuries and hours from "Offices of Dentists," "Nursing and Residential Facilities," and "Social Assistance." This adjusted rate includes hospitals, medical office buildings, home healthcare services, labs, dialysis, optometry, mental health, and so on.
3.3 Benchmark for regions with hospitals	This is the adjusted BLS rate for hospital-based regions, adjusted again to be comparable to the subset of BLS data estimated to result in accepted workers' compensation claims (based on Kaiser Permanente's experience of reported occupational incidents that result in workers' compensation claims).
1.5 Benchmark for regions that don't operate hospitals	The same process was used to arrive at an average rate of 1.5/100 FTEs for the nonhospital-based regions.

Courtesy of Kaiser Permanente

- Loss of consciousness
- Amputation or avulsion
- Second degree or worse burn
- Chemical exposure that requires medical treatment
- Compound fracture or multiple fractures
- Electrocution
- Significant laceration requiring sutures or similar treatment
- Off for more than seven consecutive scheduled shifts as a result of a work-related incident

Kaiser Permanente's reporting requirements include:

- Report serious work-related incidents involving employees, physicians, contractors, volunteers, and others working at the sites.
- Provide a detailed description of the incident.
- Do not provide identifying information about the injured worker such as employee name or employee ID number.
- Report via email to senior executives within 24 hours.

Performance Improvement

Like most healthcare organizations, Kaiser Permanente has intensified its focus on performance improvement in patient safety. This focus provides a ripe opportunity to embed worker safety practices into improvement initiatives. One example is in reducing hospital acquired pressure ulcers (HAPUs). Frontline performance improvement teams looked at a process improvement assignment to reduce an increase in skin breakdown issues with patients on their units. They assembled a clinical team consisting of management and frontline staff to fix the problem. The staff decided to increase the frequency of turning their patients by establishing a new turning schedule using two staff members to turn all patients with a Braden score initially of < 16 and then 18 at designated times and using a visual reminder to complete this activity. This project involved turning a high volume of immobilized patients at a higher frequency and using two employees for the turns. Key questions at the outset were:

- How does this change affect both patient and employee safety?
- Did involved staff consider the impact of employee safety to changes involving policies and workflows?

By considering and acting on worker safety issues, the result was an improvement in reducing HAPUs without an increase in worker injuries. Learnings include:

- Review current worker injury data for trends and opportunities
- Establish safety protocols at the beginning of all performance improvement projects for patient/employee safety
- Use hierarchy of controls when determining solutions/countermeasures
- Ensure training is adequate and appropriate
- Engage workplace safety experts as champions when initiating patient safety improvements

Digital Imaging

Another example of common ground in patient safety and workplace safety is the shift to digital imaging. Digital imaging provides higher quality data for clinicians and enhanced ability to gain expert insights by easily sharing high-quality images instantly to remote locations around the globe. For workers, it obviates the need for hazardous chemicals previously used to process film. It also reduces handling of heavy x-ray film that could contribute to ergonomic injuries. By moving to digital imaging, which was promoted primarily as a way to improve diagnoses, we have also gained worker safety benefits.

CONCLUSION

Worker and patient safety are inextricably linked. "We can't excel at patient safety without consideration of worker safety. Staff must be able to work safely if patients are to receive safe, high-quality care. When all is said and done, safety is highly behavioral, highly entropic, and highly cultural."[17] In the complex operating environment that is health care today, safety often competes with operations instead of being integrated into operations. Kaiser Permanente aims to achieve the goal of a workplace free of injuries through the implementation of a bundle of practices that are in the process of being embedded and accepted into the daily routine of healthcare workers.

References

1. Stone, P.W, & Gershon, R. R. (2009 Jul–Aug). Nurse work environments and occupational safety in intensive care units. *J Nurs Adm, 39*(7–8 Suppl),S27–S34.
2. Bureau of Labor Statistics. (2008). *Annual survey of occupational injuries and illnesses.* Retrieved from
3. Department of Health and Human Services, National Institute for Occupational Safety and Health. *Healthcare and social assistance: Advancing priorities through research and partnerships.* Retrieved from http://www.cdc.gov/niosh/docs/2009-149/pdfs/2009-149.pdf.
4. Fragala, G., & Bailey, L. (2003). Addressing occupational strains and sprains: Musculoskeletal injuries in hospitals. *AAOHN Journal, 51*(6), 252–259.
5. Charney, W., & Schirmer, J. (2007). Nursing injury rates and negative patient outcomes—Connecting the dots. *AAOHN Journal, 55*(11), 470–475.
6. Yassi, A., & Hancock, T. (2005). Patient safety—Worker safety: Building a culture of safety to improve healthcare worker and patient well-being. *Healthcare Quarterly, 8,* 32–38.
7. Institute of Medicine. (2001). *Crossing the quality chasm: A new health system for the 21st century.* Washington, DC: National Academies Press.
8. Nelson, A., Collins, J., Siddarthan, K., Matz, M., & Waters, T. (2008). Link between safe patient handling and patient outcomes in long-term care. *Rehabilitation Nursing, 33*(1), 33–43.
9. Charney, W. (Ed.). (2010). *Handbook of modern hospital safety* (2nd ed.). Boca Raton, FL: CRC Press.
10. Department of Labor, Occupational Safety & Health Administration. *Hospital eTool.* Retrieved from http://www.osha.gov/SLTC/etools/hospital/index.html.
11. Gaines, M. (2002). Caring for caregivers. *Job Safety & Health Quarterly, 13*(2), 25–27.
12. Department of Labor, Occupational Safety & Health Administration. (2008). *Safety and health case study: Countryside Care nursing home.* Retrieved from http://www.osha.gov/dcsp/success_stories/compliance_assistance/abbott/nursing_homes.html.
13. Ergonomic and Musculoskeletal Disorders, Workplace Safety and Health Topic, NIOSH. Retrieved from http://www.cdc.gov/niosh/topics/ergonomics/.
14. "Ergonomic Injuries-52 Ways to Prevent Them" Naval Safety Center, October 2006. Retrieved from http://72.3.139.6/lmpartnership/sites/default/files/4-ten-proven-practices.pdf.
15. "Ergonomics" OSHA Hospital e-Tool. Online. April 2008. Retrieved from http://72.3.139.6/lmpartnership/sites/default/files/8-eyes-on-ergonomics.pdf.
16. Bureau of Labor Statistics. Number of cases and incidence rate of nonfatal occupational injuries and illnesses for industries with 100,000 or more cases, 2010. Retrieved from http://www.bls.gov/news.release/osh.t04.htm.
17. Doug Bonacum, Vice President, Quality, Safety, and Resource Management, Kaiser Permanente.

28

IDENTIFYING AND ADDRESSING PHYSICIANS AT HIGH RISK FOR MEDICAL MALPRACTICE CLAIMS

Gerald B. Hickson, MD and James W. Pichert, PhD

INTRODUCTION

The link between patient safety and medical malpractice claims has been evaluated since the release of the Institute of Medicine's report *To Err Is Human*. The drafters of that report and patient safety experts have posited that it is the fear of potential liability that often inhibits the ability to learn from error and stifles transparency. What is also clear is that the relationships formed between patients and providers, the communication that occurs between them, and the empathy that a caregiver exhibits in the care of a patient also have a direct correlation not only to the quality of the outcome experienced by the patient but also to the likelihood of whether a claim will be asserted.

Three and a half years ago, a risk manager was notified of a malpractice claim filed against her hospital and a staff urologist.[1] The claim asserted that Dr. Urologist admitted a 36-year-old woman with severe left flank colic. A CT scan revealed a relatively large stone impacted the junction of the ureter and bladder. The patient's pain was difficult to control. She related, "I kept asking Dr. Urologist wasn't there anything else he could do? Finally, he stormed into my room and said, 'If you can't take it any longer, I'll just take you down and laser it.' He never said another word."

Dr. Urologist performed the ureteroscopy on the patient under anesthesia. The procedure was complicated by a high-grade impaction and incomplete laser fragmentation of the stone resulting in multiple fragments that dislocated back into the kidney. The doctor placed a ureteral stent and informed the patient and her husband, "Oh, there were a few little grains of sand left, but they will all pass."

Three weeks after discharge, the patient presented with urosepsis and a high-grade obstruction requiring ICU care and an urgent percutaneous nephrostomy. The malpractice claim asserted there was inadequate stone removal and no informed consent. The patient stated, "We were never given options and surely weren't told about any risk of sepsis or obstruction."

After reviewing the newest complaint, the risk manager wondered whether Dr. Urologist's practice would continue to require a lot of her attention over the coming years. She also wondered why Dr. Urologist's practice appeared to place him at risk, and whether those risks could be identified and then reduced or eliminated.

Are malpractice claims random events driven primarily by medical specialty? Or are some physicians at increased risk and, if so, is it possible to identify them by means other than simply waiting for lawsuits to accumulate? Experienced risk managers regularly recognize that certain physicians seem to have a medical malpractice dark cloud despite being well trained, highly credentialed, and even recognized as top doctors. If high-risk physicians can be identified by some malpractice proxy, how can conscientious risk managers and medical leaders make those physicians aware of their excess malpractice and patient safety risk and their personal responsibility for addressing it?[2]

In this chapter, we will present evidence showing that malpractice claims are *not* randomly distributed and most high-risk physicians can be reliably identified and intervened upon with good success. We then describe an early identification and intervention program that was used in hopes of helping Dr. Urologist *not* be one of those high-risk physicians. In addition to presenting our research data, we will share lessons and political how-tos that we have learned from implementing the process in more than 30 healthcare organizations nationally.

WHY PATIENTS FILE SUIT

Several myths distract medical professionals from dealing with their own malpractice risk. Years of hallway chatter, anecdotal lawyer stories, and the politics of tort reform have diverted leaders' attention to external causes of the malpractice problem. Because physicians are seldom provided peer-based comparison data, many believe suits are common to all who practice in their disciplines.[3] Others blame ambulance-chasing attorneys. Still others fatalistically assume malpractice claims are just a cost of doing business about which they can do little or nothing, or wrongly assume they must practice extra defensively. Understanding the empirical evidence is a first step in addressing these myths.

The magnitude of iatrogenic patient injuries was demonstrated by studies serving as the basis for the 1999 Institute of Medicine's report *To Err Is Human*.[4–8] Between 44,000 and 98,000 patients per year die as a result of medical errors. Far more patients experience long- or short-term disabilities from their care experiences. The same studies, however, established that only a relatively small percentage of patients injured by care actually file suit, perhaps less than 2%.[7,9,10] On the other hand, for every valid claim filed, two to five others are judged to be without merit.[9,11]

Several authors have asked families what prompted them to contact an attorney, a first step in filing a malpractice claim.[12,13] Respondents offered several reasons:

- Almost a quarter said money was important to cover healthcare bills or the long-term medical needs of a family member.
- More than a third reported that "jousting" (when one healthcare team member criticizes the care provided by others) promoted their claims. Among those, 60% stated they had never considered the possibility of suing until a healthcare professional (almost always a physician) suggested that the care they had received was substandard. "Dr. Surgeon stated that my infection was probably from a nurse who didn't wash her hands . . . after that, I knew what to do."[12]
- Others (20%) wanted information, reporting that no one would tell them what really happened, and many suspected a cover-up. Medical team members may well have explained reasons for unsatisfactory outcomes, but it is families, not physicians, who ultimately decide whether their information needs have been met.
- Finally, nearly 20% were driven by grief and/or anger, with a desire for revenge

or, more altruistically, to make medicine safer. One parent declared: "We didn't want Dr. OB's money; we wanted his license. We didn't want him to do this to anyone else."[12]

Are all physicians equally at risk? The next section presents evidence that lawsuits against physicians are not random but that a relatively small subset in every specialty is associated with more litigation than their peers.

MALPRACTICE CLAIMS ARE NOT RANDOM

In 1989, Sloan and colleagues examined the malpractice experiences of Florida physicians and reported that small proportions of physicians (2–8 % by specialty) were associated with disproportionate shares of claims and expenses.[14] A follow-up study demonstrated that claim experience is constant over time; that is, high malpractice risk today predicts high risk tomorrow.[15] Not to be missed is that low risk today is associated with low risk tomorrow, even for physicians who practice in what are traditionally viewed as high malpractice risk fields.

To understand why certain physicians have high claims experience, the practice characteristics of Florida obstetricians were compared. One group of obstetricians (11 % of the total) averaged one paid claim every other year during a seven-year period. Another group (20 % of the total) had no claims and practiced in the same counties as their high-risk colleagues. Medical record reviews were conducted by three experts blinded to the obstetricians' suit histories. No differences between groups were identified in patient risk factors, the obstetricians' technical or clinical competency, frequency of errors, or errors associated with adverse outcomes.[16,17]

In contrast, high-claims-experience obstetricians were associated with more patient expressions of dissatisfaction with their care. In a study involving interviews with families selected at random from Florida vital records, women, even those who had good outcomes, seeing high-claims-experience obstetricians were two to four times more likely to report concerns than patients seeing the no-claims physicians.[16–18] Specifically, patients seeing high-risk obstetricians described being treated dismissively or rudely. Others complained that their obstetrician had yelled at them, their questions were unanswered, and/or their access to their doctor was a problem. Of course, patients' statements were based on their perceptions, but these are the same perceptions that empower some people to seek an attorney whether their adverse outcome was error related or not.

BUT CAN'T YOU DO SOMETHING CONSTRUCTIVE?

Following publication of the previously described studies, our research team was challenged by a risk manager who stated, "You have described the problem, but how about doing something to address it? [Doctors and hospitals] are still getting sued." The challenge led us to ask: Do physicians with high claims experience recognize that they stand out from their peers? And if not, is it possible to make them aware? We rejected the notion of using lawsuit history as the basis for providing feedback for two reasons. First, the high-claims Florida obstetricians averaged only 0.5 suits per year of practice experience, so physicians could practice years before a pattern emerged.[17] A second problem is that most claims are judged to be without merit, so for example if Dr. Urologist were told three claims in six years is high, he might simply argue that each case was invalid or frivolous, failing to consider why his practice attracted more claims than his peers' practices. Besides, as he might continue: "Are you trying to tell me that three is significantly more than two? Come on." We concluded that a malpractice lawsuit proxy was needed, something occurring more frequently than lawsuits and linked to the reasons families sue, such as patients' complaints about their care experiences.[19]

We hypothesized that patient complaints might represent a rich source of data for quality improvement, patient safety, risk identification, and a suitable proxy for individual physician malpractice experience. After all, patients and families have a unique vantage point for providing feedback about their medical experiences and the functioning of physicians, nurses, teams, and medical systems. Such widespread surveillance can be provided by patients and families if organizations are committed to inviting comments, listening, and providing service recovery after a service failure (e.g., errors in the process and outcomes of care, miscommunication, rudeness, breaches of confidentiality, misdiagnosis, jousting, delays in diagnostic testing, and wrong or inadequate treatments).[2,19] Although Dr. Urologist and other physicians might sometimes disagree with patients' perceptions, those patients' misunderstandings imply potentially correctable defects.

SUPPORTING INFRASTRUCTURE—AN OFFICE OF PATIENT RELATIONS

The Vanderbilt Office of Patient Affairs (OPA) was established in 1990 to reliably communicate the hospital's and medical group's interest in hearing and documenting patients' stories about their healthcare experiences. Institutional policies established which complaints were to be centrally reported and which ones managed at the site of care.[2] Signs, brochures, and video messages were deployed informing patients that we wanted to hear from them. Staff at all levels were trained to assist patients in getting their messages HEARD (Hear *the patient*, Empathize, Acknowledge/Apologize *if appropriate*, Respond, and Document).[2]

INITIAL ANALYSIS OF PATIENT COMPLAINTS

As a first step in assessing if complaints might serve as a malpractice proxy, we examined our system's experience. From 1990 to 1995, Vanderbilt Patient Advocates recorded more than 8,000 complaint reports in an electronic database. Most concerns had been addressed individually, but no effort had been directed toward seeking patterns. The research team developed a convention to reliably identify location of event and associated professional(s).[19] The convention sorted complaints into six major code classes (Care and Treatment, Communication, Concern for Patients and Families, Accessibility and Availability, Safety of Environment, and Money or Payment Issues) and 34 subclasses. Each complaint was reviewed by two coders who demonstrated high interrater and test-retest reliabilities.[19] Reliabilities for identification of physicians associated with complaints were consistently high (0.96 to 0.99). The 8,324 complaint reports yielded 13,673 coded complaints (1.6 per report to a patient advocate); 2,248 were linked to an identifiable physician. The following represents examples of complaints and their major code class, similar to those associated with Dr. Urologist.

Communication:

- "I explained several times to my urologist and his staff that I have a latex allergy, but even so a latex catheter was placed in my urinary tract."
- "As I tried to talk, Dr. Urologist kept interrupting me."

Concern for Patients and Families:

- "Dr. Urologist came in yelling at me that I had 'cried wolf' [about my condition]."
- "My pets get better care and concern from my vet."

Accessibility and Availability:

- "I waited 2.5 hours today and left without being seen. I waited four hours last appointment. It's ridiculous. I just left."
- "My father hasn't seen the urologist in the three days since surgery."

Care and Treatment:

- "I reported having repeated bouts of night sweats but was not examined and

simply told twice that this just happens. To make a long story short, I had a perforated bowel."
- "I will not return to your medical group because of Dr. Urologist's incompetent treatment."

Because these are unsolicited comments, not constrained by predetermined scales on consumer satisfaction questionnaires, patients make judgments about the importance of the issues they report and identify associated providers.

Of course, just as not every dissatisfied consumer complains, neither will all patients speak up.[20] In health care, an added barrier is that patients need physicians and may believe that their current providers are the only (or best) persons to provide care. They may fear abandonment or retaliation if they complain.[20-25] Thus, the ratio of unvoiced to voiced complaints may be as high as 40 or 70 to one.[21] Like others who advocate patient empowerment or activation, we concluded that patients might effectively augment a healthcare system's surveillance of threats to safety and serve as a surrogate for malpractice risk.[26,27]

Next we learned that physician-associated complaints were highly skewed.[19] For example, many members of one 644-physician group (35%) were associated with no complaints during a six-year study period, while 9% accounted for half of all physician-associated complaints. In addition, certain subclass codes were more likely associated with high-complaint–generating physicians: "I was lied to," "the doctor made me worry," "no one would return my call," "my doctor criticized other members of the team," "there were problems with my medications."[19,28] Since physician-associated complaints were not randomly distributed, we asked if they were linked to malpractice experience, even those that appear trivial or inaccurate: "I should not have gotten such a high bill. The doctor only spent 15 minutes with my mother during her appointment—the nurse did the rest."

Logistic regression analysis identified three independent predictors of malpractice experience: physician specialty, volume of service (as measured by relative value unit [RVU][29] production), and numbers of unsolicited patient complaints.[28] Complaints proved to be of primary importance, accounting for the greatest proportion of the variance in claims with associated expenses and lawsuits. Using the identified predictors, a risk score was calculated for each cohort member, who was then sorted into one of five empirically determined predicted risk categories.[30]

Table 28.1 illustrates risk management expenses and complaints for the five groups. Physicians predicted at lowest risk comprised half the cohort but only 4% of the group's risk management expenses (awards, settlements, and costs of defense) for the six-year study. They also were associated with few patient complaints. In contrast, 103 physicians (16%) in the two highest predicted risk categories were associated with 79% of costs and a disproportionate share of complaints. Results have been replicated with 445 physicians practicing in a midwestern community medical center (Figure 28.1)[31] and confirmed in a New England medical system.[32]

Establishing the relationship between patient complaints and malpractice claims experience established the validity of the proposed proxy. The next step was to consider how best to make high-complaint physicians aware of their risk for claims. The next section provides the philosophical basis for our how-tos.

SELF-REGULATION AND PROFESSIONAL ACCOUNTABILITY

One defining characteristic of a profession is a commitment to self-regulation, meaning that members establish and enforce high standards for performance and behavior. The goals of professional self-regulation are to assure the public that members are competent and ethical, and maintain control over reputation. Self-regulation also means that

TABLE 28.1 Risk Management Expenses and Patient Complaints for Five Groupings of a Medical Center's Physicians Based on Calculated Risk Scores[30]

Predicted Risk Category	# (%)	Mean Dollars Paid Out*	Percentage of Total Dollars Paid Out	Mean Number of Complaints per MD
1 (low)	318 (49)	1	4%	2
2	147 (23)	6	13%	6
3	76 (12)	4	4%	10
4	52 (8)	42	29%	16
5 (high)	51 (8)	73	50%	42
Total	644 (100)		100%	

*Dollar value of low risk group adjusted to one. All other physician groups represented in multiples of low risk group.

Reprinted with permission from *Vanderbilt Law Review*: May 2006: 59:4,1198.

FIGURE 28.1 Patient Complaints about Physicians are not Randomly Distributed[43]

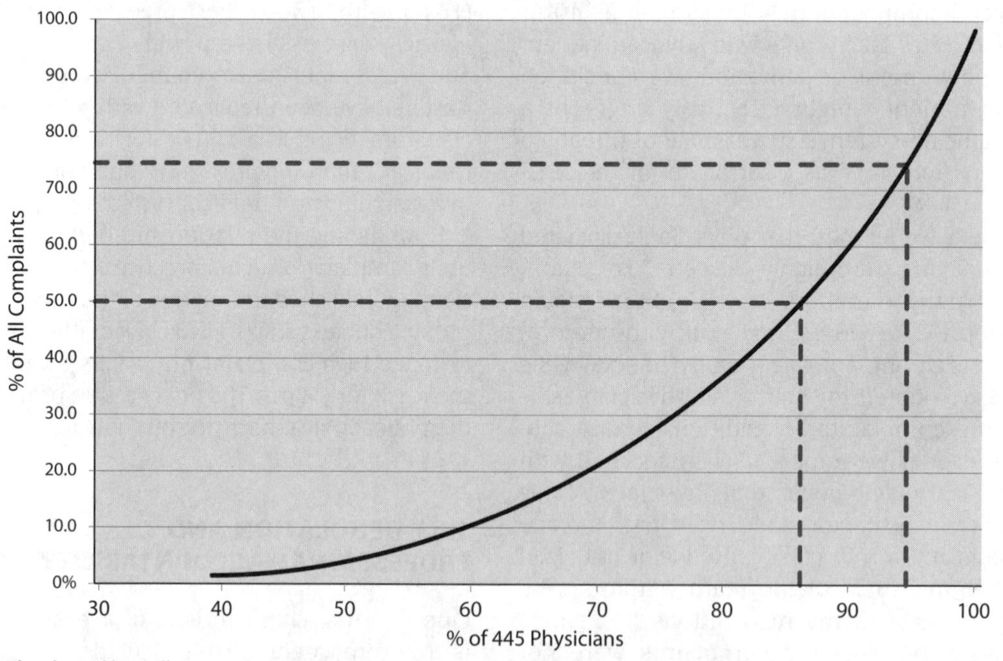

The dotted lines illustrate that 14% of study group members were associated with half of all patient complaints and that only 5% accounted for one fourth of all complaints

Hickson GB, Federspiel CF, Blackford J, Pichert JW, Gaska W, Merrigan MW, & Miller CW. Cumulative distribution of complaints by cumulative distribution of Physician Study Group based on 3291 complaints for 445 physicians 2001–2003. *Southern Medical Journal*: August 2007: 100(8):791–796.

colleagues endeavor to elevate one another's level of professionalism.[33]

Professional self-regulation occurs on at least two levels. Each individual has personal responsibility to self-monitor, seek and accept feedback, and adjust actions and practices to conform to normative standards. In other words, practitioners take care of their own practice behavior and expect colleagues to do the same. The second level of self-regulation refers to professionals' responsibility within organized groups or health systems to identify and address factors that threaten intended clinical outcomes. Each professional has a responsibility to ensure that colleagues and systems do no harm. Concerted effort to remove systemic or behavioral threats to quality must include willingness to provide feedback to others observed to behave unprofessionally or, as we have demonstrated, who are associated with disproportionate numbers of patient complaints.[33]

Unfortunately, the medical profession has had limited success in self-regulation. While participants in peer review may be motivated to ensure quality, critics have charged that peer review is often underutilized and tainted, concerned that peers may be too lenient or overzealous.[30,33,34] In our view, traditional peer review is ill-equipped and slow to identify physician behaviors that dissatisfy their patients and place themselves at increased risk for unnecessary medical malpractice suits. Peer reviewers generally are not trained to analyze whatever the data may be, with resulting large variation in performance. Participants rarely provide constructive feedback to the physician being reviewed, and communication of the outcomes to the person reviewed often occur in a quasi-adversarial setting. Traditional peer review simply does not lend itself to support nondefensive, change-related reflection so is limited in its utility for restoring the individual to the group.[30,33,34] Therefore, to achieve consensus to conduct interventions, we proposed a graduated process designed to be kinder and gentler, we obtained leadership endorsement, and we promoted physician group ownership of the process.

CHANGING PHYSICIAN PRACTICE BEHAVIORS

Can anything be done to reduce Dr. Urologist's risk? The literature about changing physician practice behavior teaches that messages must be evidence based, contain data that illustrates peer-based comparisons, be delivered by a respected peer messenger, and be repeated over time.[35–37] Messages are best delivered in a manner consistent with professional self-regulation and in a way that promotes insight, action, and accountability.[38] Consequently the research team designed a process with an associated tiered intervention strategy (Figure 28.2).[39]

As suggested by our research observations, the base of the pyramid is made up of the large proportion of physicians never or seldom associated with patient complaints. At the next level up, we suggest that whenever a complaint is recorded, the associated professional should be notified informally. In our example, patient advocates had notified Dr. Urologist about each complaint. We assumed that Dr. Urologist and others in the high-risk group would review the concern, offer service recovery, and seek to make practice adjustments as appropriate.

In some circumstances, however, our data indicate that some physicians, including Dr. Urologist, were associated with multiple complaints. Consistent with individual and group professional self-regulation, we assert that high-complaint physicians deserve and need to be made aware of their standing (Level 1 Awareness Intervention).[33,38,39] We proposed that a trained peer colleague should share the data, encouraging the high-complaint physician to reflect on the reasons for patient dissatisfaction but not provide directive or corrective advice.

Anticipating that some individuals would be unable or unwilling to respond to

FIGURE 28.2 A Tiered Approach to Promoting Professional Behavior[39]

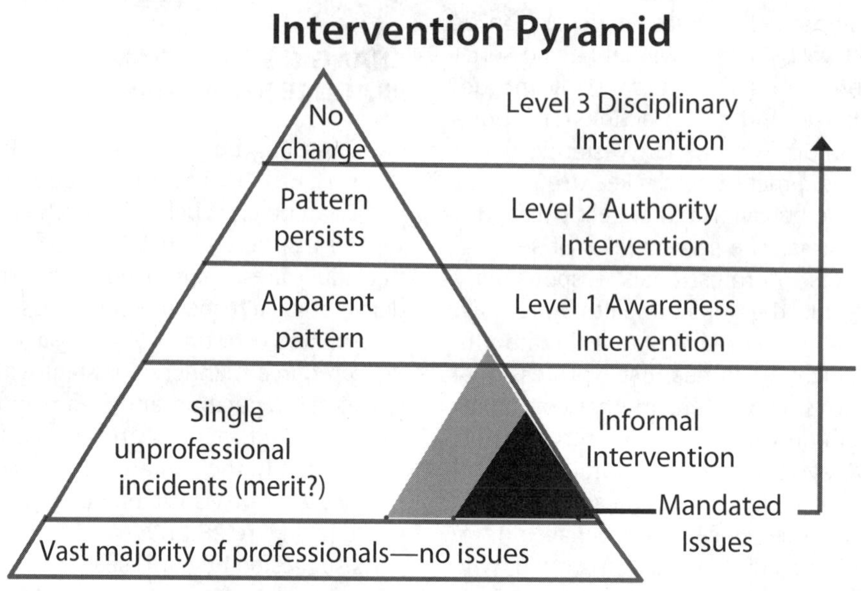

Adapted from Hickson G, Pichert JW, Webb LE, & Gabbe SG. A complementary approach to promoting professionalism: Identifying, measuring, and addressing unprofessional behaviors. *Academic Medicine*: Nov 2007: 82:(11):1040–1048.

peer-delivered messages, we proposed two authority-based interventions. Level 2 would provide the appropriate leader (chairman, chief medical officer, vice president of medical affairs) an opportunity to review the high-complaint physician's data, reflect on other sources of information about performance, and then define a plan for improvement (elements of the plan might range from coaching, a practice assessment, or a comprehensive mental health review). Level 2 interventions would include ongoing tracking of complaint data with periodic updates provided to designated leaders. The other authority intervention, Level 3, would be reserved for individuals who did not respond to the Level 2 authority-based intervention or who violated policy or legal boundaries (the gray triangle in Figure 2, those complaints/events considered most egregious).[40] These persons are referred for appropriate investigative, corrective, or disciplinary action.

THE VANDERBILT INTERVENTION PROCESS

Since implemented in 1998, 30 hospitals and medical groups have approached the CPPA (Center for Patient and Professional Advocacy at Vanderbilt University Medical Center) to establish for them an identification and intervention program, including Dr. Urologist's institution and medical group. The following section describes the eight steps for implementing the Vanderbilt tiered intervention process (Figure 28.3).

In brief, following execution of a business associate agreement (BAA), each group provides the CPPA with a physician list (names, specialties), productivity data if available, and all unsolicited complaint reports (Step 1). Complaint coding is completed and risk scores calculated for physicians practicing at the site (Step 2). Physicians with a calculated score greater than the 95th percentile for the

FIGURE 28.3 Eight Steps of the Vanderbilt Intervention Process

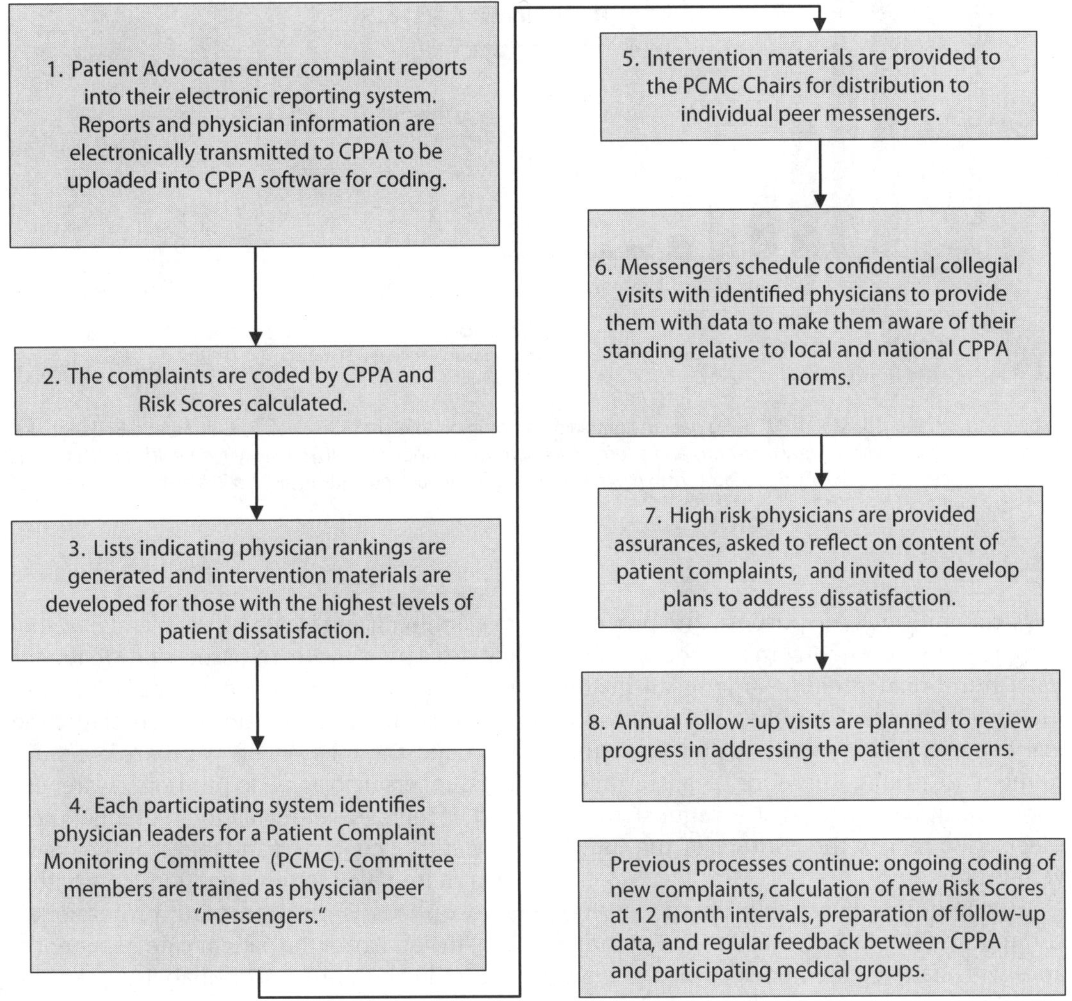

Courtesy of the Center for Patient & Professional Advocacy, Vanderbilt University Medical Center, Nashville, TN

group are identified as candidates for intervention. Intervention materials are created (Step 3) to support peer-delivered awareness (Level 1) interventions. An intervention folder is created containing a letter from the peer messenger to the high-complaint colleague, a "You Are Here" figure (Figure 28.4), a table that portrays the types of complaints voiced by patients (Table 28.2), and individual de-identified complaint narratives.

The letter prepared for a peer messenger and addressed to the high-complaint

FIGURE 28.4 Dr. Urologist's "You Are Here" Graph

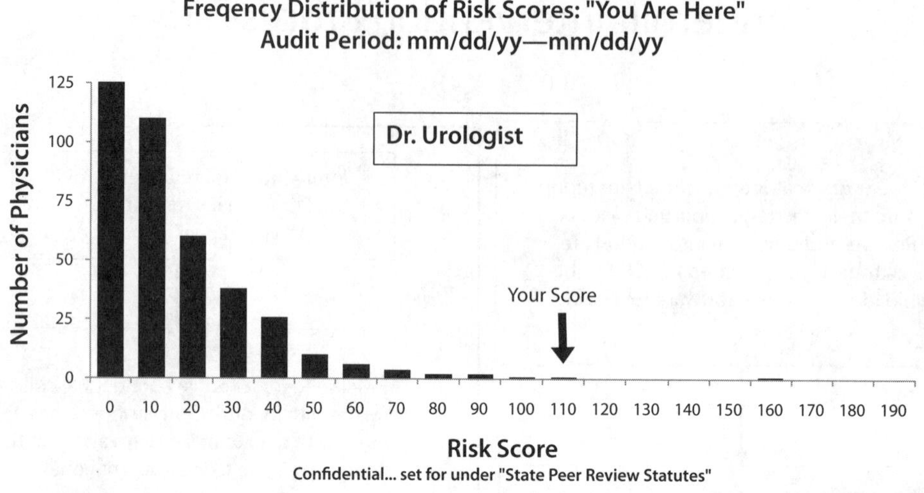

Pichert JW, Hickson GB, Moore IN. Using patient complaints to promote patient safety. Vol. 2. Culture and Redesign. In: *Advances in patient safety: New directions and alternative approaches*. Rockville (MD): *Agency for Healthcare Research and Quality*; 2008 Jul:1–10. Also available: http://www.ahrq.gov/downloads/pub/advances2/vol2/Advances-Pichert_51.pdf. Accessed April 17, 2012.

physician presents the purpose and process, local leadership endorsement, the individual's numerical ranking among all group members ("you rank number 2 of your medical center's 382 physicians and you rank number 2 among surgeons"), assurances about confidentiality, and a request for a meeting to review the content of the intervention folder.

At each site, a patient complaint monitoring committee (PCMC) is established in compliance with state requirements for peer review, and a committee chair is identified (Step 4). Committee members are nominated to be trained as peer messengers based on several criteria: drawn from various specialties, currently or recently in practice, respected by colleagues, committed to confidentiality, and willing to serve in a challenging role. We also emphasize messengers' understanding that they are just messengers and not responsible for fixing their colleagues. This qualification can be challenging for physicians accustomed to examining and weighing data, and developing a diagnosis with an associated treatment plan. But if a messenger offers a plan that does not work, the high-risk doctor can blame the plan and the messenger. We therefore want messengers who agree to promote awareness and encourage self-regulation. Potential messengers are contacted and told that they have been nominated for an important committee whose focus is on promoting professionalism, the quality of the patient care experience, and reducing unnecessary liability risk. The process is described, and they are provided three opportunities to decline participation: at the time of the initial contact, during training, and prior to the first assigned peer messenger visit. Such screening for willingness to participate results in robust committees of well-trained, committed professionals.

Messengers' own risk scores are mostly satisfactory, but, on occasion, some high-risk physicians serve successfully as messengers and, over time, as committee chairs.[30,38] The

TABLE 28.2 Example of complaint type table

Complaint Type Summary
Dr. Urologist

Audit Period: Date 1–Date 2

Complaint Type Categories	**Number of Complaints**		**Distribution of Complaints**	
	Your Complaints	**Average for Surgery**	**Your Complaints**	**Average for Surgery**
Care & Treatment	19	4.5	30.2%	39.8%
Communication	15	2.9	23.8%	25.7%
Concern for pt/family	14	1.3	22.2%	11.5%
Access/Availability	9	1.9	14.3%	16.8%
Safety of Environment	0	0.0	0.0%	0.0%
Money/Payment Issues	66	0.7	9.5%	6.2%
Total # of Complaints	**63**	**11.3**		

Total Number of Reports **Note:** each report may contain multiple complaints		
Past 48 months	**5.9**	**26**
Past 12 months	**6**	**1.7**

Courtesy of the Center for Patient & Professional Advocacy, Vanderbilt University Medical Center, Nashville, TN

identification of the right committee chairs and committee members is essential for both the effective provision of feedback to high-risk physicians and to protect the integrity of the peer feedback process.

Intervention Skills Training

PCMC members receive eight hours of training on the research background, essential steps in sharing, and how to anticipate and address common reactions, questions, and challenges. The messenger learns that sharing the data means:

- Scheduling a meeting with the identified colleague, allowing plenty of time to talk
- Reviewing contents of the letter, including rankings and assurances
- Inviting (at least with a pause) a colleague's view of her or his ranking
- Inviting the colleague to review materials
- Inviting the colleague to take time over the coming weeks to identify potential ways to address sources of patient dissatisfaction
- Expressing appreciation for the colleague's consideration and her or his contributions to the medical group

- Explaining how and when follow-up data will be provided
- Immediately after the visits, completing a debriefing report about length of visit, elements covered, perceived colleague receptivity, and potent reasons for the high risk score

Training includes demonstrations and role-play exercises with feedback during which we rehearse the importance of respecting their colleagues' professionalism and problem-solving abilities (at least initially). Once training is complete, the local chair makes messenger assignments (Step 5). Separate training for committee chairs focuses on considerations of how best to assign messengers. Data review identified that Dr. Urologist ranked #2 in his medical group. His group's messenger committee chair identified a messenger based on knowledge of committee members and Dr. Urologist.

Assignments are intended to avoid any match that might create a barrier to the intended respectful, nonjudgmental, and confidential intervention process. Therefore, the messenger committee chair avoids pairing physicians who have known conflicts of interest such as those in direct competition for patients or other resources, the presence of a poor prior relationship, or a prior or existing social relationship that makes the messenger role just too uncomfortable.

Prior to the actual intervention visit, a letter from the selected messenger to Dr. Urologist was signed and mailed, and an intervention visit was scheduled (Step 6). The goal is to prevent any recipient from asserting that the messenger walked in without providing any warning of the visit intent. At the time of the visit, the messenger delivers another copy of the information letter (in case the first had somehow gotten lost) and the aforementioned materials.

Dr. Urologist's peer messenger (a general surgeon) used the "You Are Here" graph (Figure 28.4) to illustrate how the doctor's risk score compared with other physicians' scores and to remind that many, if not most, physicians generate few or no complaints. The messenger also encouraged Dr. Urologist to review the complaint distribution table (Table 28.2) and the complaint stories as a way to gain insight into reasons for patient dissatisfaction (Step 7). Dr. Urologist then asked, "Who else knows about this? Does my chair or section chief?" His messenger accurately responded that in the initial awareness phase, only the peer messenger and local messenger committee chair are aware that the physician has been identified for intervention. His messenger reported that Dr. Urologist also challenged the validity of the complaint data, asserted that his specialty attracted challenging patients, and asked about the program's and messenger's motives. Dr. Urologist's messenger responded nondefensively to each challenge, each time simply returning to the data showing that Dr. Urologist stood out. Dr. Urologist agreed to review the materials but also asserted that "urologists should not be compared with other doctors, not even other surgeons." The visit ended with an affirmation of Dr. Urologist's importance to the medical group and a promise to return with follow-up data in 12 months (Step 8). As Dr. Urologist's messenger completed a brief post meeting debriefing form, he wondered whether this use of his time would have any effect.

Results

Prior to initiating interventions at Vanderbilt, three goals were established for assessment. First, was it was possible to recruit, train, and retain peer messengers? Would physicians agree to participate? What would they expect in return for their time and emotional energy? After their initial experiences, would they continue? A second goal was to develop insight into the process and qualitative outcomes of awareness interventions. How would high-risk physicians like Dr. Urologist respond? Would they be professional and receive the messenger well? What questions would they ask? What explanations would they offer for their high-risk status? And could messengers predict results of the intervention process? The final goal was to assess the extent to which Level 1 awareness interventions are effective in addressing sources of patient dissatisfaction and malpractice risk.

Recruiting and Retaining Messengers

Based on experience since 1998, as of this writing, the Vanderbilt team has trained more than 250 messengers. These messengers have completed more than 1,600 initial and follow-up Level 1 interventions, and only four have reportedly discontinued their service due to discomfort in the role. Anecdotally, many messengers say they are willing to try one intervention, then afterward report they are willing to do more because they felt well prepared philosophically and well supported with good data. Recent messenger comments include: "The training prepared me well. The advance letter really gets the physician thinking," "I felt well prepared (as well as possible for a first meeting) due to the training and the messenger guide," "I think this was a positive meeting, and I predict that we will see a decrease in this physician's complaint rate." Based on this experience, we concluded that messengers from diverse sites could be readily identified, they would agree (with appropriate skepticism) to receive training, and nearly all continue their service over time. We also learned that they would do so largely in support of their groups' commitment to professionalism.

The Intervention Process

With respect to the second goal, we distributed 1,511 debriefing forms (we did not use debriefing surveys early in our work); 1,406 were completed and returned (79 of these were returned stating that the physician had recently departed or was about to depart so no visit occurred), an overall return rate of 93%.

Analysis of the 1,327 completed forms revealed that initial intervention visits average just over 30 minutes in length (range = 8–90 minutes). Messengers report excellent fidelity to the eight predefined elements of the intervention process (92%). Messengers often report that high-risk physicians initially respond to the data with defensiveness, but that most are ultimately receptive and professional (75%) or at least neutral. A few, less that 4%, characterize their colleague as hostile or angry. On a few of these occasions, high-complaint physicians told their messengers to leave. One messenger reported that the high-complaint doctor flung the intervention materials against the interior office wall; we reassured the messenger that the intervention had been completed because the folder had remained in the doctor's office. Finally, a dozen high-risk doctors have refused, at least initially, to meet with a messenger after receiving the letter. Messenger committee chairs are taught to call the high-risk physician to emphasize the nonpunitive, informational reason for the visit, and to urge the doctor to reconsider. If the high-risk doctor continues to refuse, the intervention folder is delivered or mailed in a sealed envelope marked confidential with a cover note asking the doctor to review the material and offering to meet to answer questions or address issues. Anecdotally, while the number of physicians who refuse is small, this response does not appear to be predictive of subsequent outcome.

Physicians often offered multiple reasons for their high-risk status, most frequently citing: my patients or practice are somehow unique (25%), it's the system (48%), it's the nature of this work and I'm helpless to change things (10%), it's my personality and/or how I communicate (29%), and it's the high volume of patients (22%) or, like Dr. Urologist, nearly one in five were uncertain why they might stand out. The specific responses in the debriefing reports have been used over the past 10 years to continually improve the quality of the messenger training.

Intervention Results

Interventions were initiated in 1998 at Vanderbilt. More occurred elsewhere as medical centers initiated the Vanderbilt intervention program. By 2007, 336 high-complaint physicians had received an awareness visit with two subsequent years for follow-up. Overall, after being made aware of their standings and being provided follow-up data, the mean and median percentage of complaint reduction two years after the initial awareness interventions were 29% and 56%, respectively ($p < 0.001$).[38] At that time, just under 60% of physicians reduced their numbers of complaints by at least 40%. The mean and median improvements (reductions in complaints) for these responders were 78% and 79%, respectively.

As of this writing, 620 high-complaint physicians have now received one or more awareness visits (Table 28.3). Thirty-seven departed their organization within a year of the intervention and another 137 will receive their first follow-up visit over the coming months. Of the 446 for whom we have at least one year of follow-up data, 308 (69%) have improved risk scores. We divide these improved physicians into three subclasses: 203 (46%) have shown two years of improvement and achieved risk scores below the threshold for intervention. Their messengers sent them follow-up letters thanking them for their improvement and letting them know that personal visits would no longer be necessary. Another 69 (15%) reduced their risk scores by at least 15% in the previous year, and their scores are nearing or just below the threshold for intervention. Dr. Urologist is among this group (Figure 28.5). This group's messengers visited to share the data, express appreciation for the high-risk doctor's efforts, and ask what (if anything) likely contributed to the improvement. Finally, 36 (8%) reduced their risk scores by at least 15%, but their scores remain well above the intervention threshold. This latter group's messengers visited to share the data and encourage continued attention to patient concerns.

Table 28.3 shows the current standing for the remaining 134 (30%) for whom we have

TABLE 28.3 Vanderbilt intervention process results to date

Intervention Results	Number	Percentage
Total physicians with high risk scores	620	
Departed group within a year of first intervention	37	6%
First follow-up scheduled in coming months	137	22%
Total with at least one year of follow-up data	446	72%
Results for those with follow-up data	446	
Improved		
Pattern of significant improvement	203	46%
Significant improvement	69	15%
Some improvement—still needs tracking	36	8%
Subtotal	308	69%
Departed group with risk score unimproved	93	21%
Current risk score is unimproved	45	10%

Courtesy of the Center for Patient & Professional Advocacy, Vanderbilt University Medical Center, Nashville, TN

FIGURE 28.5 Dr. Urologist's Risk Scores Over Time

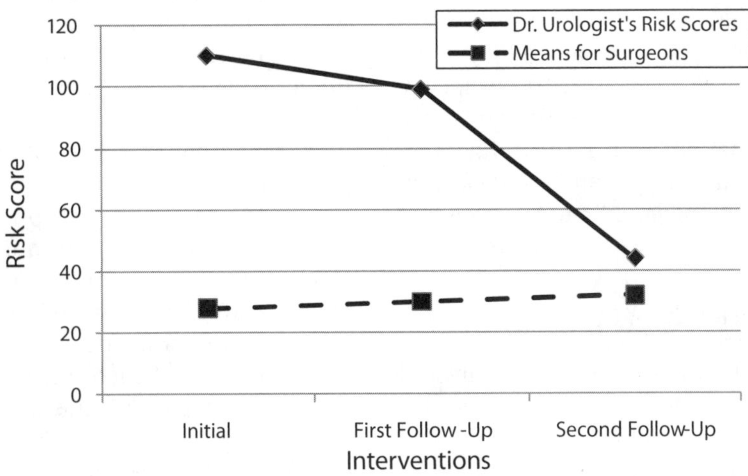

Courtesy of the Center for Patient & Professional Advocacy, Vanderbilt University Medical Center, Nashville, TN

at least one year of follow-up results and whose risk scores did not improve. Forty-eight (11%) departed their organizations; of these, 7 departed while at the Level 2 authority intervention. The rest (n = 86, 19%) have risk scores within 15% of their initial score or higher. Their messengers meet with them to report these results and, in most cases, simply remind their high-risk colleagues of the reasons for providing data and ask them to reflect on the reasons for continued patient/family dissatisfaction. The messengers may also alert them to the potential for a Level 2 intervention (with the encouragement, "but I doubt that will be necessary in your case as I know you to be an effective problem solver"). Nine of the unimproved high-risk physicians are currently in the midst of a Level 2 authority intervention. With respect to Level 2 authority interventions overall, we have follow-up information about 24: 9 (38%) subsequently improved, 8 (33%) remain unimproved and are experiencing additional authority-mandated improvement efforts tailored to their circumstances, and 7 (29%) departed their organization.

National Standings

As the numbers of physicians in our database increased and as high-complaint physicians such as Dr. Urologist asserted the uniqueness of their practices, we began to examine how risk scores might be distributed across various medical and surgical specialties and subspecialties. In one recently published study of urologists' risk scores, we constructed the distribution illustrated in Figure 28.6.[1] Dr. Urologist's scores on the distribution are highlighted. This portrayal of the data was designed to help him appreciate that he stood out even among other busy urologists, including those practicing in his urologic subspecialty. Similar curves have been published or presented at national meetings of orthopedic surgeons, emergency medicine physicians, vascular surgeons, and trauma surgeons.[41,42] All specialties' curves are similar to our repeated finding (see Figure 28.1) that many physicians are associated with no complaints or very few, but a small subset of doctors is associated with disproportionate numbers of complaints. The specialty curves address the uniqueness argument by permitting national performance comparisons for most physicians by discipline.

When Dr. Urologist complained during the first follow-up visit that he stood out locally because "urologists like me just get more complaining patients," his messenger acknowledged that urology can be difficult but then showed him Figure 28.6 to illustrate that most urologists have lower risk scores.

Claims Experience

The next question is whether peer-delivered interventions change not just complaint generation but also claims experience. The evidence to date is encouraging but not statistically conclusive. Institutions are understandably less willing to share risk management claims files, so we began with a pilot study. The pilot involved 31 Vanderbilt surgeons who were identified in 1998 as high-risk by their calculated risk scores. Following the Institutional Review Board's approval of the study as exempt from informed consent, surgeons were randomly assigned to an intervention group (physicians received awareness messages) or to a control group (no messages). Given the relatively infrequent nature of being named in risk management files with expenses (RMFEs), the study was conducted to generate data for power calculations and gain insight into the intervention process. Following the steps in Figure 26.3, surgeons in the study group received initial and follow-up interventions beginning in 1998 through 2004. RMFEs for six years preceding and subsequent to initial interventions were tracked.

FIGURE 28.6 Dr. Urologist's Risk Scores Versus Other Urologists' Scores[1]

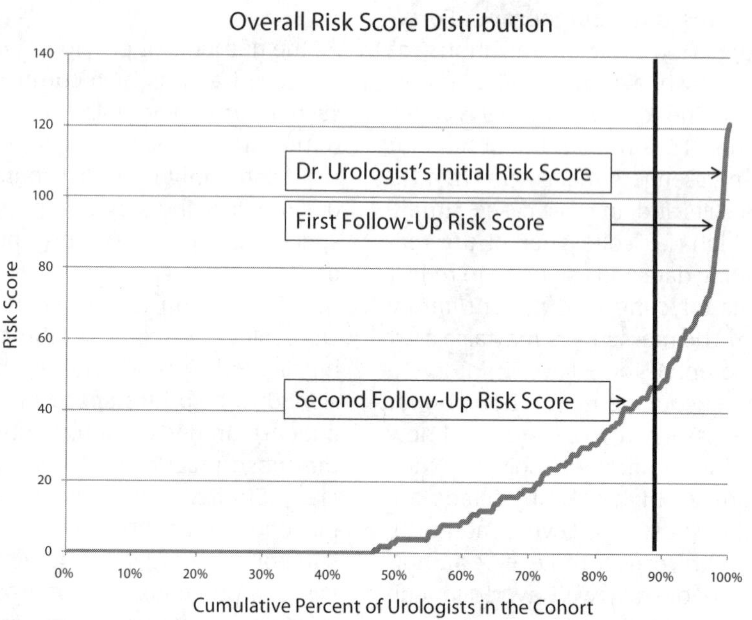

Distribution of Risk Scores Across the Overall Cohort. Right of the black dotted line represents the percent of the cohort (11%) accounting for 50% of the patient complaints (Note: Dr. Urologist's Risk Scores have been added to the published curve).

Adapted from Stimson CJ, Pichert JW, Moore IN, Dmochowski RR, Cornett MB, An AQ, & Hickson GB. Medical malpractice claims risk in urology: An empirical analysis of patient complaint data. *The Journal of Urology*: May 2010:183(5):1971–1976

FIGURE 28.7 Intervention Group Versus Control Group Risk Management Outcomes

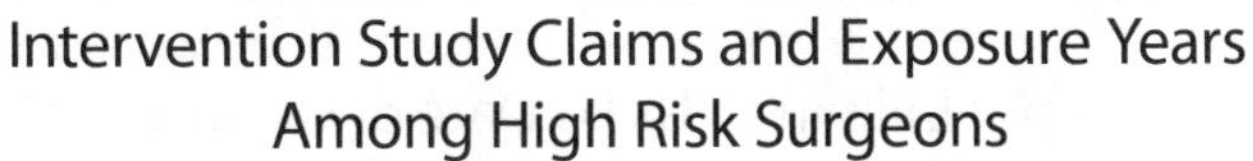

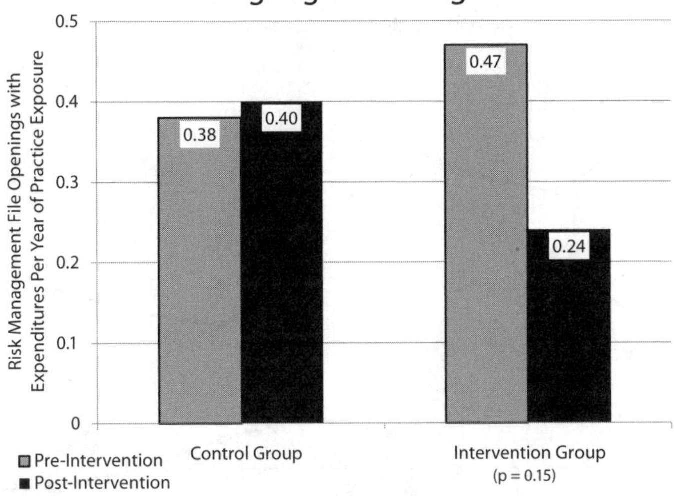

Courtesy of the Center for Patient & Professional Advocacy, Vanderbilt University Medical Center, Nashville, TN

In addition to reducing complaint numbers, the intervention group experienced almost 50% fewer RMFEs compared to no change for the control group surgeons (Figure 28.7). However, given the cohort size and frequency of risk events, the difference only constituted a trend ($p = 0.15$).

We also asked whether the peer intervention process was associated with changes in overall malpractice claims adjusted for the medical system's growth over time.[30,38] To control for institutional trends in risk management philosophy, we compared general liability (e.g., slips and falls) and professional liability claims, both adjusted for clinical volume (event per million RVUs) over time. We found a significant downward slope in Vanderbilt's professional liability claims with expenses ($t = -3.39$, $p = 0.02$), but general liability claims were unchanged. In other words, the salutary effects seem specific to professional liability actions, and the reduction does not appear to be an artifact. It is likely, of course, that both internal safety/risk/quality initiatives and external factors, such as claims frequency in the middle Tennessee area, contributed to the reductions in claims experience.

Another site, an academic medical center in a far more litigious community than Nashville, began using the Vanderbilt intervention process in 2000. That organization's lawsuit trend appears in Figure 28.8. Vanderbilt data are provided to illustrate jurisdictional differences in litigation risk. However, both institutions have experienced a similar downward trend in their claims experience.

Science and Local Politics

Creating change within medicine is a complex subject beyond the scope of this chapter. However, the science behind any proposed project is often insufficient in and of itself to promote change without a carefully crafted implementation strategy. The strategy must include creating and sustaining an understanding of need, a draft plan, a willingness to seek and respond to feedback, ongoing assessment of

FIGURE 28.8 Two Medical Centers' Lawsuit Experiences After Implementing the Vanderbilt Intervention Process

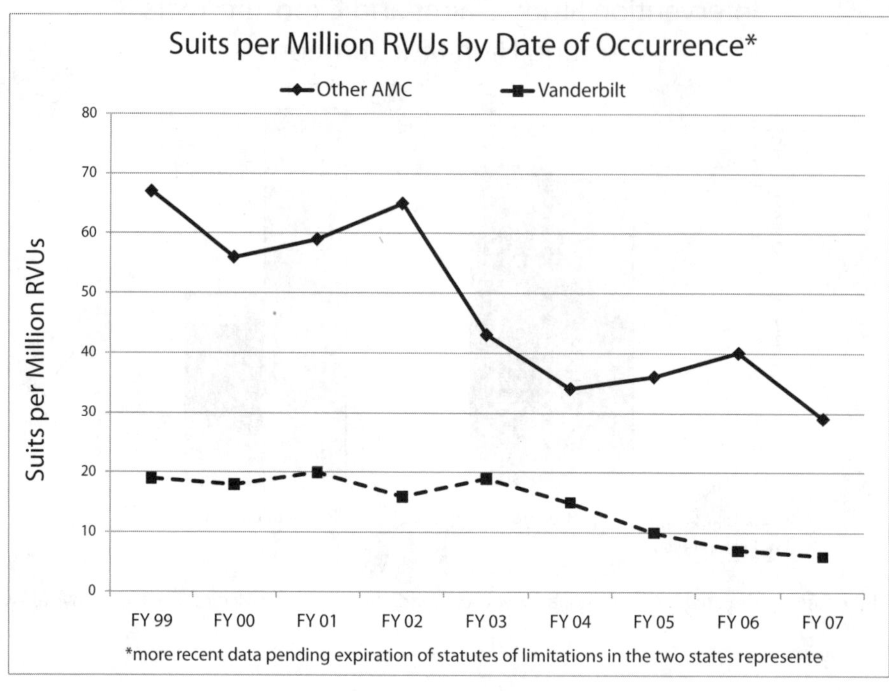

AMC = academic medical center

Courtesy of the Center for Patient & Professional Advocacy, Vanderbilt University Medical Center, Nashville, TN

performance, transparency of results, and willingness to address the unanticipated. Leaders of any medical system, whether thousand-bed academic medical centers or community hospitals, are constantly bombarded with countless good ideas. How can risk managers and other champions of change ensure their good ideas get appropriate review with some chance of adoption?

COMMUNICATING WITH LEADERS

Our first step was to focus on the notion that Vanderbilt's malpractice experience could be more systematically assessed, addressed, and redressed. Those whose professional responsibilities involve claims investigation understand that risk can be influenced, but some of their medical or hospital leadership may not. Because many leaders are data oriented and data driven, risk managers must first overcome any reluctance to share details of individual cases or group experience in properly protected venues. After all, if such information is not regularly disseminated, risk managers should not expect to gain allies in their efforts to promote quality and safety. A second challenge is that some healthcare leaders are reluctant to hear about the group's dark side or, in some locales, feel the associated costs are not worth the effort.

Consequently, we framed the need to address our malpractice problem not only in terms of financial costs but as a threat to the institution's goal of becoming the community's health system of first choice. Aligning efforts to address unnecessary risk with existing leadership priorities was key. We consistently reminded leadership that a small subset of physicians was associated with multiple alleged communication and technical errors, inadequate availability, or perceived disrespectfulness, and that these doctors were associated with adverse outcomes, consequent harm to patients, and litigation. An associated message focused on our organization's reputation: "We hear from several thousand unhappy patients and families each year. Each complaint report represents at least 50 more similarly dissatisfied individuals, all of whom share their story with 10 to 20 friends and neighbors." We raised two questions with our leadership: (1) If there were a reliable proxy for malpractice risk and if any individuals stood out, wouldn't that individual want to know?, and (2) if you had medical group members who stood out in terms of generating malpractice risk and dissatisfaction, wouldn't you want them to know?

Such messages were delivered during leadership councils, medical center medical board meetings, and faculty and department (section) meetings. Other institutions deliver similar program descriptions via internal publications and presentations by PCMC members.

As important as large group presentations are to promoting program adoption, individual and small group discussions with key leaders may be much more important. At Vanderbilt, members of our risk prevention team met individually and usually more than once, with our vice chancellor, dean, hospital and clinic operating officers, chief of staff, chief medical officer, and each department chair. Each meeting began with an expression of appreciation for their time and willingness to listen to our plan and provide feedback. We asserted that we wanted to proceed but only after we had addressed their questions. Such an approach courted the potential for many vetoes, but our philosophy was to identify issues and skeptics prior to initiating the process. Throughout, our research team aimed not to let our enthusiasm for the project outrun local buy in.

Sustaining Leadership Commitment and Support

What we learned during the individual and small group meetings ultimately resulted in the leadership commitment needed to withstand internal challenges to the process. Shortly after receiving his intervention folder, Dr. Urologist made an unannounced visit to the hospital's CEO. As he entered with his intervention folder in hand, he asked Mr. CEO whether he "was aware how inappropriate it was to single me out given how important I am to your hospital and the substantial financial contribution I make to your bottom line?" Clearly implied was a threat to take his patients elsewhere. Although perhaps with some heartburn, Mr. CEO replied: "I know about the program, and I support it. It is simply designed to give physicians a heads-up. I did not know you were identified (while thinking *somehow I am not surprised*) because the process initially is confidential. Most physicians who receive the data respond in a way to reduce their personal risk, and I trust you will as well. Have a nice day." Such unblinking leadership is critical to ongoing program effectiveness. Sustaining support also requires an active strategy. Those who provided initial endorsement and who have a right to know need to hear regular progress reports that present:

- Feedback about the numbers and quality of complaint capture and unique identification of physicians, other professionals, and units associated with complaints
- Numbers of high-risk physicians and others who have been identified and aggregate follow-up results that preserve individuals' confidentiality
- Trends in claims experience adjusted for revenue generation, patient encounters, or RVU generation

Finally, sustaining support requires intervention program leaders to anticipate, learn about, and address threats to the integrity of the process (for example, on the rare occasion when another high-risk physician barges into a leader's office). Sustaining support means taking advantage of every opportunity to provide service, data, and support to institutional leaders and PCMC chairs who request assistance in dealing with challenging circumstances. The political value of these efforts cannot be underestimated.

CONCLUSION

In conclusion, our preliminary studies (the science) and qualitative experiences (the politics) provide evidence (not proof) that the intervention program makes sense, reduces patient complaints associated with a majority of those intervened upon, and may reduce claims-related risks. In sum, a combination of science and politics has resulted in the following:

- A reliable proxy for claims (confirmed by others) permitting us to reliably identify high-risk physicians
- A tried-and-true process to make high-risk physicians aware, including the ability to acquire and process data, well-developed and tested intervention materials, substantial messenger training experience, knowledge from overseeing hundreds of interventions, and national comparison data
- A principled, graduated approach to addressing essential elements of The Joint Commission's Sentinel Event Alert #40[40]
- Ability to provide routine tracking and trending feedback using national comparison data to an organization's patient advocates about patient complaint report numbers and quality
- Ongoing, unbiased surveillance of patient complaints
- Commitment of medical leaders at Vanderbilt and other intervention sites
- Sufficient national respect to warrant demonstration projects at several of the nation's most prominent and highly ranked health systems
- Sufficient practicality for addressing perceived needs to warrant demonstration projects at unheralded but well-led hospitals and medical groups committed to professionalism and to gaining competitive advantages in their marketplace.

References

1. Stimson, C. J., Pichert, J., Moore, I. N., Dmochowski, R. R., Cornett, M. B., An, A. Q., & Hickson, G. B. (2010). Medical malpractice claims risk in urology: An empirical analysis of patient complaint data. *Journal of Urology, 183*(5), 1971–1976.
2. Hayden, A. C., Pichert, J. W., Fawcett, J., Moore, I. N., & Hickson, G. B. (2010). Best practices and advanced skills in healthcare service recovery programs. *Joint Commission Journal on Quality and Patient Safety, 36*(7), 310–318.
3. Hickson, G. B., & Entman, S. S. (2008). Physician practice behavior and litigation risk: Evidence and opportunity. *Clinical Obstetrics and Gynecology, 51*(4), 688–699.
4. Leape, L. L., Brennan, T. A., Laird, N. M., Lawthers, A. G., Localio, A. R., Barnes, B. A., Hebert, L., . . . Hiatt, H. (1991). The nature of adverse events in hospitalized patients. Results of the Harvard Medical Practice Study II. *New England Journal of Medicine, 324*(6), 377–384.
5. Brennan, T. A., Leape, L. L., Laird, N. M., Hebert, L., Localio, A. R., Lawthers, A. G., Newhouse JP, . . . Hiatt, H. H. (1991). Incidence of adverse events and negligence in hospitalized patients. Results of the Harvard Medical Practice Study I. *New England Journal of Medicine, 324*(6), 370–376.
6. Brennan, T. A., & Leape, L. L. (1991). Adverse events, negligence in hospitalized patients:

Results from the Harvard Medical Practice Study. *Perspective in Healthcare Risk Management, 11*(2), 2–8.

7. Johnson, W. G., Brennan, T. A., Newhouse, J. P, Leape, L. L., Lawthers, A. G., Hiatt, H. H., & Weiler, P. C. (1992). The economic consequences of medical injuries. Implications for a no-fault insurance plan. *JAMA, 267*(18), 2487–2492.
8. Kohn, L. T., Corrigan, J. M., & Donaldson, M. S. (1999). *To err is human: Building a safer health care system*. Washington, DC: National Academies Press.
9. Localio, A. R., Lawthers, A. G., Brennan, T. A., Laird, N. M., Hebert, L. E., Peterson, L. M., Newhouse, J. P., . . . Hiatt, H. H. (1991). Relation between malpractice claims and adverse events due to negligence. Results of the Harvard Medical Practice Study III. *New England Journal of Medicine, 325*(4), 245–251.
10. Mello, M. M., Studdert, D. M., DesRoches, C. M., Peugh, J., Zapert, K., Brennan, T. A., & Sage, W. M. (2005). Effects of a malpractice crisis on specialist supply and patient access to care. *Annals of Surgery, 242*(5), 621–628.
11. Mello, M. M., Studdert, D. M., & Brennan, T. A. (2003). The new medical malpractice crisis. *New England Journal of Medicine, 348*(23), 2281–2284.
12. Hickson, G. B., Clayton, E. W., Githens, P. B., & Sloan, F. A. (1992). Factors that prompted families to file medical malpractice claims following perinatal injuries. *JAMA, 267*(10), 1359–1363.
13. Vincent, C., Young, M., & Phillips, A. (1994). Why do people sue doctors? A study of patients and relatives taking legal action. *Lancet, 343*(8913), 1609–1613.
14. Sloan, F. A., Mergenhagen, P. M., Burfield, W. B., Bovbjerg, R. R., & Hassan, M. (1989). Medical malpractice experience of physicians. Predictable or haphazard? *JAMA, 262*(23), 3291–3297.
15. Bovbjerg, R. R., & Petronis, K. R. (1994). The relationship between physicians' malpractice claims history and later claims. Does the past predict the future? *JAMA, 272*(18), 1421–1426.
16. Entman, S. S., Glass, C. A., Hickson, G. B., Githens, P. B., Whetten-Goldstein, K., & Sloan, F. A. (1994). The relationship between malpractice claims history and subsequent obstetric care. *JAMA, 272*(20), 1588–1591.
17. Hickson, G. B., Clayton, E. W., Entman, S. S., Miller, C. S., Githens, P. B., Whetten-Goldstein, K., & Sloan, F. A. (1994). Obstetricians' prior malpractice experience and patients' satisfaction with care. *JAMA, 272*(20), 1583–1587.
18. Sloan, F. A. The injuries, antecedents, and consequences. (1993). In F. A. Sloan, P. B. Githens, E. W. Clayton, G. B. Hickson, D. A. Gentile, & D. F. Partlett (Eds.). *Suing for medical malpractice* (pp. 31–49). Chicago, IL: The University of Chicago Press.
19. Hickson, G. B., Pichert, J. W., Federspiel, C. F., & Clayton, E. W. (1997). Development of an early identification and response model of malpractice prevention. *Law and Contemporary Problems, 60*(1), 7–29.
20. Carroll, K. N., Cooper, W. O., Blackford, J. U., & Hickson, G. B. (2005). Characteristics of families that complain following pediatric emergency visits. *Ambulatory Pediatrics, 5*(6), 326–331.
21. Annandale, E., & Hunt, K. Accounts of disagreements with doctors. (1998). *Social Science & Medicine, 46*(1), 119–129.
22. Schlesinger, M., Mitchell, S., & Elbel, B. (2002). Voices unheard: barriers to expressing dissatisfaction to health plans. *Milbank Quarterly, 80*(4), 709–755, iv–v.
23. Mulcahy, L., & Tritter, J. Q. (1998). Pathways, pyramids and icebergs? Mapping the links between dissatisfaction and complaints. *Sociology of Health & Illness, 20*, 825.
24. Allsop, J., & Mulcahy, L. (2002). *Adverse events, complaints and clinical negligence claims: What do we know?* Chief Medical Officer's Advisory Group on Complaints and Clinical Negligence, Department of Health, London, UK. Retrieved from http://www.bl.dmu.ac.uk/Images/Adverse%20Events%20Report_tcm6-10832.pdf.
25. Best, A., & Andreasen, A. R. (1977). Consumer response to unsatisfactory purchases: A survey of perceiving defects, voicing complaints, and obtaining redress. *Law & Society Review, 11*, 701.
26. Vincent, C. A., & Coulter, A. (2002). Patient safety: What about the patient? *Quality and Safety in Health Care, 11*(1), 76–80.

27. Sage, W. M. (2002). Putting the patient in patient safety: Linking patient complaints and malpractice risk. *JAMA, 287*(22), 3003–3005.
28. Hickson, G. B., Federspiel, C. F., Pichert, J. W., Miller, C. S., Gauld-Jaeger, J., & Bost, P. (2002). Patient complaints and malpractice risk. *JAMA, 287*(22), 2951–2957.
29. Medicare program: Physicians Medicare fee schedule for calendar year. (1992). 56 Federal Register, 59511.
30. Moore, I. N., Pichert, J. W., Hickson, G. B., Federspiel, C. F., & Blackford, J. (2006). Rethinking peer review: Detecting and addressing medical malpractice claims risk. *Vanderbilt Law Review, 59*, 1175–1206.
31. Hickson, G. B., Federspiel, C. F., Blackford, J., Pichert, J. W., Gaska, W., Merrigan, M. W., & Miller, C. S. (2007). Patient complaints and malpractice risk in a regional healthcare center. *Southern Medical Journal, 100*(8), 791–796.
32. Stelfox, H. T., Gandhi, T. K., Orav, E. J., & Gustafson, M. L. (2005). The relation of patient satisfaction with complaints against physicians and malpractice lawsuits. *American Journal of Medicine, 118*(10), 1126–1133.
33. Hickson, G. B., Entman, S. S. (2010). Physicians influence the malpractice problem. *Obstetrics & Gynecology, 115*(4), 682–686.
34. Scheutzow, S. O. (1999). State medical peer review: High cost but no benefit—Is it time for a change? *American Journal of Law & Medicine, 25*(1), 7–60.
35. Ray, W. A., Schaffner, W., & Federspiel, C. F. (1985). Persistence of improvement in antibiotic prescribing in office practice. *JAMA, 253*(12), 1774–1776.
36. Eisenberg, J. (1986). *The reasons for doctors' practice patterns and ways to change them.* Ann Arbor, MI: Health Administration Press.
37. Soumerai, S. B., & Avorn, J. (1990). Principles of educational outreach ("academic detailing") to improve clinical decision making. *JAMA, 263*(4), 549–556.
38. Pichert, J. W., Hickson, G. B., & Moore, I. N. (2008). Using patient complaints to promote patient safety: The Patient Advocacy Reporting System (PARS). In K. Henriksen, J. B. Battles, M. A. Keyes, & M. L. Grady (Eds.), *Advances in patient safety: New directions and alternative approaches* (vol. 2, pp. 421–430). Bethesda, MD: Agency for Healthcare Research and Quality.
39. Hickson, G. B., Pichert, J. W., Webb, L. E., & Gabbe, S. G. (2007). A complementary approach to promoting professionalism: Identifying, measuring, and addressing unprofessional behaviors. *Academic Medicine, 82*(11), 1040–1048.
40. The Joint Commission. (2008). *Behaviors that undermine a culture of safety*. Sentinel Event Alert #40. Oakbrook Terrace, IL: The Joint Commission. Retrieved from http://www.jointcommission.org/SentinelEvents/SentinelEventAlert/sea_40.htm.
41. Mukherjee, K., Pichert, J. W., Cornett, M. B., Yan, G., Hickson, G. B., & Diaz, J. J. (in press). All trauma surgeons are not created equal: Asymmetric distribution of malpractice claims risk. *Journal of Trauma*.
42. Campbell, D., Cornett, M. B., Obremskey, W. T., Pichert, J. W., & Hickson, G. B. (2008). *Do orthopedists have dissimilar patient complaint profiles (and risk for litigation)?* Poster P273 presented at the annual meeting of the American Association of Orthopedic Surgeons, San Francisco, CA. Retrieved from http://www3.aaos.org/education/anmeet/anmt2008/poster/poster.cfm?Pevent = P273.
43. Hickson, G. B., Federspiel, C. F., Blackford, J., Pichert, J. W., Gaska, W., Merrigan M. W., & Miller, C. W. (2007). Cumulative distribution of complaints by cumulative distribution of Physician Study Group based on 3291 complaints for 445 physicians 2001–2003. *Southern Medical Journal, 100*(8), 791–796.

29

Medical Malpractice Litigation: Conventional Wisdom Versus Reality

Marina Karp, MJ

"Representative government and trial by jury are the heart and lungs of liberty. Without them we have no other fortification against being ridden like horses, fleeced like sheep, worked like cattle, and fed and clothed like swine and hounds."

—John Adams

Intricate matters of public policy have often been portrayed as unrealistic black and white issues by the mainstream media. Health care is no exception. In fact, the U.S. healthcare system is extraordinarily multifaceted and has been the subject of national debate for decades. The media's role in deciding *what* issues the public should care about is significant. Network executives have mastered the art of framing and reducing complex policy issues into oversimplified, 30-second sound bites. From issues as significant as waging foreign wars to inconsequential stories related to pop culture, the media has a profound influence on how people construe information. Recently, the media, specifically television news, in response to such complicated subject matter as health care, has disseminated a continuous loop of misinformation that stupefies even the most skeptical observer. Yet these unsubstantiated claims and hyperbole were reported as truth because television remains the top source for news by a majority of the public.[1] A survey conducted by the Pew Research Center for the People & the Press found that two-thirds of Americans, 66%, responded that television was their main source of national and international news.

Distortions centered on a variety of issues, from rationing and socialized medicine to death panels and tort reform.[2] The corporate media, with great success, conflated the issues and deluded the public. For instance, 59% of Americans, in response to a Kaiser public opinion poll, think the health reform law contains a government-run health plan.[3] A smaller, yet noteworthy proportion of respondents inaccurately believe myths about the legislation, including 15% of Americans who are unsure

FIGURE 29.1 Source of National and International News

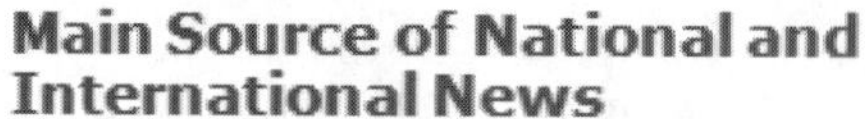

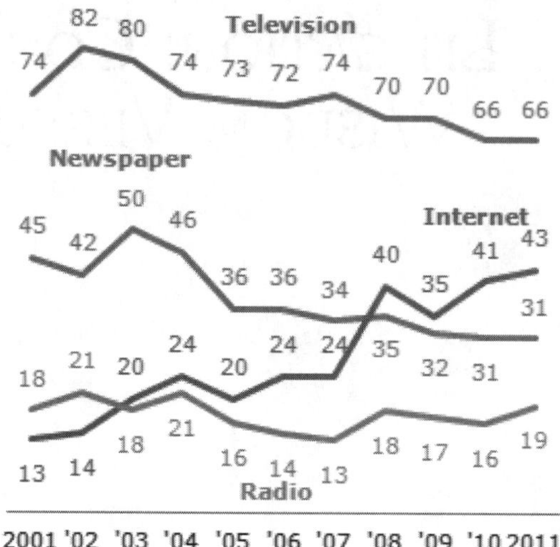

Figures do not add to 100% because of multiple responses.

Press Widely Criticized, But Trusted More than Other Information Sources: Views of the News Media: 1985–2011, September 22, 2011, the Pew Research Center For the People & the Press, a project of the Pew Research Center.

as to whether the law includes death panels, while less than half responded correctly that death panels are not included in the law.[3] The media, over the past decade, has been especially unreliable regarding issues associated with medical malpractice litigation and tort reform. The aim of this chapter is to provide an account of how the conventional wisdom related to malpractice litigation originated and evolved over time. This chapter will explore the public perception versus the reality of malpractice litigation trends. Evidence of claims filed, amounts of damage awards, and types of injuries that have warranted payments will be presented. The real crisis within the healthcare system—rates of medical errors—will be examined within the context of current litigation trends.

THE CAMPAIGN

The idea of frivolous lawsuits and restrictions on damage awards can be traced back to the 1950s.[4] The concept, while not novel, has evolved over the years, and the first major piece of legislation was enacted in 1975.[5] The Indiana state legislature was among the first to pass a strict medical malpractice law—one of the harshest in the country.[5] State legislators capped all awards and abolished punitive damages entirely.[5] Although Indiana was considered a pioneer in responding to corporate claims of frivolous lawsuits, the idea of tort reform and junk lawsuits further surfaced during the economic unrest of the mid-1980s.[6] This tumult was generally correlated with the liability insurance crisis, in which premiums for malpractice, among other types of liability coverage, skyrocketed and insurers began capriciously canceling policies, leaving many without coverage.[6] During the next decade, several states passed reforms that altered tort law, negatively impacting consumers. These "anti-consumer states," as referred to by Professor Richard Alderman, director of the Consumer Law Center at the University of Houston, provided no protection to consumers in order to gain support from big business[7] (and from practicing physicians and the American Medical Association). Consequently, the 1990s saw a surge of business-funded grassroots efforts and lobbying groups prompted by the American Tort Reform Association (ATRA).[6] Accordingly, ATRA contracted with one of the largest lobby/PR firms in the country, APCO & Associates, which built a network of local/regional tort reform advocacy organizations.[6] These organizations, called Citizens Against Lawsuit Abuse (CALA), were self-proclaimed grassroots groups, solely funded by ordinary citizens' small donations. However, investigative reports later revealed that "the money trail from many of these groups leads directly to large corporate donors, including tobacco, insurance, oil and gas, chemical and pharmaceutical companies, medical associations, and auto manufacturers."[6] The anticonsumer movement gained a foothold in 1994 during the Texas gubernatorial race.[8] Republican strategist Carl Rove devised a tactic for gubernatorial candidate George W. Bush to galvanize physicians, small businesses, and numerous healthcare industry trade groups to join the GOP by announcing his pledge to rid the civil justice system of "junk lawsuits."[9] This claim, absent any supportive data, brought in new contributors to fund future Republican candidates—at all levels of government. Rove's effective maneuvering has maintained favorable support from the healthcare industry and physicians, while the manufactured malpractice litigation crisis produced by the media has helped lobbyists shift the focus, successfully provoking major changes in state tort laws.[10]

TORT REFORM AS A NATIONAL POLICY INITIATIVE

The issue of tort reform, while a major policy initiative pursued by lobbyists and politicians, remained a relatively obscure subject among the public until the early 2000s.[5] During the 2000 presidential race, George W. Bush used his gubernatorial record of sponsoring tort reform legislation as a campaign centerpiece.[5] Subsequent to Bush's presidential appointment, he declared the need for tort reform in his 2003 State of the Union Address: "To improve our healthcare system, we must address one of the prime causes of higher cost—the constant threat that physicians and hospitals will be unfairly sued. . . . Because of excessive litigation, everybody pays more for health care, and many parts of America are losing fine doctors. No one has ever been healed by a frivolous lawsuit; I urge the Congress to pass medical liability reform."[11] Moreover, the presidential debate in 2004, when contenders John Kerry and George W. Bush sparred over the issue, officially propelled tort reform into the mainstream.[11] Since the debate, the rhetoric has only gotten more sophisticated as corporations have funded more than 100 grassroots groups and advocacy organizations committed solely to spreading the word that the civil justice system is out of control.[10] The efforts of the business community, Republican politicians, and corporate lobbyists have paid off because there are now more than 30 states with restrictions on both punitive damages and noneconomic damages.[12]

- Thirty-three states have reformed punitive damages law; one state had reforms struck down as unconstitutional and has not enacted additional reforms.[12]
- Twenty-three states have modified the rules for awarding noneconomic damages; four states have had reforms struck down as unconstitutional and have not enacted additional reforms.[12]

In a speech in Little Rock, Arkansas, on January 26, 2004, President George W. Bush said,

"One of the major cost drivers in the delivery of health care are these junk and frivolous lawsuits."[13] Bush further contended that "[r]ising malpractice insurance premiums and needless medical procedures ordered up out of fear of lawsuits cost federal taxpayers 'at least' $28 billion a year in added costs to government medical programs."[13,14] Despite Bush's inflated figures related to defensive medicine, the Congressional Budget Office (CBO) issued its own analysis and concluded that the study "was not a valid basis for projecting total costs of defensive medicine."[15] Even further, the CBO applied the same methodology used in the study of Medicare patients hospitalized for two types of heart disease to a broader set of ailments and found no evidence that restrictions on tort liability reduce medical spending.[15]

Again, in 2005, Bush stumped on the issue of tort reform.[16] Speaking in front of a room full of physicians, Bush asserted: "What I'm here to do is say as clearly as I can—the United States Congress needs to pass real medical liability reform this year."[16] He further stated that large malpractice awards have increased the cost of health care so much that doctors across the country have begun to "close their doors or scale back on services."[16] The movement to restrict injured patients from holding wrongdoers accountable for their negligence gained tremendous momentum over the past decade. In fact, President Obama, in his 2011 State of the Union Address, remarked that he would be willing to discuss "medical malpractice reform to rein in frivolous lawsuits."[17]

CONVENTIONAL WISDOM

It is no surprise that the public believes that predatory trial lawyers have plagued the civil justice system with junk suits intended to trick juries into awarding excessively large payments to undeserving plaintiffs. The results of a recent nationwide Rasmussen poll found the following attitudes concerning malpractice litigation and tort reform:

- More than half (57%) of voters nationwide favor limiting the amount of money a jury can award a plaintiff in a medical malpractice lawsuit. Only 29% disagree, and 14% are not sure.[18]
- Just under half (47%) believe that restricting jury awards for medical malpractice lawsuits will significantly reduce the cost of health care in the United States, 28% disagree, and 25% are not sure.[18]
- Just under half of U.S. voters (48%) say it is too easy to sue a doctor for medical malpractice in the United States today.[18]

REALITY OF MALPRACTICE LITIGATION

A review of the literature, government agency studies, and year-over-year statistics has demonstrated that the public has a fundamentally flawed perception of malpractice litigation and tort reform.[19] The figures discussed below illustrate these stark gaps in perception versus reality. The evidence substantiates that there is no explosion of malpractice claims and the injuries suffered by victims of negligent care are hardly frivolous. Public Citizen's Congress Watch conducted an analysis of data from the federal government's National Practitioner Data Bank (NPDB), the Department of Health and Human Services, and A.M. Best, which in fact revealed that in 2010 the "prevalence and cost of medical malpractice litigation were at their lowest levels on record."[20] The analysts found that between 2000 and 2010, healthcare spending rose 90%, while medical malpractice payments fell 11.9%.[20] Thus, the rising costs of care cannot be explained by the current trend in malpractice litigation.[20] The total number of paid claims in 2010 was 9,894 (Figure 29.2), with the average claim payment totaling $336,437 (Figure 29.3).[21] The payments allotted to injured victims in 2010 amounted to 0.13 of 1% of national healthcare costs.[20]

Additionally, the number of malpractice payments made on behalf of doctors decreased 5% from 2009 to 2010 (Figure 29.4), denoting

FIGURE 29.2 Number of Paid Medical Malpractice Claims, 2010

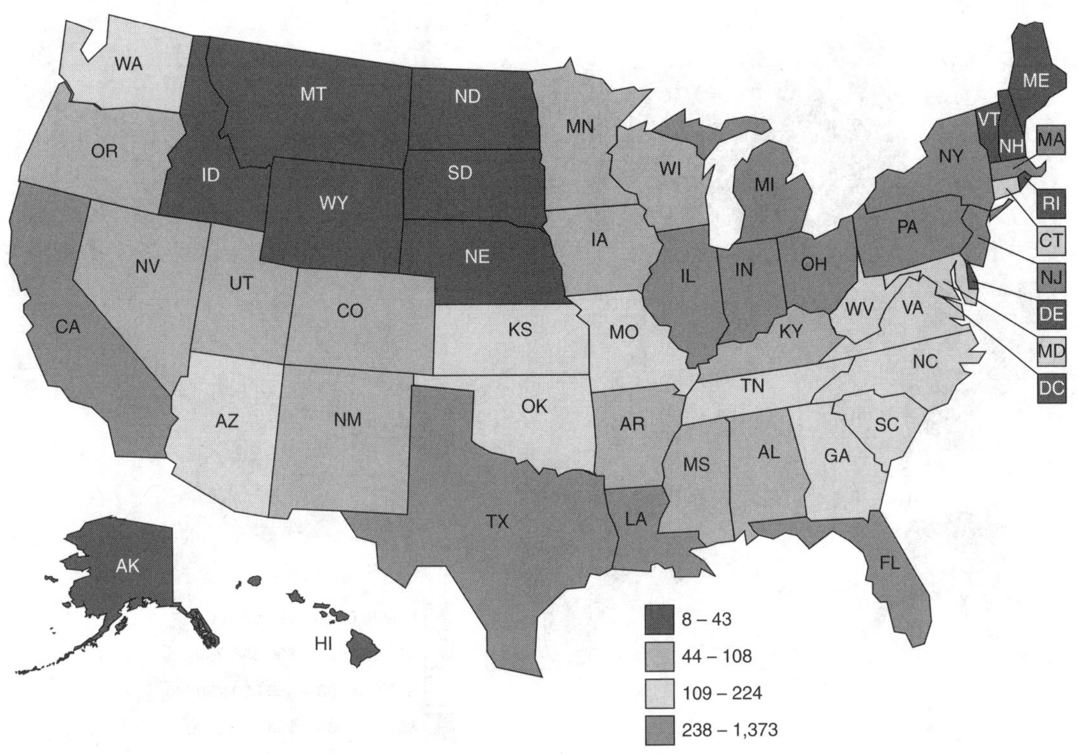

Number of Paid Medical Malpractice Claims, 2010, statehealthfacts.org, The Henry J. Kaiser Family Foundation, December 2010. This information was reprinted with permission from the Henry J. Kaiser Family Foundation.

the seventh straight year that the number of payments has fallen.[20] Peculiarly, the total liability insurance premiums declined from 2007 to 2009, but reductions in premiums have not matched reductions in litigation payments.[20] Specifically, payments made on behalf of doctors in 2009 for medical malpractice negligence were 8.7% lower in unadjusted dollars than in 2000; however, liability insurance premiums for doctors were 56.2% higher in 2009 than in 2000.[20] Additional data illustrate that of the 10,772 medical malpractice payments in 2009, nearly two-thirds (64.5%) compensated for negligence that resulted in a significant permanent injury, major permanent injury, quadriplegia, brain damage, the need for lifelong care, or death.[20] Even more notable, the dollar value of payments for these adverse outcomes accounted for an even higher proportion—more than four-fifths (82.1%) of the total value of malpractice payments.[20] As Figure 29.5 represents, approximately 47% of the malpractice payments compensated victims and families for negligence resulting in death, quadriplegia, brain damage, or injuries requiring lifelong care.[20]

THE REAL PROBLEM

The campaign to restrict damage payments to injured victims has prevailed in shaping public opinion, state legislation, and congressional

FIGURE 29.3 Total Dollars in Paid Claims

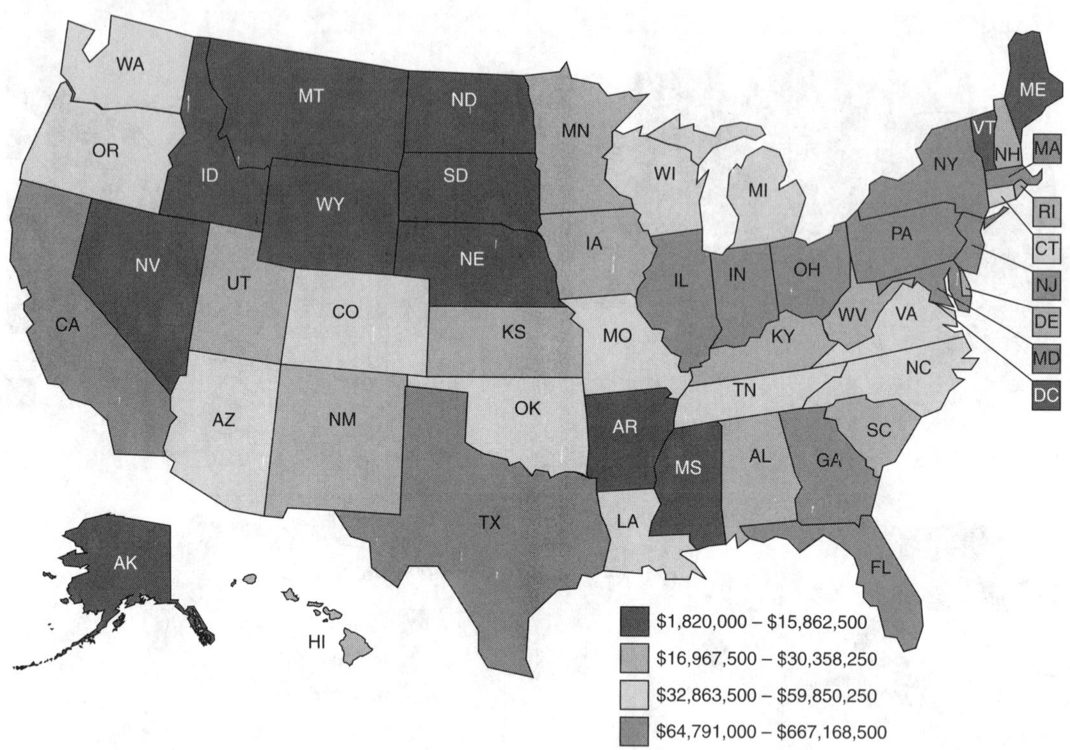

Payments on Medical Malpractice Claims, 2010, statehealthfacts.org, The Henry J. Kaiser Family Foundation, December 2010. This information was reprinted with permission from the Henry J. Kaiser Family Foundation

proposals.[22] Although the evidence repudiates the widespread perceptions about malpractice litigation, the numbers have not been the subject of any mainstream media discussion. The heated arguments have resulted in misconceptions and a general lack of understanding of the issues. The strategic omission of facts and lack of intelligent analysis have masked a more important problem within the healthcare industry—medical error.[23]

The most cited study documenting the incidence of the rate of medical errors includes the 1999 Institute of Medicine's (IOM) report *To Err Is Human*. The study concluded that 44,000–98,000 patients were dying every year because of preventable medical errors.[24] This landmark study provoked thought, prompted questions, and impelled a pursuit of accountability within hospitals. Medical error rates have since, although not consistently, been monitored and studied. More recently, findings have indicated that rates of error and adverse outcomes have not significantly declined over time. The findings from the Department of Health and Human Services and hospitals in the state of North Carolina have indicated that error rates have not decreased despite the drop in litigation.[20] The Department of Health and Human Services Inspector General published

FIGURE 29.4 Number of Medical Malpractice Payments Made on Behalf of Physicians, 1991–2010

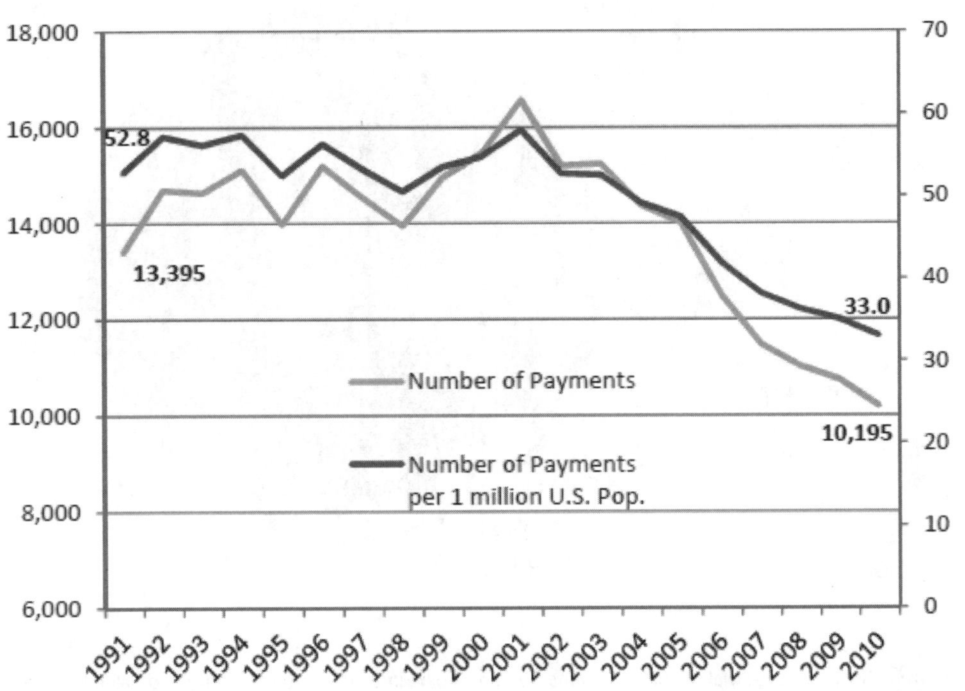

Public Citizen (2011). Medical Malpractice Payments Declined Again in 2010: Both Frequency and Value Fell To Lowest Levels on Record by Most Measures. Data Source: National Practitioner Data Bank; U.S. Census. http://www.citizen.org/documents/NPDB-2010.pdf. Accessed December 14, 2011.

a report that concluded that one in seven Medicare patients experienced a serious adverse event during their hospital stays in 2008.[25] Specifically, 13.1% of Medicare patients experienced an adverse event resulting in the four most serious categories of patient harm.[25] In one month, 1.5% of Medicare patients experienced an event that contributed to their deaths, which equates to 15,000 patients in a single month.[25] The study also revealed that 44% of the medical errors were preventable, which resulted in a key recommendation from the Inspector General: The "need for hospitals to significantly reduce the incidence of adverse events, as many of the events identified were preventable."[25]

Another recent study sought to address the uncertainty as to whether any improvements have been made in the safety of patients at the state level.[26] The investigators analyzed whether the "statewide rates of harm" in North Carolina have been decreasing over time.[26] The reviewers identified 588 harms from 2,341 patient admissions (25.1 harms per 100 admissions).[26] The analysis confirmed "no significant changes in the overall rate of harms per 1000 patient-days or the rate of preventable harms."[26]

Information detailing medical error rates has been recorded since the mid-1970s.[27] Preventable medical error rates have not significantly decreased over time.[27] Perhaps the "real problem is too much medical malpractice, not too

FIGURE 29.5 Total Value of Payments by Injury Type, 2010

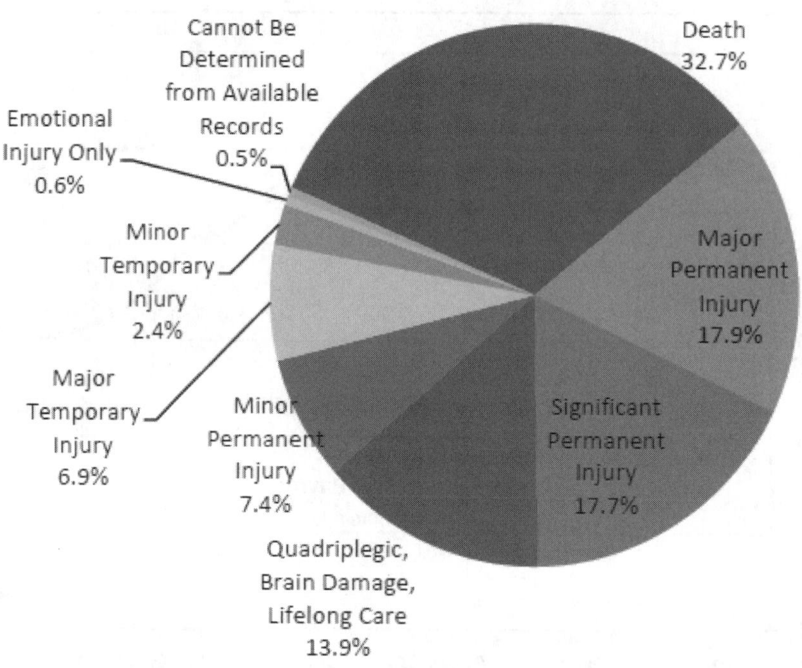

Public Citizen (2011). Medical Malpractice Payments Declined Again in 2010: Both Frequency and Value Fell To Lowest Levels on Record by Most Measures. Data Source: National Practitioner Data Bank. http://www.citizen.org/documents/NPDB-2010.pdf. Accessed December 14, 2011.

much litigation."[27] The strategy employed by "organized interests" of downplaying the impact of patient harm as a result of preventable medical error while overestimating the rate of malpractice litigation, has proven effective in swaying a majority of the public.[27] Despite decades of deceptive practices, we should not despair because research has indicated that a "far less financially vested group" is emerging and gaining attention.[29] The patient advocacy and safety movement has been promoting a completely different set of policies and principles.[28] The advocacy group has employed a radical approach, that is, one that identifies the root cause of the problems associated with malpractice litigation.[28] The aim of their efforts is to "significantly lower the amount of actual medical malpractice, errors and negligence that result in harm" that occur in health care.[28] Initially, it will be necessary to dispel myths linked with malpractice claims, including that the civil justice system is inundated with malpractice suits, a majority of which are baseless; the risk of litigation prompts an equal amount of defensive medicine practices; and patients are eager to sue doctors.[28]

Additionally, advocates promote a new culture—one of transparency that will incentivize exposure of patient harm and preventable errors.[28] The veil of secrecy will no longer be accepted. Proponents will facilitate in the implementation of policies that will prompt collaboration, while ensuring safeguards for the full disclosure of error. Human beings, even physicians, are fallible and inevitably subject to misjudgments and mistakes. However, each incident, if disclosed and addressed, can be a chance to uncover and change harmful habits and techniques while advancing knowledge. The creation of an open, honest culture will result in a seismic shift in the way care is delivered—an ambitious, yet achievable goal. To think otherwise would be detrimental to all those toiling in the trenches.

CONCLUSION

The Bill of Rights included in the United States Constitution guarantees the people the right to hold accountable their offenders in both criminal and civil matters. Specifically, the Seventh Amendment provides: "In Suits at common law, where the value in controversy shall exceed twenty dollars, the right of trial by jury shall be preserved, and no fact tried by a jury, shall be otherwise re-examined in any Court of the United States, then according to the rules of the common law."[29] This fundamental right has been stripped from many citizens because state legislatures have altered tort laws and unjustly restricted payment amounts for those victimized by the healthcare industry. The elimination of individual liberties is dangerous, and once the liberty is taken away, it becomes nearly impossible to regain.

Tort reform is hardly the answer to combat malpractice. The corporate interests, physician groups, and politicians have upheld tort reform as the solution to malpractice litigation. This type of response will only further burden victims of harm caused by negligence. The hype over tort reform has overshadowed thoughtful discussion and what is certain to remedy the problem of litigation—reduce malpractice.[30]

> *"The best defense against a claim, after all, is that no damage has occurred."*
>
> **—Randall Bovbjerg**

References

1. Pew Research Center for the People & the Press. (2011, September 22). *Press widely criticized, but trusted more than other information sources: Views of the news media: 1985–2011*. Retrieved from http://www.people-press.org/2011/09/22/press-widely-criticized-but-trusted-more-than-other-institutions/. Accessed May 15, 2012.
2. Pearle, L. (2007, May 2). *I'm being sued for what?* ABC News Law & Justice Unit. Retrieved from http://abcnews.go.com/TheLaw/story?id=3121086&page=1.
3. The Henry J. Kaiser Family Foundation. (2011, February 5). *Pop quiz: Assessing Americans' familiarity with the health care law*. Retrieved from http://www.kff.org/healthreform/upload/8148.pdf
4. The literature traces the origins of restricting the amount of damages awarded to a patient (plaintiff) from a jury dating back to the 1950s (although not called "tort reform").
5. Mencimer, S. (2006). *Blocking the courthouse door: How the Republican Party and its corporate allies are taking away your right to sue*. New York, NY: Free Press. Although this book does not provide an account of the story of Frank Cornelius, his role was critical in the passage of the Indiana state law restricting damages paid to injured patients.
6. Deal, C., & Doroshow, J. (2003, August 3). *The CALA files: The secret campaign by big tobacco and other major industries to take away your rights*. Center for Justice and Democracy and Public Citizen. Retrieved from http://centerjd.org/content/cala-files-secret-campaign-big-tobacco-and-other-major-industries-take-away-your-rights.

   Although this paper does not explore the causes that may have contributed to the "liability insurance crisis," the authors cite numerous studies revealing that the so-called crisis was instigated by the insurance industry's abuse of underwriting practices. [Note from authors: The research for this report includes a massive accumulation of documents made public during the state attorneys general litigation against the tobacco industry in the late 1990s that was specially analyzed for this report. The data revealed that "big tobacco" spent millions of dollars a year (and in at least one year $15 million) supporting ATRA, state CALAs, and other activities to weaken tort laws in many states. For instance, in 1995, big tobacco allocated $5.5 million for ATRA, more than half of ATRA's budget. In some cases, CALAs, such as the one in Louisiana, were virtually created by the tobacco industry. Tobacco money has gone directly to ATRA, APCO, and state organizations. It has also been indirectly funneled to the cause through law firms such as the Washington, DC, firm Covington & Burling, trade associations, and lobbyists. The industry's Tobacco Institute also played an instrumental role through its State Activities Division. In the 1980s, big tobacco's efforts were instrumental in the passage of legislation immunizing the industry against product liability claims in New Jersey and California.]

7. Savage, D. G. (2004, September 22). The race for the White House: Texans still at odds over Bush's legal reforms. *LA Times*. Retrieved from http://articles.latimes.com/2004/sep/22/nation/na-texas22.
8. Texas Archival Resources Online. An inventory of press office speech files at the Texas state archives, 1986, 1989–2000, Texas Governor George W. Bush. Retrieved from http://www.lib.utexas.edu/taro/tslac/40090/tsl-40090.html.
9. Saladoff, S. (Director). *Hot coffee*. [HBO Documentary Films Summer Series Premiered: June 27, 2011].
10. Mencimer, S. (2005, May 5). *The fake crisis over lawsuits: Who's paying to keep the myths alive?* The Alicia Patterson Foundation. Retrieved from http://aliciapatterson.org/stories/fake-crisis-over-lawsuits-whos-paying-keep-myths-alive.
11. State of the Union Address of George W. Bush to the Joint Session of Congress. (2003, January 28). Retrieved from http://legacy.c-span.org/Transcripts/SOTU-2003.aspx.
12. American Tort Reform Association (ATRA). (2011, June 30). Tort Reform Record. Retrieved from http://www.atra.org/sites/default/files/documents/record_12-22-11.pdf.
13. Bush, G. W. (2004, January 26). *President Bush calls for medical liability reform*. Speech before the Baptist Health Medical Center in Little Rock, Arkansas. Retrieved from http://georgewbush-whitehouse.archives.gov/news/releases/2004/01/20040126-3.html.

    Bush relied on a 1996 paper, authored by Stanford economists Daniel P. Kessler and Mark McClellan. McClellan, an economist and a physician, served as Bush's senior White House policy director for health care and was subsequently appointed as the head of the Food and Drug Administration.
14. Kessler, D., & McClellan, M. (1996). Do doctors practice defensive medicine? *Quarterly Journal of Economics, 355*, 353–390.

    Specifically, the study estimated that states with any of four restrictions (caps on noneconomic or total damages, prohibitions on punitive damages, no automatic addition of prejudgment interest, and offsets for collateral-source benefits) lowered spending for inpatient care by between 5% and 9% in the year following the patients' initial admission for either diagnosis. However, the study also found that a second set of tort restrictions (caps on contingent fees for plaintiffs' attorneys, deferred payment of some or all damages, restrictions on joint-and-several liability, and public compensation funds for patients) tended to increase spending by between roughly 2% and 3%, at least in the short run. Those results were unexplained.
15. FactCheck.org, Annenberg Public Policy Center of the University of Pennsylvania. (2004, January 29). President uses dubious statistics on costs of malpractice lawsuits: Two congressional agencies dispute findings that caps on damage awards produce big savings in medical costs. Retrieved from http://www.factcheck.org/president_uses_dubious_statistics_on_costs_of.html.
16. Gonzalez C. (2005, January 5). U.S. President George W. Bush delivers tort reform address in Madison County. *The Madison Record*. Retrieved from http://www.madisonrecord.com/news/138396-president-bush-transcripts-of-tort-reform-address.
17. State of the Union Address of Barack Obama to the Joint Session of Congress (2011, January 26). Retrieved from at http://abc

news.go.com/Politics/State_of_the_Union/state-of-the-union-2011-full-transcript/story?id = 12759395.
18. Rasmussen Reports. (2009, June 17). *48% say it's too easy to sue doctors, 44% favor caps on jury awards*. Retrieved from http://www.rasmussenreports.com/public_content/business/general_business/june_2009/48_say_it_s_too_easy_to_sue_doctors_44_favor_caps_on_jury_awards.
19. Rasmussen Reports. (2009, December 2). *Voters favor tort reform by two-to-one margin*. Retrieved from http://www.rasmussenreports.com/public_content/politics/current_events/healthcare/november_2009/voters_favor_tort_reform_by_two_to_one_margin.
20. Public Citizen's Congress Watch. (2011, May). *Medical malpractice payments declined again in 2010: Both frequency and value fell to lowest levels on record by most measures*. Retrieved from http://www.citizen.org/documents/NPDB-2010.pdf.

    Premiums' share of overall health costs in 2009 was lower than in any year since NPDB began collecting data on medical malpractice payments.
21. Kaiser Family Foundation. *Number of paid medical malpractice claims, 2011*. Retrieved from http://www.statehealthfacts.org/comparemaptable.jsp?ind = 436&cat = 8.
22. Rivoli, D. (2011, July 8). *House committee passes bill aimed at frivolous suits*. Law360. Retrieved from http://www.law360.com/articles/256795/house-committee-passes-bill-aimed-at-frivolous-suits.

    The bill, the Lawsuit Abuse Reduction Act, cleared the U.S. House committee 20–13. If passed into law, it would undo the changes to civil procedure instituted in 1993 that gave leeway to judges in deciding sanctions and penalties.
23. Bovbjerg, R. R. (2006). Beyond tort reform: Fixing real problems. *Indiana Health Law Review, 3*, 3.
24. Kohn, L. T., Corrigan, J. M., & Donaldson, M. S. (Eds.) (1999). *To Err Is Human: Building a Safer Health Care System*. Washington, DC: National Academies Press.
25. Department of Health and Human Services, Office of Inspector General. (2010, November). *Adverse events in hospitals: National incidence among medicare beneficiaries*. Retrieved from http://oig.hhs.gov/oei/reports/oei-06-09-00090.pdf.
26. Landrigan, C. P., Parry, G. J., Bones, C. B., Hackbarth, A. D. Goldmann, D. A., & Sharek, P. J. (2010). Temporal trends in rates of patient harm resulting from medical care. *New England Journal of Medicine, 363*, 2124–2134. Retrieved from http://www.nejm.org/doi/full/10.1056/NEJMsa1004404.

    A 2010 study of patients treated in North Carolina hospitals found that 18% of patients suffered adverse events and 63% of these harms were avoidable. Of the adverse events, 2.4% caused or contributed to a patient's death.
27. Baker, T. (2005). *The medical malpractice myth*. Chicago, IL: University of Chicago Press.
28. Mahar, M. (2011, March 11). *Instead of tort reform, why not focus on reducing actual malpractice?* Health Beat. Retrieved from http://www.healthbeatblog.com/2011/03/instead-of-tort-reform-why-not-focus-on-reducing-actual-malpractice.html.
29. U.S. CONST. amend. VII, § 1.
30. Bovbjerg, R. R. (1986). Medical malpractice on trial: Quality of care is the important standard. *Law & Contemporary Problems, 49*, 321.

30

Quality and Safety Education for Nurses: Integrating Quality and Safety Competencies into Nursing Education

Gwen Sherwood, PhD, RN, FAAN, Louise LaFramboise, PhD, RN, Connie Miller, PhD, RN, and Bethany Robertson, DNP, CNM, NM

Nurses have the responsibility of constant surveillance of hospitalized patients and so spend the most time with patients. In ambulatory settings, nurses coordinate care among multiple disciplines. As nurses guide and plan patient care, they are increasingly accountable for leading in quality and safety both for the care they deliver and to improve the systems in which they work. As healthcare organizations have responded to the Institute of Medicine's reports that exposed poor communication, lack of care coordination, and gaps in health professions education related to quality and safety, nurses are increasingly recognized for their potential to champion applications of new safety and improvement science to improve care outcomes.

Public awareness of quality and safety issues in health care stemming from the Institute of Medicine's Quality Chasm series of reports[1,2,3] helped stimulate widespread initiatives for change. Rapid responses among regulatory agencies prompted immediate quality and safety improvement projects, which organizations were not always prepared to implement and which nurses and other disciplines often were not prepared to lead.[4] To address this gap, the 2004 IOM report charged 21st century health professionals to be prepared to focus on safety by delivering patient-centered care in interprofessional teams based on evidenced-based standards with continuous quality improvement enhanced by application of informatics;[5] application of these six competencies can help mitigate healthcare errors, assure care coordination, and improve care outcomes. However, analysis of health professions educational curricula revealed few opportunities for achieving the competencies.

The purpose of this chapter is to describe the changes in nursing education led by the Quality and Safety Education for Nursing (QSEN) project to meet the challenges as healthcare organizations transition to a new accountability for quality and safety.[2] We will describe key attributes of the six competencies for integrating into nursing education, as well as a 15-school learning collaborative that piloted implementation and outcomes assessments. We include two exemplars from the collaborative to illustrate integration of the competencies and how faculty and students achieved the competency objectives.

QUALITY AND SAFETY EDUCATION FOR NURSES (QSEN)

The Quality and Safety Education for Nurses (QSEN) project has become a strategic voice in defining, piloting, and implementing quality and safety competencies to transform prelicensure and graduate nursing education.[6,7,8] Led by Professor Linda Cronenwett at the University of North Carolina at Chapel Hill, the QSEN project was launched in 2005 and funded by the Robert Wood Johnson Foundation. The commitment and will to improve nursing education as a bridge to improve nursing care quality has led a renaissance in transforming nursing curricula and educational standards, ignited by a Pilot School Learning Collaborative to demonstrate the successful integration of quality and safety.

The purpose of QSEN is to integrate quality and safety work into nursing-role identity so that it is a part of their daily work; nursing care is based on a framework of quality and safety so that nurses ask the kind of questions about the care they deliver that leads to improving quality outcomes and patient safety from a systems perspective.

DEFINING THE COMPETENCIES

The QSEN project team first defined the competencies identified by the Institute of Medicine (IOM) that are essential for all health professionals: patient-centered care, teamwork and collaboration, evidence-based practice, quality improvement, and safety and informatics.[5] A national expert panel and advisory board representing each of the IOM competencies, innovative pedagogies, key education and professional organizations, nursing executives, and physician accrediting groups reached consensus on definitions of the six competencies shown in Figure 30.1.[6] Each competency was described with the knowledge, skills, and attitudes (KSAs) for each so that faculty could employ innovative approaches to curricula integration based on their school's philosophy and framework of teaching. Faculty may use multiple avenues to achieve the competencies, such as threading throughout the curriculum, embedding in simulated learning scenarios, integrating into clinical learning experiences, facilitating through postclinical conference reflections, developing narrative pedagogies, and other innovative teaching approaches.[9]

These six competencies extend traditional views of nursing by incorporating new quality and safety science adapted from high-performance industries.[10] The competencies are interrelated and together form a composite view of quality and safety practice. The competencies have explicit knowledge, skills, and attitudes for prelicensure educational entry programs including diploma, associate degree nursing, and baccalaureate programs.[6] Higher-level knowledge, skills, and attitudes describe application in graduate nursing education consistent with the practice requirements and environment for advanced practice nursing as approved by the National Organization of Nurse Practitioner Faculty (NONPF) (www.qsen.org).[7,8,11]

Patient-Centered Care

Patient-centered care is expanding the traditional basis for nursing. The KSAs expand the focus to include the patient and their family as central to decision making about their care accomplished by including them as valuable team members and safety allies.[12] Patients and families can help identify and prevent errors, which can also be used as opportunities to provide information to them about their care. For example, it should be regarded as a warning sign of potential error when patients and their families question the accuracy of medication administration.[13] Nurses are cautioned to stop to investigate correct administration and to offer patient education information if orders have changed. Recognizing and respecting the uniqueness of

FIGURE 30.1 Definitions of the Six Quality and Safety Competencies[6,7,8]

1. Patient-centered care: Recognize the patient or designee as the source of control and full partner in providing compassionate and coordinated care based on respect for the patient's preferences, values, and needs.
2. Teamwork and collaboration: Function effectively within nursing and interprofessional teams, fostering open communication, mutual respect, and shared decision making to achieve quality patient care.
3. Evidence-based practice: Integrate best current evidence with clinical expertise and patient/family preferences and values for delivery of optimal health care.
4. Quality improvement: Use data to monitor the outcomes of care processes and use improvement methods to design and test changes to continually improve the quality and safety of healthcare systems.
5. Safety: Minimize risk of harm to patients and providers through both system effectiveness and individual performance.
6. Informatics: Use information and technology to communicate, manage knowledge, mitigate error and support decision making.

patients, appreciating their values and beliefs, and mindfully listening are key to patient-centered care.

Interprofessional Teamwork and Collaboration

Interprofessional teamwork is a contributing factor in 70% of medical errors, yet few health professions schools offer learning experiences that bring multiple health professions students together to be prepared for working together in complex practice environments.[5] Teamwork and collaboration are built from developing self-awareness, transformational leadership, and interactional skills based on emotional intelligence.[14] Complex care requires coordination across disciplines, such as physicians, pharmacists, and others involved in a patient's care to communicate[15] through briefings (planning), huddles (problem solving), and debriefings (process improvement) designed in the TeamSTEPPS program.[16]

Evidence-Based Practice

The continuing evolution of knowledge development requires skills in asking critical questions to search for the latest evidence to support practice decisions. Nursing care standards are written to include sources and levels of evidence by applying a model of evidence-based practice. The first step is assessing and defining the clinical issue with specific questions and then researching the current state of knowledge about the problem identified. Systematic review of the literature concludes with a synthesis of application in clinical practice. For each situation, the clinician must ask how the evidence fits within patient-centered care for the particular patient and family and then must evaluate the outcomes. Questions to ask for evidence-based practice include: Why did I choose the care plan I am following? What is the level of evidence for the care I am providing? What questions should I ask about the care I am giving?

Quality Improvement

Nurses spend more time with patients than any other provider, which offers situational awareness for identifying quality gaps and safety lapses that can be addressed through continual improvement initiatives and searches for the evidence to support care standards. Nurses increasingly lead data collection on nurse-sensitive quality indicators, as well as other quality markers, and help design quality improvement initiatives to close gaps.[17] Healthcare organizations match their own quality data with industry benchmarks among peer institutions to identify areas for improvement. Nurses, as well as new graduates, need knowledge and skills for choosing and implementing quality-improvement tools, combining quality data with current literature, and designing and implementing evidence-based standards to improve care.

Safety

New safety science challenges traditional views of safety that focused on managing bed rails, the five rights of medication safety, and other ways nurses manage the individual patient's environment. In health care, near misses and adverse and sentinel events have been viewed as single occurrences with a single patient, unlike in other high-performance industries in which a single event impacts a large number of people, such as an airplane crash that generates much public attention. The aviation industry works with the federal government with a reporting system that aggregates sentinel events and near misses for broader analysis of system issues. Health care lacks a similar aggregate reporting system in part because of the complexity of multiple interacting factors, but this enables process and system issues to remain undetected with the same error repeated.

Workers at times develop "work arounds" to overcome lack of available resources, staff shortages, or barriers to completing a task; that is, they find shortcuts to standard methods to complete their work in ways that may compromise safety and quality. Analysis of the situation may indicate the need for a process change.[17,18] Other high-performance industries, such as aviation, nuclear power, and railway, have applied new quality and safety science to dramatically improve safety outcomes. Formal reporting requirements aggregate data on errors, near misses, and poor outcomes from across the industry so that repeated system issues can be detected, analyzed, and changed to establish new evidence-based procedures that may build in checks and balances to prevent occurrences. Tubing misconnection is an example of a potential error that can be addressed as a system change; misconnections are a preventable but frequently occurring error because portals can be mismatched when a patient has multiple invasive tubes for medications and discharge of bodily fluids. Root-cause analysis of tubing misconnections may reveal the need to change equipment purchases that prevent mismatching or that provide a color coding system as an alert to avoid misconnecting tubes and ports.[19]

Implementing new safety science from other industries shifts how healthcare errors are viewed and managed and is at the heart of the changes recommended.[20] Historically, blame was assigned to the individual who was believed to have caused the error. Applying Reason's error model is part of a just culture organizational framework that goes beyond reporting errors and investigates errors through root-cause analysis and like errors can be aggregated to reveal the need for system changes to prevent future occurrences.[21] Staff trained in risk management conduct meetings with individuals involved in all stages of the event to identify each step leading to the error and to define steps to prevent future occurrences. Transparency is a key component of a just culture in which patients and families are kept informed of what happened. Individual accountability remains to be attentive to potential error and to report near misses and adverse events, but the emphasis shifts to safe reporting as a learning tool and to help patients and families have answers to their questions about the event.

Informatics

Competence in informatics enables nurses to manage and design electronic health records, search literature and other sources to determine best practices that establish evidence-based standards to guide practice, implement quality-improvement strategies, and utilize decision support resources.

While none of the competencies are discrete concepts alone, all are interrelated to provide quality and safe care. This is particularly evident in considering informatics, which is an essential skill undergirding each competency and safety science that provides a philosophical foundation for integration into curricula. These new views of safety are essential to realize the significance of applying each competency.

DEFINING THE GAP BETWEEN NURSING CURRICULUM AND GOALS FOR NURSING PRACTICE

The project team had anecdotal evidence contrary to the high rate of inclusion reported in the survey and designed a series of focus groups to be able to have discussions with nurse educators. The QSEN project team assessed the level of current integration of the competencies in nursing curriculum using an electronic survey of the U.S. baccalaureate nursing schools and a select sample of associate degree nursing programs.[10] Based on the definitions of the competencies, the majority of the schools reported they teach the competencies in some way in their curriculum, although evidenced-based practice, quality improvement, and informatics were less likely to be included, faculty were less comfortable teaching, and students less likely to have achieved. Focus groups with faculty, administrators, and new graduates revealed very different responses. In the focus groups, the knowledge, skill, and attitude (KSA) objectives that described each competency[6] were presented to participants for their initial view. Project leaders led focus groups of deans, directors, and faculty of nursing schools at several large nursing conferences, this time presenting not only the definitions but also distributing the KSAs (165 total for the six competencies). Upon examination of the KSAs, faculty identified a gap in what they know to teach and expectations for new graduates that were developing in practice.[10] The project team recognized the need for evidence that the KSAs could be successfully integrated into curricula and evidence of teaching strategies that demonstrated student achievement. Thus Phase II was designed to pilot how the competencies could be integrated into nursing education and practice.

PILOT SCHOOL LEARNING COLLABORATIVE

The question emerged whether faculty could lead their schools in the proposed education transformation so that nurses are able to think differently about quality and safety in their practice. The project expert panel designed a learning collaborative to pilot the integration of the competencies into nursing curricula.[8] Fifteen schools were selected from a call for proposals; schools had a year to complete concept mapping of their curricula to determine gaps between the KSA objectives and what they were currently teaching and complete pilot projects that were presented to all the pilot schools at the year-end workshop. Many designed faculty development experiences to enable faculty to work within the full scope of quality and safety science.[22] Results of the collaborative and examples of their presentations are available at www.qsen.org, the project's Web site. Two exemplars are included in this chapter to illustrate the pilot school initiatives.

Student Evaluation Survey

Graduating students in the pilot school learning collaborative completed a student evaluation survey to determine their self-assessed levels of achievement for the 165 KSAs in their nursing program, the manner in which they were instructed, and their attitudes about the importance of learning the competencies.[23] Although there was wide variability reported among the schools, the majority of the 595 students who completed the survey felt that quality and safety knowledge and skills were addressed adequately in their nursing programs. Teamwork and collaboration and quality improvement were ranked as the lowest concentration for content. The highest rated skills were assessing pain, ability to communicate care provided and needed in handoffs, and effective use of strategies to reduce risk of harm to self or others. Students wanted more experience with knowing how to use quality improvement tools, locate evidence reports for clinical practice guidelines, and evaluate the effect of practice changes derived from quality improvement initiatives. Students recognized the value of the QSEN competencies and the implications for changing practice.

Delphi Survey

Barton et al.[24] completed a Delphi survey to determine placement of the KSAs in the curriculum as a result of questions raised by the pilot collaborative learning schools. With 18 faculty from the pilot schools participating, the results of the Delphi survey created a developmental approach moving from beginning to advanced levels of competencies to guide faculty in placing the KSAs in their curriculum. Patient-centered care and safety competencies are most appropriate for early introduction, evidence-based practice and informatics are best spread evenly throughout the curriculum, and teamwork and collaboration and quality improvement are more suited for intermediate and advanced placement in the curriculum. Consistent and progressive exposure was recommended for reinforcement in practice habits in all phases of learning experiences.

Pilot School Exemplars

EXHIBIT 30.1 Teaching the QSEN Competencies: A Pilot School Learning Collaborative Exemplar, University of Nebraska School of Nursing

Connie Miller and Louise LaFromboise

At the University of Nebraska School of Nursing, we used our year in the 15 School Pilot Learning Collaborative to focus on safety. Nurses play a vital role as champions for safe, efficient patient care. Nursing education is responsible for providing opportunities to acquire the knowledge and skills needed to provide safe, quality care. In a recent systematic review of the literature, Wong, Etchells, Kuper, Levinson, and Shojania[1] identified that, while it is common to include both didactic and experiential components (mainly consisting of chart audits) for teaching quality and safety, study findings failed to demonstrate changes in learners' behaviors or potential patient benefits.

Clearly, experiential components must take a more active form than simply reviewing charts for potential errors. One example is provided by Voss et al. (2008),[2] who engaged residents in a curriculum that included, among other things, root cause analysis and human factors analysis. Active learning strategies were incorporated to help residents examine perceptions about individual actions and to complete a root cause analysis of a case selected from the residents' own experiences. Findings indicated the experiential curriculum shifted residents' thinking about patient safety to a systems-based approach.

As participants in the QSEN Pilot School Learning Collaborative, we based our project on the safety competency. Recognizing the importance of experiential learning in shifting how students view the healthcare system, a root cause analysis exercise was incorporated into the senior-level critical care nursing course. The analysis was completed on a near miss because near misses are considered to be an opportunity for proactive analysis[3] of potential system failures and development of countermeasures.[4]

Exemplar

- To begin, all students in the course received classroom content on root cause analysis (RCA) in a leadership course they take concurrently with the critical care course.

EXHIBIT 30.1 Teaching the QSEN Competencies: A Pilot School Learning Collaborative Exemplar, University of Nebraska School of Nursing (*Continued*)

- Midway through the semester, the experiential component of a RCA was initiated with one clinical group. Each of eight students in the clinical group was required to conduct a literature search and read an article on RCA.
- In addition, faculty assigned two readings[5,6] that explained the purpose and process of RCA. Students were then asked to engage in a discussion during a clinical conference about RCA using information from the students' articles and the assigned articles.
- During the next clinical conference, the mock RCA took place using the near miss case provided below. For review of the case, students were assigned the roles of primary nurse, lead nurse, lead pharmacist, and floor pharmacist. The other four students were observers to the process. During the mock RCA, the observers made notes about the exchange that took place between the four healthcare professionals, taking special notice of nonverbal communication, ineffective communication techniques, and effective, constructive communication.
- A debriefing was conducted after the RCA, which focused on the six-step process outlined by.[5]

Near Miss Case

A nurse is caring for a 64-year-old male who is 36 hours post myocardial infarction. The patient requires ventilator support to maintain adequate oxygenation and a dopamine infusion to maintain an adequate blood pressure. The admixture of dopamine is 400 mg in 500 ml of normal saline. The floor pharmacist is responsible for preparing the dopamine infusion. The nurse informs the floor pharmacist at 0700 that the patient will require a new dopamine infusion at approximately 0730. The nurse then proceeds to conduct morning assessments and complete required documentation on the two patients assigned to her. Meanwhile, the pharmacist delivers the dopamine to the patient's room without speaking to the nurse. The intravenous infusion pump alerts the nurse to an empty I.V. fluid bag at 0745. The nurse hurriedly grabs the newly delivered dopamine bag, quickly removes the existing bag, and spikes the bag with the existing tubing. She resets the volume to be infused on the pump, but prior to beginning the infusion realizes that this admixture is dopamine 800 mg/500 ml of normal saline. She immediately changes the pump to reflect the correct solution concentration thereby preventing the administration of twice the amount of dopamine that is required by the patient. The situation was reported to both the lead nurse and the lead pharmacist, and appropriate documentation was completed.

Upon completion of the experiential component for the selected clinical group, all students in the course were asked to take part in focus group discussions. Focus groups were composed of individual clinical groups. Students were asked to read and discuss the outcomes of a case study related to a patient who had an amputation due to treatment error. Content analysis of discussions related to the case were conducted. Discussions in the groups of students who received only the classroom content for RCA focused heavily on blaming and lesser on lack of communication and resource seeking. Discussions in the clinical group that had the experiential component with the mock RCA in addition to the classroom content focused on safety, problem-solving systems, and lack of communication.[7] Durham and Sherwood[8] support the importance of an experiential component for promoting student incorporation of the quality and safety concepts that are vital to safe patient care so that we incorporate these lessons about experiential learning to help students master other QSEN competencies.

References

1. Wong, B. M., Etchells, E. E., Kuper, A., Levinson, W., & Shojania, K. G. (2010). Teaching quality improvement and patient safety to trainees: A systematic review. *Academic Medicine, 85*(9), 1425–1439.
2. Voss, J. D., May, N. B., Schorling, J. B., Lyman, J. A., Schectman, J. M., Wolf, A. M. D., . . . Plews-Ogan, M. (2008). Changing conversations: Teaching safety and quality in residency training. *Academic Medicine, 83*(11), 1080–1087.

(*continues*)

EXHIBIT 30.1 Teaching the QSEN Competencies: A Pilot School Learning Collaborative Exemplar, University of Nebraska School of Nursing (*Continued*)

3. Mick, J. M., Wood, G. L., & Massey, R. L. (2007). The dood catch pilot program. Increasing potential error reporting. *Journal of Nursing Administration, 37*(11), 499–503.
4. Kanse, L., van der Schaaf, T. W., Vruland, N. D., & Van Mierlo, H. (2006). Error recovery in a hospital pharmacy. *Ergonomics, 49*(5–6), 503–516.
5. McDonald, A., & Leyhane, T. (2005). Drill down with root cause analysis. *Nursing Management, 36*(10), 26–32.
6. Williams, P. M. (2001). Techniques for root cause analysis. *Baylor University Medical Center Proceedings, 14*(2), 154–157.
7. Miller, C., & LaFramboise, L. (2009). Student learning outcomes after integration of quality and safety education competencies into a senior-level critical care course. *Journal of Nursing Education, 48*(12), 678–685.
8. Durham, C. J., & Sherwood, G. D. (2008). Education to bridge the quality gap: A case study approach. *Urologic Nursing, 28*(6), 431–453.

EXHIBIT 30.2 Faculty Development Exemplar, Emory University

Bethany Robertson

Selected as one of the 15 schools in the QSEN Pilot Learning Collaborative, we focused on the competencies of teamwork and collaboration, as well as quality improvement. To accomplish our goal we chose to strategically influence faculty development around quality improvement within the School of Nursing. To focus on teamwork and collaboration, we developed faculty development workshops and endowed lectureships within the School of Nursing, as well as engaged members of the Health Sciences Center as volunteer facilitators to assist with our interprofessional team training for undergraduate healthcare professionals.

Across the Health Sciences

As part of our work as a QSEN pilot school, we chose the competency of teamwork. To close the quality chasm, team development must occur in both the academic and practice arenas, and the design of the team training pilot program developed at Emory is aimed at this goal. Our overarching objective is to change the academic culture from a silo experience whereby each discipline is learning completely separated from one another to one of integration with the hopes of changing the culture and expectations around interprofessional learning and subsequently teamwork in the professional environment.

From the perspective of enhancing student knowledge around teamwork in the academic arena, we developed a pilot interprofessional team training event for approximately 200 senior nursing and third-year medical students using TeamSTEPPS as the educational framework for team concepts. The original pilot curriculum included a large group lecture, TeamSTEPPS videos, and a simulation activity.[1] The curriculum design provided for a large group lecture to create a shared understanding of the event's objectives, as well as to emphasize how interprofessional learning, particularly teamwork skills, is critical to their professional development and linked to patient outcomes. The small group provided an opportunity for interactive activities, and simulation provided an opportunity for students to demonstrate a shared goal across all disciplines (e.g., taking care of patients) and facilitated the development of relationships as one student to another. To provide a large group of students with a 10-person small group experience required recruitment and training facilitators. We requested volunteers across the health sciences, as well as from members of our health system. The goal was to expose the 40 facilitators who responded to the science of teamwork and its role in patient safety, as well as to provide an opportunity to work with other members of the healthcare team in a different environment. Two facilitators led each small group; pairing was done deliberately, with each member representing a different discipline. Each facilitator attended a two-hour facilitator training session that focused on how to systematically influence the students' perceptions about teamwork but also those of practicing healthcare professionals.

EXHIBIT 30.2 Faculty Development Exemplar, Emory University (*Continued*)

While this was a pilot project, this interprofessional team training development has occurred annually since 2008. The student numbers doubled as the project expanded to include all the disciplines in the health sciences center: physician assistants, physical therapists, medical imaging, anesthesia assistants, nursing, and medicine, and the number of facilitators now includes well over 100. Additionally, we have expanded the frequency of this activity into both the fall and spring semesters; each cohort now has more than the single experience.

Faculty development to improve knowledge and attitudes around teamwork occurred during a two-hour facilitator session, which focused on the larger vision of quality improvement work, primarily utilizing work from the Institute of Medicine and TeamSTEPPS.[2–4] The design was based on the "learn one teach one" philosophy; facilitators would teach students, in a coaching fashion, what they learned to their small student groups. Ample and well-structured resources were provided to facilitators to help them understand their facilitator role, as well as small group content. Feedback from facilitators was high posttraining in both satisfactions with the facilitator training and perceived level of relevance.

Within the School of Nursing

Within the School of Nursing, we chose to strategically align all opportunities for communicating information to faculty about quality improvement particularly focused on the QSEN KSAs, over a two-year period. We mapped content across our endowed lectures and faculty development events to focus on the quality and safety movement, starting with a broad overview (macrosystem) and ending with the unit-based influences (microsystem). Focused dialogue is interspersed at both Bachelors of Science in Nursing (BSN) and Masters of Science in Nursing (MSN) faculty meetings. Our efforts began in the fall of 2008 with the Jower's lecture, an endowed lecture focused on quality and safety, with Linda Cronenwett, principal investigator on the QSEN project, as the guest speaker. Students and faculty were encouraged to attend to gain insights into the broader movement behind QSEN, and those who did not attend were required to view the videotaped lecture. The first faculty development occurred several months following this lecture, which all faculty were strongly encouraged to attend. The dean of the School of Nursing introduced QSEN and its role in revolutionizing nursing education, followed by an inspiring presentation by a clinical nurse specialist from Emory Healthcare sharing her team's success story with implementing the ventilator assisted pneumonia bundle, demonstrating quality improvement in action. The concurrent breakout sessions that followed discussed curricula integration of QSEN KSAs with tracks for BSN and MSN faculty. Although at this early stage of QSEN the graduate-level KSAs had not been fully developed, we felt it was appropriate to begin the introduction and dialogue around the QSEN competencies at all levels. The afternoon session was the first of the facilitator training sessions for the interprofessional team training event (described above), allowing for School of Nursing faculty and others to participate. A concurrent session was provided for MSN faculty who had missed the morning session and who were not going to participate in the interprofessional event as a facilitator.

A similar pattern was used in the fall of 2009. While our efforts in the fall of 2008 focused more on the broad view of quality and safety, our subsequent focus was on how QSEN competencies manifest themselves in the everyday work of nurses. Our endowed lecture provided another opportunity to invite a notable expert in the area of quality and safety, Marjory Godfrey, whose work focuses on the microsystem and how performance improvement is essential to improved patient care. A faculty development event that followed continued the focus on quality improvement work occurring on units at Emory Healthcare. Collaboration with Emory Healthcare's chief quality officers provided an opportunity for them to lead this special session, sharing the impact of quality and improvement in action and its effect on patient outcomes.

(*continues*)

EXHIBIT 30.2 Faculty Development Exemplar, Emory University (*Continued*)

Lessons Learned

Embarking on faculty development in the area of quality improvement needs innovation and deliberate strategy, meaning the ways in which we engage faculty need to be experiential, focused, relevant, and descriptive. Strategy for deployment and change needs to be clearly developed with methods to measure success. Utilization of change management sciences is highly recommended because the true aim is to change the way people think about and do their work of teaching the next generation of healthcare professionals, many of whom have been doing it the same way for well over 40 years. Quality improvement has been a rapid development in health care, and it is easy to forget that many providers may not readily adapt to the new paradigm of quality and safety. Having key faculty lead the initiative initially is a sound strategy; however, if there is not a deliberate plan for the "train a trainer" approach, the champions will quickly become the "owners" of this work. While quality improvement work and teaching it can indeed become the focus of a faculty's life work, quality and safety must ultimately become the framework that underpins all of our educational endeavors.

References

1. Robertson, B., Atallah, H., Kaplan, B., Higgins, M., Lewitt, M. J., & Ander, D. S. (2010). The use of simulation and a modified TeamSTEPPS curriculum for medical and nursing student team training. *Simulation in Healthcare, 5*, 332–337.
2. Institute of Medicine. (2001). *Crossing the quality chasm: A new health system for the 21st century*. Washington, DC: National Academies Press.
3. Institute of Medicine. (2003). *Health professions education: A bridge to quality*. National Academies Press.
4. King, H. B., Battles, J., Baker, D. P., Alonso, A., Salas, E., Webster, J., . . . Salisbury, M. (2008). *TeamSTEPPS: Team strategies and tools to enhance performance and patient safety*. Retrieved from http://www.ahrq.gov/downloads/pub/advances2/vol3/Advances-King_1.pdf.

REACHING A TIPPING POINT

The work of QSEN has contributed to a renaissance in nursing education scholarship. Educators in academia and practice settings are engaging in new approaches to education, as well as experiencing satisfaction from value-based nursing care.[25] The motivation and joy from doing work well is a basic desire and value among those who choose nursing as a profession. Working in systems that embrace quality and safety as core values attracts and retains workers.[26] The competencies have been integrated into educational essentials for baccalaureate education[27] and for advanced practice nursing,[28,29] and thus have influenced nursing education policies.

The current focus is on educator development and assessment of the impact of QSEN. To achieve quality and safety goals requires educator development in these six quality and safety competencies to be able to lead integration both in academic and clinical settings.[25] Innovative partnerships between practice settings and schools of nursing can design human patient simulation exercises and redesign clinical learning opportunities that facilitate mastery of the competences.[9] Collaboration across settings for research and evaluation studies can help determine applicability in varied settings to assess the universality of the six competencies defined by the IOM and QSEN project. Working to improve quality and safety outcomes not only addresses our moral commitment to do no harm but also contributes to a healthy work environment that increases worker satisfaction and retention. Through education, nurses can lead integration of quality and safety competencies and experience the joy from helping patients improve healthcare outcomes.

References

1. Kohn, L., Corrigan, J., & Donaldson, M. (Eds.). (2000). *To err is human: Building a safer health system*. Washington, DC: National Academies Press.
2. Committee on Quality of Health Care in America, Institute of Medicine. (2001). *Crossing the quality chasm: A new health system for the 21st century*. Washington, DC: National Academies Press. Retrieved from http://www.nap.edu/catalog.php?record_id=10027.
3. Institute of Medicine. (2003). Health professions education: A bridge to quality. Washington, DC: National Academies Press. Retrieved from http://www.nap.edu/catalog.php?record_id=10681#toc.
4. Sherwood, G., & Drenkard, K. (2007). Quality and safety curricula in nursing education: Matching practice realities. *Nursing Outlook, 55*(3), 151–155.
5. Institute of Medicine Committee on the Health Professions Education Summitt. (2004). In A. C. Greiner & E. Knebel (Eds.), *Health professions education: A bridge to quality*. Washington, DC: National Academies Press.
6. Cronenwett, L., Sherwood, G., Barnsteiner, J., Disch, J., Johnson, J., Mitchell, P., Sullivan, D. T., & Warren, J. (2007). Quality and safety education for nurses. *Nursing Outlook, 55*, 122–131.
7. Cronenwett, L., Sherwood, G., Pohl, J., Barnsteiner, J., Moore, S., Taylor Sullivan, D., Ward, D., & Warren, J. (2009). Quality and safety education for advanced practice nursing practice. *Nursing Outlook, 57*(6), 338–348.
8. Cronenwett, L., Sherwood, G., & Gelmon, S. (2009). Improving quality and safety education: The QSEN Learning Collaborative. *Nursing Outlook, 57*(6), 304–312.
9. Day, L., & Smith, E. L. (2007). Integrating quality and safety content into clinical teaching in the acute care setting. *Nursing Outlook, 55*(3), 138–143.
10. Smith, E., Cronenwett, L., & Sherwood, G. (2007). Quality and safety education: Prelicensure nursing educator views. *Nursing Outlook, 55*(3), 132–137.
11. Pohl, J., Savrin, C., Fiandt, K., Beauchesne, M., Drayton-Brooks, S., Scheibmeir, M., . . . Werner, K. E. (2009). Quality and safety in graduate nursing education: Cross-mapping QSEN graduate competencies with NONPF's NP core and practice doctorate competencies. *Nursing Outlook, 57*(6), 349–354.
12. Sherwood, G., & Hicks, R. (2010). Quality and safety in nursing education (QSEN). In B. Cherry & S. Jacobs (Eds.), *Contemporary nursing: Issues, trends and management* (5th ed., pp. 464–476). New York, NY: Elsevier.
13. Aspen, P., Walcott, J., Bootman, L., & Cronenwett, L. (Eds.) and the Committee on Identifying and Preventing Medication Errors. (2007). identifying and preventing medication errors. Washington, DC: National Academies Press.
14. Horton-Deutsch, S., & Sherwood, G. (2008). Reflection: An educational strategy to develop emotionally competent nurse leaders. *Journal of Nursing Management, 8*, 946–954.
15. Barnsteiner, J., Disch, J., Hall, L., Mayer, D., & Moore, S. (2007). Promoting interprofessional education. *Nursing Outlook, 55*(3), 144–153.
16. King, H. B., Battles, J., Baker, D. P., Alonso, A., Salas, E., Webster, J., . . . Salisbury, M. *TeamSTEPPS™: Team strategies and tools to enhance performance and patient safety*. Retrieved from www.ahrq.gov/downloads/pub/advances2/vol3/Advances-King_1.pdf.
17. Hall, L. W., Moore, S. M., & Barnsteiner, J. H. (2008). Quality and nursing: Moving from a concept to a core competency. *Urologic Nursing: Special Topic Issue on Quality, 28*(6), 417–425.
18. Page, A. (2004). *Keeping patients safe: Transforming the work environment of nurses*. Institute of Medicine, Board on Health Care Services. Washington, DC: National Academies Press.
19. Simmons, D, Graves, K. (2008). Tubing misconnections—a systems failure with human factors: lessons for nursing practice. *Urol Nurs, 28*(6), 460–464.
20. Reason, J. (2000). Human error: Models and management. *BMJ, 320*(7237), 768–770.
21. Marx, D. (2001). *Patient safety and the "just culture": A primer for health care executives*. New York, NY: Columbia University. Retrieved from http://www.unmc.edu/rural

/patient-safety/tools/Marx%20Patient%20Safety%20and%20Just%20Culture.pdf.

22. Armstrong, G., Sherwood, G., & Tagliareni, E. (2009). Quality and safety education in nursing (QSEN): Integrating recommendations from IOM into clinical nursing education. In T. Valiga & N. Ard (Eds.). *Clinical nursing education: Critical reflections* (pp. 207–226). New York, NY: National League for Nursing Press.
23. Sullivan, D. T., Hirst, D., & Cronenwett, L. (2009). Assessing quality and safety competencies of graduating pre-licensure nursing students. *Nursing Outlook, 57*(6), 323–331.
24. Barton, A., Armstrong, G., Preheim, G., Gelmon, S., & Andrus, L. (2009). A national Delphi to determine developmental progression of quality and safety competencies in nursing education. *Nursing Outlook, 57*(6), 313–322.
25. Thornlow, D., & McGuinn, K. (2010). A necessary sea change for nurse faculty development: Spotlight on quality and safety. *Journal of Professional Nursing, 26*(2), 71–81.
26. Ulrich, B., Woods, D., Hart, K., Lavandero, R., Leggett, J., & Taylor, D. (2007). Critical care nurses' work environments value of excellence in beacon units and magnet organizations. *Critical Care Nurse, 27*, 68–77.
27. American Association of Colleges of Nursing. (2009). *The essentials of baccalaureate education for professional nursing practice*. Washington, DC: American Association of Colleges of Nursing.
28. American Association of Colleges of Nursing. (2008). *The essentials of master's education for professional nursing practice*. Washington, DC: American Association of Colleges of Nursing.
29. American Association of Colleges of Nursing. (2008). *The essentials of doctor of nursing practice*. Washington, DC: American Association of Colleges of Nursing.

Acknowledgment

Quality and Safety Education for Nurses is funded by the Robert Wood Johnson Foundation.

Linda R. Cronenwett, University of North Carolina at Chapel Hill, is principal investigator.

31

Supporting a Culture of Safety: The Magnet Recognition Program

Katherine A. Pischke-Winn, MBA, RN, Karen M. Stratton, PhD, RN, NE-BC, Kathleen Ferket, RN, MSN, APN, and Wendy Tuzik Micek

BACKGROUND

The 2010 Institute of Medicine's (IOM) *The Future of Nursing: Leading Change, Advancing Health* report states a "promising field of evidence links nursing care to high quality of care for patients, including protecting their safety; nurses are crucial in preventing medication errors, reducing rates of infection, and even facilitating patients' transition from hospital to home" (p. 3).[1] In fact, nursing has been called the gatekeeper of patient safety. Our physician colleagues recognize and honor nursing for the vital role nurses play in patient safety. However, keeping patients safe is not discipline specific. Patient safety involves timely communication and coordination of care, interdisciplinary teamwork, and a constant vigilance and mindfulness of the potential dangers within our complex, high-risk healthcare environment. Nurses assume a "wingman" role in averting errors, in advocating for patients, and in improving the healthcare system. Around the clock, nurses are the closest to the patient and therefore are in a unique position to ensure patient safety.[2]

The 2010 Institute of Medicine report, sponsored by the Robert Wood Johnson (RWJ) Foundation, mentions the American Nurse's Credentialing Center's (ANCC) Magnet recognition program as advancing nursing excellence and leadership. Based on rigorous criteria, Magnet status recognizes high standards related to quality and nursing practice.[1] According to ANCC, "the full expression of the Magnet forces embodies a professional environment guided by a strong, visionary nursing leader who advocates and supports development and excellence in nursing practice" (p. 244).[1] Like any pursuit of excellence, the Magnet program "elevates the reputation and standards of the nursing profession."[3] Aiken and colleagues'[4] research associates the characteristics of Magnet hospitals with higher levels of satisfaction among patients and lower mortality rates.

This chapter will illustrate how hospital staff who have achieved or are striving for Magnet recognition build a culture of empowered, professional nurses who focus on quality outcome measures, innovations in practice, and a patient-centered environment whose primary goal is keeping patients safe.

INTRODUCTION

The timeless writings of Florence Nightingale's *Notes on Nursing*[5] continue to inspire and guide nurses more than 100 years after her death. Nightingale created the philosophy of the nurse as the patient and family advocate. As an advocate, nurses help assure safe care through standards as basic as hand washing to decrease infections. Nurses not only wash their own hands, but they speak up so that others wash their hands to protect patients. Similarly, nurses get involved through professional development. They use evidence to offer solutions and make improvements, conduct research, use data to help change massive health systems, engage in lifelong learning, strive for continual improvements, and publish their findings and opinions. Nurses reach out to other healthcare professionals, academia, the business community, government officials, consumers, and philanthropies to transform the profession and improve patient care and outcomes.

More than 100 years after Ms. Nightingale's writing, the ANCC created the Magnet recognition award to acknowledge healthcare organizations that demonstrate nursing excellence. The criteria for Magnet recognition echoed some of the same standards Ms. Nightingale championed. From its origins in the 1980s, the Magnet award has grown to epitomize outstanding patient care in a safe, high-quality environment, with demonstrated superior clinical outcomes.[6] Magnet hospitals provide consumers with the ultimate benchmark in measuring expected quality of care. Magnet facilities show better outcomes than non-Magnet facilities as evidenced by a decrease in patient mortality.[7] Evidence continues to grow that the Magnet program leads to improved patient safety and improved patient outcomes.

The seminal IOM report, *To Err Is Human*, found that medical errors kill between 44,000 and 98,000 people in U.S. hospitals each year.[8] The IOM recommends that healthcare organizations create environments in which the culture of safety is an explicit organizational goal, a top priority, and driven by leadership.[9] In response to the IOM recommendations, healthcare organizations began the process of studying the elements of a patient safety culture and how to make that culture and organization safe for patients.[10] Healthcare leaders have asked, "How will we know when we have created a culture of safety within our hospitals?"[11] After all, a culture entails not just written rules but beliefs, attitudes, and behaviors.[9] For the desired culture of safety, the Magnet standards lay out a framework, which includes operationalizing concepts such as workplace empowerment and transformational leadership.

CULTURE OF SAFETY DEFINITION

A first step in determining if an institution has a culture of safety is to define safety culture. In their chapter titled, "What exactly is patient safety?," Emmanuel and colleagues[12] used the definition from the Agency for Healthcare Research and Quality (AHRQ):

> Patient safety is a discipline in the health care sector that applies safety science methods toward the goal of achieving a trustworthy system of health care delivery. Patient safety is also an attribute of health care systems; it minimizes the incidence and impact of, and maximizes recovery from, adverse events.

A CULTURE OF SAFETY

The goal of patient safety is to create a healthcare system that minimizes the occurrence and impact of adverse events and maximizes recovery from any such event.[12] Healthcare organizations now understand that people make errors most often due to system breakdowns, not because of individual incompetence, and *blame* has a toxic effect.[13] Errors can be reduced by redesigning systems using human factor principles.[14] Mistakes can be reduced through design features such as standardization; simplification; training physicians and nurses to work better in teams, including pharmacists in patient rounds; fully disclosing information about errors and near misses; and encouraging and rewarding individuals who report safety issues.[15]

A culture of patient safety means developing a high-reliability organization. The 2001 AHRQ white paper, *Making Health Care Safer*,[16] cites four common traits among organizations with a culture of safety:

- Acknowledgment of the high-risk, error-prone nature of an organization's work
- Blame-free environment where individuals are able to report errors and close calls without punishment
- Expectations of collaboration across ranks to seek solutions to vulnerabilities
- Willingness on the part of the organization to direct resources to address safety concerns

Frankel and colleagues[15] discuss the tools to achieve high reliability in patient safety: development of a fair and just culture, collaborative team behavior, and leadership engagement. The three together comprise a cornerstone necessary for a comprehensive patient safety plan. Critical to a culture of safety is leadership, intelligently conducted walk rounds, and using frontline provider insights to directly influence operational decisions. Equally critical is systematic reinforced training in both teamwork and effective communication, integrated into all operations.[15] These "three concepts, developed and applied concurrently, weave a supporting framework for the effective implementation of new technologies and evidence-based practices" (p. 1707[15]; see Figure 31.1).

Patient safety is one of the core components of quality health care.[17,18] In subsequent reports, the IOM pointed out the critical role nursing plays in providing safe care, and it identified healthcare essential management practices required for a healthy patient safety culture:[1] creating and maintaining trust throughout the organization, having an adequate number of healthcare workers, developing openness in regard to reporting and preventing errors, involving workers in decision making pertaining to work design and work flow, and actively managing the process of change.[1] Nursing has 24-hour accountability for hospitalized patients. The physician gatekeeper metaphor, "nursing is the gatekeeper of patient safety," may reflect nurses' responsibility to coordinate communication and teamwork among the interdisciplinary team.

In terms of communication, Magnet-recognized hospitals are more likely to support decision making that coordinates the whole unit, down to the end provider of care—the staff nurse. Magnet hospitals also have an influential, powerful nurse executive; they promote professional nursing practice; and they provide superior patient care and have low mortality rates.[6]

Hospital safety has been found to closely parallel aviation safety due to the high reliance on team-based roles.[19–21] Improvements in aviation safety are attributed to improved crew coordination, communication, and decision making. Aviation culture encourages individuals to step forward and share their stories about adverse events.[13] The Magnet recognition program acknowledges the autonomous nurse who confidently advocates for patients and shares stories in the form of exemplars that speak to the standards of professional excellence found in the Magnet sources of evidence.

In 2010, Sammer and colleagues[9] conducted a comprehensive meta-analysis of the literature on culture of safety in U.S. hospitals. The goal was to develop a common typology,

FIGURE 31.1 Determinants of High Reliability in Health Care (abbreviated).[15]

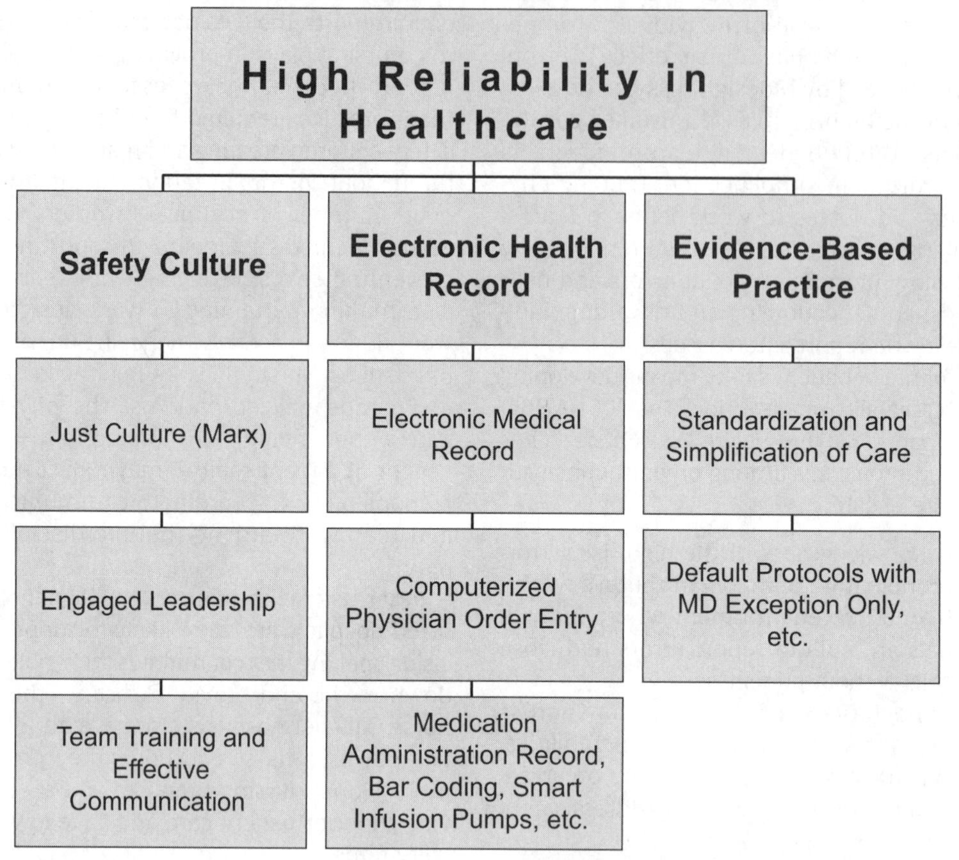

Adapted from "Fair and Just Culture Team Behavior, and Leadership Engagement: The Tools to Achieve High Reliability" by A. S. Frankel, M. W. Leonard, and D. Denham. 2006. *Health Research and Education Trust, 41*:4, p. 1692. Copyright 2006.

identify key concepts of a patient safety culture, and define a conceptual model for such a culture. Their findings identified a broad range of safety culture properties that were organized into seven subcultures (Table 31.1). These key subculture concepts for a culture of patient safety are mirrored in some of the important components of the current Magnet recognition program.

SAFETY AND NURSE ADVOCACY

Registered nurses (RNs), by their very standards and licensure, care and advocate for the patient. RNs are licensed by the state they practice in, and every RN licensure act includes a statement or definition on nurse advocacy. The American Nurses Association (ANA) code of ethics for nurses includes in its Provision 3: "The nurse promotes, advocates for, and strives to protect the health, safety, and right of the patient" (p. 23).[22] However, many barriers can prevent advocacy at even the best institutions. Nurses at Magnet-recognized organizations have created a culture whereby staff identify and work to overcome barriers to patient safety. Barriers can include:

TABLE 31.1 Definitions of patient safety subcultures

Subculture	Definition
Leadership	Leaders acknowledge the healthcare environment is high risk and seek to align vision/mission, staff competency, and fiscal and human resources from their decisions to the front line.
Teamwork	A spirit of collegiality, collaboration, and cooperation exists among executives, staff, and independent practitioners. Relationships are open, safe, respectful, and flexible.
Communication	An environment exists where an individual staff member, no matter what his or her job description, has the right and the responsibility to speak up on behalf of a patient.
Evidence Based	Patient care practices are based on evidence. Standardization to reduce variation occurs at every opportunity. Processes are designed to achieve high reliability.
Learning	The hospital learns from its mistakes and seeks new opportunities for performance improvement. Learning is valued among all staff, including the medical staff.
Just	A culture that recognizes errors as system failures rather than individual failures and, at the same time, does not shrink from holding individuals accountable for their actions.
Patient Centered	Care is centered around the patient and family. The patient is not only an active participant in his or her own care but acts as a liaison between the hospital and the community.

Adapted from "What is Patient Safety Culture? A Review of the Literature" by C. E. Sammer, K. L. Lykens, K. P. Singh, D. A. Mains, and N. A. Lachan, 2010. *Journal of Nursing Scholarship, 42*(2), p. 157–163. Copyright 2010 by Sigma Theta Tau International.

- Regulatory issues—There is a scope of practice limitations from state to state; in many cases, nurses are not always allowed to practice in accordance with their professional training.
- Structural flaws in nursing education—Entry into practice is at different levels of education, such as diploma, associate's degree, Bachelor of Science in Nursing (BSN), or Master of Science in Nursing (MSN); these discordances cause much confusion within nursing, for hiring practices, and with the general public.
- Difficulty in transitioning from school to practice—Nursing does not require an internship or residency from education to practice; hence, healthcare organizations must absorb the cost of a transition to practice and nursing has no established transition standards.
- Work environment—A report by the American Association of Critical-Care Nurses[22] identified six standards for a healthy work environment: skilled communication, true collaboration, effective decision making, appropriate staffing, meaningful recognition, and authentic leadership. The six AACN healthy work environment standards are remarkably similar to Sammer's seven subcultures of safety.[9] However, many hospitals continue to have hostile work environments, horizontal and vertical violence (bullying), and a pecking order among physicians, nurses, and the interdisciplinary team.

- Senior leadership—Leaders may emphasize the bottom line over safety. Despite the changing focus on aligning reimbursement with quality patient outcomes (the National Quality Forum's "never events"),[23] strategies more often concentrate on remedial education and chart audits as opposed to developing and supporting the core competencies for a culture of patient safety.

In many hospitals, these barriers continue to challenge the creation of a culture of safety. Nurses are usually the largest workforce at any hospital, and their goals and priorities can be very influential. The journey to achieving Magnet recognition helps the entire organization focus on a healthy work environment, and quality and safety outcomes.

THE MAGNET RECOGNITION PROGRAM

During a nursing shortage in the 1980s, some hospitals were able to create nursing practice organizations that served as "magnets" for professional nurses. These hospitals could attract and retain nurses who provided a higher level of quality, safe patient care. They had higher quality scores, lower mortality rates, innovative nursing practices, and happy, motivated nurses. These initial Magnet organizations were studied, and, through research, specific elements of nursing practice were identified that were thought to lead to best practices and best patient outcomes.[24] These elements were seen as essential to providing quality, safe patient care and became known as the "forces of magnetism." The Magnet award started with eight forces and by 2005 had grown to fourteen forces. The forces (Table 31.2) are standards that need to be present throughout every patient care unit within the organization.

The Magnet recognition program has been called the "gold seal" for excellent nursing care. The award is bestowed for four years and a requires an annual report, and the bar for nursing staff is raised every year so that continual improvements are made, including increased focus on nursing research, ongoing interdisciplinary collaboration, continuing education through national specialty certifications and advanced degrees, continual input into executive decisions, and strategic involvement in community education, events, and meetings with key stakeholders. Since August 1990, *U.S. News & World Report* ranks the best hospitals in the United States, and one of the nine ranking categories is Magnet recognition.[25]

In 2008, ANCC embedded the 14 Magnet forces into five model components, and it placed *an even stronger* emphasis on measureable nursing outcomes in which quality and safety are entrenched. Becoming a Magnet organization requires a rigorous process of organizational assessment against national benchmarks, with every patient care unit consistently demonstrating above-midline quality scores. Nursing leadership needs to be transformational, which is crucial for the ability to empower and help transform staff and the organization. The goal of transformation is a culture of patient-centered accountability where relationships with professional colleagues are mutually respectful and nursing is viewed on a par with all other disciplines. Magnet standards require hospital-wide adherence to core principles such as shared decision making, practice based on evidence, a professional practice model, self-confidence, and peer review.

Attaining Magnet recognition requires a rigorous transformation process that usually takes three to five years. The organization must make a conscious decision to invest the time and energy to apply for and then work toward Magnet recognition. While structures and processes for the work of nursing create the infrastructure for excellence, the outcomes of the infrastructure are essential to a culture of innovation and improvements.[3]

Before a hospital applies to ANCC for Magnet status, it should begin integrating the basic principles of shared decision making,

TABLE 31.2 Selected standards for the 14 forces of ANCC's Magnet recognition program

1. **Quality of Nursing Leadership.** Transformational, knowledgeable, strong risk-takers, willing to advocate for staff. CNO serves at the executive level.	8. **Consultation & Resources.** Consultation includes advance practice nurses and peer support is available & used.
2. **Organizational Structure.** Flat. Decentralized departments, unit-based decision-making. Strong nurse representatives in committees throughout organization. Nursing leader serves at the executive level.	9. **Autonomy.** Permitted & expected to practice autonomously consistent with professional standards as members of a interdisciplinary team. Independent judgment expected & encouraged.
3. **Management Style.** Shared Decision-making. Involve staff at all levels throughout organization. Feedback from staff encouraged & valued.	10. **Nurses in the Community.** Strong community presence. Strong outreach programs that meet & improve the health of the community.
4. **Personnel Policies and Programs.** Competitive salaries & benefits. Creative & flexible staffing models. Staff input into personnel policies. Opportunities for professional growth & promotion.	11. **Nurses as Teachers.** Nurses incorporate teaching in all aspects of practice. Involved in educational activities.
5. **Professional Model of Care.** Nurses have responsibility, accountability & authority in their patient care. Coordinate care with support & resources from the organization.	12. **Image of Nursing.** Nurses viewed as essential to the hospital's delivery of patient care services.
6. **Quality of Care.** Measured in outcomes. Nurses believe they provide high-quality care to patients & it's seen as an organizational priority.	13. **Interdisciplinary Relationships.** Positive, strong, & collegial. Mutual respect among all disciplines.
7. **Quality Improvement.** Viewed as educational and continuous. Staff participate in the QI process.	14. **Professional Development.** Career development, advanced formal education & life-long learning.

Adapted from "Executive Master of Science in Nursing Program: Incorporating the 14 Forces of Magnetism" by J. Thomas and D. Herrin, 2006, *Journal of Nursing Administration, 38*(2), p. 65. Copyright 2005 by the American Nurses Credentialing Center.

evidence-based practice, and a professional practice model. ANCC uses a multifaceted system of evaluation to assess Magnet excellence. The evaluation includes collecting detailed demographic information from the organization and reviewing a comprehensive, written document that reflects how the organization met all the program requirements—a document that sets forth the sources of evidence.

The sources of evidence are told in stories or exemplars, and empirical outcomes provide the proof of excellence in quality and safety. If the document, which includes feedback from public comment and community stakeholders, meets the standards for the first level of review by trained, independent appraisers, the ANCC conducts a site evaluation with staff, physicians, and community members. The site visit verifies and expands on the written application. The appraisers complete the document review and site visit, prepare summary reports, and submit the reports to the Commission on Magnet Recognition (COM) for final deliberation.[3] Eight to 12 weeks after the site visit, the organization is usually informed if they have earned Magnet recognition.

PATIENT SAFETY AND THE MAGNET RECOGNITION PROGRAM SYNERGIES

Many of the Magnet guiding principles and forces directly correlate with a culture of safety: leadership, evidence-based practice, shared decision making, staff empowerment, professional practice nursing model, teamwork, communication, collegiality, patient centeredness, continual quality improvement, and continual learning. Several of the Magnet forces are similar to Sammer's seven subcultures required for a culture of safety and AACN's healthy work environment guidelines.[9] While there are currently fewer than 400 hospitals that are Magnet designated or redesignated (four are international), hundreds are on the Magnet journey, working to change their organizational culture to one of exemplary professional practice with consistent high standards and outstanding patient outcomes. With the maturing of the Magnet model into the current five model components, there is an even greater emphasis on measurable empirical outcomes including patient safety.

With the 2008 Magnet model, ANCC embedded the 14 forces into five model components: Transformational Leadership, Structural Empowerment, Exemplary Professional Practice, New Knowledge, Innovation and Improvements, and Empirical Quality Outcomes. While structure and process create the infrastructure for excellence, quantitative and qualitative measures of outcomes for the patient, nurses, organizations, and consumers now have a much greater emphasis. Outcomes have to be measured and reported at the individual unit, department, population, or organizational level. The original 14 forces are grouped into the five model components as shown in Table 31.3.

For first time Magnet applicant organizations submit data and narratives for 88 sources of evidence, and ANCC places a heavier emphasis on transformational leadership, structural empowerment, and exemplary professional practice in their document and site visit scoring. The Magnet award is conferred for four years with demographic information sent yearly to ANCC. An interim report is submitted midway between designations (year two), which includes a quality report card containing all of the nursing clinical quality outcome measures, as well as patient and nursing satisfaction data. Magnet redesignation is a rigorous process, and the bar continues to be raised in terms of nursing research, quality outcomes, and outreach to the community and Magnet journey organizations.

The Magnet program is based on four foundational documents:

- American Nurses Association (ANA) Scope and Standards of Practice (2010)
- ANA Scope and Standards for Nurse Administrators (2010)
- ANA Nursing's Social Policy Statement: The Essence of Nursing (2010)
- ANA Guide to the Code of Ethics for Nursing: Interpretation and Application (2010)

These ANA documents are the standards for nursing practice. After *To Err Is Human* was published, nursing realized that national agencies such as the National Quality Forum (NQF), AHRQ, and the IOM were all working to improve patient safety and the efforts of these agencies were in ideal alignment with the Magnet recognition program.

Armstrong and Laschinger's 2009[21] study on Magnet hospital characteristics and workplace empowerment found that when leaders empower nurses through professional standards, professional practice, and leadership support, nurses will fully engage in creating a consistent culture of safety; in fact, patient lives may depend on empowered hospital nurses. Aiken and colleagues (2000)[6] found that Magnet hospitals had patient mortality

TABLE 31.3 Magnet model® components aligned with the 14 Magnet® forces

2008 Model Component	2005 Force Number and Title
Transformational Leadership	1. Quality of Nursing Leadership
	3. Management Style
Structural Empowerment	2. Organizational Structure
	4. Personnel Policies and Procedures
	10. Community and the Organization
	12. Image of Nursing
	14. Professional Development
Exemplary Professional Practice	5. Professional Models of Care
	8. Consultation and Resources
	9. Autonomy
	11. Nurses as Teachers
	13. Interdisciplinary Relations
	6. Quality of Care: Ethics, Patient Safety, and Quality Infrastructure
New Knowledge, Innovation, and Improvements	6. Quality of Care: Research and Evidence-Based Practice
	7. Quality Improvements
Empirical Quality Outcomes	6. Quality of Care: Outcomes

Adapted from "Recognizing Nursing Excellence. Application Manual: Magnet Recognition Program®" by the American Nurses Credentialing Center, 2008, p. 3. Copyright 2008 by the American Nurses Credentialing Center.

rates that were 7% lower than those at non-Magnet hospitals. This finding highlights the effects of nursing leadership and staff nurse performance in Magnet versus non-Magnet hospitals. A recent study[26] examined the role between hospital nursing leadership styles and 30-day mortality rates in 90 acute care hospitals in Alberta, Canada. High emotional intelligence and relational skill sets define a resonant leader. The resonant leadership style, defined in the Magnet program as transformational, was significantly related to lower patient mortality after controlling for patient demographics, co-morbidities, and organizational factors.

A CULTURE OF PATIENT SAFETY AND MAGNET

Knowing and understanding the characteristics that define a safety culture can be elusive. A safety culture encompasses beliefs, attitudes, and behaviors.[9,27] Sammer found that a framework of the concept "culture of safety" included seven "safety subcultures." Table 31.4 includes the Magnet characteristics that exemplify those safety subcultures.

To illustrate the application of the safety typology and ANCC Magnet model component framework provided in Table 31.4, each safety subculture identified by Sammer et al.[9] will be

TABLE 31.4 Safety subculture, safety culture properties & Magnet® characteristics

Safety Subculture	**Safety Culture Properties**	**Magnet Component** **Magnet Force** **Magnet Characteristic**
Leadership	Accessibility priority Change management resources Commitment role model Executive rounds support Governance vigilance Open relationships Visibility Physician engagement vision/mission	Transformational leadership Structural empowerment Shared decision making Autonomy Interdepartmental relationships Leaders at every level Servant leadership
Teamwork	Alignment Deference to expertise wherever found Flattened hierarchy Multidisciplinary/multigenerational Mutual respect Psychological safety Readiness to adapt/flexibility Supportive Watch each other's back Standardization, protocols, checklists, and guidelines Technology, automation	Structured empowerment Interdisciplinary relations Code of conduct Safer surgery program Image of nursing
Communication	Assertive/speak up Bottom-up approach Clarity Hands off Linkages between executives and front line for resolution and feedback Safety briefings/debriefings Structured techniques/SBAR, time-out, read back	Professional practice model Care delivery model AHRQ culture of safety survey High alert "red rules"
Evidence-Based Practice	Best practices High reliability/zero defects Outcome driven Science of safety	Exemplary professional practice Evidence-based nursing practice Structure-process-outcome

TABLE 31.4 Safety subculture, safety culture properties & Magnet® characteristics (*Continued*)

Safety Subculture	Safety Culture Properties	Magnet Component Magnet Force Magnet Characteristic
Learning	Awareness/informed Celebrate success/rewards Data driven Education and training, including physicians Learn from mistakes Evaluate, monitor, and feed back Performance improvement Proactive Root cause analysis (RCA) Share lessons learned	Mindfulness Daisy Award Steps program—novice to expert Career development/trajectory Professional development Continuing education programs Peer review
Just	Blame free Disclosure Nonpunitive reporting Systems—not individuals Trust	Best practices committee Anonymous reporting Supportive (RN–RN interaction, RN–MD interaction) Flat hierarchy Zero tolerance for disruptive behaviors
Patient Centered	Community/grassroots involvement Compassion/caring Empowered patients/families Exemplary patient care Focus on patients Formal participation in care Health promotion Informed patients/families Patient stories	Definition of community served End-of-life communication and care Patients on hospital boards Patient satisfaction scores and stories Mission/vision Bedside rounds Patient handoffs Community involvement Nurses as teachers Patient engagement with rounds Magnet stories

Adapted from "What is Patient Safety Culture? A Review of the Literature" by C. E. Sammer, K. L. Lykens, K. P. Singh, D. A. Mains, and N. A. Lachan, 2010. *Journal of Nursing Scholarship, 42*(2), p. 157–163. Copyright 2010 by Sigma Theta Tau International.

described and followed by a Magnet exemplar that represents the specific safety subculture characteristic. Exemplars are stories that Magnet nurses use to describe their journey to excellence.

Leadership and a Culture of Safety

Essential to a culture of safety is leadership. Without leadership, safety efforts will be fragmented and inconsequential.[28] Executive and senior leadership and the governing body play a key role in designing, fostering, and nurturing a safety culture. Leadership is needed to define accountability.[29] Engaged leaders drive the culture by designing strategy and building structures that guide the safety process and outcomes.[30]

Leaders commit to safety as the top business priority. Safety is a precondition, not a competing goal, and it is a responsibility of the system, not individuals. Employees are encouraged to speak up. At-risk behavior is not condoned. A leader's presence is felt; leaders "round" on patient care areas and talk with staff and patients. Leaders press for system improvements that maintain quality and reduce the variability in the delivery of healthcare services.[17]

The Magnet recognition program begins with transformational leadership, which is essential to excellence at the patient's bedside. In terms of patient safety, leaders empower the staff nurse to use his or her professional autonomy to advocate for and protect the patient. Transformational leaders at all levels of the organization convey a strong sense of advocacy and support on behalf of staff and patients.[3] Transformational leaders inspire, motivate, and become "servant leaders" to staff. Their relationship with staff is built on trust, collaboration, and accountability, some of the same core principles of a safety culture.

Transformational leaders encourage staff to voice their opinions and take part in decision making. Such empowerment of staff can begin in a structured, shared governance model, by which leaders develop and support autonomous patient advocates. Empowerment is important for patient safety, and nurse managers are ideally positioned to create positive work conditions that nurture empowerment.[31] Critical to a culture of safety are engaged leaders who support a robust error-and-near-miss reporting system, which is critical to every culture of safety.[30,32] While a culture of safety begins with the CEO, it has to be driven just as strongly by the chief nursing officer (CNO) because historically nurses are the professionals who most often report adverse events and safety issues.

Staff nurses are key clinical leaders for patient safety because they are the end-line providers of nursing care. They can "stop the line" or call a "time-out" to avoid risky, unsafe, or uncertain practices among all providers. Staff nurses notice latent, subtle practices that have the potential for harm; if nurses are empowered and supported, they step forward, speak up, and demonstrate their role in a culture of safety. A Magnet nurse is an empowered, mindful patient advocate committed to providing consistently safe patient care.

Leadership Exemplars and Safety

The following stories are sources of evidence from Magnet-recognized organizations where all nurses consider themselves leaders and play an essential role in ensuring a culture of safety.

Visibility, Accessibility, and Communication

Input from direct-care nurses is used to improve the work environment and patient care. Feedback provided by direct-care nurses is taken very seriously because as end providers of care, they must ensure patient safety. There is an unwavering commitment on the part of the CNO and nurse managers to seek and listen to the voices of nurses, and this is the very fabric of nurses' shared governance structure. The CNO and other leaders throughout the organization demonstrate a servant leader philosophy and fully recognize and understand that a healthy, safe work environment for the patient and employee cannot be created and sustained without feedback and participation from direct-care nurses.

The overall organizational construct and our shared governance structures and processes are essential in soliciting feedback from direct-care staff to improve the work environment and optimize clinical outcomes. Direct-care nursing staff are encouraged and supported to participate in unit-based, shared governance teams, as well as in the various corporate councils. Examples of structures and processes by which input from direct-care nurses is used to improve the work environment and patient care follow.

The Guiding Excellent Motivated Staff (GEMS) council is a primary structure for the process of garnering input from direct-care nurses. The GEMS council consists of nurses representing every department where nurses are on staff. GEMS serve as ambassadors and provide direct feedback to the CNO and other nursing leaders. On an annual basis, the CNO engages nurses at all levels, including direct-care nurses, in nursing town hall meetings. The data from the GEMS meetings and town halls often spark an improved work environment or enhanced care delivery.

Yearly, the hospital participates in the National Database for Nursing Quality Indicators (NDNQI) Nurse Satisfaction Survey. In 2009, the survey garnered responses from 81% of eligible direct-care nurses, and while the hospital nurses scored in the top quartile for RN job enjoyment, there are times when the survey results have also demonstrated unit-based, as well as organizational, opportunities for improvement. Feedback from direct-care nurses has been invaluable in developing appropriate action plans targeted at improving the work environment and enhancing patient care and safety.

In 2008, the CNO acted to recognize improvements in the work environment and in patient care by establishing the Center for Clinical Affairs. The Center rests on four pillars—professional practice, professional development, research, and patient care support; each pillar is considered distinct and yet all are complementary. Each pillar has a director responsible for operations and programmatic development, but the real synergy related to the Center for Clinical Affairs comes through collaboration with the staff. Direct-care nurses interact with members from the Center to advance nursing practice in the pillar areas of evidence-based practice, professional development, research, and quality improvement. Two years ago, the Center for Clinical Affairs focused on two key initiatives involving refinements to the nursing quality dashboard and the patient acuity system. The dashboard serves to educate nurses at all levels about quality and to update staff on a quarterly basis concerning current measurement status for each indicator; thus the dashboard drives a focus on quality at the staff nursing level. The refinement of the patient acuity classification was based on input from direct-care nurses relative to the need to better align human and financial resources for safe, quality patient care.

Leading Indicators

At another Magnet organization, the CNO and clinical leaders developed significant tactics supporting the strategic key result areas of health outcomes. Particular emphasis was placed on achieving the top decile in the Center for Medicare & Medicaid Services (CMS) bundles that track the effectiveness and efficiency of evidence-based care related to acute myocardial infarctions (AMI), congestive heart failure (CHF), surgical care improvement project (SCIP), and pneumonia; obtaining The Joint Commission Disease Specific Certification for Primary Stroke Care, Heart Failure and Ventricular Assist Device; and enhancing the medical center's Cancer and Neuroscience Institutes. Strategic planning and development of focused tactics yielded significant achievements in all key result areas and have enhanced effectiveness and efficiency as the following summary of outcomes illustrates.

As the medical center met or exceeded the targets for the four CMS bundles—AMI, heart failure, pneumonia, and SCIP—it dramatically improved clinical outcomes. For each of the CMS bundles, the medical center significantly improved operations through the application of leading indicator methodology. The leading indicator check sheet is a visual prompt placed during admission at the front of the patient's chart, allowing nursing to concurrently monitor the clinical care processes, ensuring compliance to achieve perfect care. This sheet is updated and completed by any healthcare provider involved in the patient's care. Each opportunity for improvement is thoroughly investigated, and leaders report compliance to the staff weekly. When indicators are not met, action plans are developed to analyze the process and list the steps staff will take to meet the indicator. Executive leadership has set clear goals, and leaders require ongoing feedback on performance measures.

Implementation of the leading indicator methodology led to improved compliance over a 30-month period, with perfect care provided by frontline staff: heart failure performance increased from 71% to 90%, AMI care performance increased from 89% to 100%, pneumonia care performance increased from 32% to 96%, and SCIP performance measures increased from 51% to 94%. Quality care outcomes have steadily increased and have held the gain. Also, the medical center received The Joint Commission's Disease Specific Care Certification for Primary Stroke Care, Heart Failure and Ventricular Assist Device.

These outstanding improvements are attributed to devoted and accountable teams. Compliance and success were driven by standardization of processes, creation of innovative tools, partnering with existing clinical committees, and education of the nursing staff. Concurrent chart reviews and interventions have all led to improvements in the processes. The nurses continue to receive feedback from the monitoring and understand the impact of noncompliance on measures. Executive leadership's focus on improvement and holding staff accountable for the measures was crucial to the improvement process.

TEAMWORK AND A CULTURE OF SAFETY

A second critical safety subculture is teamwork. Patient safety advocates have long recognized that the vast majority of errors are caused not by individual lapses but by system problems.[10,29] A major cause of system problems is the complexity of the modern healthcare environment. Systems always change because new information arrives, demands compete for a worker's time, workers must perform when fatigued, and stress pervades the hospital system. Staff errors can be reduced only if systems are improved. Basic to patient safety and fundamental to improved teamwork is to stop the blame game and become a cooperative, supportive team.

As mentioned above, health care has learned from aviation, long considered a high-risk yet reliable industry. Aviation developed a model for organizational safety in which teamwork encompasses all disciplines and generations, who communicate openly across ranks, layers, and individuals.[33,34] Communication is key; AHRQ and Institute for Healthcare Improvement (IHI) studies have shown that poor communication is the leading cause of medical errors.[35]

Safety depends on implementation of a unified interdisciplinary system of physicians, nurses, and all other healthcare personnel who talk with each other daily about the realities of practice and patient care. The march to Magnet recognition restructures nursing organizations in a way that helps speed up the behavior changes that create a new culture—focusing on the patient and family and their outcomes. When clinicians cooperate, they advance toward improving and maintaining patient safety. Again, the march to Magnet provides a structure and time frame, usually a number of years, for clinical team leaders and multidisciplinary committees to collaborate more fully around patient care to meet a component requirement.

Magnet recognized organizations have flattened hierarchical structures where every employee is recognized and valued. The image of a nurse is that of a strong professional; nurses speak up for patients and themselves, and are involved as equals in the care of patients. Examples of interdisciplinary teamwork in Magnet organizations are interdisciplinary patient rounds, safer surgery programs where all members of the surgical team start with a time-out and can stop the process at any time, implementing a standard code of conduct for physicians and all employees, and the hospital pharmacy and therapeutics committee where nurses share responsibilities and integrate improvements.

Teamwork Exemplars and Safety

The following exemplars are sources of evidence from Magnet-recognized organizations where nurses consider themselves part of a high-functioning, collaborative, interdisciplinary team and play a vital role in ensuring a culture of safety.

Speaking Up: The Case of the Missing Lap Sponge

At one of the on-the-Magnet-march organizations, during a long, complicated, high-risk organ transplant surgery that included a change-of-shift nursing team in the middle of the surgery, both the scrub and circulating nurses declined to hand closing sutures to the attending surgeon because their count of lap sponges (8 × 12 sponge with a metal tag on one end) was off by one. While the circulating nurse continued to recount sponges, including opening up garbage bags in an attempt to find the errant sponge, the scrub nurse (per policy) called for an abdominal flat-plate x-ray in an attempt to locate the missing sponge. The first x-ray was read as nothing being found in the abdomen, but the sponge count remained off by one. The surgeon called for the closing sutures a second time, but again the nurses would not hand the sutures over and a second abdominal x-ray was requested. The second x-ray showed a "shadow" but nothing definitive; all the while the circulating nurse was recounting sponges through the numerous procedure garbage bags. For a third time, the surgeon called for the closing sutures, and the nurses would not hand over the sutures but asked for a third flat-plate abdominal x-ray. The third time was the charm because the x-ray revealed a fist-sized, balled-up, blood-soaked sponge, adhered to the posterior side of the liver. The sponge was quickly removed and the closing sutures were given to the surgeon. The metal tag, usually identified on an x-ray had gotten twisted and buried in the middle of the blood-soaked, balled-up lap sponge and was undetectable on x-ray.

What makes this story of teamwork in the operating room (OR) even more remarkable is the operating room team members included four different ethnic cultures, which at times experienced teamwork issues due to their cultural variations, including deference to hierarchy. The nurses were Asian females, the attending surgeon was a middle-European male, the male residents were from Arabian countries, and the anesthesiologist was an American-born male. In refusing to hand the closing sutures, the nurses adhered to safer surgery policies but went against their cultural instincts of subservience to physicians and males. While the situation was fraught with tension and risk, all personnel in the OR remained respectful, never became disruptive, and treated the incident as business as usual.

The nurses received the institution's "Stick Your Neck Out" award and were celebrated at a breakfast attended by perioperative staff, surgeons, the CNO, CEO, the hospital director of risk and safety, and the nursing director of quality and safety. Their story was featured in the internal nursing newsletter, P.E.N. (*Professionalism and Excellence in Nursing*), and inspired other nurses to take the risk of speaking up, no matter the situation, to keep patients out of harm's way. The patient's outcome: discharged six days postoperatively, "feeling better than I have in years." The nurses in the OR exhibited personal courage and trust in the culture that, no matter the outcome, finding the sponge or making a lap sponge count mistake, they would be supported because their intention was not to disrupt the surgery but to help to provide a culture of safety.

Handoff Tool

Another exemplar shows how teamwork guarded patient safety at a Magnet institution; this exemplar describes a handoff tool. A survey conducted on one unit at a large children's hospital in the Midwest ranked handoffs/transfers as the greatest safety risk. Nursing staff further explored this topic and decided to see how this concern could be addressed through the creation of a safer handoff tool to be used for all pediatric patients. The nurses applied the Comprehensive Unit Based Safety Program (CUSP) methodology. The project followed basic steps educating staff on how easily errors occur, conducting safety surveys, prioritizing improvements, implementing and evaluating the changes, and reassessing the unit safety culture. A multidepartmental team was formed with clinical staff from various shifts that ultimately created a revised handoff tool that would accompany all patients from the pediatric ED and pediatric oncology clinic to the inpatient unit. During the data collection period, out of 438 patients who came to the unit, only 38 arrived without the handoff tool. No patient safety events were reported by the participating units. The staff also have reported an 83% improvement in teamwork between the units. This program has empowered frontline clinicians to identify a safety concern close to them and create a successful solution.

Human Factors and Teamwork

A third teamwork exemplar comes from a Magnet organization that opened additional surgical-services operating suites. Transition into the new space was successful because of planning and preparation spearheaded by nurses. The process began with a core team of direct-care nurses and nursing leaders participating in the Association of periOperative Registered Nurses (AORN) National Conference; they attended presentations and spoke with vendors. An interdisciplinary team made site visits to Chicago metro hospitals to discuss workflow patterns, evaluate surgical equipment, and assess perioperative environmental design. As a result of this work, the team was actively involved in selecting important technology, including booms and lights so that high-risk patients occupied a safe environment.

COMMUNICATION AND A CULTURE OF PATIENT SAFETY

Communication is another vital characteristic and an integral subculture of patient safety.[32,34,36] Too often communication between various healthcare professionals around clinical care is discipline specific rather than interdisciplinary.[29] Collaborative communication is built on mutual respect for all team members. Communication remains the number one issue in patient safety.[35] Investigations into adverse events have found that, while all communication between disciplines is important, communication between nurses and physicians is vital for patient outcomes.[37]

In his 1994 classic study on communication between nurses and physicians in intensive care units (ICUs), Shortell and his colleagues[38] examined four elements of communication:

- Openness—the extent to which nurses believe they can speak to physicians without fear of repercussions
- Timeliness—the degree to which nurses believe that information about patient care is relayed promptly to physicians
- Accuracy—the extent to which nurses believe that the information conveyed to them by physicians is accurate

- Understanding—the extent to which nurses believe that communication on the unit is effective and comprehensive

These elements are especially important for patient safety in the complex, fast-paced ICU environment. Physicians and nurses vary in their ideas about what constitutes good communication.[37] In the march to Magnet, many organizations work on improving communication among teams, especially the nurse–physician relationship.

Manojlovich's[37] research in a Magnet organization showed that, as timeliness of communication increased, the prevalence of pressure ulcers decreased. The meta-analysis by Sammer and colleagues[9] showed that a culture of safety requires assertive language such as, "I need clarity," and structured language such as "read backs," which clarifies and confirms verbal orders and test results.

Time-outs structure communication among team members prior to an invasive procedure to verify the correct procedure at the correct body site is being performed on the correct patient.[39] Another communication structure is the handoff between care providers to ensure information and the plan of care are transferred cohesively between shifts, departments, and units.[32,36] Briefings and debriefings are valued communication tools at several Magnet organizations.

Openness, trust, and honesty are key components to staff engagement. Engagement is defined as "a situation in which employees enjoy their work, contribute enthusiastically to meeting goals, and feel a sense of belonging and commitment to the organization."[40] When managers and executives provide feedback and close the loop with frontline staff, they let staff know their input and communications are heard and acknowledged. This feedback builds trust and openness—both important aspects of a culture of safety. Communication needs to be dynamic and open; nurses tend to use silence instead of voice when dealing with physicians.

When organizations build electronic communication, they must also consider human factors. For example, simple dissemination of clinical practice guidelines, which supports consistent patient outcomes, does not necessarily result in their application; attention to human-factor design elements significantly improved guideline compliance in one hospital.[14] When using an electronic medical record, human factors such as simplicity, standardization in design, and efficiency can make for successful adherence to the guidelines because they are perceived as easy to use and add value to the provider.

While SBAR communication (**S**ituation, **B**ackground, **A**ssessment, and **R**ecommendation) between peers and the interdisciplinary team is more common, highly reliable organizations use an iterative communication process called "sense-making," which cuts across hierarchical boundaries. Sense-making fosters understanding between parties so that failures are averted; it involves a five-step process known as STICC:[37]

- Situation—"Here's what I think we face."
- Task—"Here's what I think we should do."
- Intent—"Here's why."
- Concern—"Here's what we should keep our eyes on."
- Calibrate—"Now talk and push back; tell me if you don't understand, cannot do it, or see something I do not."[41]

This form of contributory communication requires feedback among various disciplines and is in the best interest of the patient because the open nature of the conversation is directed toward the best possible outcome.

Interdisciplinary relationships are one of the forces of Magnetism, and collegiality is considered an outgrowth of collaboration with physicians and other allied health disciplines. Collaborative working relationships and professional, mutually respectful communication are expected in a Magnet organization, and the expectation is based on the premise that all members of the healthcare team contribute essentially to clinical outcomes.[3] Conflicts and disruptive behaviors can erode patient safety, so conflict management strategies are in place and used effectively. Strategies may include a multidisciplinary code of conduct, training on crucial conversations, or coaching and role modeling collaborative behaviors.

Communication Exemplars and Safety

The following stories are sources of evidence from Magnet-recognized organizations where nurses actively communicate with each other and with a collaborative, interdisciplinary team. This communication plays a vital role in ensuring a culture of safety.

Safety Alert: GEM 4000 Blood Gas K+ Results

When a laboratory blood gas instrument failed, management attempted to prevent patient harm by circulating an SBAR communication memo to all clinical staff (see Table 31.5).

Nursing Communication Handoff Tool

Another exemplar of improving communication at a Magnet organization is the 5P Handoff Communication tool developed to promote continuity of care and foster a collaborative, interdisciplinary process. Information based on risk occurrence reports and recent AHRQ patient safety results identified an opportunity to improve the handoff communication process. Nursing's Practice Council examined the current handoff process and implemented recommendations for improvement. Accurate standardized handoff communication improves safety, and The Joint Commission requires it to comply with National Patient Safety Goal #2.

The multidisciplinary team included, as chair, an advanced practice nurse who was the patient safety manager; representatives from nursing (Emergency Department [ED], Medical/Surgical, Critical Care, Pediatrics,

TABLE 31.5 SBAR communication memo

To all Physicians, Nurses, and Clinical Practitioners:

S-Situation: The manufacturer of the GEM 4000 Blood Gas Instrument has identified an issue in which falsely lowered, erroneous K+ results on a blood gas analysis can occur.

B-Background: We have been notified by our Instrumentation Laboratory GEM 4000 blood gas vendor that occurrences of **falsely lowered K+ results** (potential negative bias of 0.6 to 1.2 mmol/L) can occur on patient blood analysis, leading to erroneous results with potentially severe impact to patient treatment. The event is considered rare based on an internal investigation that identified an incidence rate of 0.0013% (1 out of 77,000 samples) from an estimated 1.7 million sample results. Results in the 1.2 mmol/L range are considered remote, but potentially serious if they do occur.

A-Assessment: While the potential incident rate of occurrence is rare, we must assure that all reported blood gas result analyses are accurate and valid and will not lead to inappropriate diagnosis and/or treatment of our patients. The medical center's laboratory system should always be the preferred choice for any orders requesting a plasma K+ analysis.

R-Recommendation: The Pulmonary Function Lab will be electronically blocking the reporting of K+ results on all analyzed blood gases effective immediately. This will eliminate the possibility for potentially erroneous results to be reported and/or documented on any patient within the medical center. All physician orders for a K+ should be processed and analyzed via the hospital laboratory department. It is our expectation that a software upgrade to correct this situation will take place on October 10th and the K+ analyses on blood gases will be available again beginning on October 11th.

We apologize for any inconvenience this may cause.

Thank you,

The Pulmonary Function Laboratory

Operating Room [OR], Post-Anesthesia Care Unit [PACU], and Day Surgery Center); representatives from Allied Health (Physical Therapy [PT], Cardiac Catherization Lab, Imaging, Cardiodiagnostics); and representatives from Clinical Education and Risk Management. Objectives for the team included evaluating the existing handoff process, reviewing the current handoff policy and tools used, identifying opportunities for improvement, implementing the revised process, and developing a process to measure success.

To guide the team, an interdisciplinary work plan was created. The team met every week for six weeks, at which time an open forum was held for discussion between the direct-care nurses and other disciplines as to what data the handoff tool should contain to provide the safest and most effective handoff for the inpatient, outpatient, and transport staffs. Between team meetings, feedback was received from nurse leaders and direct-care nurses, as well as from ancillary support staff.

The tool was named the 5P Passport because it is used as the patient travels from one area to another and it outlines key elements of the patient's care essential for ensuring continuity of care and patient safety during transport. This standardized handoff prescribes a "real-time, interactive process of passing patient-specific information from one caregiver or team to another for the purpose of ensuring continuity and safety of the patient's care." The handoff communication policy stipulates that the handoff key elements include the following:

- Patient—the name of the patient to whom the handoff applies
- Plan—what is to happen next
- Purpose of the plan—the desired outcome
- Problems—what is known to be different, unusual, or complicating about the patient
- Precautions—what could be expected to be different, unusual, or complicating about the patient

The tool was piloted on selected patient care units. Educational meetings were held with the piloting units and the patient transportation departments. The tool was piloted for several months on several units, at the end of which a feedback survey was collected from the piloting units. The outcomes of the pilot program provided useful information regarding the essential information needed for an interdisciplinary handoff. This information was used in collaboration with information systems staff to create a real-time patient handoff tool in the electronic medical record to accompany patients, ensuring safe and effective patient care. In one division, the Pediatric Respiratory Therapy Unit Council created a 5P video based on the game show "Deal or No Deal," which was shared as a best practice with the Practice Council members and distributed to all clinical managers to be shown at staff meetings.

EVIDENCE-BASED PRACTICE (EBP) AND A CULTURE OF PATIENT SAFETY

A culture of safety is exhibited by healthcare organizations that use evidence-based best practices and standardized processes, protocols, checklists, and guidelines.[11,17,42,43] Evidenced-based practice is the conscientious integration of the best research evidence with clinical expertise and patient preferences. For many years, nuclear power and aviation industries have been consultants to healthcare leaders who studied safety principles and safety models. For example, aviation uses a checklist prior to every flight to ensure the complicated working of the aircraft, its systems, and, its crew are ready and working.[44] However, is it possible that patient safety may be more complicated than air or nuclear safety because healthcare systems involve countless disciplines and a culture of safety must change multiple behaviors on both ends of the spectrum, from the patient to each administrator and every provider?

Peter Pronovost and the World Health Organization (WHO) introduced standardized checklists for safer surgeries and checklists in intensive care units (ICUs) to lessen the infection rates.[45] Standardizations, checklists, and best practices are difficult to implement due to the long-held medical model of physician autonomy and the "art" of medicine. Physicians push back from "cook-book medicine" and resist guidelines and checklists. However, as new generations of physicians are trained, they are more comfortable using evidence-based guidelines, checklists, time-outs, and best practices.[46]

Over the past decade, colleges of nursing have been embedding evidence-based practice in nursing curricula at both the graduate and undergraduate levels. Materials available to nurses to study for national certification exams are evidence based. However, for some of the more experienced and seasoned nurses, practicing based on evidence is a new concept. To fill that educational gap, hospitals have had to develop evidence-based education programs. The 2008 Magnet model placed an even stronger emphasis on nurses using both evidence-based best practices and measureable outcomes to determine how the practices impact patient care and/or systems.

Evidence-Based Practice Exemplars and Safety

The following exemplars are sources of evidence from Magnet-recognized organizations where nurses actively and consistently use evidence and measure outcomes of care to determine the end effect on patient care. Basing practice on evidence plays an essential role in assuring a culture of safety.

Institute for Healthcare Improvement (IHI) Patient Flow Initiative

One Magnet hospital recognized that quality of care was impacted depending on whether patients were placed in holding patterns, managed by off services, boarded in the ED or PACU, or subject to delayed medical or surgical admissions. The hospital made a commitment to improve practice using a systemwide approach. They formally engaged the Institute for Healthcare Improvements (IHI) as an external consultant to develop a patient flow plan specific to their hospital. In partnering with IHI on the initiative *Optimizing Patient Flow: Moving Patients Smoothly Through Acute Care Settings*, they better understood how patient safety, hospital revenue, staff satisfaction, and patient satisfaction were negatively impacted when patients, information, and materials did not move through the hospital in a timely and efficient manner.

A steering committee was formed, with the CNO as the administrative sponsor, and included three interdisciplinary work groups (from the OR, ED, and in-patient nursing); the committee's mission was to address flow in their respective clinical areas. The work groups were challenged to always consider the patient's unique perspective and patient safety as the guiding principle when making recommendations for improving structures and processes. The groups each followed the same objectives, including minimizing waits, optimizing handoffs, identifying and eliminating barriers to flow, and focusing organizational energy on accomplishing these goals while eliminating unnecessary aspects of the process identified as waste.

In keeping with a systemwide approach, patient-flow initiatives were rolled out across the hospital to all in-patient nursing units. Early in the day, the in-patient nursing units began participating in a daily bed huddle to plan for each day's admissions and discharges. This huddle allowed nurses to determine both demand and capacity on their units and then formulate plans to better match capacity to demand. This activity involved both unit-based and hospital-wide bed huddles. The organization's peak flow census plan was revised to include a tiered approach, with each department having responsibility for implementing a department-specific plan during peak census levels. The role and availability of the hospital's capacity coordinators was further defined and expanded to support efforts to improve patient flow. These efforts were parlayed into two valuable tools for improvement:

- A uniform interdepartmental tool for requesting and communicating data necessary for in-patient admission from the ED
- A standardized set of orders for patients admitted from the ED

One key aim of the initiative was ensuring patients were discharged earlier in the day. The bed huddles engaged stakeholders to do what was appropriate to increase efficiency. By using the time of patient discharge as a quantitative measure, the staff identified what improvements were making a difference. Outcomes show the hospital is making the right improvements in improving patient flow. Figure 31.2 represents overall patient flow improvements. As a result of targeted improvements, the peak discharge times have moved from later in the day to earlier in the day, and discharge rates appear to be consistently high through 3:00 p.m.

Through collaboration with the IHI, the hospital realized that improvements require changes but not all changes bring improvement. With the help of internal experts and the IHI as external consultant, the hospital targeted the changes that were most likely to result in improvement. They also realigned teams so that, rather than focusing on a particular service area, the focus groups now look at either input, throughput, or output.

This important work continues today and is currently focused on identifying specific barriers impacting patient flow surrounding admission from the ED to an in-patient nursing unit. Once barriers are identified, future plans call for developing strategies to overcome these barriers, interdisciplinary education of all stakeholders, and an evaluation method to measure success of the project.

Postpartum Depression Program

At one Magnet organization, a comprehensive project demonstrated that nurses can

FIGURE 31.2 Discharge Times Comparison, 2008

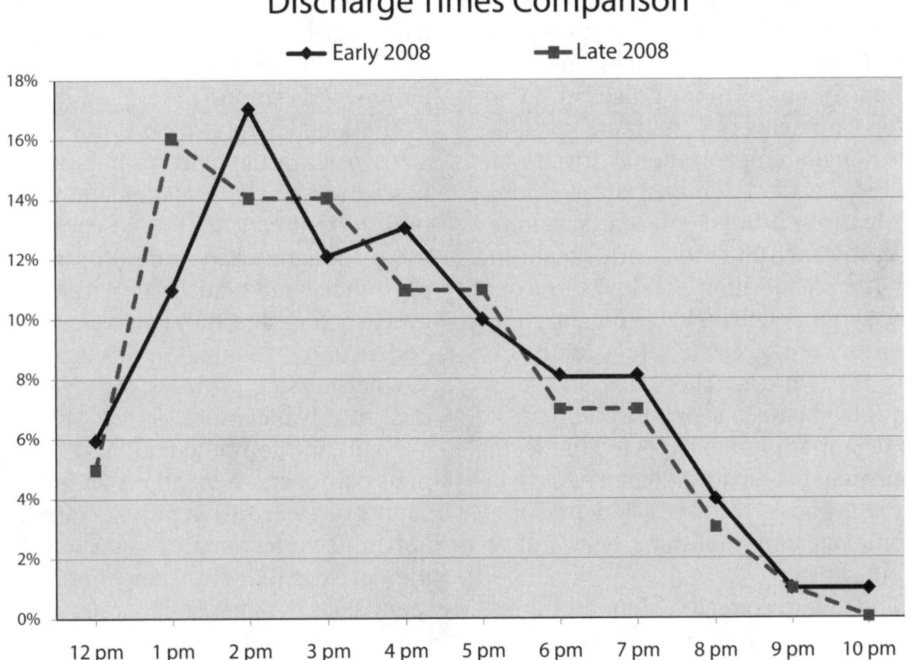

autonomously translate evidence into practice and enhance patient care. This demonstration came about via the postpartum depression (PPD) program that was implemented with the Women and Infants Department. In 2007, a nurse saw an opportunity to impact nursing practice and improve patient outcomes for women experiencing the overwhelming complication of postpartum depression. She evaluated various depression screening tools; tested them in this environment, which has a very short length of stay; and implemented a screening program to detect risk of postpartum depression. This program has been embraced by all the clinicians with results that are saving lives. This dedicated nurse proceeded to take the program to another level by coordinating a postpartum adjustment support team with regular meetings held at the medical center.

LEARNING AND A CULTURE OF PATIENT SAFETY

Another key concept of patient safety is a culture of continual learning within the organization. Learning from mistakes and using performance improvement processes to advance the care delivery system create safety awareness and an organizational drive to improve.[32,35,47] Leaders demonstrate a willingness to learn and build internal structures and processes such as a robust error-reporting system. The organization also looks to external sources from highly reliable organizations with a history of successful safety cultures so they can learn at a quicker pace. In the interest of advancing the nursing profession, Magnet organizations are expected to mentor other nurses and hospitals; this mentoring includes sharing best practices, safety practices, and exemplars, and publishing results of research outcomes.

Learning cultures create safety awareness among staff and physicians and promote an environment of learning through educational opportunities.[9,32] Many of the education programs (continuing education) are offered to an interdisciplinary audience who enrich the postpresentation discussions. Organizations that have access to a simulation lab use the lab venue to develop lifelike simulations for real-life learning. Education and training should include a basic understanding of (1) the science of safety, (2) what it means to be a high-reliability organization, (3) the value of a safety culture assessment, and (4) the performance improvement process, including rapid cycle testing of change or a "work-out."[9,11,30]

Organizations that continually learn from mistakes and near misses should be transparent in reporting key safety indicators with results posted and updated in a timely, meaningful manner.[9,11,30,48] Hospitals that are data driven learn from failures, near misses, and successes. In learning cultures, failures and near misses are investigated using root cause analysis (RCA).[9,30,42] As hospitals with learning cultures mature, all workers become proactive; they anticipate and identify potentially unsafe processes and speak up to prevent errors. Sharing lessons learned is part of a continual evaluation of the evolving learning process. Finally, a learning culture celebrates and rewards success.[30,49]

The Magnet recognition program emphasizes orientation and on-boarding of new hires, in-service education, continuing education, formal education, and career development.[3] Magnet nurses develop professional portfolios and plan career trajectories. At every career stage, they stress lifelong learning and value personal and professional growth. Magnet nursing provides competency-based clinical advancement, as well as resources to maintain competency. Magnet organizations demonstrate programs and resources to support career development, formal education, and professional certification, including the development of leadership and management skills. Magnet staff nurses inform leadership about topics needed for education and competencies.

Learning Exemplars and Safety

The following story is a source of evidence from a Magnet-recognized organization where nurses and the organization learn from errors, near misses, and others' successes. A culture of continual learning is an essential function in ensuring a culture of safety.

Commitment to Professional Development

This Magnet organization strives to create a culture in which nurses advance the profession. One such mechanism is through the support provided to nurses at all levels of the organization to become nationally certified.

Whether certification is required or voluntary, it is seen as an opportunity that affords nurses professional growth and financial rewards, such as recognition, reimbursement, salary increases, and career advancement opportunities, as well as the opportunity for personal growth. The following graphic summary in Figure 31.3 represents the organization's four-year journey related to efforts at establishing and sustaining a culture that values certification.

Good Catches: Engaging Frontline Staff in Patient Safety

Patient safety is essential to exemplary professional practice and is everyone's responsibility; however, finding a creative way to support staff engagement is challenging. A "Good Catch" reporting program was implemented at a large midwestern medical center. The objectives of the program are to encourage staff recognition and reporting of near-miss events, and direct staff actions that will intercept adverse events, thus preventing errors from reaching the patient. Reportable events included medication errors and fall prevention, among others.

The program was implemented using a friendly competitive Baseball World Series theme with three leagues, and it was clearly defined as a nonpunitive reward program. Monthly communication was sent to individual units; it described the staff's Good Catch and provided safety-culture language. Recognition to individuals was a key factor for success. During National Patient Safety Week, the medical center held an event to share safety accomplishments and celebrate the Good Catch winners. This development of a Good Catch program has led to a nonpunitive

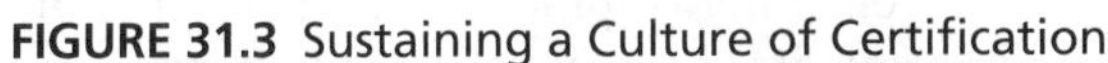

FIGURE 31.3 Sustaining a Culture of Certification

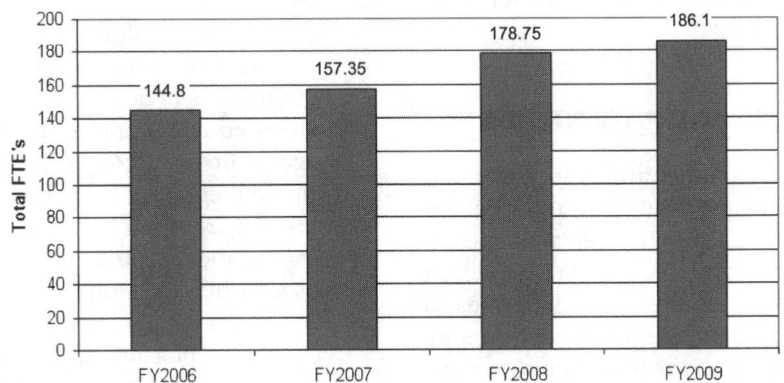

Reprinted from Northwest Community Hospital Magnet re-Application, 2010. Copyright, Northwest Community Hospital, 2010.

environment that "hardwires" a culture of safety at the sharp end of patient care.

As part of the Good Catch program, all near misses are evaluated and trended, and prompt action is taken to prevent any immediate danger to patients and staff. An example is the Neonatal Intensive Care Unit (NICU) staff nurse who identified an incorrect dosage of a heparin floor-stock vial, which was immediately removed from stock. As a result of this event, the pharmacy director worked with her teams in the removal of all heparin floor stock in the NICU and the other pediatric departments. In another case, an advanced practice nurse prompted the investigation of a product by reporting the potential for catheter rupture in a new "Power Port a cath needle." A team, led by the manager of phlebotomy and venous access, assessed patient safety risk and developed education on the distinguishing features of the Power Port. The education is now provided during Port-a-Cath classes and during the adult unit based orientation classes.

Outcomes have included an increased awareness of patient safety events, opportunities to spread the program to other areas, and ability to form interdisciplinary partnerships with pharmacy, lab, and radiology, among others. The near-miss reporting has identified system processes that can be improved to minimize risk of injury to patients. Data trends have shown that over three years of the Good Catch program, error reporting has increased 65%.

JUST CULTURE AND PATIENT SAFETY

A just culture is another important subculture for patient safety. Justice is often depicted as a blind-folded figure holding a balance. In health care, one side of the scale is individual accountability; the other side is the healthcare system.[49] Marx[50] describes determining whether errors are individual failures or system failures by asking four questions:

1. Was the care provider's behavior malicious?
2. Was the care provider under the influence of a substance?
3. Was the care provider aware he or she was making a mistake?
4. Would two of three of the care provider's peers make the same mistake?

A key component of a just culture is trust.[51] It is a blame-free, error-reporting, nonpunitive environment.[20,32] To nurses, the perception that they work in a fair and just culture is very important. Historically, the nursing profession was treated as being on the low end of health care's hierarchy and given less respect than physicians and other disciplines. As nursing improves its image through formal education, national certifications, and Magnet recognition, nurses will perceive a just culture only when they receive the same respect as all healthcare disciplines.

Despite efforts to remove punitive healthcare work environments, evidence suggests they still exist.[52] In fact, nursing literature is rife with articles on hazing, horizontal and vertical violence (bullying), and blame. When an error occurs, nursing staff fear repercussion from managers and peers and negative consequences, including job loss or criminal prosecution if reported.[52,53] Creating cultures of nonpunitive reporting, strong interdisciplinary collaborative practices, and systems improvements helps organizations develop a just culture.[29]

Creating a just culture requires transparency in error disclosure and having no secrets. In matters of patient safety, everyone is treated as an equal, including top admitting physicians. Errors are openly discussed, and information regarding near misses and errors flows freely. Transparency builds trust within the organization. A just culture learns from disclosure while individual accountability for improvements is maintained.

All members of a just culture are mindful of their behaviors and work together to get the job done right. Disruptive behaviors are not tolerated. Nurse leaders liberate their staff to always do the right thing and openly discuss challenges and barriers in current work processes. Nurse leaders see that staff are heard when they speak up, and those leaders promote mindfulness in seeking errors.

One of the requirements of a Magnet nurse is to engage in professional peer review. Nursing peer review facilitates a culture of safety when it analyzes medical errors to eliminate future adverse events. Peer review is consistent with evidence-based professional standards and helps to identify improvements in systems and processes.[54] A peer review process can identify strengths and opportunities for improvements in nursing care and staff performance by comparing these with evidence-based standards of nursing practice. In 2008, ANCC determined that peer review was a component of being a professional nurse and attaining Magnet recognition. Developing an objective, nonjudgmental peer review process for professional nurses is an element of the march to Magnet recognition.

Just Culture Exemplar and Safety

The following story, Just Culture Decision Matrix, is a source of evidence from a Chicago metro, Magnet-recognized organization where nurses and the organization worked toward creating a fair and just culture.

The medical center implemented a just culture to support and strengthen the reporting of patient safety events based on the *just culture* term coined by David Marx. The term was, in turn, based on James Reason's research into the management of human error and system failure.[55] The goal was to apply the just culture matrix during patient safety investigations that involve staff and thereby to ensure a more just manner of responding to patient safety–related errors. It emphasizes error reporting for learning purposes and establishes a consistent and balanced approach to process redesign or corrective action when safety incidents occur. The matrix allows the organization to build staff accountability for their actions but not for flawed systems; it creates a nonpunitive reporting environment. The matrix uses four tests to answer questions about an individual's actions, motives, and behavior at the time of a safety incident:

- Deliberate Harm Test—Identifies cases where harm was intended
- Incapacity Test—Identifies whether ill health or substance abuse caused or contributed to an incident
- Foresight Test—Examines whether protocols and safe working practices were adhered to
- Substitution Test—Identifies deficiencies in training, experience, or supervision, as well as ineffective or nonexistent protocols

The matrix is a decision model that assists leaders and human resource management to investigate incidents and respond appropriately. It promotes a culture in which errors are brought forward so that everyone may learn, fix system errors, and correct unhealthy norms. The organization's just culture decision matrix is depicted in Figure 31.4.

PATIENT-CENTERED CARE AND A CULTURE OF SAFETY

"A patient centered environment embraces the patient and family as the sole reason for the hospital's existence" (p. 163).[9] Patient centeredness promises to value the patient by providing a caring, healing environment during the hospitalization. Patient centeredness also promotes health and well-being by building a trusting relationship between patients and families with their providers; this trust building includes always being honest with the patient throughout the continuum of care. Patient centeredness should be a core value of the business of health care and is one of the six aims of the 2010 IOM report.[1] The medical staff and all employees should make every effort to focus on the patient and offer the patient an exemplary experience marked by caring and compassion.[56]

Patient-centered care responds to each patient's wants, needs, and preferences; it

FIGURE 31.4 Just Culture Decision Matrix

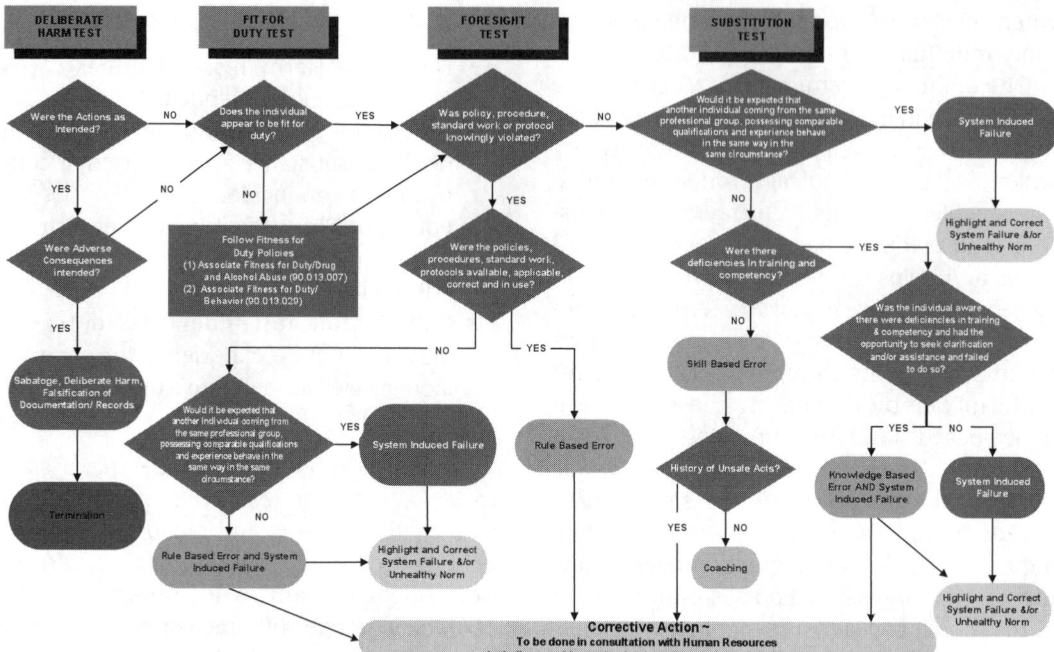

Reproduced from "Managing the Risks of Organizational Accidents" by James Reason, 2003. Ashgate Publishing Group: Burlington, VA; p. 191–222; and "Managing the Maintenance Error: A Practical Guide" by James Reason & Alan Hobbs (2003). Ashgate Publishing Group: Hampshire, England.

encompasses qualities of compassion, empathy, and responsiveness, and it gives patients abundant opportunities to be informed and involved in medical decision making.[57] Hospitals with a patient-centered environment support providers who care and attend to the patient's physical and emotional needs; and they ensure adequate and appropriate staffing, a documented Magnet characteristic. Patient-centered care requires a full, informed consent for all procedures and engaged communication about treatment options.

A patient-centered hospital empowers patients to be partners in their care decisions. Hospitals share their patient-centered vision with their community, which allows the community to feel a sense of pride and ownership of their hospital.[42] The 2001 IOM report, *Crossing the Quality Chasm*, highlights the importance of patient centeredness by suggesting hospitals partner with patients and families to improve each individual patient's experience in treatment.[18] Patient-centered hospitals use the collective voice of patients, who are uniquely informed participants of the healthcare system, to make the system truly responsive to those receiving care.

Patient stories are used to put a face on system failures that have caused serious adverse events. Stories enhance the richness of description and create an environment where discussion can lead to safety action.[58,59] When errors occur, the emphasis needs to be on the patient and family impacted by the mistake. Full disclosure of medical errors is aligned with being patient centered. "The ethically embarrassing debate over disclosure of injuries to patients is, we strongly hope, drawing to a close. . . . Few health care organizations now question the imperative to be honest and forthcoming with patients following an injury" (p. 1385).[60]

To achieve Magnet recognition, nursing must focus on measurable patient outcomes. The organization must have a facility-wide approach for proactive risk assessment and error management. Nurses have to describe the nursing structures and processes that support a culture of patient safety. Under the model component, Exemplary Professional Practice, Magnet organizations highlight their quality measures, which must be above the mean when compared to a national benchmark.

At Magnet hospitals, nurse-sensitive quality indicators must outperform the mean of the national database used. Measurable quality outcomes that are evaluated include patient falls, nosocomial pressure ulcers, patient restraint use, ventilator acquired pneumonia (VAP), blood stream infections, urinary tract infections with a Foley catheter, pediatric I.V. infiltrations, and other specialty-specific, nationally benchmarked indicators. Patient satisfaction with nursing care, measured against a national benchmark, must be shown over a two-year period for every unit and must be above the mean. Research has shown that happy nurses equals better patient outcomes, so staff nurse satisfaction, also compared to a national benchmark, must be above the mean. The Magnet-recognition program places great emphasis on exemplary professional practice, which measures various aspects of patient quality and safety, including national patient safety goals.

Patient-Centered Care Exemplars and Safety

The following stories are sources of evidence from Magnet-recognized organizations where nurses and the organization have placed the patient and family at the center of all work. Patient centeredness is an essential characteristic of a culture of safety.

Patient Hourly Rounding

Changing the culture of the units to become more patient centered was the ultimate goal, and the safety culture was enhanced with the education of hourly rounding. Education was completed with the hourly rounding video developed by the chief nurse executive. This new practice was reinforced when the leader rounded with each staff member to ensure competency, understanding, and expert delivery; rounds focused on "pain, position and potty." The hourly rounding competency checklist and feedback are now shared in weekly newsletters and shift-change huddle-ups.

Patient Safety Manager Rounds

To ensure that safety had a voice and remained at the top of everyone's mind, the medical center created a patient safety manager who is responsible for oversight and leadership of the culture of safety initiative hospital-wide. The patient safety manager is a key participant in many of the patient safety site and system teams, including environment of care, patient identification, the critical event review team, and the patient safety council, a multidisciplinary group of clinicians who meet monthly to oversee the medical center's patient safety program.

A culture of safety is assured by integrating all relevant processes, functions, and services. The patient safety manager implemented patient safety rounds, a strategy to garner information on barriers and opportunities for improvement to create a safer environment for the patient. In support of these rounds, the manager developed two standard lists of questions: one for staff interviews and one for patient/family interviews. Any concerns regarding safety issues and findings are presented to the patient safety council. One major outcome of these rounds was the development of a new Code H sign for patient rooms. The Code H process was developed in accordance with The Joint Commission's National Patient Safety Goal, requiring the organization to educate the patient and family on available reporting methods for concerns related to care, treatment, and services. The Code H process includes a dedicated phone line for patients and families to call if there are concerns about the patient's condition. The Code H sign provides the patient and family direction on when they should activate the Code H process.

Working with Community Organizations to Improve Outcomes

Another Magnet hospital created a unique partnership with an external organization, WINGS (Women in Need Growing Stronger), a community agency dedicated to victims of domestic violence. Expertise from the staff at WINGS was essential in assisting staff with the development of policies, education, and protocols to help nurses at all levels to identify issues of domestic violence and offer services for employees, patients, and the community. Key accomplishments included development of:

- An interdisciplinary team for assessment and planning
- An educational program for 25 nurse champions who represent the clinical spectrum
- A hospital-wide domestic-violence screening tool for staff, utilizing the hospital clinical computer system, with the expectation of screening 100% of patients on admission
- A domestic violence brochure for the community and hospital staff with translations in Spanish, Russian, and Polish
- Creation of a new position in the hospital: domestic violence site coordinator

The Magnet framework enabled the team to bring the message of domestic violence prevention from the hospital setting to the community, from coworkers to neighbors, which enhanced the message of patient safety across the continuum of care.

As demonstrated in the preceding exemplar stories, the Magnet recognition program clearly promotes and sustains a culture of safety. However, although Magnet recognition is bestowed by ANCC (a nursing award), it is in fact an organizational award because only good collaboration and interdisciplinary work will achieve it. The classic Donabedian[61] framework of structure, process, and outcomes (the right structures produce the right processes, which produce the right outcomes) has been used as an analogy in aligning the Magnet program with patient safety: Patient safety, to be a successful core goal, also needs organizational collaboration. Magnet recognition provides the structure which promotes empowerment for nurse gatekeepers to champion an environment of care that continually promotes patient safety.

CONCLUSION

In 2004, the Institute of Medicine Quality Chasm Series, "Patient Safety: Achieving a New Standard of Care," recommended the development of patient safety systems to achieve acceptable patient safety standards. Eight years later, healthcare professionals continue to work collaboratively to improve safety in hospitals, and the nursing profession (the largest healthcare workforce) is leading many patient safety initiatives. A prime example is the National Database of Nursing Quality Indicators (NDNQI), a national nursing registry and database that tracks the performance of more than 22 measures of nurse-sensitive outcomes in hospitals.[62] These outcome measures are used to study the impact of hospital nursing care on patient quality and safety, with a growing body of evidence that links the availability and quality of nursing care to prevention of many adverse events (IOM, 2010).[1] Patient-centered, evidence-based data are fundamental to the building of comprehensive patient safety systems; yet without a culture of safety embedded into an organization, data may not be used to transform healthcare delivery.

The structure and rigor of the Magnet recognition program process, particularly the emphasis on empirical outcomes, has helped nurses and organizations focus on patient safety. One of the greatest challenges is sustaining the necessary characteristics of a Magnet organization and a culture of safety. The Magnet award is bestowed for a four-year period, and ANCC raises the bar for each redesignation; no organization is allowed to rest on its laurels. This continual aspiration for excellence in Magnet designation supports the goals of continual improvements in maintaining an organization's culture of patient safety.

Finally, in 2006, Dr. Pronovost and colleagues asked, "How will we know when we have created a culture of safety" (p. 1988)?[11] The structures embedded in the Magnet recognition program help a hospital develop as an evidence-based, patient-centered, reliable organization with strong leadership, as well as with empowered, collaborative staff who communicate well and work together as a team—a learning environment on a constant quest to improve patient outcomes, and one that supports a fair and just culture. Patient safety serves as the core guiding principle in the development of Magnet organizations. The Magnet journey helps nursing and the entire healthcare team advance a strong culture of patient safety.

References

1. Institute of Medicine. (2010). *The future of nursing: Leading change, advancing health*. Committee on the Robert Wood Johnson Foundation, Initiative on the Future of Nursing. Washington, DC: National Academies Press.
2. Newhouse, R., & Poe, S. (2005). *Measuring patient safety*. Sudbury, MA: Jones & Bartlett.
3. American Nurses Credentialing Center (ANCC). (2008). *Application manual: Magnet recognition program*. Retrieved from http://www.nursecredentialing.org/.
4. Aiken, L., Clarke, S., Sloane, D., Sochalski, J., & Silber, J. (2002). Hospital nurse staffing and patient mortality, nurse burnout, and job dissatisfaction. *JAMA, 288*(16), 1987–1993.
5. Nightingale, F. (1860). *Notes on nursing: What it is, and what it is not*. New York, NY: Appleton & Co.
6. Drenkard, K. (2009). The Magnet® imperative. *The Journal of Nursing Administration, 39*(7/8), S1–S2.
7. Aiken, L., Havens, D. S., & Sloane, D. (2000). The Magnet® nursing services recognition program: A comparison of two groups of Magnet hospitals. *American Journal of Nursing, 100*, 26–36.
8. Kohn, L., Corrigan, J., & Donaldson, M. (2000). *To err is human: Building a safer health system*. Washington, DC: National Academies Press.
9. Sammer, C., Lykens, K., Singh, K., Mains, D., & Lackan, N. (2010). What is patient safety culture? A review of the literature. *Journal of Nursing Scholarship, 42*(2), 156–165.
10. Leape, L., Berwick, D., & Bates, D. (2002). What practices will most improve safety? Evidence-based medicine meets patient safety. *JAMA, 288*(4), 501–507.
11. Pronovost, P., Holzmueller, C. G., Needham, D. M., Sexton, J. B., Miller, M., Berenholtz, S., . . . Morlock, L. (2006). How will we know patients are safer? An organization-wide approach to measuring and improving safety. *Critical Care Medicine, 34*(7), 1988–1995.
12. Emmanuel, L., Berwick, D., Conway, J., Combes, J., Hatlie, M., Leape, L., . . . Walton, M. (2008). What exactly is patient safety? In K. Henriksen, J. B. Battles, M. A. Keyes, & M. L. Grady (Eds.), *Advances in patient safety: New directions and alternative approaches* (Vol. 1). Rockville, MD: Agency for Healthcare Research and Quality.
13. Helmreich, R. (2000). On error management: Lessons from aviation. *BMJ, 320*, 781–785.
14. Reingold, S., & Kulstad, E. (2007). Impact of human factor design on the use of order sets in the treatment of congestive heart failure. *Society for Academic Emergency Medicine, 14*(11), 1097–1105.
15. Frankel, A., Leonard, M., & Denham, C. (2006). Fair and just culture, team behav-

ior and leadership engagement: The tools to achieve high reliability. *Health Research and Educational Trust, 41*(4), 1690–1709.

16. Agency for Healthcare Research and Quality (AHRQ) (2001). *Making health care safer.* White Paper. Retrieved from http://www.innovations.ahrq.gov/.
17. Clarke, J., Lerner, J., & Marcella, W. (2007). The role for leaders of health care organizations in patient safety. *American Journal of Medical Quality, 22*(5), 311–318.
18. Institute of Medicine Committee on Quality of Health Care in America. (2001). *Crossing the quality chasm: A new health system for the 21st century*. Washington, DC: National Academies Press.
19. Sexton, J., Thomas E., & Helmreich, R. (2000). Error, stress, and teamwork in medicine and aviation: Cross sectional analysis. *BMJ, 320*, 745–749.
20. Pronovost, P., Weast, B., Holzmueller, C., Rosenstein, B., Kidwell, R., Haller, K., . . . Rubin, H. (2003). Evaluation of the culture of safety: Survey of clinicians and managers in an academic medical center. *Quality and Safety in Healthcare, 12*(6), 405–410.
21. Armstrong, K., & Laschinger, H. (2009). Structured empowerment and Magnet hospital characteristics as predictor of patient safety climate. *Journal of Nursing Care Quality, 24*(10), 53–62.
22. American Nurses Association (ANA) (2010). *Guide to the code of ethics for nurses: Interpretation and application*. Retrieved from www.nursesbooks.org.
23. American Association of Critical-Care Nurses. (AACN). (2005). *Standards for establishing and sustaining a health work environment: A journey to excellence*. Retrieved from http://www.aacn.org/WD/HWE/Docs/HWEStandards.pdf.
24. Thomas, J., & Herrin, D. (2008). Executive master in science in nursing program: Incorporating the 14 forces of magnetism. *The Journal of Nursing Administration, 38*(2), 64–68.
25. Comarow, A. (2010). Best hospitals. *U.S. News & World Report*. Retrieved from www.usnews.com.
26. Cummings, G. G., Mididzi, W. K., Wong, C. A., & Estabrooks, C. A. (2010). The contribution of hospital nursing leadership styles to 30-day patient mortality. *Nursing Research, 59*(5), 331–339.
27. Strauss, A., & Corbin, J. (1998). *Basics of qualitative research: Techniques and procedures for developing grounded theory*. Thousand Oaks, CA: Sage.
28. Leape, L. L., & Berwick, D. M. (2000). Safe health care: Are we up to it? *BMJ, 320*, 725–726.
29. Connor, M., Ponte, P., & Conway, J. (2002). Multidisciplinary approaches to reducing error and risk in a patient care setting. *Critical Care Nursing Clinics of North America, 14*, 359–367.
30. Yates, G., Bernd, D., Sayles, S., Stockmeyer, C., Burke, G., & Merti, G. (2005). Building and sustaining a system-wide culture of safety. *Journal of Quality and Patient Safety, 31*(12), 684–689.
31. Moore, S., & Hutchinson, S. (2007). Developing leaders at every level: Accountability and empowerment actualized through shared governance. *The Journal of Nursing Administration, 37*(12), 564–568.
32. Blake, S., Kohler, S., Rask, K., Davis, A., & Naylor, D. (2006). Facilitators and barriers to 10 National Quality Forum safe practices. *American Journal of Medical Quality, 21*(5), 323–334.
33. Association of Peri-Operative Registered Nurses (AORN). (2006). AORN guidance statement: Creating a patient safety culture. *Journal on Quality and Patient Safety, 32*(12), 672–675.
34. Hansen, M., Durbin, J., Sinkowitz-Cochran, R., Vaughn, A., Langowski, M., & Gleason, S. (2003). Do no harm: Provider perceptions of patient safety. *Journal of Nursing Administration, 33*(10), 507–508.
35. Weinstock, M. (2007). Can your nurses stop a surgeon? *Hospitals and Health Networks*, 38–46. Retrieved from: www.hhnmag.com.
36. Rapala, K., & Kerfoot, K. (2005). From metaphor to model: The clarion safe passage program. *Nursing Economics, 23*(4), 200–203.
37. Manojlovich, M., Antonakos, C., & Ronis, D. (2009). Intensive care units, communication between nurses and physicians, and patients' outcomes. *American Journal of Critical Care, 18*(1), 21–30. doi.10.4037ajcc2099353.
38. Shortell, S. M., Zimmerman, J. E., Rousseau, D. M., Gillies, R. R., Wagner, D. P., Draper, E. A., Knaus, W., & Duffy, J. (1994). The performance of intensive care units: Does good

management make a difference? *Medical Care, 32*(5), 508–525.

39. The Joint Commission. (2009). *Joint commission standards*. Retrieved from http://www.jointcommission.org/standards_information/standards.aspx.
40. Daft, R. L. (2010). *Management* (10th ed.). Mason, OH: South-Western University, Cengage Learning.
41. Sutcliffe, K., Lewton, E., & Rosenthall, M. (2004). Communication failures: An insidious contributor to medical mishaps. *Academy of Medicine, 79*(2), 186–194.
42. Apold, J., Daniels, T., & Sonneborn, M. (2006). Promoting collaboration and transparency in patient safety. *Journal on Quality and Patient Safety, 32*(12), 672–675.
43. Frankel, A., Gandhi, T. K., & Bates, D. W. (2003). Improving patient safety across a large integrated health care delivery system. *International Journal for Quality in Health Care, 15*(Suppl 1), 31–40.
44. Frankel, A., & Haraden, C. (2004). Shuttling toward a safety culture: Healthcare can learn from probe panel's findings on the Columbia disaster. *Modern Healthcare, 34*(1), 21.
45. Gawande, A. (2010). *The checklist manifesto: How to get things right*. London, UK: Profile Books.
46. Sammer, C., Lykens, K., & Singh, K. (2008). Physician characteristics and the reported effect of evidence-based practice guidelines. *Health Services Research, 43*(2), 569–581.
47. Farrell, V., & Davies, K. (2006). Shaping and cultivating a perioperative culture of safety. *AORN Journal, 84*(5), 857–860.
48. McDonald, T., Helmchen, L., Smith, K., Centomani, N., Gunderson, A. Mayer, D., & Chamberlin, W. (2010). Responding to patient safety incidents: The seven pillars. *Quality and Safety in Health Care*. doi:10.1136/qshc.2008.031633.
49. Kaissi, A. (2006). An organizational approach to understanding patient safety and medical errors. *Health Care Manager, 25*(4), 292–305.
50. Marx, D. (2008). Patient safety and the "just culture": A primer for health care executives. *Medical Event Reporting System for Trans fusion Medicine*. Retrieved from http://mers-tm.org/.
51. AORN. (2002). Retrieved from http://www.jointcommission.org/assets/1/18/RWJ_Future_of_Nursing.pdf.
52. Vogelsmeier, A., & Scott-Cawiezell, J. (2007). A just culture: The role of nursing leadership. *Journal of Nursing Care Quality, 22*(3), 210–212.
53. Weissman, J. S., Annas, C. L., Epstein, A. M., Schneide, E. C., Clarridge, B., Kirle, L., . . . Ridley, N. (2005). Error reporting and disclosure systems: Views from hospital leaders. *JAMA, 293*, 1359–1366.
54. Diaz, L. (2008). Nursing peer review: Developing a framework for patient safety. *Journal of Nursing Administration, 38*(11), 475–479.
55. Reason, J. (2003). *Managing the risks of organizational accidents*. Burlington, VT: Aldershot.
56. Rose, J. D., Thomas, C. S., Tersigni, A., Sexton, J. B., & Pryor, D. (2006). A leadership framework for culture change in health care. *Joint Commission Journal on Quality and Patient Safety, 32*(8), 433–442.
57. Berntsen, K. J. (2006). Implementation of patient centeredness to enhance patient safety. *Journal of Nursing Care Quality, 21*(1), 15–19.
58. McDonald, T. (2009). Presentation: Tragedy strikes—What's next?: Setting up a full disclosure program. Chicago, IL: University of Illinois at Chicago.
59. Morath, J., & Leary, M. (2004). Creating safe spaces in organizations to talk about safety. *Nursing Economics, 22*(6), 344–354.
60. Leape, L., & Berwick, D. (2005). Five years after *To err is human*: What have we learned? *JAMA, 293*, 2384–2390.
61. Donabedian. A. (1966). Evaluating the quality of medical care. *Milbank Quarterly, 44*, 166–206.
62. Institute of Medicine. (2010). The future of nursing: Leading change, advancing health. Committee on the Robert Wood Johnson Foundation, Initiative on the Future of Nursing. National Academies Press. Washington, DC. Retrieved from http://www.jointcommission.org/assets/1/18/RWJ_Future_of_Nursing.pdf. Accessed May 23, 2012.

32

TEACHING PHYSICIANS TO PROVIDE SAFE PATIENT CARE

Dennis O'Leary, MD and Lucian Leape, MD

PREFACE

First do no harm. This centuries-old admonition—attributed to Hippocrates in the fourth century BC—was directed to physicians, presumably both as practitioners and as teachers.[1] It was more prophetic than anyone could have imagined. And it could today be directed to any healthcare professional, any provider organization, or indeed any country responsible for the design and delivery of health care for its citizens.

This is because history shows that Hippocrates's admonition—at least in terms of outcomes—has largely been ignored. Thus, in the 1850s, Florence Nightingale is heard complaining vehemently about the unsafe patient care circumstances at the Crimean War front.[2] In the same era, Ignaz Semmelweis challenges his colleagues to wash their hands to prevent puerperal sepsis and is committed to a mental institution.[3] Semmelweis's urgings would be very much in place today because the simple failure of healthcare practitioners to wash their hands now accounts for tens of thousands of healthcare-associated infections each year. And finally, there is Ernest Amory Codman setting forth his end results thesis in 1910, wherein he frames the obligation of physicians to study the outcomes of the care they provide, take action to remedy their errors, and make public their results.[4] For his cutting-edge posture, Codman was ostracized by his colleagues, died a pauper, and is buried in an unmarked grave in Boston.

A number of decades would pass before efforts were undertaken to actually study and codify the depth and scope of the patient safety problem. This work began with the Harvard Medical Practice Study in the 1980s, which found that 4% of hospitalized patients were injured and that two-thirds of those injuries were preventable.[5] In 1999, the Institute of Medicine's report *To Err Is Human* extrapolated from this work and a subsequent study to estimate that there were between 44,000 and 98,000 preventable deaths in the United States each year.[6] Although these figures were challenged by skeptics, subsequent similar studies and reports in the United Kingdom, Canada, Denmark, New Zealand, and Australia, among others, found much higher rates, which led the World Health Organization to conclude that serious preventable adverse events occur—on average—during one out of every 10 patient hospitalizations in developed countries around the world.[7]

Recognition of the gravity of the continuing patient safety problem has led to improvement initiatives in many countries. In the United States, the National Patient Safety Foundation has worked with stakeholder groups for over a decade to advance patient safety learning and bring forward new solutions.[8] The Agency for Healthcare Research and Quality has invested in defining measures to assess patient safety and in the development of its Patient Safety Improvement Corps.[9] The National Quality Forum has certified a series of safe practices and is leveraging their implementation.[10] The Joint Commission has issued a set of National Patient Safety Goals and requires compliance with these requirements for accreditation purposes.[11] The Institute for Healthcare Improvement has launched two major national campaigns to inspire thousands of hospitals to adopt specified safe practices.[12] And there is more.

Nevertheless, health care in this country remains unsafe. Although no one intends to harm recipients of care, healthcare practitioners and provider organizations unwittingly harm and sometimes cause the death of patients every day. For example, the Centers for Disease Control and Prevention conservatively estimates that there are at least two million hospital-acquired infections each year and that these infections lead to approximately 90,000 deaths.[13] Medication errors harm 1.5 million people each year, 400,000 of these in hospitals.[14] Twenty percent of hospitals fail to conduct time-outs before surgery, an effort known to be important in preventing the remarkably frequent occurrences of wrong-site surgery.[15] Further, almost twice as many hospitals do not have effective processes for timely reporting of critical test results. And there are many more examples.[15]

As other industries have learned, achieving safety in the work environment requires much more than implementing new rules and procedures. It requires the development and sustainment of cultures of safety that engender trust and embrace reporting, transparency, and disciplined practices. It also requires an atmosphere of respect among the healthcare disciplines and a fundamental ability of all practitioners to work together in teams. And it begs the need for practitioners, particularly physicians, who have the knowledge, skills, and attitudes necessary to support, and even lead, the creation and perpetuation of cultures of safety.

In all fairness, there are other significant barriers to improving patient safety. These include the current flawed payment system whose "rewards" sometimes undermine safety improvement efforts while failing to pay for others; the existing dysfunctional medical liability system, which chills reporting of adverse events and their underlying causes; apparent public policy confusion over the treatment of reported or discovered adverse healthcare events; and long-delayed and probably still insufficient federal investment in electronic health records.

Thus, the need to address health professional education is not the only patient safety improvement challenge that this country faces, but many believe that it is the foremost challenge among equals. For if these other barriers are overcome and health professional education remains unchanged, meaningful improvements in safety cannot and will not happen. Simply stated, health professional education needs to be redesigned to equip students with the knowledge, skills, and attitudes they need to function safely and effectively in healthcare delivery in the 21st century. While this need exists across the health professions, it is most compelling in medical education because the actions of physicians and their decisions largely determine the care that all other healthcare professionals provide.

EXECUTIVE SUMMARY

Healthcare delivery continues to be unsafe despite major patient safety improvement efforts over the past decade. The Lucian Leape Institute (LLI) Roundtable on Reforming Medical Education (hereafter referred to as LLI Roundtable) concluded that substantive improvements in patient safety will be difficult to achieve without major medical education reform at the medical school and residency-training program levels. Medical schools must not only assure that future physicians have the requisite knowledge, skills, behaviors, and attitudes to practice competently but are also prepared to play active roles in identifying and resolving patient safety problems. These competencies should become fully developed during the residency-training period.

Medical schools today focus principally on providing students with the knowledge and skills they need for the technical practice of medicine but often pay inadequate attention to the shaping of student skills, attitudes, and behaviors that will permit them to function safely and as architects of patient safety improvement in the future. Specifically, medical schools are not doing an adequate job of facilitating student understanding of basic knowledge and the development of skills required for the provision of safe patient care, namely, systems thinking, problem analysis, application of human factors science, communication skills, patient-centered care, teaming concepts and skills, and dealing with feelings of doubt, fear, and uncertainty with respect to medical errors.

In addition, medical students all too often suffer demeaning experiences at the hands of faculty and residents, a phenomenon that appears to reflect serious shortcomings in the medical school and teaching hospital cultures. Behaviors like these that are disruptive to professional relationships have adverse effects on students, residents, nurses, colleagues, and even patients. Students frequently tend to emulate these behaviors as they become residents and practicing clinicians, which perpetuates work environments and cultures that are antithetical to the delivery of safe, patient-centered care.

After the chapter, the recommendations set forth by the LLI Roundtable appear as an appendix.

INTRODUCTION

Recent studies in multiple countries—stimulated by the Institute of Medicine's (IOM) *To Err Is Human* report in 1999—have found pervasive patient safety problems in hospitals and other healthcare settings around the world.[6,16–19] Although awareness of this problem is growing dramatically, there has been uneven and slow progress in improving patient safety since the issuance of the IOM report.[20,21]

Among the challenges involved in achieving tangible improvements in patient safety, none is more daunting than the need for major alterations in the educational preparation of health professional students.[22] While this need exists across the health professions, it is most compelling in medical education.[23]

Medical education in the United States needs to be substantially restructured to enhance the development of skills, behaviors, and attitudes that students will need as practicing physicians. These include—in addition to the crucial ability to manage clinical and scientific information—understanding of the basic concepts of human dynamics, patient safety, and systems theory, and the development of basic management, communication, and teamwork skills. To do this, it will be necessary for medical schools to reduce the current intensity of their focus on the acquisition of scientific and clinical facts, and for residency training programs to emphasize and assure the application of these new skills, attitudes, and behaviors on a continuing basis.

Over the past 10 years, the IOM, the Accreditation Council for Graduate Medical Education (ACGME), and the American Board of Medical Specialties (ABMS) have formulated concise sets of desired practitioner competencies.[22,24,25] Notably, these priorities almost uniformly focus on the acquisition of knowledge, skills, and attitudes that support desired behaviors.

These well-informed directions suggest that medical schools need to sharpen their focus on teaching concepts that underlie the behaviors for which future physicians will be held accountable and that teaching should be undertaken in an interdisciplinary fashion and capitalize on the rapidly expanding applications of simulation as a teaching tool. This approach could also benefit from utilization of the case study method—a proven method for integrating knowledge in U.S. business schools—as an integral part of the medical education process.

Because of the current lack of emphasis on patient safety education and training, today's medical schools are producing square pegs for our care system's round holes. Medical education must change to meet the needs of an increasingly complex and vulnerable system-based healthcare delivery system. A strategy is also needed for retraining those physicians whom the system has already produced. This is especially important in light of the fact that they are the mentors and role models for our future physicians.

The type of medical education reform necessary to improve patient safety in this country requires the buy in and coordination of a variety of important stakeholders. It is these stakeholders who largely made up the composition of the LLI Roundtable. The LLI Roundtable discussed the current shortcomings of U.S. medical education with respect to patient safety, what medical education ideally should become in the future, and what strategies should be deployed to achieve the desired changes in medical education. This white paper is the culmination of these discussions.

PART I. THE NEED FOR MEDICAL EDUCATION REFORM

Square Pegs

One of the principal conclusions reached in the IOM's *To Err Is Human* report is that the major underlying cause of adverse health events is poorly designed systems—specifically, patient care processes—as opposed to negligent individual performance.[6] The implication of this insight is that physicians, healthcare managers, nurses, pharmacists, and others should work together in teams to identify and redesign flawed patient care processes to prevent human error from actually reaching patients to harm them. A major reason this is not happening is that physicians and other healthcare professionals have not received appropriate education and training to prepare them to function in teams to carry out this critically important work.[22,26]

The typical medical school curriculum exemplifies the problem. Little or no instruction is provided in engineering concepts applicable to systems thinking, safety science, the science of improvement, human factors, leadership, and teamwork.[27] Few or no opportunities are offered for applied experience in examining the patient care processes that constitute everyday practice in the real world of health care. Graduates too often lack the knowledge and interpersonal skills to relate well and communicate effectively with coworkers, meet patient needs, and deal with their own feelings of doubt, fear, and uncertainty.[23] Yet, these are precisely the knowledge and skills that most people consider essential for a physician. This awareness and these capabilities need to be embedded in the teaching of every student from the beginning of medical school.

The problem is compounded by the current focus in medical education on "courses" and content in a world of exploding medical knowledge that simply cannot be captured by a medical school curriculum, let alone by an individual medical student. In the alternative, there is much to be said for the development of skills in utilizing informatics—as recommended by the IOM—that would permit students to acquire much relevant knowledge and information on an as-needed, just-in-time basis.[28] Such an approach becomes particularly compelling in light of the reality that approximately half of the information provided to students in medical school will eventually be proven to be wrong.

Emerging Issues in Health Care

Medical education underwent a major transformation in its structure and curricula following release of the Flexner Report in 1910.[29] Many believe we are at a similar transformational moment now. While health care has changed dramatically over the past few decades, medical education has struggled to keep up.[30] Even more wrenching changes are under way, and emerging challenges will require rethinking both the content and the methods used to prepare medical students. These include changes in the organization of medical care, the changing role of the physician, the exponential increase in medical knowledge, and the increasing involvement of patients in their care.

Changes in the Organization of Medical Care

The U.S. healthcare system was designed primarily for episodic inpatient and outpatient care, but it now needs to adjust to a significant and still progressing shift in emphasis from acute care to chronic disease management. Today, the care for patients with chronic diseases is typically provided by multiple specialists, with or without a primary care coordinator, who work with other practitioners to provide the care and support required by these patients. In this context, the autonomous physician model of care is not only becoming obsolete, it is hazardous because it exposes patients to increased risks associated with transitions, handoffs, and communication failures. A different model—one that emphasizes collaborative practice and interprofessional teamwork—is needed.[31] In this model, patients with chronic diseases become the collective responsibility of stable teams, which have established role definitions and communication patterns, agreed-on goals for their patients, and clear strategies not only for achieving these goals but also for engaging patients and their families to become their own primary care providers. Healthcare organizations—including hospitals, nursing homes, outpatient services, and home health programs, among others—will face a growing need to become increasingly integrated to support this new model of care delivery.

The Changing Role of the Physician

In the face of growing demands for better coordinated and integrated care, the roles of physicians are changing.[32] Although the medical home model calls for primary care doctors to be the decision makers and managers of all healthcare resources for patients, nurses and other practitioners may play central care coordinator roles in other models.[33] The chronic care model, the most widely accepted model for managing patients with chronic diseases, calls for physicians to work in interprofessional teams with nurses, pharmacists, and others to better coordinate and integrate the use of healthcare resources both in inpatient and outpatient settings and in the community.[31] In any event, doctors will certainly require improved management and team skills to collaborate with specialists, nurses, pharmacists, therapists, and other practitioners across various inpatient, outpatient, and residential settings.

Increasing Medical Knowledge

It is impossible for doctors to master or even read all of the emerging medical information being published every week, even in their own specialty.[34] Doctors require different skill sets other than to just be able to absorb large quantities of information. They need to recognize that they must be lifelong learners who seek continual improvement in the care they provide to patients. In addition, they must realize the value of information technology in helping them deliver up-to-date, evidence-based care and be able to use information technology tools to find pertinent literature, review guidelines, calculate patient risk factors, and apply clinical pathways. They also need to critically appraise important studies and use literature to answer important clinical questions.

Increasing Patient Involvement in Their Own Care

Physicians must also learn how to involve patients in their own care in a more direct manner than they ever have previously. Patients are becoming more engaged consumers of health care, seeking medical information on the Internet and second opinions on treatment plans more frequently than ever before.[35,36] Patient consumer groups are forming to give patients a more active voice. Patients are also increasingly using disease self-management tools, and personalized health records are becoming more common.[37] Efforts to let patients have easy computer access to all of their medical records are also under way. Increased openness, transparency, and patient engagement are key aspects of improving patient safety. Physicians need to facilitate and lead these efforts, be able to communicate effectively with patients, be knowledgeable about their needs, and know what resources are available. Indeed, physicians must learn to have patients as partners in their own care.

Other emerging challenges in health care with implications well beyond reforming medical education can be cited. For physicians to meet these challenges and work effectively in a changing healthcare system, they must be able to work in and manage systems, manage large amounts of information, communicate effectively with patients and coworkers, and place patients' needs first. Most importantly, they need to feel they have the skills necessary to provide good care and adapt to new challenges.

When Things Go Wrong

We now realize that when a serious patient safety misadventure occurs, there are two victims. The first of course is the patient. The second—less frequently recognized—is the practitioner who was at the sharp end of the failed care delivery process (i.e., the person who actually committed the act that harmed or killed the patient).[38,39]

The practitioner becomes a victim because likely she or he is commonly providing care in a "shame and blame" environment that has little tolerance for patient care failures attributable to human error. Further, the practitioner—if a physician—has been acculturated in an education and training environment that views the physician as being at the top of the care hierarchy and therefore the accountable party.[40] In this framework, all good outcomes are attributable to the individual physician and, similarly, all bad outcomes are the fault of the physician. Such perceptions quite clearly overlook the roles of other healthcare team members and the importance of flawed patient care processes that permitted the physician's error to actually reach and harm the patient.[41]

The upshot of physician demoralization in the wake of a serious adverse event is an individual who may be psychologically unable to participate in the ensuing analysis, diagnosis, and resolution of the failed patient care process(es).[38] For example, she or he may have little insight into what really happened and be unable to empathize and communicate effectively with the injured and frightened patient.[42] She or he may lack the knowledge and skills necessary to work with other team members to investigate the occurrence and analyze and redesign the relevant care processes to prevent similar circumstances from recurring in the future. This in a nutshell is the problem at hand.

The Medical Education Culture

Much of what is right and wrong with medical education can be traced to the organizational—school and teaching hospital—cultures in which education and training are provided. Outside of the military, healthcare settings are among the most hierarchical in American society. In these settings, students, residents, nurses, pharmacists, and other healthcare workers are often intimidated by physicians and reluctant to question decisions or offer alternative views.[43] These are the frameworks in which student values, attitudes, and behaviors are shaped.

The science content–packed curriculum reinforces these frameworks by its emphasis on the acquired knowledge and primacy of the individual physician and his or her judgment. This leaves little room in the curriculum for developing the skills, attitudes, and behaviors needed for collaborative practice and for the provision of safe care.[44] Culture change comes slowly to medical schools and teaching hospitals because the underlying cultural beliefs and values are intertwined with long-standing traditions and behaviors that pervade the medical school and teaching hospital continuum.

One might argue that much of what constitutes the medical school culture is good or, if not good, harmless enough. But there are elements of this culture that are not harmless. For example, the creation of professional egocentricity is a problem because it inhibits team building across disciplines and fails to acknowledge that most care is provided by teams of individuals, some of which are not led by physicians. Shortcomings in achieving cultures of safety in teaching hospitals and other care delivery settings are widely recognized and are the subject of ongoing improvement efforts by The Joint Commission and the Institute for Healthcare Improvement, among others.[11,45]

One of the more serious problems at the school and hospital levels is that some student clinical experiences are dehumanizing. This is sometimes seen as an element of what has been referred to as the "hidden curriculum."[44] Simply put, students assimilate the values, behaviors and attitudes of their mentors. Most often these are positive experiences, but occasionally students are exposed to and adopt unprofessional behaviors. In a survey of third-year medical students, student observation of and accommodation to unprofessional behaviors progressively increased during the first five months of clerkships.[46] Initially critical of these behaviors, students increasingly perceived them to be appropriate as training progressed and steadily began to emulate them.

An anonymous survey of 1,853 third- and fourth-year medical students in 1992 and 1993 at six Pennsylvania medical schools also found disheartening results.[47] Ninety-eight percent of students had heard physicians refer derogatorily to patients; 61% had witnessed what they believed to be unethical behavior by other medical team members, and, of these students, 54% felt like accomplices. Many students reported dissatisfaction with their actions and ethical development: 67% had felt badly or guilty about something they had done as clinical clerks, and 62% believed that at least some of their ethical principles had been eroded or lost. Controlling for other factors, students who had witnessed an episode of unethical behavior were more likely to have acted improperly themselves for fear of poor evaluations. Moreover, students were twice as likely to report erosion of their ethical principles if they had behaved unethically for fear of poor evaluation or to fit in with "the team."

More worrisome still are the student accounts of disrespectful behavior and abuse on the part of faculty. The survey of graduating medical students conducted annually by the Association of American Medical Colleges (AAMC) finds significant numbers of medical students who feel that they have experienced some form of abuse or disrespectful behavior during their education and training.[48] For the most recent five-year period for which data are available (2004–2008), the number of students who answered yes to having been "publicly belittled or humiliated" ranged from 12.7% to 16.7%, with nonwhite and female respondents reporting higher rates.[49] Approximately half of these students report the frequency of such abuse as occurring "Occasionally," while a much smaller fraction (5%) report these events as occurring "Frequently." The most common sources of this abuse were clinical faculty and residents (66% and 67%, respectively), followed by smaller but significant percentages of nurses and patients (multiple responses to this question allowed). Abusive behavior can be as subtle as making a student feel foolish for asking a question or as overt as throwing surgical instruments in the operating room. Some may argue that an overall 12 to 17% rate of abusive and disrespectful behavior over the four-year medical school experience is not so extraordinary, but the rate ranges far higher in some schools. Even then, it is hard to imagine any successful industry or company that tolerates abusive behavior at any level.

To capture some examples of the problem of abusive and disruptive behavior, a medical student member of the LLI Roundtable solicited anonymous stories from medical students who had experienced disruptive or abusive behavior. A sampling of these poignant stories is provided in Table 32.1.

Disruptive, abusive, and disrespectful behaviors are more than simply a problem in communication between two individuals.[50] Such behaviors create a culture of fear and intimidation, diminish individual and collective pride and morale, impair learning, and sap joy and meaning from work. This is the stuff of which shame and blame environments are made. Further, disruptive and abusive behaviors are contagious.[46] Abused students, residents, and nurses perpetuate dysfunctional healthcare organization cultures by modeling the demeaning and disrespectful behaviors to which they were exposed and passing these behaviors along to the next generation of learners.

Breaking this cycle and changing this culture of fear and intimidation to a culture that facilitates and reinforces learning is the responsibility of organization leaders. In education and training settings, these are primarily medical school deans, teaching hospital CEOs, department chairs, and residency program directors.

Selecting for What?

Medical schools have long sought to attract the best and the brightest to become future physicians, and they have largely succeeded in this endeavor. But today there are growing questions as to whether this description of what is desired in a medical school applicant is sufficient.

At the initial international gathering of the Patients for Patient Safety program of the World Alliance for Patient Safety in London several years ago, a spontaneous comment ignited a consensus among the patient attendees that what they want their physicians to be is not the best and the brightest.[51] What these patients—many of whom had personally suffered the consequences of preventable adverse events—wanted was doctors who are competent, listen to patients, are empathetic and compassionate, and communicate effectively with patients. Their message was simple: there is more to being a good physician than academic achievement.

Over the past decade, medical school interest in selecting for interpersonal skills and attributes that reflect the concepts of professionalism has been growing. The most prominent effort in this regard has been the development and application of a multiple mini-interview (MMI) process at the Michael DeGroote School of Medicine at McMaster University.[52] The MMI consists of brief interviews of each applicant student at a series of at least nine structured clinical examination stations at which the applicant is presented with scenarios that require him or her to discuss a health-related issue with an interviewer. In this process, applicants literally rotate through a group of individual interviewers who cover domains such as ethics, professionalism, and interpersonal relationships, among others. MMI results over the past six years have demonstrated high correlations both with clinical performance and with national licensing examination results. The MMI process is now used widely in Canadian medical schools and in some U.S. schools.

Just as relevant in the selection process is the avoidance of potential students with serious psychosocial disorders and other undesirable traits. Too often, these individuals,

TABLE 32.1 Disrespectful or Abusive Behavior Examples Observed or Experienced by Medical Students

Example 1. Two second-year medical students spent an afternoon observing surgery in the OR as part of a medical school course. The chief surgical resident assigned the students to a corner of the room with instructions to be quiet and not touch anything. After the students had washed their hands and moved to their assigned place, the attending surgeon noticed them and yelled: "Who are you? What are you doing in this OR? When you come into an OR you introduce yourself to the surgeon. And why are you standing there? Go stand in that (pointing to a different) corner."

Example 2. One third-year medical student was scrubbed in for a case, observing and occasionally assisting the surgeon. At one point, she noticed the surgeon pulling a retractor in a way that seemed to indicate that the surgeon wanted her to take over retracting. As she reached to grab the retractor, the surgeon, who apparently didn't want her assistance, slapped her hand out of the field instead of verbally instructing her to remove her hand.

Example 3. From a female third-year medical student on surgery rotation: "I had an attending who told me he was excited that I would be a grad student the following year because I would technically *not* be a med student anymore. Then he specifically said that he was thinking some very non-PC things in his head once he learned about this—to my face. Made me feel very uncomfortable."

Example 4. From a third-year medical student on OB/GYN rotation: "I was instructed to observe a hysterectomy, but when I arrived to the OR, the doctor looked at me with disdain and told me to stand in the far corner and not mess anything up. So, I perched myself atop a small step-stool in the back corner of the room, and I spent the next three hours squinting from across the room, completely unable to see anything except for blue-gowned backs.

"Suddenly, the doctor called out, 'You, over there!' I looked over in surprise—me? Apparently, there was no one available to pull out the catheter, and they beckoned for me to approach the table. I cautiously approached, and before I could even begin, the doctor sharply barked, 'DON'T mess this up for me!' Shaking, I followed her instructions and managed to remove the catheter without contaminating the sterile field. 'Now, GET OUT of the way!' she yelled. I couldn't see behind me, and in a small tremulous voice, I asked, 'Is it okay to move backwards, I can't see anything behind me?' Raising her voice up a notch, she yelled, 'Just GET OUT!' I took several hasty steps backwards, and my arm grazed lightly against the side of a table holding sterile instruments—mind you, no where *near* the tabletop, where the instruments lay, but just on the side curtain—and a nurse shrieked, 'She contaminated the whole sterile field!' With fury, the doctor looked up and spat, 'F--- you!' I blinked, and stared right back at her—really, did she just actually say that? Although I didn't feel sad at all—only mad as hell—tears rushed to my eyes in a visceral response to all of the shouting. The instant that the curse left her lips, I could tell that she regretted it, but you can't take back something like that, so the words hung awkwardly in the air, hovering over all of our heads for the rest of the procedure.

She tried to make up for it, sending arbitrary, irrelevant compliments in my direction, and the nurse patted me on the shoulder several times and tried to appear motherly and compassionate. But, what I remember most strongly from the experience—what I *still* cannot believe—is the fact, despite their palpable remorse, no one ever said, I'm sorry."

Courtesy of the Lucian Leape Institute at the National Patient Safety Foundation.

once admitted to medical school, become those difficult-to-extrude problem students who continue to slip through the system to become problem doctors. All of this begs the need for more effective applicant screening mechanisms. Some progress has been made in developing formal personality screening methods, but greater efforts are needed in developing and/or refining appropriate tools.[53]

Core Competencies: The Missing Link

In 2003, the Institute of Medicine issued a sharply critical report on health professions education that outlined five core competencies that all health professionals should be able to demonstrate.[22] Although the report did not single out the medical profession, the text of the recommendations made clear that medical education was very much front of mind as the core competencies were developed. Most would agree that the core competencies suggested by the IOM are rather straightforward. They include the following:

- The provision of patient-centered care
- The ability to work in interdisciplinary teams
- Employment of evidence-based practices
- Application of quality improvement concepts
- Utilization of informatics

Six years later, there are serious questions as to whether the competencies of today's graduating physicians fully meet any of these objectives. Perhaps even more to the point, we should ask why the IOM found it necessary to frame such basic recommendations. For example, if physicians are not providing patient-centered care, what kind of care are they providing? Or if physicians are not practicing evidence-based medicine, what kind of medicine are they practicing? These are not silly questions. They are compelling acknowledgments of serious problems.

The provision of patient-centered care is of course not so simple.[54] It involves working with the patient as a partner and often as shared decision maker, the ability to develop long-term relationships with patients that underpin the successful management of chronic conditions, and cultural and racial sensitivities, among others. The dimensions of patient-centered care also include the ability to communicate at the patient's level of understanding, the willingness and ability to provide timely and effective relief of pain, and the simple ability to listen and actually hear the patient.[55] Finally, physicians need to grasp what the experiences of illness and hospitalization are like from the perspective of the patient. How much time and effort are being devoted to developing these and other related skills in medical schools today? And, as important, how well do student role models—the faculty and residents—perform against these expectations?

Teamwork is another competency often overlooked at the medical school level.[22] Many schools seem to think that this set of skills should be developed at some point following medical school graduation and thus miss multiple opportunities for interdisciplinary education and training with nursing, pharmacy, and other types of students. This omission is even more striking today in the face of the expanding array of teamwork simulation exercises. The hard reality is that delivering effective care in a variety of clinical settings is all about the ability of the participants to work together as a team.

The failure to employ evidence-based practices across the continuum of patient care is a long-standing problem that will be further challenged by the emerging comparative effectiveness initiatives.[56] The schools have a clear role in teaching students to become scholarly critics of accepted practices and of the clinical literature. Such training should also include the development of at least a basic understanding of the Cochrane criteria and their application.[28]

The application of quality improvement (QI) concepts encompasses a multidimensional set of skills.[57] In its most basic applications, however, quality improvement is about understanding the fundamental roles of measurement. These include problem identification, the setting of priorities for improvement interventions, and the eventual determination as to whether a QI intervention has been successful.

Since most students today enter medical school with at least a fundamental appreciation of informatics and its applications, this fifth and final basic problem area is one that has the potential to solve itself over time. But the schools have a role to play as well. The medical school faculty have traditionally placed their heaviest curricular emphasis on the transmittal of what some view as excessive amounts of fact-based information to students. Today, that may be occurring at the expense of developing skills and behaviors that are of at least equal importance in the preparation of the complete physician. Thus, medical schools could become part of this solution by rebalancing their current curricular emphases and teaching students how to utilize existing informatics capabilities to acquire much of the information they need when they need it (just in time) to support effective clinical decision making.

What is notable about the foregoing five competencies is that they describe desired behaviors and skills as opposed to particular knowledge bases. This strong behaviors and skills emphasis is further reflected in an additional set of physician-specific core competencies that have been promulgated by the ACGME and ABMS.[24,25] These competencies, which build on those set forth by the IOM, include the following:

- **Patient care.** The ability to provide patient care that is compassionate, appropriate, and effective for the treatment of health problems and the promotion of health
- **Medical knowledge.** Demonstration of knowledge of established and evolving biomedical, clinical, epidemiological, and social–behavioral sciences, as well as the application of this knowledge to patient care
- **Practice-based learning and improvement.** Demonstration of the ability to investigate and evaluate the care of one's own patients, to appraise and assimilate scientific evidence, and to continuously improve patient care based on constant self-evaluation and lifelong learning
- **Interpersonal and communication skills.** Demonstration of interpersonal and communication skills that result in the effective exchange of information and collaboration with patients, their families, and health professionals
- **Professionalism.** Demonstration of a commitment to carry out professional responsibilities and adhere to ethical principles
- **Systems-based practice.** Demonstration of an awareness of and responsiveness to the larger context and system of health care, as well as the ability to call effectively on other resources in the system to provide optimal care

Importantly, these competencies are those that residents completing training and physicians maintaining board certification will be expected to demonstrate on a continuing basis. For medical schools, this places the pressure for education and training reform much closer to home, especially since the Liaison Committee on Medical Education (LCME), for its part has not yet moved to establish core competencies for graduating physicians. Rather, this task has been left to the determination of the individual medical schools.

Educational Content and Methods Through a Different Prism

Experts agree that patient safety is predominantly about the proper design of healthcare systems and patient care processes. This thesis was the main thrust of the IOM's *To Err Is Human* report and is now widely accepted in the healthcare community. In the engineering community, this has never been news at all.[6]

Unfortunately, system design failures continue to translate into preventable patient deaths every day. Thus, one would expect that teaching the prevention of iatrogenic patient deaths would be among the highest priorities in medical schools, but sadly it is not. Missing in part, or totally, from the typical medical school curriculum is substantive attention to safety science, systems thinking, the science of improvement, human factors, and, as previously noted, teamwork.[58] In the clinical setting, those who will be called upon to analyze, diagnose, and redesign flawed patient care processes are those whose work is most affected by these processes—physicians, nurses, pharmacists, and other health professionals. Today, these individuals are unable to fix what they do not understand. Tomorrow, that must—with some urgency—change.

The need to understand basic error science and human factors science and their applications bears particular mention.[59,60] For the student, this is an important opportunity to learn, in an applied fashion, about the interactions among systems, individuals, and their environments. If nothing else, this experience should provide significant insights into cognitive dissonance, human fallibility, and the importance of being humble. Students who gain a basic understanding of human factors theory should, for example, come to appreciate the significance of sleep deprivation and fatigue in the generation of errors.

Of equal importance is the art of communication, which has already been referenced as one of the ACGME/ABMS core competencies. In The Joint Commission's Sentinel Event Database, the most common underlying cause of serious adverse events resulting in death or permanent loss of bodily function is communication failure.[61] Communication failures come in many forms—failure to recognize language or health literacy barriers to patient/family understanding, failure to read back verbal orders, failure to transmit important patient information when handing a patient over to the care of another physician, untimely reporting of critical test results, and inappropriate use of abbreviations in writing patient orders, among others.

Communication skills are often found wanting when physicians need to talk with a patient and/or a patient's family following a preventable adverse event.[62] What most patients and patient families want is an acknowledgment that a preventable adverse event occurred, a commitment to thoroughly investigate what happened, a commitment to take appropriate steps to prevent future occurrences, and an apology. That, however, may prove to be a tall order for a physician lacking specific training in the development of communication skills, especially those relating to apology.

Some medical schools have taken initial steps to incorporate some of this fundamentally different content into their curricula, but this is proving to be no small challenge.[63] First, this content is as much or more about the acquisition of appropriate skills, attitudes, and behaviors as it is about acquiring new knowledge. Thus, substantive evaluation of students in this realm involves approaches that require the student to demonstrate observed mastery of these concepts in simulated or other clinical settings or through other emerging evaluation methods.

In addition, relatively few faculty are skilled in teaching patient safety–related content, and such educational efforts are all too often not valued by other faculty, department chairs, and even the dean.[64] Further, students who do develop patient safety awareness, knowledge, and skills may find themselves ignored or put down by faculty when they try to apply these new competencies.

Meanwhile, some schools are beginning to introduce students to faculty from other relevant disciplines such as engineering and management. Similarly, case studies and simulation applications are beginning to be used for skill development in some schools. However, such exposures are today most notable for being the exceptions.

PART II. WHAT CHANGES ARE NEEDED

Creating the Right Culture

Culture is defined as the customary beliefs, values, and behaviors shared by members of a group (e.g., the faculty of a medical school). The challenge involved in changing culture is embodied in this definition. Beliefs, values, and behaviors are difficult to change because they are often intertwined with long-established professional traditions and reward systems. This does not mean that culture change is impossible, but such change does require unwavering leadership engagement and persistence. Culture change is a journey, not a specific action or set of actions.

Much has been written about the key characteristics of the ideal patient safety culture in hospitals.[65-67] These include strong leadership (including the setting of the right examples: "walking the talk"), organization competence in care process design and redesign, transparency, active engagement of patients and their families in patient care and problem-solving processes, resource investment that tracks the organization's cultural objectives, and reward mechanisms that encourage and incent desired behaviors, among others. Such characteristics also include the "psychological safety" for clinicians and others to report errors while, at the same time, not tolerating deliberate unsafe acts by individuals (sometimes referred to as a *just culture*).[68,69] Most of these descriptors apply to the medical school and teaching hospital cultures as well.

Leadership

Views vary widely as to the power and authority of the medical school dean to achieve major change across the school. However, the changes we envision cannot happen without leadership by the dean. Some also worry about the diffusion of leadership in many medical schools. But that diffusion can be a strength if consensus is achieved among those who have leadership roles (e.g., department chairs) in determining what the school's goals, values, and priorities should be in the new healthcare climate. The same accountabilities apply to teaching hospital CEOs and hospital staff leaders.

The top leadership priority should be to create a culture of learning at all levels. This means, among other considerations, that teaching skills are highly valued and that teachers consistently emphasize that patients come first. In this context, students and indeed residents provide care to patients primarily in furtherance of their education as opposed to the simple provision of service. In addition, there is mutual respect among all of the participants in the education and patient care processes ("the members of the team") and zero tolerance for confirmed egregious abusive and disruptive behaviors that demean and dehumanize the educational experience of those who stand low in the hierarchy.

Faculty Competencies

Most faculty members work conscientiously to keep up with and acquire new knowledge that is relevant to their responsibilities, but the emergence of the priority to teach patient safety content and skills is a challenge of a different kind. This is primarily because the teaching of skills and behaviors requires the application of nontraditional educational approaches and evaluation methods. Schools need to identify or acquire faculty who are expert in teaching patient safety. Such faculty may include non-MD doctorate-level individuals who have expertise in human factors, safety science, or communications, among other areas.

At the same time, it is important to be aware that patient safety applications pervade all of medicine's domains. This means that almost all schools and teaching hospitals will need to face up to the need for a broad-based effort to educate all or most of the current faculty on the basics of patient safety. At a minimum, this continuing education initiative needs to address the science of safety, systems theory and analysis, care process evaluation and redesign, human factors, teamwork, communication skills, and error disclosure and apology. Development of such knowledge and skills will permit the faculty themselves to become creators and integrals of high-reliability clinical environments.

Safe Reporting of Adverse Events

If students are to be taught about patient safety and the importance of the learning and eventual change that comes from analyzing adverse events, it is essential that they become facile and feel comfortable ("safe") in identifying, reporting, and discussing preventable adverse events and other patient safety problems with their peers and the faculty. In so doing, students may also find meaningful opportunities to become engaged in the teaching hospital's patient safety initiatives.

All of this requires a receptive, concerned, and supportive faculty and a hospital environment that embraces the characteristics of an ideal or "just" patient safety culture. That specifically also includes the provision of support to those—students, residents, faculty, and other caregivers—who have been directly involved in a preventable adverse occurrence, as well as a willingness to share adverse event root cause analysis findings and improvement actions taken across the organization. Such a culture may actually ease the tension between individual accountability and a sense of safety to report errors and create opportunities for learning and constructive remediation.

Recognition and Rewards

One of the greatest needs in today's academic health centers is stronger emphasis on and rewards for teaching skills. To all appearances, the idealized and longed-for "master teacher" is more an imagined figment than a reality in many medical schools. That simply must change, especially in anticipation of the important new responsibilities that need to be placed on the shoulders of the faculty. Existing recognition and rewards systems could serve this need if properly applied. This would include enhanced financial support (salary level, staff resources) for those who devote themselves primarily to teaching activities, modification of promotion pathways to recognize teaching skills and achievements, and the creation of mechanisms to validate the importance of the work of the teaching faculty.

In this schema, the opportunities exist both to reward particular efforts such as interdisciplinary teaching and to exclude from teaching activities those who marginalize themselves by virtue of their behavior, their unwillingness to be further educated, their ineffectiveness as teachers, or other dissonant expressions of "academic freedom." Being afforded the opportunity to teach students should be regarded as a privilege that is maintained through ongoing commitment and demonstrated excellence in performance. In the end, every teacher must be the kind of physician we want our students to become.

Resource Investment

In the world of academe, as elsewhere, money talks. The investments made by medical school leaders in the educational enterprise are unambiguous statements of priorities. Enhancing patient safety teaching capabilities is a critical need, and it will require new resources. These are likely to include new faculty, an investment in existing faculty education, new curricular materials, and new training and evaluation capabilities, such as simulation laboratories and observed structured clinical examination (OSCE) capabilities.

Recommendation 1. Medical school and teaching hospital leaders should place the highest priority on creating learning cultures that emphasize patient safety, model professionalism, enhance collaborative behavior, encourage transparency, and value the individual learner.

a. Medical school deans, teaching hospital leaders, and other faculty should work to eliminate hierarchical authority gradients that intimidate others and stifle teamwork.
b. Medical school deans, teaching hospital leaders, and other faculty should emphasize that professionalism means, among other things, demonstrating mutual respect and nontolerance for abusive or demeaning behaviors.
c. Medical school deans and teaching hospital CEOs should declare and enforce a zero tolerance policy for confirmed egregious disrespectful or abusive behaviors on the part of faculty, staff, residents, and students.
d. Medical school deans and teaching hospital CEOs should serve as role models

for treating students with respect and dignity.

e. Medical school deans should elevate the importance of patient safety among the faculty.

Recommendation 2. Medical school deans and teaching hospital CEOs should launch a broad effort to emphasize and promote the development and display of interpersonal skills, leadership, teamwork, and collaboration among faculty and staff.

a. Medical school deans and teaching hospital CEOs should set behavioral expectations for both faculty and students.
b. Every teacher must be the kind of physician we want our students to become.

Recommendation 3. As part of continuing education and ongoing performance improvement, medical school deans and teaching hospital CEOs should provide incentives and make available necessary resources to support the enhancement of faculty capabilities for teaching students how to diagnose patient safety problems, improve patient care processes, and deliver safe care.

a. Medical schools should identify or acquire faculty who are expert in teaching patient safety ("master teachers").
b. All faculty must acquire sufficient patient safety knowledge and skills to permit them to function as effective student role models.
c. Medical schools should cast the patient safety intellectual investment as a scholarly activity and meaningfully reward the effective teaching of patient safety skills.
d. The end goal must be a cadre of faculty, residents, and students who are capable of contributing to the creation of high-reliability systems.

Recommendation 4. The selection process for admission to medical school should place greater emphasis on selecting for attributes that reflect the concepts of professionalism and an orientation to patient safety.

a. Although medical schools generally have highly effective selection processes, greater emphasis should be placed on selecting for interpersonal skills that promote patient safety, such as mindfulness, compassion, empathy, collaboration, and effective communication.
b. Screening tools to identify sociopathic tendencies and undesirable behavioral traits in candidates for admission should be further refined and/or developed and applied.
c. Medical schools should carefully monitor student behavior and intervene early if there are displays of unprofessional or maladaptive behavior.

Rebalancing the Curricular Equation

Medical schools have done an excellent job of providing students with the knowledge and related skills they need for the technical practice of medicine. However, the new and still evolving care environment requires more than this in the contemporary physician. One need look no further than the IOM and ACGME/ABMS competencies to recognize the deficiencies in the skill and behavior sets of many physicians today.[24] What is needed in today's medical school curriculum is concentrated attention to the task of helping students begin to develop the skills and behaviors described by the IOM, ACGME, and ABMS. These competencies constitute at least a partial road map to future curriculum reform.

Also missing is in-depth attention to patient safety and its improvement. The critical content, skills, and behaviors that relate to patient safety substantially overlap with and mirror the IOM and ACGME/ABMS competencies. This is evident, for example, in the emphasis of the competencies on mindfulness, patient-centered care, teaming, and interpersonal and communication skills. In addition, students need support in learning how to manage stress and conflict resolution and how to deal with feelings of doubt, fear, and uncertainty when they are involved in an adverse event.[70] In sum, the priority for and provision of safe care is an integral part of being a good doctor.

The elemental nature of patient safety education has profound implications for curricular design. Teaching of patient safety needs to begin on day one of medical school and be extended throughout the four-year medical school experience. Basic dimensions of patient safety—such as safety improvement science, systems theory and analysis, human factors concepts, and teaming—need to be addressed in defined, separate coursework—most reasonably as a first-year "basic science." However, it is equally important that patient safety concepts be embedded in all teaching activities, including the traditional basic sciences. Formal classroom teaching should be the prelude to the development of desired skills and behaviors that are both taught and modeled by the faculty—an approach that has potential applications well beyond the teaching of patient safety.[71]

A discussion of what constitutes an appropriate patient safety curriculum is beyond the scope of this paper. However, several detailed patient safety curricula have been or are being developed. The most elaborate of these is the *Patient Safety Curriculum Guide for Medical Schools*, which was developed under the aegis of the WHO World Alliance for Patient Safety.[72] In addition, the Institute for Healthcare Improvement (IHI) has created an electronic Open School whose quality and safety improvement curriculum is being progressively expanded.[73] The enthusiastic reception that has greeted this initiative has led to the rapid creation of multiple medical school-based "chapters" of the School—a clear index of the hunger of medical students for this kind of knowledge.

A more encompassing approach to patient safety curriculum development has been taken by the Patient Safety Educational Project (PSEP).[74] This international collaboration of primarily Australian and American educators has developed an educational framework that is geared more generally to the patient safety learning needs of all types of healthcare workers. Finally, the Telluride Interdisciplinary Roundtable, sponsored by the University of Illinois at Chicago (UIC) and the Southern Illinois University School of Medicine (SIU), has developed general curricular principles and identified essential elements of an effective patient safety curriculum.[71] The orientation of these latter patient safety curriculum development efforts is clearly multidisciplinary and underlines the importance of medical school leadership in identifying interdisciplinary education and training opportunities as the foundation for future teamwork development activities.

The bridging of education and training across professional schools also raises the possible desirability of inviting contributions to the medical school curriculum from related academic disciplines such as engineering, sociology, and management. These disciplines, at the least, offer content and skill development enrichment capabilities that are highly germane to patient safety teaching. There are other examples as well.

Recommendation 5. Medical schools should conceptualize and treat patient safety as a science that encompasses knowledge of error causation and mitigation, human factors concepts, safety improvement science, systems theory and analysis, systems design and redesign, teaming, and error disclosure and apology.

a. Opportunities should be identified to integrate other relevant disciplinary teaching that relates to patient safety—such as engineering, management, and sociology—into the medical school curriculum.

Teaching Methods

The medical school lecture hall is not going to disappear as a teaching venue anytime soon, nor should it. Basic science and clinical lectures provide the core knowledge that underpins clinical insight and judgment, diagnostic acumen, and sound decision making at the bedside. The conveyance of basic knowledge is also, as noted previously, prelude to development of important skills and behaviors that will permit physicians to function as architects of quality and safety improvement in the future.

However, there are other existing venues that could and should evolve to become effective patient safety teaching forums. Classic among these is the traditional Morbidity and Mortality (M and M) Conference.[75] Though long a symbol of medicine's old shame and blame culture, M and M conferences offer the opportunity for thoughtful review and analysis of real patient safety occurrences and for the active participation of students, residents, and other healthcare professionals, such as nurses and pharmacists, in this process. Exploration of team functioning (or malfunctioning) is another potential by-product of such discussions.

Another teaching vehicle relatively new to the medical school setting but long a staple of business school teaching is the use of case studies. This problem-based learning approach capitalizes on engaging the student as an active learner and is particularly effective in teaching analytic skills. Such skills are fundamental to the systematic review of factors that did contribute or may have contributed to preventable adverse events (root cause analysis) and to the dissection and redesign of potentially flawed patient care processes (failure mode and effects analysis).

The McMaster Medical School (Ontario, Canada) provides a unique example of an educational system based on active learning around clinical problems.[76] The intent is to train physicians to be problem solvers and lifelong learners who consistently demonstrate the abilities to work in multidisciplinary teams and to communicate effectively with their patients. McMaster does not evaluate students through traditional examinations but rather utilizes a system that emulates actual physician practice. Primary emphasis is placed on the student's self-assessment and assessments by his or her peers. SIU is another longtime user of the problem-based learning method.

Role-playing models such as crew resource management (CRM) teach still other important skills and behaviors.[77] These include leadership, situational awareness, teamwork, and communication skills, particularly across authority gradients. CRM has its origins in the National Aeronautical and Space Administration (NASA) and is required training for commercial pilots in many countries. UIC is among those educational institutions that have developed a CRM training model.

Role-playing and other methods for teaching problem solving also lend themselves well to interprofessional training. The sharing of experiences among student professionals—particularly those training in medicine, nursing, and pharmacy—early in their education and training is an especially effective way for student physicians, nurses, and pharmacists to develop team skills, as well as respect for the contributions of other team members on whom they will necessarily rely in the future.[22]

A further important teaching dimension is offered by the growing range of simulation applications.[78–80] Simulation has established uses in teaching both basic skills, such as management of respiratory function and cardiovascular hemodynamics, and advanced clinical skills, such as management of difficult airways, tension pneumothorax, pulmonary embolism, and shock. In the medical school setting, simulation offers a significant number of potential applications in error prevention, assessment of clinical and safety-related competencies, and the development of skills in performing a wide variety of procedures. The old approach to teaching procedures—See one, Do one, Teach one—is antithetical to safe, patient-centered care. Simulation provides the opportunity for one to see as many as one would like, do as many as are necessary to demonstrate procedural competence, and leave the teaching to experts. Indeed, some argue that students should not "practice" on patients until they are found to be competent for each and every procedure that entails risk to a patient (e.g., spinal tap, drawing of arterial blood, placement of a central line).

OSCE has been used as a basic element of both medical education and evaluation for a number of years. Its principal applications have been to assess clinical skills and reasoning. The process uses individuals who are trained to respond to questions and behaviors in standardized fashions. However, OSCEs can also be adapted to testing student assimilation of safety concepts. An OSCE station that addressed communication and management of prescription errors was introduced in 2003 at Mayo Medical School as part of the school's quality improvement curriculum.[81] Key learning identified through this application included the effective use of root cause analysis, the value of collaboration with pharmacists, and enhanced ability to communicate with patients about prescription errors.

Last but certainly not least is the potential role of patient stories in teaching important patient safety concepts and interpersonal skills to medical students. These poignant and all-too-real life experience descriptions truly bring home the significance of patient safety learning and situational awareness. For their part, patients and their families are more than willing, even eager, to share their experiences in furtherance of the goal of continual improvement in patient safety.

Recommendation 6. The medical school experience should emphasize the shaping of desired skills, attitudes, and behaviors in medical students that include, but are not limited to, the IOM and ACGME/ABMS core competencies—such as professionalism, interpersonal skills and communication, provision of patient-centered care, and working in interdisciplinary teams.

a. Desired patient safety skills, attitudes, and behaviors should be subject to the same intensity of teaching and testing as basic and clinical science content.
b. In addition to appropriate lectures, the patient safety educational experience should include the use of case studies, role playing, and patient stories.
c. Student competence to perform procedures should be developed through simulation models to the extent possible to avoid placing patients at risk.
d. Students should be provided training experiences that involve working with students from other professional disciplines, such as nursing and pharmacy.
e. The acquisition of relevant patient safety knowledge and skills should be evaluated in simulated settings, such as through the use of observed clinical examinations.
f. Students should be encouraged to develop and/or participate in patient safety projects under appropriate faculty guidance.
g. Medical school deans and teaching hospital CEOs should assure the adequacy of resources necessary to the support of patient safety education and training (e.g., simulation capabilities, including both facilities and personnel).

One Continuous Pathway

The inevitable focus on "courses" in the medical school curriculum tends to distract from the ultimate overarching goal of producing physicians who are fully prepared to enter graduate medical training. That transition should ideally be seamless, as should the transition of students from college to medical school. With regard to the latter, there is much to be said for the arguments set forth by Dienstag that medical schools waste too much precious time in the preclinical years on elementary basic science education and that colleges need to devote greater efforts toward creation of coursework that integrates the relevant science preparation needed by premedical students.[82] This was in fact one of the principal conclusions reached in the recent Association of American Medical Colleges (AAMC) and Howard Hughes Medical Institute (HHMI) study, titled "Scientific Foundations for Future Physicians."[83] Suffice to say, this is one of several potential initiatives that could help to decompress the medical school course traffic jam and assure a sharper focus on producing the right end product—a good doctor.

What is needed is some linear connectivity between a point late in the student's premedical preparation and his or her entrance into graduate medical education and, more to the point, some reliable guideposts for measuring or otherwise determining whether important developmental milestones are being met as the student progresses through the medical education process. In this regard, the IOM and ACGME/ABMS competencies are necessary but not sufficient. What is missing is the articulation of a set of expected medical school competencies by the LCME. That is, what do we expect the graduating medical student/physician to be able to do?

It is beyond the scope of this paper to frame a potential set of desired medical student competencies at the conclusion of, and indeed at selected milestones along, the medical education process, but such a document would be immensely valuable. It would logically identify key themes or emphases—such as patient centeredness, patient safety applications, teamwork, communication skills, and professionalism—that should be emphasized throughout the curriculum and the medical student experience. It should as well set forth expected clinical competencies that complement those framed by the IOM, ACGME, and ABMS and underscore the need to weigh the development of important skills and behaviors at at least the same level of importance as the acquisition of medical knowledge. We would then begin to graduate classes of physicians who are consistently prepared in their abilities not only as clinicians but also as mentors and teachers of patient safety.

From there, the baton passes to the residency training programs and their overseer, the ACGME, whose accreditation process is framed around its core competencies, and then finally to the ABMS and its various certification boards and to the purveyors of continuing medical education (CME)—medical school and teaching hospitals—who operate in this regard under the aegis of the Accreditation Council for Continuing Medical Education (ACCME). The development of patient safety knowledge and skills should be made available as discrete continuing education activities, and the principles of patient safety should be integrated into the broad range of CME courses. Eventually, these CME activities should reinforce and strengthen the knowledge and skills of practitioners who have had patient safety education and training in medical school and their residencies. And in the near term, CME could become a core mechanism for furthering the education of the thousands of current practitioners who never had the opportunity to develop patient safety competencies as part of their medical school education and residency training.

Recommendation 7. Medical schools, teaching hospitals, and residency training programs should ensure a coherent, continuing, and flexible educational experience that spans the four years of undergraduate medical education, residency and fellowship training, and lifelong continuing education.

a. Patient safety curricular content and experiences should be longitudinal to the extent possible and be linked to desired competencies that support the provision of safe, patient-centered care.
b. The concept of patient-centered care should be introduced in the first year of medical school and be reinforced throughout the educational continuum.
c. Medical schools should assure that graduating medical students are properly grounded in patient safety concepts and their applications in preparation for entry into residency training.
d. Residency training program patient safety education and training efforts should build on medical school education and training preparation to provide a truly graduate patient safety training experience.
e. Continuing medical education efforts supported by the medical school and/or the teaching hospital should provide

ongoing enhancement of learners' patient safety knowledge and skills that promote and enable contemporary patient safety practices.

* * *

Responsibilities for moving the foregoing recommendations forward lie primarily with medical schools and teaching hospitals and their leaders. In medical schools, leaders include the dean and his or her senior staff, department chairs, and other faculty leaders. In teaching hospitals, those leaders include the CEO and his or her senior staff, the ACGME designated institutional officer (DIO), department chairs, and residency program directors.

Defining and measuring success with respect to these recommendations will be challenging, as is often true for patient safety interventions. To begin with, the impacts of the progressive implementation of these recommendations will likely not be felt—let alone be measurable—for at least a decade. In addition, the success or failure of public policy makers in addressing such key issues as payment reform and medical liability reform will also have a great deal to do with the ultimate achievement of tangible and measurable improvements in patient safety. There is more than sufficient evidence that effective implementation of each of the foregoing recommendations will have intrinsic value in itself, and such implementation efforts can certainly be measured. Further, if the LCME does establish specific terminal competencies for graduating medical students, student success in demonstrating these competencies will be measurable as well. Indeed, the ACGME is already far along in developing measurement strategies for assessing resident achievement of the ACGME/ABMS competencies.

PART III. STRATEGIES FOR CHANGE

Accreditor Opportunities

Today, there is apparent growing interest among medical school faculty and students in understanding and teaching patient safety. Many of the current efforts involve limited courses, but some schools are pursuing much more aggressive and elaborate patient safety education and training initiatives. However, the progress is uneven at best and still nonexistent in some schools even though the urgency to train physicians to become patient safety problem solvers and leaders is great. Strategies need to be formulated to leverage acceleration of the desired changes set forth in this paper. Among the potential strategies, modernization of the LCME and ACGME standards appears to offer the greatest opportunity to create substantive positive change.

The accreditation status of medical school programs that provide education and training leading to the MD degree is determined by the LCME, which is the only entity recognized by the U.S. Department of Education to assume this responsibility.[84,85] The LCME is jointly sponsored by the AAMC and the Council on Medical Education of the American Medical Association. LCME accreditation is required for medical schools to receive federal grants for medical education and to participate in federal loan programs. Most state licensure boards require that medical schools be LCME accredited as a condition for licensure of their graduates. Finally, school accreditation by the LCME is required to permit the school's students to take the United States Medical Licensing Exam (USMLE) and to matriculate into residency training programs accredited by the ACGME. The accreditation process requires medical schools to provide assurances that their graduates exhibit *general* (emphasis added) professional competencies that are appropriate for entry to the next stage of their training and that serve as the foundation for lifelong learning and proficient medical care.

One of the more significant changes in the LCME standards in recent years has been the creation of a new standard on the learning environment (MS-31-A).[85] However, the new standard does not mention organization culture and the important characteristics that positive cultures need to bring to the support of constructive learning environments (see

Recommendation 1). Nor is there explicit mention of the vital importance of leadership in creating these facilitative cultures and learning environments. In this regard, it is notable that The Joint Commission has recently issued a new standard that holds healthcare organization leaders accountable for creating and maintaining a culture of safety and explicitly charges them to "address disruptive behavior of individuals working at all levels of the organization, including management, clinical and administrative staff, independent practitioners, and governing body members."[86] The responsibilities of deans and department chairs, and other faculty leaders in assuming a similar leadership role should be made explicit in the LCME standards.

Second, the previously articulated need to introduce patient safety teaching early in the medical education curriculum and to extend its applications throughout the curriculum frames a strong case that the LCME standards should make patient safety education an explicit curriculum requirement. This recommendation is tendered in full recognition of the significant number of scholarly priorities that compete for attention in medical school curricula. Nevertheless, the fundamental importance of patient safety in medical care is at least as great as the importance accorded to other specific content areas that have been singled out in the LCME standards as explicit curriculum requirements. These include behavioral and socioeconomic subjects (at standard ED-10), culturally competent care (at standards IS-16 and ED-21), clinical and translational research (at standard ED-17-A), common societal problems (at standard ED-20), medical ethics and human values (at standard ED-23), and eight basic sciences by individual name (at standard ED-11).[85]

Finally, as previously stated, the time is now opportune for the LCME to set forth expected terminal competencies for graduating medical students. At present, the LCME standards simply require the medical schools to develop school-specific objectives that guide the development of "competencies that the profession and the public expect of a physician" (at standard ED-1-A).[85] By contrast, the ACGME/ABMS competencies (see Part I), developed in 1999, today provide the basic underpinning of the ACGME accreditation process.[24,25] This would seem to be a desirable evolution for the LCME accreditation process as well. Indeed, the previously referenced (in Part II) AAMC/HHMI report issued in the spring of 2009 notes that "[t]he shift from defining required courses to articulating competencies is becoming increasingly widespread in education" and goes on to describe in detail separate series of recommended competencies both for medical school graduates and for entering students.[83] This is not to suggest that these specific competencies should necessarily be adopted in total by the LCME. However, they constitute a logical starting point for an important process that might logically also draw upon or link to the ACGME/ABMS competencies and address the basic patient safety skills and behaviors described in this paper as well.

The ACGME is the principal evaluator and accreditor of medical residency programs in the United States.[87] Established in 1981, the ACGME includes among its member organizations the American Board of Medical Specialties, the American Hospital Association, the American Medical Association, the Association of American Medical Colleges, and the Council of Medical Specialty Societies. The standards framework that it has established includes detailed sets of institutional requirements and common program requirements.[88] In addition, the ACGME has 26 residency review committees, which may set additional expectations for each of 26 specialty training programs.[87]

The ACGME could also have a profound effect on both student education and resident training through expansion of its institutional requirements and its common program requirements and through its institutional review and residency review committees. Specifically, ACGME standards should set forth expectations for the creation of cultures of safety and learning similar to those suggested for the

LCME above. Again, because development and maintenance of these cultures are leadership driven, the accountabilities of teaching hospital CEOs, ACGME designated institutional officers, and residency program directors in this regard need to be explicitly stated. In addition, the ACGME standards could and should develop behavioral and patient safety competency requirements for attending physicians who serve as faculty and mentors for both residents and students.

Recommendation 8. The LCME should modify its accreditation standards to articulate expectations for the creation of learning cultures having the characteristics described in Recommendation 1 previously, to establish patient safety education—having the characteristics described herein—as a curricular requirement, and to define specific terminal competencies for graduating medical students.

a. The cultural expectations might best be addressed at standard MS-31-A.
b. The establishment of patient safety instruction as a curricular requirement could be addressed either in the institutional setting standards chapter or in the educational program standards chapter, perhaps best at standard ED-7.
c. The definition of medical student terminal competencies might best be addressed at standard ED-1-A.

Recommendation 9. The ACGME should expand its common program requirements to articulate expectations for the creation of learning cultures having the characteristics described in Recommendation 1, to emphasize the importance of patient safety-related behavioral traits in residency program faculty, and to set forth expected basic faculty patient safety competencies.

a. A fundamental expectation for all residency program faculty should be that they display competency in interpersonal skills, leadership, teamwork, and collaboration.
b. Residency programs should define program faculty patient safety competencies as including the ability to demonstrate basic knowledge about error causation and mitigation, human factors concepts, safety improvement science, systems theory and analysis, systems design and redesign, teaming, and error disclosure and apology.
c. The adequacy of residency program learning cultures and faculty safety-related competencies should be addressed in the annual program and faculty evaluations.

Recommendation 10. The LCME and the ACGME should direct particular attention to the adequacy of the patient safety-related preparation of graduating medical students for entry into residency training.

Monitoring and Public Reporting on Medical School Performance

A number of medical schools are beginning to move forward on many of the necessary changes in medical education that are discussed in this paper (see Table 32.2). One would hope that others will follow. But hope is far from sufficient when the stakes are this high. Some ongoing credible mechanism is needed to monitor school progress toward, and, later, maintenance of achievement of, the objectives set forth herein.

The LCME generally conducts its accreditation reviews of individual medical schools every eight years.[84] These searching evaluations include the gathering of student views on the environment and the quality and effectiveness of the educational experience, but this information is simply integrated into the evaluation process and not otherwise disseminated or made public. The AAMC conducts a survey of graduating medical students each year, and results are provided to the individual medical schools, but again, school-specific results are not publicized.[48]

TABLE 32.2. Medical Schools That Have Begun to Implement Changes Recommended in This Report

Case Western Reserve University School of Medicine
Dartmouth Medical School
Duke University School of Medicine
Mayo School of Graduate Medical Education
Michigan State College of Human Medicine
Northwestern University Feinberg School of Medicine
Ohio State College of Medicine
Southern Illinois University School of Medicine
Tufts University School of Medicine
University of California San Francisco School of Medicine
University of Central Florida College of Medicine
University of Chicago Pritzker School of Medicine
University of Connecticut School of Medicine
University of Illinois College of Medicine at Chicago
University of Kentucky College of Medicine
University of Michigan Medical School
University of Minnesota Medical School
University of Missouri School of Medicine
University of Nebraska College of Medicine
University of North Carolina School of Medicine
University of South Florida College of Medicine
University of Virginia School of Medicine
Vanderbilt University School of Medicine

Courtesy of the Lucian Leape Institute at the National Patient Safety Foundation.

The LLI Roundtable believes that focused evaluations of medical schools should be undertaken on an annual basis and that the school-specific results should be made public. These evaluations would assess medical school education and training priorities, school effectiveness in shaping desired student behaviors and competencies, and the creation of school and teaching hospital cultures that support patient safety.

The evaluation dimensions would include quantitative and qualitative measures of formal education on patient safety and healthcare quality in the classroom and in simulated experiences that facilitate application of related knowledge and skills, clarity and enforcement of behavioral norms that foster treatment of students with dignity and respect, strength of faculty development programs; safety culture of the teaching environments, whether students are permitted and encouraged to report errors and harms that they observe, harmonization of all four years of medical school around a patient safety education platform, fulfillment of interprofessional education opportunities, and "psychological safety" (i.e., whether the student can safely speak up and/or question authority). Performance would be evaluated against standardized metrics, and publication of the evaluation results would be done in a fashion consistent with the transparency and accountability objectives reflected above.

Recommendation 11. A survey of medical schools should be developed to evaluate school educational priorities for patient safety, the creation of school and teaching hospital cultures that support patient safety, and school effectiveness in shaping desired skills, attitudes, and behaviors.

a. The evaluation should include:
   - Quantitative and qualitative measures of formal education on patient safety in the classroom and in simulated experiences that facilitate application of related knowledge and skills.
   - Clarity and enforcement of behavioral norms that foster treatment of students with dignity and respect.
   - Strength of faculty development programs.

- Safety culture of teaching environment.
- Whether students are permitted and encouraged to report errors and harms that they observe.
- Harmonization of all four years of medical school around a patient safety educational platform.
- Fulfillment of interprofessional education opportunities.
- "Psychological safety" (i.e., whether the student can safely speak up and/or question authority).

b. Specific metrics need to be developed for each of these evaluation dimensions.

c. The survey should be administered annually, and its results should be publicly reported.

Textbooks and Testing

One of the reasons for the low to nonexistent profile of patient safety in medical schools is its low to nonexistent profile in medical textbooks utilized by medical students. The same may be said for the various written and other examinations to which medical students are subjected. The content of these education and evaluation vehicles makes potent statements as to what is considered important in medicine.

Student facility in utilizing the Internet and other media to supplement their learning can help to bridge the patient safety visibility gap. Indeed, the extraordinary uptake of the IHI Open School curricular offerings in a relatively brief period of time dramatizes what is possible.[73] Meanwhile, efforts need to be undertaken to connect other major purveyors of safety knowledge and skills—the Agency for Healthcare Research and Quality, The Joint Commission, the National Quality Forum, the National Patient Safety Foundation, and the Veterans Administration National Center for Patient Safety—with medical students. That is the responsibility both of these organizations and the medical schools. There is also a compelling need for a single source textbook that addresses patient safety and quality improvement content and competencies. Most of all, patient safety content needs to be integrated into other widely used medical textbooks.

Examination content is an even more powerful vehicle for capturing the intellectual attention of both medical schools and their students. To this end, the National Board of Medical Examiners (NBME), which, together with the Federation of State Medical Boards, prepares the United States Medical Licensure Examination (USMLE), is currently investing in the development of competency-based examinations that presumably will provide effective ways to assess analytic and other skills.[89] This could and should be a major opportunity for putting testing for patient safety knowledge and skills on the map. Similarly, the American Board of Medical Specialties, the parent body of the certification boards for the major medical specialties, is developing a patient safety module.[90] The content of this module should eventually find expression in the various board certification examinations.

Meanwhile, on the front end of the testing process, the Medical College Admission Test (MCAT) is currently undergoing development of what will become its fifth iteration.[91] That version, expected to be introduced no earlier than 2013, "will consider recent calls for new information about applicants' mastery of natural sciences and humanities content; behavioral and social sciences and humanities content; and professional competencies like cultural competence, communication skills, and professionalism."[92] This too appears to be an opportunity to accentuate the importance of foundational patient safety concepts such as systems theory and applications, human factors concepts, and error causation for those who are seeking entrance to medical school.

Financial Incentives

Titles VII and VIII of the Public Health Service Act authorize the annual awarding of programmatic grants to support health professional education.[93] Title VIII focuses predominantly on nursing professionals, while Title VII funds are available to medical, dental, and other professional schools. The general purposes of these titles are to increase the numbers of healthcare professionals, improve the distribution of these professionals to underserved areas, and provide education and training opportunities for more minority professionals. However, there have been multiple instances over the past 40 years where funding under these titles was provided to assist schools in improving or enhancing their curricula.[94] Since preventable adverse events rank at least eighth (and probably higher) among causes of death in the United States, a strong case can be made that patient safety is a major public health issue and that patient safety education and training should be made a high priority for funding under both Titles VII and VIII. Since Title VII and Title VIII funding has now dwindled to a few hundred million dollars a year, a compelling case can also be made for new stimulus money under these titles to address this critically important public health priority. The recommendations set forth in this paper would provide a ready-made framework for evaluating the impacts of such programmatic funding.

At the state level, largely discretionary funding of varying levels is provided to a substantial number of medical schools. Many of these states have existing and/or new high-priority patient safety initiatives (e.g., the mandatory reporting of "never events"). Current state funding levels create significant opportunities for interested states to further their safety-related public health priorities through leveraging implementation of the medical education reforms recommended in this paper.

The same proposition applies to the Medicare Indirect Medical Education (IME) funds that are used to support graduate medical education.[95] Here, the funding is in excess of $5 billion per year. Medicare policy tensions do exist over the question as to whether the IME funds are actually supporting patient care or medical education activities. These exist because the payment of Medicare funds is theoretically supposed to be limited to support for patient care. However, it is perhaps time to declare that this money is indeed supporting medical education and then describe the important opportunity this presents for leveraging changes in undergraduate and graduate medical education that will improve patient safety.

Recommendation 12. Financial, academic, and other incentives should be utilized to leverage desired changes in medical schools and teaching hospitals that will improve medical education and make it more relevant to the real world of patient care.

a. The federal government should commit existing and new Title VII funds to support patient safety education and training in medical schools, and should use the recommendations set forth in this paper as the framework for evaluating the success of this programmatic initiative.
b. States that provide significant funding to medical schools within their borders should consider making such funding contingent upon demonstrated satisfactory performance against the recommendations of this paper that are the responsibility of medical schools.
c. Continued access to federal funds to support residency training programs should similarly be tied to demonstrated satisfactory performance against the recommendations of this paper that are the responsibility of teaching hospitals.
d. Efforts should be launched to develop a textbook that focuses primarily on patient safety content and competencies, and to integrate relevant patient safety content into other standard medical textbooks.
e. Relevant patient safety-related content should be included in the fifth iteration of the MCAT, which is currently under development.
f. Standardized postadmission external tests (e.g., those developed by the NBME) should emphasize knowledge and analytic skills relevant to patient safety to

redirect the intellectual attention of both medical schools and students to this important knowledge and skills.

* * *

Responsibilities for Recommendations 8 and 9 belong to the LCME and ACGME, respectively, and for Recommendation 10, to the LCME and ACGME together. For Recommendations 11 and 12, responsibilities for pursuing implementation will lie principally with the Lucian Leape Institute itself.

CONCLUSION

Twenty-four centuries is a long time for a significant problem to finally come to a head, but medical care has come a long way since Hippocrates implored physicians to "do no harm." The remarkable advances since then, especially those of the past century, have saved countless lives and enhanced the quality of life for millions of people who otherwise would have died or suffered the prolonged effects of disease and injury. Ironically, however, these advances have also given cover to a problem that continues to pervade medical care: the thousands of preventable adverse events that kill and maim patients every day.

But changes are occurring that give us new hope. We have now just come to the 10th anniversary of the release of the IOM report *To Err Is Human*.[6] That report was remarkable not only for shredding the secrecy that had long enshrouded the patient safety problem but also for its boldness in framing the problem and suggesting logical, if challenging, solutions. While some observers and analysts have expressed disappointment about the apparent lack of progress over the past decade in addressing what was and still is a "top ten" cause of death in the United States, the level of awareness of this issue among the public, health professionals, and provider organizations is now stunning, and the hunger for solutions—indeed for being part of the solution—is growing rapidly. The question has, with seeming suddenness, become not whether to invest in patient safety improvement but rather what changes need to be made and what strategies need to be pursued to make them happen. Today, we are seeing this awareness and, in fact, a new commitment to change among policy makers, health professionals, healthcare executives, and health professional schools, among others.

What is most striking, though, are the changes occurring in medical education. Five years ago, a Joint Commission initiative to promote the introduction of patient safety education and training into the curricula of medical, nursing, pharmacy, and healthcare administration schools failed to gain any traction within any of these disciplines. Today, at least some aspects of patient safety are being taught in over half of the nation's medical schools, and perhaps as many as 20% of medical schools are in the process of adopting and pursuing many of the recommendations set forth in Part II of this paper. That is indeed good news. However, the bad news is that most medical schools are lagging well behind where they should be in embracing patient safety education and training. The challenges inherent in this effort are admittedly daunting, but the stakes are high and the urgency is great.

This white paper seeks to underscore this urgency and makes explicit recommendations for leaders in medical education and teaching hospitals who must become part of this solution. Even under the best of circumstances, it will take years to create a critical mass of patient safety-competent physicians. But each physician who fully grasps the multiple dimensions of patient safety is one more physician likely to find humility in the challenge and therefore likely to provide safe care to his or her patients. Even more important, each such physician will have the potential to be a much-needed leader who, in collaboration with others, can help develop positive organization cultures and patient safety solutions. When this happens across the profession, we will be able to lay to rest the concerns of Hippocrates and other leaders over the centuries who have recognized that the first obligation to patients is not to harm them.

References

1. Smith, C. M. (2005). Origin and uses of primum non nocere—Above all, do no harm! *Journal of Clinical Pharmacology, 45*(4), 371–377.
2. Joint Commission on Accreditation of Healthcare Organizations. (1999). *Florence Nightingale: Measuring hospital care outcomes*. Oakbrook Terrace, IL: Joint Commission on Accreditation of Healthcare Organizations.
3. Thompson, M. (1949). *The cry and the covenant*. New York: Garden City Books.
4. Codman, E. A. (1996). *A study in hospital efficiency*. Oakbrook Terrace, IL: Joint Commission on Accreditation of Healthcare Organizations.
5. Leape, L. L., Brennan, T. A., Laird, N., Lawthers, A. G., Localio, A. R., Barnes, B. A., . . . Hiatt, H. (1991). The nature of adverse events in hospitalized patients. Results of the Harvard Medical Practice Study II. *New England Journal of Medicine, 324*(6), 377–384.
6. Kohn, L. T., Corrigan, J., & Donaldson, M. (Eds). (1999). *To err is human: Building a safer health system*. Washington, DC: National Academies Press.
7. Donaldson, L. J., & Fletcher, M. G. (2006). The WHO World Alliance for Patient Safety: Towards the years of living less dangerously. *Medical Journal of Australia, 184*(10 Suppl), S69–S72.
8. National Patient Safety Foundation. http://www.npsf.org/.
9. U.S. Department of Health and Human Services, Agency for Research and Healthcare Quality. (2007, April). *Patient safety improvement corps*. Retrieved from http://www.ahrq.gov/About/psimpcorps.htm.
10. National Quality Forum. http://www.qualityforum.org/.
11. The Joint Commission National Patient Safety Goals. http://www.jointcommission.org/patientsafety/nationalpatientsafetygoals/.
12. Institute for Healthcare Improvement. http://www.ihi.org/ihi.
13. Centers for Disease Control and Prevention: Healthcare Infection Control Practices Advisory Committee. http://www.cdc.gov/hicpac/pubReportGuide/publicReportingHAI.html.
14. Bootman, J. (2006). *Preventing medication errors*. Washington, DC: National Academies Press.
15. Joint Commision National Patient Safety Goals Compliance Data. http://www.jointcommission.org/PatientSafety/NationalPatientSafetyGoals/NPSG_Compliance_Data.htm.
16. Aiken, L. H., Clarke, S. P., Sloane, D. M., Sochalski, J. A., Busse, R., Clarke, H., . . . Shamian, J. (2001). Nurses' reports on hospital care in five countries. *Health Aff (Millwood), 20*(3), 43–53.
17. Forster, A. J., Asmis, T. R., Clark, H. D., Al Saied, G., Code, C. C., Caughey, S. C., . . . Ottawa Hospital Patient Safety Study. (2004). Ottawa Hospital Patient Safety Study: Incidence and timing of adverse events in patients admitted to a Canadian teaching hospital. *Canadian Medical Association Journal, 170*(8), 1235–1240.
18. Wu, A. W., & Johansen, K. S. (1999). Lessons from Europe on quality improvement: Report on the Velen Castle WHO meeting. *Joint Commission Journal on Quality Improvement, 25*(6), 316–329.
19. Drosler, S. E., Klazinga, N. S., Romano, P. S., Tancredi, D. J., Gogorcena Aoiz, M. A., Hewitt, M. C., . . . Kelley, E. (2009). Application of patient safety indicators internationally: A pilot study among seven countries. *International Journal for Quality in Health Care, 21*(4), 272–278.
20. Leape, L. L., & Berwick, D. M. (2005). Five years after *To Err Is Human*: What have we learned? *JAMA, 293*(19), 2384–2390.
21. Wachter, R. M. (2010). Patient safety at ten: Unmistakable progress, troubling gaps. *Health Aff (Millwood), 29*(1), 165–173.
22. Greiner, A. C., & Knebel, E. (2003). *Health professions education: A bridge to quality*. Washington, DC: Institute of Medicine.
23. Swick, H. M., Szenas, P., Danoff, D., & Whitcomb, M. E. (1999). Teaching professionalism in undergraduate medical education. *JAMA, 282*(9), 830–832.
24. Batalden, P., Leach, D., Swing, S., Dreyfus, H., & Dreyfus, S. (2002). General competencies and accreditation in graduate medical

education. *Health Aff (Millwood), 21*(5), 103–111.

25. American Board of Medical Specialties: MOC competencies and criteria. http://www.abms.org/Maintenance_of_Certification/MOC_competencies.aspx.
26. Grumbach, K., & Bodenheimer, T. (2004). Can health care teams improve primary care practice? *JAMA, 291*(10), 1246–1251.
27. Sandars, J., Bax, N., Mayer, D., Wass, V., & Vickers, R. (2007). Educating undergraduate medical students about patient safety: Priority areas for curriculum development. *Medical Teacher, 29*(1), 60–61.
28. Greenes, R. A., & Shortliffe, E. H. (1990). Medical informatics. An emerging academic discipline and institutional priority. *JAMA, 263*(8), 1114–1120.
29. Flexner, A. *Medical education in the United States and Canada*. (1910). New York: The Carnegie Foundation for the Advancement of Teaching.
30. Cooke, M., Irby, D. M., Sullivan, W., & Ludmerer, K. M. (2006). American medical education 100 years after the Flexner report. *New England Journal of Medicine, 355*(13), 1339–1344.
31. Bodenheimer, T., Wagner, E. H., & Grumbach, K. (2002). Improving primary care for patients with chronic illness: The chronic care model, Part 2. *JAMA, 288*(15), 1909–1914.
32. Blumenthal, D., & Epstein, A. M. (1996). Quality of health care. Part 6: The role of physicians in the future of quality management. *New England Journal of Medicine, 335*(17), 1328–1331.
33. Sia, C., Tonniges, T. F., Osterhus, E., & Taba, S. (2004). History of the medical home concept. *Pediatrics, 113*(5 Suppl), 1473–1478.
34. Hunt, R. E., & Newman, R. G. (1997). Medical knowledge overload: A disturbing trend for physicians. *Health Care Manage Review, 22*(1), 70–75.
35. AcademyHealth. (2007). *Improving quality health care: The role of consumer engagement*. Princeton, NJ: Robert Wood Johnson Foundation.
36. Coulter, A., & Rozansky, D. (2004). Full engagement in health. *BMJ, 329*(7476), 1197–1198.
37. Ball, M. J., Costin, M. Y., & Lehmann, C. (2008). The personal health record: Consumers banking on their health. *Studies in Health Technology and Informatics, 134*, 35–46.
38. Wu, A. W. (2000). Medical error: The second victim. The doctor who makes the mistake needs help too. *BMJ, 320*(7237), 726–727.
39. Scott, S. D., Hirschinger, L. E., Cox, K. R., McCoig, M., Brandt, J., & Hall, L. W. (2009). The natural history of recovery for the healthcare provider "second victim" after adverse patient events. *Quality and Safety in Health Care, 18*(5), 325–330.
40. Holm, S. (1995). The medical hierarchy and perceived influence on technical and ethical decisions. *Journal of Internal Medicine, 237*(5), 487–492.
41. Thomas, E. J., Sexton, J. B., & Helmreich, R. L. (2003). Discrepant attitudes about teamwork among critical care nurses and physicians. *Critical Care Medicine, 31*(3), 956–959.
42. Murray, D., & Enarson, C. (2007). Communication and teamwork: Essential to learn but difficult to measure. *Anesthesiology, 106*(5), 895–896.
43. Shostek, K. (2007). Developing a culture of safety in ambulatory care settings. *Journal of Ambulatory Care Management, 30*(2), 105–113.
44. Hafferty, F. W., & Franks, R. (1994). The hidden curriculum, ethics teaching, and the structure of medical education. *Academic Medicine, 69*(11), 861–871.
45. Institute for Healthcare Improvement. *Develop a culture of safety*. Retrieved from http://www.ihi.org/IHI/Topics/PatientSafety/SafetyGeneral/Changes/Develop+a+Culture+of+Safety.htm.
46. Reddy, S. T., Farnan, J. M., Yoon, J. D., Leo, T., Upadhyay, G. A., Humphrey, H. J., & Arora, V. M. (2007). Third-year medical students' participation in and perceptions of unprofessional behaviors. *Academic Medicine, 82*(10 Suppl), S35–S39.
47. Feudtner, C., Christakis, D. A., & Christakis, N. A. (1994). Do clinical clerks suffer ethical erosion? Students' perceptions of their ethical environment and personal development. *Academic Medicine, 69*(8), 670–679.
48. Association of American Medical Colleges (AAMC). *Graduation questionnaire*. Retrieved from http://www.aamc.org/data/gq/.
49. Prescott, J. (2009). (AAMC). Personal communication.

50. Porto, G., & Lauve, R. (2006). Disruptive clinician behavior: A persistent threat to patient safety. *Patient Safety and Quality Healthcare, 3*, 16–24.
51. O'Leary, D. (2005). Comments made during Patients for Patient Safety Program of the World Alliance for Patient Safety in London.
52. Eva, K. W., Reiter, H. I., Trinh, K., Wasi, P., Rosenfeld, J., & Norman, G. R. (2009). Predictive validity of the multiple mini-interview for selecting medical trainees. *Medical Education, 43*(8), 767–775.
53. Salvatori, P. (2001). Reliability and validity of admissions tools used to select students for the health professions. *Advances in Health Sciences Education, 6*(2), 159–175.
54. Stewart, M., Brown, J. B., Weston, W. W., McWhinney, I. R., McWilliam, C. L., & Freeman, T. R. (1995). *Patient centered medicine: Transforming the clinical method*. Thousand Oaks, CA: Sage.
55. Davis, K., Schoenbaum, S. C., & Audet, A. M. (2005). A 2020 vision of patient-centered primary care. *Journal of General Internal Medicine, 20*(10), 953–957.
56. Davidoff, F., Haynes, B., Sackett, D., & Smith, R. (1995). Evidence-based medicine. *BMJ, 310*(6987), 1085–1086.
57. Kritchevsky, S. B., & Simmons, B. P. (1991). Continuous quality improvement. Concepts and applications for physician care. *JAMA, 266*(13), 1817–1823.
58. Cuff, P. A., & Vanselow, N. A. (2004). *Improving medical education: Enhancing the behavioral and social science content of medical school curricula*. Washington, DC: Institute of Medicine.
59. Carayon. P. (Ed.). (2006). *Handbook of human factors and ergonomics in health care and patient safety*. Mahwah, NJ: Lawrence Erlbaum.
60. Karsh, B. T., Holden, R. J., Alper, S. J., & Or, C. K. (2006). A human factors engineering paradigm for patient safety: Designing to support the performance of the healthcare professional. *Quality and Safety in Health Care, 15*(Suppl 1), i59–i65.
61. The Joint Commission. *Sentinel events*. Retrieved from http://www.jointcommission.org/SentinelEvents/.
62. Kaldjian, L. C., Jones, E. W., & Rosenthal, G. E. (2006). Facilitating and impeding factors for physicians' error disclosure: A structured literature review. *Joint Commission Journal on Quality and Patient Safety, 32*(4), 188–198.
63. Halbach, J. L., & Sullivan L. L. (2005). Teaching medical students about medical errors and patient safety: Evaluation of a required curriculum. *Academic Medicine, 80*(6), 600–606.
64. Gosbee, J. W., Williams, L., & Dunn, E. (2006). Teaching the teachers of patient safety: A progress report. *ACGME Bulletin*, September, 15–19.
65. Pronovost, P., & Sexton, B. (2005). Assessing safety culture: Guidelines and recommendations. *Quality Safe Health Care, 14*(4), 231–233.
66. Gershon, R. R., Karkashian, C. D., Grosch, J. W., Murphy, L. R., Escamilla-Cejudo, A., Flanagan, P. A., . . . Martin, L. (2000). Hospital safety climate and its relationship with safe work practices and workplace exposure incidents. *American Journal of Infection Control, 28*(3), 211–221.
67. Singer, S. J., Gaba, D. M., Geppert, J. J., Sinaiko, A. D., Howard, S. K., & Park, K. C. (2003). The culture of safety: Results of an organization-wide survey in 15 California hospitals. *Quality Safe Health Care, 12*(2), 112–118.
68. Marx, D. (2001). *Patient safety and the "just culture": A primer for health care executives*. New York: Columbia University.
69. Frankel, A. S., Leonard, M. W., & Denham, C. R. (2006). Fair and just culture, team behavior, and leadership engagement: The tools to achieve high reliability. *Health Services Research, 41*(4 Pt 2), 1690–1709.
70. Mosley, T. H. Jr., Perrin, S. G., Neral, S. M., Dubbert, P. M., Grothues, C. A., & Pinto, B. M. (1994). Stress, coping, and well-being among third-year medical students. *Academic Medicine, 69*(9), 765–767.
71. Mayer, D., Klamen, D. L., Gunderson, A., & Barach, P. (2009). Designing a patient safety undergraduate medical curriculum: The Telluride Interdisciplinary Roundtable experience. *Teaching and Learning in Medicine, 21*(1), 52–58.
72. World Health Organization. (2009). *WHO patient safety curriculum guide for medical schools*. Geneva, Switzerland: World Health Organization.
73. Institute for Healthcare Improvement (IHI). *IHI Open School for health profession-*

als. Retrieved from http://www.ihi.org/IHI/Programs/IHIOpenSchool/.

74. *Patient safety education project*. Retrieved from http://patientsafetyeducationproject.org/index.php.
75. Kravet, S. J., Howell, E., & Wright, S. M. (2006). Morbidity and mortality conference, grand rounds, and the ACGME's core competencies. *Journal of General Internal Medicine, 21*(11), 1192–1194.
76. Blake, J. M., Norman, G. R., & Smith, E. K. (1995). Report card from McMaster: Student evaluation at a problem-based medical school. *Lancet, 345*(8954), 899–902.
77. Helmreich, R. L., Merritt, A. C., & Wilhelm, J. A. (1999). The evolution of Crew Resource Management training in commercial aviation. *International Journal of Aviation Psychology, 9*(1), 19–32.
78. Weller, J. M. (2004). Simulation in undergraduate medical education: Bridging the gap between theory and practice. *Medical Education, 38*(1), 32–38.
79. Issenberg, S. B., McGaghie, W. C., Hart, I. R., Mayer, J. W., Felner, J. M., Petrusa, E. R., . . . Ewy, G. A. (1999). Simulation technology for health care professional skills training and assessment. *JAMA, 282*(9), 861–866.
80. Ziv, A., Wolpe, P. R., Small, S. D., & Glick, S. (2003). Simulation-based medical education: An ethical imperative. *Academic Medicine, 78*(8), 783–788.
81. Varkey, P., & Natt, N. (2007). The Objective Structured Clinical Examination as an educational tool in patient safety. *Joint Commission Journal of Quality Patient Safety, 33*(1), 48–53.
82. Dienstag, J. L. (2008). Relevance and rigor in premedical education. *New England Journal of Medicine, 359*(3), 221–224.
83. Association of American Medical Colleges and Howard Hughes Medical Institute. (2009). *Scientific foundations for future physicians*. Washington, DC: AAMC and HHMI.
84. Liaison Committee on Medical Education (LCME). *Overview: Accreditation and the LCME*. Retrieved from http://www.lcme.org/overview.htm.
85. Liaison Committee on Medical Education (LCME). (2008). *Function and structure of a medical school*. Washington, DC: LCME. Retrieved from http://www.lcme.org/functions2010jun.pdf.
86. Youssi, M. D. (2002). JCAHO standards help address disruptive physician behavior. *Physician Executive, 28*(6), 12–13.
87. Accreditation Council for Graduate Medical Education. Retrieved from http://www.acgme.org/acWebsite/home/home.asp.
88. *ACGME institutional requirements*. (2007). Retrieved from www.acgme.org/acWebsite/irc/irc_IRCpr07012007.pdf.
89. National Board of Medical Examiners. http://www.nbme.org/index.html.
90. *ABMS patient safety improvement program*. Retrieved from http://www.abms.org/Products_and_Publications/pdf/ABMS_Patient_Safety_Combined_Syllabus_092008.pdf.
91. AAMC: Medical College Admission Test (MCAT). Retrieved from http://www.aamc.org/students/mcat/.
92. MR5: 5th Comprehensive Review of the MCAT Exam. http://www.aamc.org/students/mcat/mr5/start.htm.
93. U.S. Department of Health and Human Services: Public Health Service Act. http://www.fda.gov/RegulatoryInformation/Legislation/ucm148717.htm.
94. U.S. Government Accountability Office. *Health professions education programs: Action still needed to measure impact*. (2006). Washington, DC: GAO. Retrieved from http://www.gao.gov/new.items/d0655.pdf.
95. Centers for Medicare and Medicaid Services. *Acute inpatient PPS*. Retrieved from http://www.cms.hhs.gov/acuteinpatientpps/07_ime.asp.

Appendix 1

Setting the Right Organization Context

Health care has undergone a major sea change over the past two decades. As these changes and the complexities of health care have escalated, patient safety problems have become increasingly evident, and medical education and training institutions have found themselves struggling to keep up with the need to ensure that student physicians are properly equipped with the skills, attitudes, knowledge, and behaviors (i.e., patient safety competencies) that will make them capable of becoming part of the patient safety solution. This need constitutes a major challenge to medical schools and teaching hospitals, and particularly their leaders and faculty, to develop their own competencies to guide their charges in learning to manage a new "disease state."

Recommendation 1. Medical school and teaching hospital leaders should place the highest priority on creating learning cultures that emphasize patient safety, model professionalism, enhance collaborative behavior, encourage transparency, and value the individual learner.

Recommendation 2. Medical school deans and teaching hospital CEOs should launch a broad effort to emphasize and promote the development and display of interpersonal skills, leadership, teamwork, and collaboration among faculty and staff.

Recommendation 3. As part of continuing education and ongoing performance improvement, medical school deans and teaching hospital CEOs should provide incentives and make available necessary resources to support the enhancement of faculty capabilities for teaching students how to diagnose patient safety problems, improve patient care processes, and deliver safe care.

Recommendation 4. The selection process for admission to medical school should place greater emphasis on selecting for attributes that reflect the concepts of professionalism and an orientation to patient safety.

STRATEGIES FOR TEACHING PATIENT SAFETY

Medical schools have done an excellent job of providing students with the knowledge and related skills they will need for the technical practice of medicine. However, the new and still evolving care environment requires more than this with respect to patient safety. The elemental nature of patient safety education has profound implications for future curricular design. The teaching of patient safety needs to begin on day one of medical school and be extended throughout the four-year medical school experience and beyond by becoming embedded in all teaching activities. It is equally important to understand that patient safety education is much more than the absorption of concepts and knowledge and requires particular attention to the acquisition of desired skills, attitudes, and behaviors. This is because the long-term intent is that these skills, attitudes, and behaviors become an integral part of the physician's professional way of life.

Recommendation 5. Medical schools should conceptualize and treat patient safety as a science that encompasses knowledge of error causation and mitigation, human factors concepts, safety improvement science, systems theory and analysis, system design and redesign, teaming, and error disclosure and apology.

Recommendation 6. The medical school experience should emphasize the shaping of desired skills, attitudes, and behaviors in medical students that include, but are not limited to, the Institute of Medicine and Accreditation Council for Graduate Medical Education (ACGME)/American Board of Medical Specialties (ABMS) core competencies—such as professionalism, interpersonal skills and communication, provision of patient-centered care, and working in interdisciplinary teams.

Recommendation 7. Medical schools, teaching hospitals, and residency training programs should ensure a coherent, continuing, and flexible educational experience that spans the four years of undergraduate medical education, residency and fellowship training, and lifelong continuing education.

LEVERAGING CHANGE

There is today apparent growing interest among medical school faculty and students in understanding and teaching patient safety. Many of the current efforts involve limited courses, but some schools are pursuing much more aggressive and elaborate patient safety education and training initiatives. However, the progress is uneven at best and still non-existent in some schools, while the urgency to train physicians to become patient safety problem solvers and leaders is great. This requires attention to formulating strategies that are likely to leverage acceleration of the desired changes set forth in this paper. Among the potential strategies, modernization of the Liaison Committee on Medical Education (LCME) and ACGME standards appears to offer the greatest opportunity to create universal substantive positive change. In addition, public monitoring of school efforts in making these changes is another potentially strong lever. Other opportunities exist as well.

Recommendation 8. The LCME should modify its accreditation standards to articulate expectations for the creation of learning cultures having the characteristics described in Recommendation 1 above, to establish patient safety education—having the characteristics described herein—as a curricular requirement, and to define specific terminal competencies for graduating medical students.

Recommendation 9. The ACGME should expand its Common Program Requirements to articulate expectations for the creation of learning cultures having the characteristics described in Recommendation 1, to emphasize the importance of patient safety–related behavioral traits in residency program faculty, and to set forth expected basic faculty patient safety competencies.

Recommendation 10. The LCME and the ACGME should direct particular attention to the adequacy of the patient safety–related preparation of graduating medical students for entry into residency training.

Recommendation 11. A survey of medical schools should be developed to evaluate school educational priorities for patient safety, the creation of school and teaching hospital cultures that support patient safety, and school effectiveness in shaping desired student skills, attitudes, and behaviors.

Recommendation 12. Financial, academic, and other incentives should be utilized to leverage desired changes in medical schools and teaching hospitals that will improve medical education and make it more relevant to the real world of patient care.

LUCIAN LEAPE INSTITUTE AT THE NATIONAL PATIENT SAFETY FOUNDATION

The Lucian Leape Institute was formed in 2007 to provide thought leadership and a strategic vision for improving patient safety. Composed of thought leaders in patient safety, the Institute functions as a think tank to identify new approaches to improving patient safety and to encourage key stakeholders to assume significant roles in advancing patient safety.

The initial work of the Institute has focused on identifying and framing vital transforming concepts that require system-level attention and action. The five concepts identified to date include medical education reform, active consumer engagement in all aspects of health care, transparency as a practiced value in everything we do, integration of care within and across healthcare delivery systems, and restoration of joy and meaning in work. These concepts are described in the Institute's first work product, "Transforming Healthcare: A Safety Imperative," recently published in *Quality and Safety in Healthcare.** Fulfilling the objectives embodied in these five concepts is critical to moving the national patient safety agenda forward; it is clear that this will require profound changes in the culture and structure of our healthcare system. Expert roundtables will be convened to address each of these transforming concepts.

This white paper addresses the first major concept—medical education reform. The problem analysis and recommendations set forth herein are the result of in-depth deliberations by an Expert Roundtable on Reforming Medical Education that included a broad array of medical education leaders, students, patients, representatives from key organizations, experts from related fields, and members of the Institute. The Roundtable met in extended sessions in Boston in October 2008 and June 2009. This report describes the consensus achieved regarding the current state of medical education, what medical education should ideally become, and what strategies should be used to leverage desired changes in medical education.

*Transforming Healthcare: A Safety Imperative. Leape L, Berwick D, Clancy C, et al., for the Lucian Leape Institute at the National Patient Safety Foundation. *Qual Saf Healthcare.* Dec 2009;18(6):424–428. Available at: http://qshc.bmj.com/content/18/6/424.full

NATIONAL PATIENT SAFETY FOUNDATION

The National Patient Safety Foundation has been diligently pursuing one mission since its founding in 1997—to improve the safety of the healthcare system for the patients and families it serves. NPSF is unwavering in its focus on uniting disciplines and organizations across the continuum of care, championing a collaborative, inclusive, multistakeholder approach. NPSF is an independent, not-for-profit 501(c)(3) organization based in Boston, Massachusetts.

ROUNDTABLE ON REFORMING MEDICAL EDUCATION INVITED EXPERTS

Richard M. J. Bohmer, MD, MBA
Harvard Business School

Jordan Bohnen
Student, Harvard Medical School & Harvard Business School

Alvin Calderon, MD, PhD, FACP
Virginia Mason Medical Center

Christine Cassel, MD, MACP
American Board of Internal Medicine & ABIM Foundation

John R. Combes, MD
AHA Center for Healthcare Governance

Joanne Conroy, MD
Association of American Medical Colleges

Colleen Conway-Welch, PhD, RN, CNM, FAAN, FACNM
Vanderbilt University School of Nursing

David Davis, MD
Association of American Medical Colleges

Linda Emanuel, MD, PhD
Northwestern University Kellogg School of Management

Peter (Jeff) Fabri, MD, PhD
University of South Florida College of Medicine

Liz Frank
Patient, Dana-Farber Cancer Institute

David Gaba, MD
Stanford University School of Medicine

Rosemary Gibson, MSc
Robert Wood Johnson Foundation

Anne Gunderson, Ed.Dc, GNP
University of Illinois College of Medicine at Chicago

Frank Hartmann
Roundtable Facilitator
Harvard Kennedy School

Rich Hawkins, MD, FACP
American Board of Medical Specialties

Ruth Horowitz, PhD
Accreditation Council for Continuing Medical Education

Michael Howell, MD, MPH
Beth Israel Deaconess Medical Center

William Iobst, MD
American Board of Internal Medicine

Hal B. Jenson, MD, MBA
Alliance of Independent Academic Medical Centers

Debra Klamen, MD, MHPE
Southern Illinois University School of Medicine

Kim Edward LeBlanc, MD, PhD
Federation of State Medical Boards

John Ludden, MD, FACPE
Tufts University School of Medicine

Kenneth Ludmerer, MD
Washington University in St. Louis

David Mayer, MD
University of Illinois College of Medicine at Chicago

Donald Melnick, MD
National Board of Medical Examiners

David Nash, MD, MBA
Jefferson Medical College

Marlene Nusbaum, PhD
Patient, Dana-Farber Cancer Institute

Jay Perman, MD
University of Kentucky College of Medicine

Ingrid Philibert, PhD, MBA
Accreditation Council for Graduate Medical Education

Sandra Potthoff, PhD
University of Minnesota School of Public Health

John Prescott, MD
Association of American Medical Colleges

Philip Schneider, MS, FASHP
University of Arizona College of Pharmacy at the Phoenix Biomedical Campus

Richard Schwartzstein, MD
Beth Israel Deaconess Medical Center

Carl Sirio, MD, FACP, FCCP, FCCM
American Medical Association

Prathibha Varkey, MD, MPH, MHPE
Mayo Clinic

Steven Wartman, MD, PhD, MCAP
Association of Academic Health Centers

Saul Weingart, MD, PhD
Dana-Farber Cancer Institute

Kevin Weiss, MD, MPH
American Board of Medical Specialties

Marina Zeltser
Student Member, American Medical Student Association

MEMBERS OF THE LUCIAN LEAPE INSTITUTE AT THE NATIONAL PATIENT SAFETY FOUNDATION

Lucian L. Leape, MD
Chair, Lucian Leape Institute
Adjunct Professor of Health Policy, Harvard School of Public Health

Donald M. Berwick, MD, MPP
President & CEO, Institute for Healthcare Improvement

Carolyn M. Clancy, MD
Director, Agency for Healthcare Research and Quality

James B. Conway, MS
Senior Vice President, Institute for Healthcare Improvement

Paul A. Gluck, MD
Immediate Past Chair, NPSF Board of Directors

James A. Guest
President, Consumers Union

David M. Lawrence, MD
Chairman & CEO (retired), Kaiser Foundation Health Plan, Inc., and Kaiser Foundation Hospitals

Julianne M. Morath, RN, MS
Chief Quality and Safety Officer, Vanderbilt University Medical Center

Dennis S. O'Leary, MD
President Emeritus, The Joint Commission

Paul O'Neill
Former Chairman & CEO, Alcoa, 72nd Secretary of the US Treasury

Diane C. Pinakiewicz, MBA
President, Lucian Leape Institute, President, National Patient Safety Foundation

REVIEWERS

John Gosbee, MD, MS
University of Michigan Health System
Red Forest Consulting, LLC

Ben-Tzion Karsh, PhD
University of Wisconsin Madison College of Engineering

Thomas Nasca, MD, MACP
Accreditation Council for Graduate Medical Education

Robert Wears, MD
University of Florida College of Medicine, Jacksonville

NPSF STAFF

David Coletta
Vice President, Strategic Partnerships & Communications

Thomas Isaac, MD
Lucian Leape Institute Fellow

Elma Sanders, PhD
Communications Manager

Manisha Shah, MBA, RCP
Vice President, Programs

Anita Spielman
Director, Information Resources and Research

The Lucian Leape Institute at the National Patient Safety Foundation gratefully acknowledges **The Doctors Company Foundation** for its generous support of the LLI Expert Roundtable on Reforming Medical Education and of the publication and dissemination of this white paper.

The Lucian Leape Institute at the National Patient Safety Foundation offers sincere thanks to the many organizations that have generously supported the work of the Institute since its inception in 2007 and recognizes in particular the significant support provided by the following partners:

Hospira
McKesson
The Doctors Company Foundation

33

Improving the Safety of the Medication Use Process

David A. Ehlert, PharmD and Steven S. Rough, MS

Although there is a substantial body of literature describing medication errors and preventable adverse drug events, historically, medication safety has not been a topic that generated much attention. Medication errors were often thought to be a result of human lapses, rather than system failures. Efforts to improve the reporting of medication errors were often met with resistance by hospital administrators and risk management departments. However, the release of the Institute of Medicine's (IOM) report *To Err Is Human: Building a Better Health System* in November 1999 has helped to foster the development of a national agenda for reducing errors and improving patient safety.[1] With estimates of 44,000 to 98,000 deaths annually due to medical errors, and more than 7,000 deaths per year due to medication errors alone, this IOM report has heightened awareness and has stimulated many healthcare organizations to develop strategies to address the situation. In March 2001, the Institute of Medicine released *Crossing the Quality Chasm: A New Health System for the 21st Century*.[2] This was the second and final report of the Committee on the Quality of Health Care in America. Whereas the first IOM report focuses largely on patient safety, the second report has a broader focus and provides strategic direction for redesigning the healthcare delivery system for the 21st century.

Rather than waiting for healthcare institutions to address the issue of medication safety on their own, many healthcare purchasers and payers are demanding that hospitals and health systems implement specific safeguards to maximize the safety of the medication use process. For instance, the Business Roundtable, an association of chief executive officers of leading corporations, recently unveiled its Leapfrog Group initiative.[3] This consortium of more than 135 employers and other major healthcare purchasers collectively provides health benefits to more than 33 million Americans. The Leapfrog Group is attempting to leverage this purchasing power to ensure that hospitals and health systems appropriately address the medical and medication error problems. The Leapfrog Group proposed three initial hospital safety measures that will facilitate comparisons that can be used to help determine which hospitals and facilities the companies contract with for their employees. The group estimates that their initial three improvements—computerized prescriber order entry (CPOE), staffing intensive care units with board-certified intensivists, and evidence-based hospital referral—could save up to 58,000 lives per year and prevent 522,000 medication errors if implemented by all nonrural hospitals in the United States.

Groups other than healthcare purchasers are beginning to mandate that healthcare facilities focus on improving medication safety. Since July 2001, The Joint Commission has had standards focused on improving patient safety and reducing medical and medication errors.[4] These initial standards require hospitals to foster a conducive, nonpunitive environment that encourages error identification and reporting. Hospitals also are required to inform patients and their families about the results of care, including unanticipated outcomes, and to aggregate patient safety-related data to identify risk to patients. In January 2003, the first six Joint Commission national patient safety goals became effective. For instance, goal 2 is to improve the effectiveness of communication among caregivers. Included in that goal is the implementation of a process for taking verbal or telephone orders that requires a verification "read-back" of the complete order by the person receiving the order. Also included in goal 2 is the development of a list of unacceptable abbreviations, symbols, and order-writing conventions.

The general public's interest in and awareness of the risk of medication errors and adverse drug events is also increasing. A survey conducted by the Kaiser Family Foundation and the Agency for Healthcare Research and Quality indicated that quality of care is the biggest concern in choosing a health plan.[5] Although few Americans use comparative quality information to help them make their healthcare choice (because of a lack of quality information and the fact that approximately 40% of Americans have no choice in health plans), most Americans believe that information about medical errors would tell them a lot about the quality of physicians. The general public is more concerned about serious errors or mistakes happening when they receive health care than when they fly on airlines. Furthermore, 73% of those surveyed reported that the government should require healthcare providers to report all serious medical errors to make sure this information is publicly available.

The purpose of this chapter is to provide some background on the medication safety problem, to provide very practical examples of how a health system is responding to this problem, and to identify best practices for maximizing medication safety.

BACKGROUND

Terminology

Medication misadventures, medication errors, adverse drug events (ADEs), and *adverse drug reactions* (ADRs) are terms that are frequently used to describe medication-related occurrences. However, these terms cannot be used interchangeably. According to a consensus definition reached by the National Coordinating Council for Medication Error Reporting and Prevention (NCCMERP), a medication error is "any preventable event that may cause or lead to inappropriate medication use or patient harm while the medication is in the control of the healthcare professional, patient, or consumer. Such events may be related to professional practice, healthcare products, procedures and systems including: prescribing; order communication; product-labeling; packaging and nomenclature; compounding; dispensing; administration; education; monitoring; and use."[6] Analysis of the literature reveals that there is considerable variability in how medication error occurrences are defined. For instance, the first IOM report defined an error as the failure of a planned action to be completed as intended or the use of a wrong plan to achieve an aim.[1] The key components of these definitions are that medication errors are preventable, they do not always cause patient harm, and they can be caused by errors in planning (e.g., prescribing), not just errors in execution (e.g., administering the drug to the wrong patient).

The majority of medication errors are not adverse drug events. An ADE is defined as an injury from a medicine (or lack of intended medicine). In a study by Bates and coworkers, only 0.9% of medication errors resulted in ADEs.[7] The death of an infant from a 10-fold overdose of morphine (because the morphine order did not include a leading zero) is an example of a medication error that resulted in an adverse drug event (preventable adverse drug event). Adverse drug reactions are a subset of ADEs. The World Health Organization (WHO) defines an adverse drug reaction as "any response that is noxious, unintended, or undesired, which occurs at doses normally used in humans for prophylaxis, diagnosis, therapy of disease or modification of physiological function."[8] The majority of adverse drug reactions are not preventable; however, preventable adverse drug reactions do occasionally occur. For instance, red man syndrome from rapid administration of vancomycin could be considered a preventable adverse drug reaction (i.e., a medication error and an adverse drug reaction). Figure 33.1 illustrates the relationships among the different types of medication misadventures.

The Incidence of Medication Misadventures

The exact incidence of medication errors and adverse drug events is unknown and varies from one study and from one institution to another. Medication error rates depend on the methodology and intensity of surveillance used to detect them. Because many medication errors do not cause patient harm, many errors go undetected. Furthermore, spontaneous reporting, one of the most common methods for detecting medication errors, fails to identify the majority of medication-related occurrences. Therefore, it is nearly impossible to ascertain the true incidence of medication errors. Nevertheless, a variety of different methodologies have been used within the medical literature in an attempt to quantify and estimate the true incidence of medication errors and adverse drug events.

The Harvard Medical Practice Study, in which over 30,000 records were randomly selected from 51 New York hospitals, indicated that drug complications were the most common type of adverse event.[9,10] Nearly 20% of the injuries that prolonged hospitalization or produced patient disability were due to the use of medications. Of these drug-induced adverse events, 20% were judged to be due to negligent care.

In a different study that used an intensive, multidisciplinary surveillance process of self-reporting and extensive chart review, Bates and colleagues found that an average of 1.4 medication errors occurred for every admission at Brigham and Women's Hospital.[7] Stated differently, they found that there were 311 medication errors for every 1,000 patient-days (or 530 medication errors per 10,070 orders). Of the 530 medication errors identified during the study, only 0.9% actually caused patient harm and resulted in an ADE.

FIGURE 33.1. The relationships among the different types of medication misadventures[6,30]

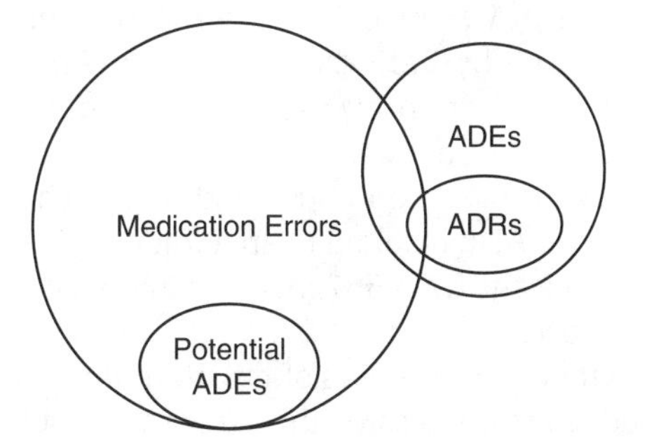

Other methodologies for detecting medication errors and adverse drug events have been used with success. For instance, integration of computerized detection programs into hospital information systems has been shown to be of utility. The reported ADE rates (per 1,000 patient-days) in four different publications, each using different error reporting and detection methods, ranged from 0.2% using a voluntary self-reporting system to 21% when a system of chart review and computerized screening was used.[11–14] The computerized detection programs screen for signs of potential ADEs such as abrupt medication discontinuation orders, antidote ordering (e.g., naloxone, flumazenil, diphenhydramine), and certain abnormal laboratory values.

Financial Impact

Medication misadventures result in significant consumption of resources in the form of increased lengths of stay, increased cost of care, rework time, patient costs (e.g., patient suffering, lost productivity), and malpractice claims. Using a decision analysis model, Johnson and Bootman estimated that the annual cost of drug-related morbidity and mortality in the ambulatory setting was $76.6 billion.[15,16] These authors estimated that almost 60% of the costs attributable to drug-related morbidity and mortality were preventable.

Other studies have focused more on the inpatient setting and have utilized prospective, case-control designs to estimate the additional resource consumption resulting from ADEs. For instance, Classen and coworkers found that each ADE increased the mean length of stay (LOS) by 3.23 days and the mean cost of hospitalization by $4,655.[17] In a different study, Bates and colleagues used a nested case-control design and found that each preventable ADE resulted in an additional LOS of 4.6 days and a $5,857 increase in hospitalization costs.[18]

Although the results of the aforementioned studies are impressive, the studies were not designed to take into consideration the amount of rework time and other costs (e.g., malpractice costs, costs to the patient) associated with ADEs, potential ADEs, and medication errors. For instance, although most medication errors do not result in patient harm, they frequently result in a significant amount of rework time (e.g., telephone calls for order clarification, tracking down missing doses).

The Medication Use Process

The medication use process encompasses all areas of medication use and is a highly complex, multidisciplinary process. In its simplest form, the medication use process consists of five domains: purchasing/inventory management; prescribing/medication determination; medication preparation, dispensing, and counseling; medication administration; and patient monitoring/assessment. Some medication use process models ignore the purchasing/inventory management phase. However, there are countless examples of medication errors and adverse drug events that could have been prevented by better purchasing/inventory management practices. Removing dangerous products (e.g., concentrated potassium chloride, hypertonic saline) from patient care areas is an example of an inventory management function that because of some highly publicized cases has only recently become standard practice.

Thinking of medication use in terms of a multistep process or system is critical to being able to understand and develop strategies to improve medication safety (Tables 33.1 and 33.2). It is also essential to have an understanding of which phases of the medication use process are associated with the most medication errors and ADEs. Bates and coworkers used a four-phase medication use model to categorize the potential and preventable ADEs that were detected using an intensive surveillance process.[13] These four phases were ordering, transcription, dispensing, and administration. In this study, the majority of preventable and potential ADEs occurred in the ordering and administration phases (49%

TABLE 33.1 Common Sources of Medication Error

Ambiguous orders	Incorrect drug selected
Drug device use	Incorrect patient
Environmental stress	Insufficient drug information
Errors in communication/miscommunication of drug orders	Insufficient information about other drugs patient is on (therapeutic duplication)
Error-prone abbreviation	Insufficient laboratory information
Illegible handwriting	Known allergy
Improper dose	Limited patient education
Incomplete orders	Limited staff education
Incomplete/insufficient monitoring	Look-alike or sound-alike drugs
Incomplete patient information/patient information unavailable	Poor communication

TABLE 33.2 Common Strategies for Preventing Errors in Each Phase of the Medication Use Process

Purchasing/Inventory Management

Purchase products from different manufacturers (if possible) for products with similar packaging.

Streamline order procurement process; use bar code restocking. Routine expiration date checking system is in place.

Dangerous products such as concentrated solutions (e.g., potassium chloride, hypertonic saline) are not stored in patient care areas.

Ordering/Prescribing

Implement computerized prescriber order entry.

Computer system is utilized for documentation of drug allergies and screening profiles for allergies or cross-sensitivities.

Allergy information is clearly documented in the chart and is readily retrievable (e.g., including allergy information on top of all inpatient medication ordering forms).

Forcing functions are printed on inpatient order forms or on prescription pads.

Maximize use of preprinted order sets for frequently prescribed orders.

Preprinted forms undergo multidisciplinary development and review.

A list of prohibited dangerous abbreviations is incorporated into employee training programs and order forms.

Orders such as "resume pre-op medications" or "resume home medications" are prohibited.

Verbal or telephone orders from prescribers who are on-site in the hospital are used only in true emergencies or during sterile procedures when ungloving and ungowning are impractical.

(*continues*)

TABLE 33.2 Common Strategies for Preventing Errors in Each Phase of the Medication Use Process (*Continued*)

Pharmacist obtains complete drug history, including all prescription, OTC, and herbal/alternative therapies, illicit drug use, and immunization status.

Incorporate a pharmacist on the patient care units.

Ensure sufficient access to current drug information resources.

Circulate physician-directed newsletters.

Implement electronic medical records.

Laboratory results are available at time of prescribing.

Verbal orders for chemotherapy are never used.

Doses are adjusted for specific populations (e.g., pediatrics, elderly, patients with renal and/or hepatic impairment).

Dispensing

Automatic counting machines are used when filling prescriptions.

Entering information into the allergy field is a required function that cannot be bypassed before entering the order.

Pharmacy computer system screens medication profile against known allergies for potential problems or cross-sensitivities.

Bar-coded medication selection exists.

Dose-range checking is a feature of the pharmacy computer system.

Alerts are built into the computer software regarding look-alike/sound-alike drugs.

Products with look-alike drug packaging or look-alike drug names are stored separately, not alphabetically.

Alternatively, look-alike and sound-alike drugs are flagged on the shelf.

Pharmacy order entry shall occur prior to nursing staff access in automated dispensing systems.

Administration

High-risk medication policies and procedures are in place.

All inpatient drug orders are reviewed by a pharmacist before being administered. If unable to be verified by a pharmacist, an independent double-check system is utilized.

Medication administration records are available at the bedside.

Medications should not be removed from their containers in advance of the time they are to be administered.

Limit the variety of devices and equipment. Eliminate free-flow infusion pumps.

Point-of-care technology that features bar coding is used to verify patient identity.

Patient wristband is verified before each medication is administered.

TABLE 33.2 Common Strategies for Preventing Errors in Each Phase of the Medication Use Process (*Continued*)

Monitoring
Provide educational brochure with tips patients can use to prevent errors in the inpatient and ambulatory setting.
Educate patients about new drug therapy prior to administration of the first dose. Incorporate monitoring parameters into preprinted orders.
Miscellaneous
Improve training on the medication use process/system and how and when to report medication errors (incorporate into new employee orientation; incorporate into competency programs). Make sure training is consistent across all disciplines.
Communicate to staff about known medication errors from outside organizations. Educate staff about strategies to prevent medication errors.
Improve interdisciplinary communication. Embrace a nonpunitive culture.
Ensure an adequate work environment (e.g., sufficient light).
Develop computerized event monitoring that screens for signals that an error may have occurred.
Provide psychological support and counseling to professionals involved in an error.
New products should be screened for their error potential before being added to the formulary.
When drugs with heightened error potential are identified during the formulary review process, standardized order forms, prescribing guidelines, and/or some other limitations on use are instituted before initial use.
For recently approved formulary drugs that have been on the market less than 6 months, the literature is scanned to identify published errors or adverse drug reactions that may have been reported.

and 26%, respectively). The dispensing and transcription phases were associated with 14% and 11% of the preventable and potential ADEs, respectively. When only medication errors that caused patient harm were considered (i.e., preventable ADEs), 56% occurred during the ordering phase, 34% during administration, 6% during transcription, and 4% during dispensing. These data suggest that system changes aimed at improving the ordering and administration phases of the medication use process are likely to have the greatest impact on reducing medication errors and preventable ADEs. The high incidence of preventable ADEs in the ordering phase is one of the major reasons why a well-designed CPOE system is touted as being so critical to improving the safety of the medication use process.

The study by Bates and colleagues also confirmed that errors were more likely to be intercepted if they occurred early in the process.[13] If errors occurred later in the medication use process, they were far less likely to be detected, as evidenced by the fact that no administration errors were intercepted in this study. This finding, coupled with the fact that the administration phase had the second highest incidence of preventable ADEs, reinforces the need for appropriate double checks in the administration process and, if possible, the use of point-of-care bar code scanning technology to build another layer of protection into the medication use system.

Although a macro-level view of the medication use process has been presented thus far, more complicated models of the process do exist. The medication use system in hospitals is inherently complex, often containing more than 100 steps with multiple handoffs. Flowcharting the existing medication use process lays the foundation for a systems approach to medication errors and preventable adverse drug events. Flowcharting the process also helps to illustrate weaknesses and unnecessary steps in the existing system and can help identify the multiple points in the system where breakdowns could occur and cause errors.

Systems Approach

Historically, medical and medication errors have been viewed as individual human failure. Punishing individuals for their mistakes was, and in some cases still is, common. Consequently, many healthcare practitioners are reluctant to report their mistakes or the errors of coworkers. However, a medication error is rarely the result of just one individual. It usually is the end result of a chain reaction of events that is fueled by faulty system design. Poor systems not only contribute to and make errors more likely, but can also make errors more difficult to detect and correct.

In developing a systems approach to reducing medication errors and preventable ADEs, it is important to understand the concepts of active and latent error. Active errors are usually visible because they occur on the "sharp end" (i.e., on the front lines of practice). Consequently, active errors generally garner the most attention and are the ones that tend to result in punishment and reprimand of healthcare professionals. However, even more important than active errors are latent errors. Latent errors are far more insidious than active errors and can include faulty design, bad management decisions, and poorly structured systems. Latent errors tend to occur on the "blunt end" and are difficult to associate with individual practitioners because their effects are not immediately felt. Often, latent error is inadvertently introduced into the system as a consequence of other decisions or changes in the system.

Latent errors are a real threat to organizations and their medication safety campaigns because they are difficult to detect and because they can result in several types of active errors. Therefore, to have a meaningful impact on the safety of the medication use system, latent error and failure need to be aggressively sought out and eliminated.

Because human beings are a key component of the medication use process, it is inevitable that mistakes will occur. One way to maximize the safety of the medication use system is to make it difficult for individuals to commit errors by building in double checks and other redundancies to ensure that any errors that do occur are detected and corrected before they reach the patient. It may be helpful to think of medication errors using an analogy of Swiss cheese. This analogy has been described elsewhere.[19] Each layer of safeguards and double checks in the medication use process can be thought of as a slice of Swiss cheese. Ideally, these layers of defense would be impenetrable; however, in actual practice, the defenses are usually flawed and contain one or more holes.

Even though safer systems tend to have more safeguards and layers of defense (i.e., slices of cheese), errors can still occur when a series of failures align to produce disaster. The *Challenger* disaster is an example of a situation in which several faults aligned to produce tragic results. By themselves, the unexpected cold weather or the brittle O-ring seals would not have caused the accident; however, the combination of these occurrences along with the presence of other contributing factors resulted in tragedy.

Another way to improve the safety of the medication use process is to incorporate human factors principles whenever possible. Human factors research in the healthcare setting has only recently begun to develop. Other industries, such as the nuclear power industry and the airline industry, have done an excellent job of examining why humans make mistakes and developing strategies to prevent them. Some of the core concepts and principles that have resulted from research in preventing errors in other industries include simplifying and standardizing processes; reducing reliance on memory; using constraints and forcing functions; improving information access; decreasing reliance on vigilance; increasing feedback; reducing handoffs; and sensibly using protocols. One way to think of human factors is to consider a statement eloquently articulated by James Reason: "We can't change the human condition, but we can change the condition under which humans work."

Medication Error Reporting

Obtaining accurate data on where medication errors and preventable ADEs occur in the system and ascertaining what system factors contributed to the error are critical to being able to develop strategies to minimize and prevent similar occurrences in the future. All too often, the reported medication error rate is only a small fraction of the actual medication error rate within an institution. The invisible, or unreported, errors tend to reflect the near misses and other potential ADEs that do not cause patient harm either because of chance or because they are detected before they reach the patient. These unreported or underreported errors are some of the most critical errors because understanding why they occurred and developing strategies for preventing similar occurrences in the future can lead to substantial improvements in the safety of the medication use process.

There are a number of reasons why healthcare professionals are reluctant to report actual and potential medication errors. The most common reason cited for not reporting incidents was that it was unnecessary—either the circumstances of the case did not warrant reporting or else the healthcare professional did not feel that incident reporting ultimately improves the quality of patient care.[20] Other common reasons given for not reporting errors include lack of time to complete a report when an incident is discovered, fear of discipline or other repercussions, the perception that only severe incidents require reporting (i.e., there is no need to report near misses), and a lack of familiarity with the reporting process.

Although a large portion of this chapter focuses on a health system's approach to improving medication safety, the literature has demonstrated that errors occur in all practice settings (e.g., hospitals, physician offices, emergency departments, nursing homes). Many of the error prevention strategies discussed in this chapter apply to nearly every practice setting.

TECHNOLOGY

The term *technology* refers to anything that is used to replace routine or repetitive tasks previously performed by people, or which extends the capability of people. The term *automation* refers to any technology, machine, or device linked to or controlled by a computer and used to do work. Automation can be designed to streamline and improve the accuracy and efficiency of the medication use process. All automation is technology, but the inverse is not necessarily true.

Although information technologies and automated medication systems are widely used in health systems and are integral components of the first IOM report and the Leapfrog Group recommendations, very little data are available regarding their impact on patient safety. The only exception to this is computerized prescriber order entry (CPOE) with computerized clinical decision support. Other technologies, such as using robotic technology to fill medication doses, bar coding of medications, automated dispensing devices, and computerized medication administration records, are much more widely implemented than CPOE systems, yet their reported impact on reducing medication errors and preventable ADEs is variable at best. Implementing new technology can create major infrastructure changes that introduce new sources of error, and some vendors market their products without sufficient testing or without being able to fully implement the technology as advertised. Nevertheless, all of these systems intuitively show promise in their potential to reduce medication error. If properly integrated, all of these systems should ultimately improve patient safety and will likely be incorporated into most medication use systems of the future.

Technology has the potential to reduce medication errors by reducing complexity, simplifying and standardizing processes, avoiding over-reliance on memory, and improving efficiency. However, technology by itself will rarely prevent medication errors. Rather, it must be effectively integrated into the existing medication use system and appropriately managed for it to positively affect patient safety. In fact, if technology is not used properly, it can prolong a system of errors and introduce dangerous new ones. Implementing technology within a previously suboptimal manual system will most often yield a suboptimal automated system. Without a comprehensive system to ensure that patients are getting their drugs and dosages correctly and on time, errors will continue to occur. In anticipation of the implementation of new technology, policies and procedures must be modified to ensure that a safe and proper infrastructure continues to exist for medication purchasing, ordering, preparation, dispensing, administering, and monitoring. After all, technology does not preclude the need for safety checks and verification for appropriateness.

Health systems are often unrealistic in what they expect from technology. Technology can instill a false sense of security, leading to carelessness by healthcare professionals. For instance, healthcare professionals often neglect to exercise sound double- and triple-check procedures with medications obtained from automated dispensing devices because of an over-reliance on the technology. To avoid such problems, it is critical that all personnel be adequately educated so that they understand that technology cannot completely substitute for human safety checks. Additionally, managers must make certain that staff levels are not overly reduced in response to system automation and that staff are not forced to work at a pace that precludes the ability to deliver safe and effective health care. With all technology, it is absolutely critical that appropriate quality control systems exist to ensure its accurate and safe use.

This section briefly describes the advantages, disadvantages, and issues surrounding the use of several existing technologies that (if appropriately deployed) can help improve the safety of the medication use process. This section describes only those technologies thought to have the greatest potential impact on patient safety, and is not designed to be inclusive. More extensive reviews of automated technologies and their impact on the medication use process exist elsewhere.[21]

Desired Features for Reducing Errors

There is little doubt that the innovative and appropriate use of technology within the medication use process can significantly improve patient safety. Furthermore, it is reasonable to draw four conclusions about information technology and automation as they apply to preventing medication errors.

1. The use of bar-coded medications should be maximized throughout the medication use process, including the administration and documentation phase of the process.
2. Information technologies can be used to analyze and prevent medication errors. For instance, sophisticated pharmacy or CPOE systems may be integrated with patient-specific laboratory and nursing clinical documentation systems to identify adverse drug events and medication errors when they occur. Analyzing data from such integrated systems will provide better data for trends analysis than existing manual medication error reporting systems, thus enabling the development of systems for measuring and managing adverse drug events

and the clinical and economic implications thereof. Additionally, potential errors identified by electronic prescribing and point-of-care scanning devices could be analyzed for common problems to facilitate minimization and elimination of recurring root causes of potential errors within organizations.

3. Automated dispensing systems, especially those incorporating the use of bar code technology, have the potential to improve medication dispensing accuracy and patient safety.
4. Aggressive implementation of CPOE will improve patient safety, as long as the system incorporates appropriate computerized decision support and is properly designed, implemented, and maintained.

Decentralized Automated Dispensing Devices

Decentralized automated dispensing systems, sometimes referred to as unit-based dispensing cabinets, are secure storage cabinets capable of handling most unit-dose and some bulk (multiple-dose) medications.* These devices are typically connected via a real-time interface to the hospital's pharmacy computer system in an attempt to maintain control over drug dispensing. Automated dispensing devices were originally installed in hospitals in the late 1980s and early 1990s to provide increased control over controlled substances and floor stock medications in patient care areas. In addition to their traditional uses, many hospitals now use these devices for storing and dispensing nearly all medication doses, thereby eliminating the manual medication cart-fill and delivery process.

The primary focus of these automated dispensing systems is to provide prompt, real-time availability of medications for nurses and patients. They can also help to improve controlled substance accountability, increase productivity, improve charge capture and documentation accuracy, and reduce pharmacy and nursing labor costs. However, the impact of these decentralized automated dispensing systems on medication errors is less clear. Decentralized dispensing devices are increasingly incorporating bar code labeling and scanning into the replenishment process, thus improving restocking accuracy and potentially improving medication safety. Also, the use of automated dispensing systems can result in pharmacists not having to check manually filled medication carts and first doses and can result in the redeployment of pharmacists to patient care units to engage in clinical activities that optimize the safety and efficacy of medication use.

As with any technology, there is the potential for increased errors associated with the use of automated dispensing systems. For instance, purchasing an insufficient number of cabinets may preclude an institution's ability to maintain a truly efficient system, resulting in a higher potential for product selection and administration errors. Despite increasing pressure from The Joint Commission and other interested parties, most organizations have yet to link their pharmacy computer systems to cabinets in such a way that restricts nurses from obtaining medications that are not ordered for patients. Other medication administration safety concerns with automated dispensing devices include the following:

- Nurses may retrieve an incorrect medication because of open access to all drugs in a drawer.
- Carelessness or lack of verification of drug labels may occur because of a belief that the system is computerized and therefore not susceptible to errors (or the belief that the pharmacy placed the drug there and the pharmacy does not make mistakes).
- Changing the location of the drug in the cabinet may cause errors because

*Examples of automated dispensing systems currently on the market include Pyxis, AcuDose, OmniCell, and Sure-Med.

the healthcare professional may choose drugs from particular locations by habit rather than verifying each drug's identity.

- Drugs may be stocked in the wrong pocket either because one or more doses inadvertently fell into the wrong slot or because of a pharmacy restocking error.

Conflicting reports exist in the literature on the impact of automated dispensing devices on medication error rates.[22-24] Unfortunately, significant capital investments have been made in these systems without full evaluation of the operational changes needed to ensure that efficiency goals were met without compromising patient safety. Regardless of whether state regulations exist to ensure safe use of automated dispensing systems, it is extremely important that every organization develop, enforce, and continuously improve multidisciplinary policies and procedures to ensure patient safety, accuracy, security, and confidentiality. Table 33.3 provides an extensive list of guidelines and considerations for the safe use of decentralized automated dispensing systems.

Centralized Robotics for Dispensing Medications

Centrally located automated dispensing devices are designed to automate the entire process of medication dispensing, including medication storage, dispensing, restocking, and crediting of unit-dose medications.* An interface must be created with the pharmacy information system to provide the centralized dispensing device with access to each patient's medication profile. Bar coding of medication doses allows dispensing accuracy to approach 100% with centralized robotics technology. Thus, as long as a patient-specific computerized medication profile is maintained in an accurate and timely manner, pharmacists may be freed from medication-checking duties.

The centralized robotic system was traditionally used exclusively to dispense unit-dose bar-coded medications for scheduled medication cart filling; however, several organizations have recently expanded the use of this technology to include automation of first-dose dispensing. Another recent expanded use of this technology is its ability to pick medication doses to be restocked in decentralized automated dispensing cabinets. This has the potential to reduce medication administration errors by improving restocking accuracy.

Potential advantages of robotics include reducing pharmacy labor costs; eliminating certain technical tasks of pharmacists, allowing for their redeployment to perform clinical activities; and improving medication dispensing accuracy. No published data are available on these advantages, but in one unpublished study a robot decreased the dispensing error rate from 2.9% to 0.6%.[25] However, this improved dispensing accuracy has never been proved to result in improved patient safety since nurses still have open access to all robot-dispensed medications after they are distributed to patient care areas.

Perhaps the greatest advantage of implementing robotic technology is that all doses dispensed by the robot are bar coded, thus facilitating the implementation of point-of-care drug administration and documentation scanning systems. However, the necessity for bar codes on all medications dispensed by the robot has the potential to introduce new error into the medication use system. Although some manufacturers provide bar-coded medications, most unit-dose medications must be accurately repackaged and bar coded by the pharmacy department.

In addition to the automated dispensing devices that exist for hospitals, dispensing systems for ambulatory and retail pharmacies

*The two most prevalent systems on the market are Robot-Rx (McKesson) and the ATC-212 and ATC-Profile (Automed Technologies, Inc.). Other centralized automated dispensing systems exist, but currently are in the alpha- and beta-testing stages.

TABLE 33.3 Guidelines for Safe Use of Decentralized Automated Dispensing Systems

Agree with the vendor on a documented preventive maintenance schedule that does not disrupt workflow.
Any high-risk medications stocked in devices should be accompanied by an alert system for nurses (such as a maximum-dose prompt).
Carefully select stored drugs based on the needs of the patient care unit, patient age, diagnosis, and staff expertise.
Conduct monthly expiration date checks, concomitantly verifying inventory accuracy. Configure devices to provide single-dose (or single-drug) access whenever possible, focusing such control on high-risk medications and controlled substances. Develop an ongoing competency assessment program for all personnel who use or affect the system, including direct observation and random restocking accuracy audits, as well as observation of dispensing accuracy as part of the assessment.
Develop a system to remove all recalled medications.
Develop clear, multidisciplinary system downtime procedures that are included in an ongoing competency program.
Develop strict safety criteria for selecting medications that are (and are not) appropriate for storing in devices.
Develop systems to account for narcotic waste, and routinely audit controlled substance dispenses versus patient orders and medication administration records.
Do not stock look-alike and sound-alike drugs in the same open-access drawer.
Have strict security procedures to limit unauthorized access.
Place allergy reminders for specific drugs such as antibiotics, opiates, and NSAIDs on appropriate drug storage pockets, or have them automatically appear on the dispensing screen.
Require all personnel to attend formal training and demonstrate competency prior to assigning them access to the system.
Require nurses to return medications to a return bin, never back to the original storage pocket or location.
Require pharmacist medication order review and approval before administration of the first dose of medication (profile dispensing), and limit medications in which profile dispensing may be overridden.
Use open-access drawers only for stocking drugs with low potential for causing patient harm if administered in error.
Whenever possible, use bar coding capabilities for restocking medications and for retrieval.
With few exceptions, maximize use of unit-dose medications in ready-to-administer form.

that automate the filling of individual patient prescriptions exist.* Adoption of these technologies in community pharmacies has been limited by their high cost and space requirements. Nevertheless, the advantage of these automated dispensing devices for ambulatory pharmacies is that medication dispensing errors are reduced by automating manual tasks such as counting, pouring, and filling. Furthermore, most of these technologies offer visual imaging systems that help the pharmacist verify the appropriateness of the medication being dispensed.

*Some of the systems on the market are Baker Cells (McKesson), QuickScript (Automed Technologies), Optifill II (Automed Technologies), and Pharmacy 2000 (McKesson).

Point-of-Care Bedside Medication Charting Systems and Bar Coding

Point-of-care technology enables caregivers to enter and retrieve patient-specific data in an electronic format at the bedside. Advanced portable medication scanners are used by nurses at the point of care to electronically verify and document medication administration.* Some of the devices utilize wireless handheld personal digital assistant (PDA) technology to increase their portability. The point-of-care technology receives real-time patient information and medication profiles from the pharmacy computer system, usually by way of a radio frequency network. When a medication order is initiated, modified, or discontinued in the pharmacy computer system, the order information is updated into the point-of-care system. For all scheduled doses, the device alerts the nurse when it is time to administer the medication.

To ensure accurate medication administration and documentation, these point-of-care systems require the scanning of three items prior to medication administration: the bar code on the medication dose, the caregiver's unique bar code (often on the nurse's name badge), and the patient's unique bar code identifier (often a wristband). These point-of-care systems ensure the "five R's" of medication administration: right patient, right drug, right dose, right time, and right route. When the nurse scans the medication he or she is planning to administer, that medication is electronically compared to the patient's medication profile. These point-of-care systems can identify incorrect and omitted medications and alert the nurse in real time if a physician has cancelled or changed a patient's medication order. This technology offers the potential to dramatically reduce the risk of drug administration errors. Organizations that have implemented this technology report that between 5% and 10% of all doses scanned result in one of the following discrepancies: wrong patient, wrong drug, wrong dose, wrong time, or wrong route.

Although improvements are being made in point-of-care patient information systems and electronic medication administration records (MARs), effectively implementing these systems can be costly and complicated. Major limitations to implementing point-of-care technology include the following:

- The cost of the devices is high.
- All medications must be bar coded to achieve the optimal safety benefit (usually requiring labor-intensive and potentially error-prone repackaging in the pharmacy).
- Commercial products are still at a very early stage of development.
- Nursing workflow redesign issues exist.
- Elaborate interfaces between information systems are necessary to ensure accurate patient records on the point-of-care system.
- Installation of a dedicated radio frequency network within the hospital may be incompatible with certain patient monitoring devices in the hospital.

These stated limitations and incompatibilities have limited the use of point-of-care technologies in many healthcare settings.

Because one of the major limitations of point-of-care technology is bar coding all medications, a cursory understanding of the information contained in a bar code is necessary. A bar code is simply a method of encoding numbers and letters by using a combination of bars and spaces with varying widths stacked side by side in such a way that the scanner interprets the rows as data. Each bar code has specific identification encoded in it, and those data are used by a computer/scanner to look up all specific information associated with the code. Bar codes on medications contain specific information about that drug, including but not limited to the product name, dose, dosage, form, route of administration, expiration date, and lot number. A critical component of a bar code

*Some of the systems on the market are AcuScan-Rx, Autros, Bridge Medical Medication Management System, BD-Rx, and PYXISVERI5.

system is the scanner's ability to quickly and accurately interpret the bar code data, which depends on two criteria: the quality of the bar code print on the product and the symbology of the bar code. The space available on most unit-dose packages is limited, yet some manufacturers have been able to successfully bar code these products.

Bar coding of drugs would seem to be useful for reducing errors because it can help to rapidly ensure that the drug at hand is actually the intended one. The major barrier to implementing bar codes on all medications is the lack of consensus among pharmaceutical manufacturers on the appropriate approach for adding bar coding to unit-dose product labels. Currently, no universal standard bar code symbology has been adopted for medications. However, in August 2000, the National Coordinating Council for Medication Error Reporting and Prevention (NCCMERP) organized a meeting of pharmacy organizations, information technology vendors, pharmaceutical manufacturers, and other interested parties to facilitate a dialogue for developing a standardized bar code symbology. The NCCMERP later disseminated a white paper entitled *Promoting and Standardizing Bar Coding on Medication Packaging: Reducing Errors and Improving Patient Care*. In 2002, the Food and Drug Administration worked to further develop a proposal that would require a bar code on the label of all drug and biological products for human use. Then, in early 2003, Pfizer announced that it would place bar codes on each of its unit-of-use packaged products. However, until standards exist for bar coding, the ability of many scanning devices to accurately scan all products may be severely limited. Symbology standardization within health care is essential in order for bar code technology to be applied successfully throughout the medication use process.

Computerized Prescriber Order Entry

CPOE is a system in which prescribers enter medication and other orders (e.g., laboratory and radiology) for patients via an electronic software application. CPOE probably has the greatest potential of any technology for reducing medication errors. However, for a CPOE system to prevent errors other than those due to illegible handwriting, the system must have the following critical characteristics:

- Relevant patient-specific information (e.g., demographic data, laboratory and diagnostic test results) must be readily available at the time of prescribing or order entry.
- Drug–drug interaction, drug-allergy, drug–laboratory, drug contraindication, and maximum/minimum dosing alerts for potentially serious mistakes must be provided. These alerts must be carefully established so that they are not easily overridden. Furthermore, the sensitivity of these alerts must be set such that clinically insignificant alerts are minimized. Otherwise, if prescribers are frequently alerted with nonsignificant warnings, they may become desensitized to all alerts and may then miss the clinically significant warnings.
- The selection of standard order sets (medication use algorithms and guidelines for high-risk patient populations) should be automated at the point of prescribing.
- The system must be efficient and easy to use. If the system is too complex and it takes too long to learn all the nuances and intricacies, physician compliance with implementing and maximizing the use of the CPOE system will suffer.

Although ideal, systems that fulfill these criteria are uncommon. One published study[26] demonstrated that serious medication errors fell 55% following implementation of a CPOE system, while the rate of all errors fell 83% in another study.[27] Most inpatient physician order entry systems currently on the market provide the benefit of improved prescription legibility and medication turnaround time, but they are inefficient in that they often require a high level of pharmacist intervention, including reentering of medication orders. Although such systems may result in the reduction of some errors by simply computerizing the process, they do not provide the physician with the necessary clinical information and decision support at the point of decision making that would result in the greatest impact on error reduction. Literature documenting the "efficient" use of computerized prescriber medication order entry systems is limited. Most successful systems have been home-grown and have not achieved the theoretical safety benefits of an integrated system that incorporates pharmacy, laboratory, and other patient-specific clinical information into one database. Some commercially available pharmacist computer order entry systems exist that provide some of the ideal capabilities listed earlier, but commercially available integrated systems for physicians are in the very early stages of development.

A few guidelines for maximizing the likelihood of successful implementation of an inpatient physician order entry system include the following:

- Use a unique prescriber order entry system, *not* a modified pharmacist order entry system. Physicians generally do not think like pharmacists, nor will they have the time to pay attention to the high level of detail required in most pharmacy order entry systems.
- Identify physician project champions at a very high level in the organization and involve them in the decision-making and planning process from the very beginning.
- Set realistic time frame expectations and make sure the implementation team is multidisciplinary.
- Pay close attention to the process and the flow of information in the proposed CPOE system.
- Plan on 5 or more years of system development and enhancement after the product is initially piloted.
- Do not be discouraged by initial dissatisfaction among physicians, and do not interpret initial negative reactions as failure. Physician transition may be easier in a teaching hospital versus a private or nonteaching hospital. More experienced physicians are sometimes less eager to embrace the change unless they can enter orders from their office during the course of the day as test results become available for their inpatients. In teaching hospitals, resident physicians are generally more adaptable and can usually be required to make the change.

Over the past few years, great strides have been taken to improve ambulatory CPOE technologies. Many physicians are using PDA-based prescribing devices to directly link themselves with dispensing pharmacies at the time the prescription is written. These systems essentially replace the traditional paper prescription pad. The capabilities of these systems include fast prescription processing with few keystrokes, online claim submission within 20 seconds, provision of generic alternatives, dosing and allergy alerts, prescribing histories, and plan-specific formulary recommendations and therapeutic alternatives (many systems contain formulary information from nearly 800 plans).

Medication Use Process Strategic Plan Within a Health System

Historically, automation had to result in proven cost reduction, quality improvement, improved service, and increased efficiency to be deemed successful. Although expense continues to be one of the major barriers to implementing new technologies, the 1999 IOM report and other news media have persuaded many organizations to invest heavily in new technologies that improve patient safety. For example, Allina Health System in Minneapolis, Minnesota, has committed $25 million to the development and implementation of an integrated CPOE and bar-coded medication administration system over the next 5 years. Integrated health systems should not view automation and technology as a means to an end, but rather as a series of sophisticated tools to help them optimize the medication use process. The value achieved by implementing new technology within organizations depends primarily on three factors: the efficiency of the system being replaced, the level of detail applied to managing and making the most of the system following implementation, and cooperation between departments to ensure the success of the system.

Within most hospitals, there is consensus that the inpatient medication use process should be automated, but there are many questions and much debate as to the best way to automate the process. There is no right or wrong answer, and any of the previously discussed approaches can succeed or fail, depending on how well they are managed. Suggested characteristics of an ideal system will likely include patient care and safety benefits, responsiveness to customer needs, cost-effectiveness, and ability to leverage the purchase of other existing and pending technologies. It is very important that decision makers evaluate the clinical, cost, and safety advantages and disadvantages of competing technologies, as well as safety claims made by the manufacturer, before reaching a final purchase decision. Table 33.4 lists ideal features to ensure patient safety throughout the medication use process, regardless of which automated technologies are employed.

TABLE 33.4 Desired Safety Features for Incorporating Technology into the Medication Use Process

All actions and usage on a system must be reportable in an easily reviewed format, including identification of the user, the medication, the patient for whom the drug was dispensed, and the time of the transaction.
At medication administration, one system must be able to identify and document the medication, person administering the medication, and patient by utilizing bar code technology.
Hospital admit/discharge/transfer and medication order entry computer systems should be interfaced with automation devices to provide caregivers with warnings about allergies, interactions, duplications, and inappropriate doses at the point of dispensing and/or administration.
Information necessary to properly manage patient care must be accurate, accessible, and timely.
Pertinent patient- and medication-specific information and instructions entered into pharmacy and/or hospital information systems should be available electronically at the point of care (administration), and the system should prompt the nurse to record pertinent information before administration may be documented.
Real-time systems integration should exist from the point of prescribing (order entry) through dispensing and through documentation of medication administration.
The system must accommodate bar-coded unit-dose medications and utilize the bar code capability for drug restocking, retrieval, and administering medications.
The system should force users to confirm their intention whenever medications are accessed or administration is attempted outside of the scheduled administration time or dosage range. Such events should be signaled visibly or audibly for the user, and all such events should be electronically documented and reported daily for follow-up.
The interface with the pharmacy computer system should allow the nurse to view and access only those medications that have been ordered for the specific patient.
The nurse should be electronically reminded when a medication dose is due (and by a different mechanism when it is past due).
User access should be restricted to a unique user identification code and password, or a unique bar code.

MAXIMIZING MEDICATION USE SAFETY WITHIN AN INTEGRATED HEALTH SYSTEM: THE UNIVERSITY OF WISCONSIN HOSPITAL AND CLINICS MODEL

The University of Wisconsin Hospital and Clinics (UWHC) is an integrated health system that consists of UW Hospital, UW Children's Hospital, UW Comprehensive Cancer Center, University Community Clinics, University Physicians and Physicians Plus, Unity Health Plans, and Chartwell Wisconsin. The hospital is a 471-bed academic tertiary medical center. UW Hospital consistently ranks among the finest academic medical centers in the country, with centers of excellence in organ transplant, hematology/oncology, ophthalmology, HIV, and critical care. There were nearly 130,000 patient-days in fiscal year 2002, with an average daily census of about 390 patients (not including observation patients).

Approximately 214 full-time equivalents work within the Department of Pharmacy at the University of Wisconsin Hospital and Clinics. Comprehensive pharmacy services are provided at UWHC 24 hours a day. On weekdays, there are eight decentralized pharmacy teams, with 14 pharmacists covering these teams on the first shift and 9 pharmacists covering on the second shift. Weekend and holiday staffing features fewer teams and fewer pharmacists to offset the decreased patient volume. The night shift features one central pharmacist and one decentralized pharmacist who covers the ICUs and all hospital codes.

Decentralized pharmacy services are provided to every patient. The highest priority of decentralized pharmacists is to ensure safe and appropriate medication use. In addition, pharmacists assist in education and research and assist with quality improvement and cost-containment initiatives. Pharmacists perform a number of valuable clinical services on a daily basis, including medication admission histories, participation in daily work rounds with the different medical teams, therapeutic drug monitoring (e.g., renal dosing, pharmacokinetics, IV-to-oral conversion, antibiotic streamlining), and patient discharge counseling.

Through the years, the Department of Pharmacy at UWHC has taken great pride in being at the forefront of technological innovation and novel improvements in the medication use process. The hospital was one of the first in the country to fully implement a unit-of-use system in the late 1960s. In 1993, UWHC was the second hospital in the United States to implement a robotic cart-fill system that automated, streamlined, and improved the accuracy of the cart-fill process. In the current dispensing and distribution process, medications not filled by the robot are prepared in unit-of-use doses in the central pharmacy or in the sterile products area located within the central pharmacy. Narcotics as well as all floor stock and as-needed (PRN) medications are stored and dispensed from automated dispensing systems located in the patient care units.

The provision of safe, rational, and cost-effective therapy was a component of the pharmacy department's mission well before the first IOM report was released. With the release of that report and subsequent reports offering best-practice recommendations (e.g., the Advisory Board's *Prescription for Change* series), members of the pharmacy department have given multiple presentations to senior hospital administrators comparing the hospital's existing medication use system with best-practices recommendations found in the literature. The UWHC pharmacy department has found these presentations to be an excellent way to improve awareness of senior management and secure the necessary buy-in to make medication safety a hospital-wide initiative and priority. Benchmarking an organization's medication use processes with best practices described in the literature is also extremely valuable in that it helps identify areas for improvement.

There are several unique elements of the UWHC medication use process and hospital information system that are believed to make them extremely safe. These elements were in place well before the Institute of Medicine released its 1999 report and include the following:

- Pharmacist-conducted admission histories and discharge counseling for every patient.
- Unit doses of virtually all medications, including individual patient-specific doses of oral and injectable products, are prepared by the pharmacy.
- Pharmacy-maintained medication administration record (MAR) using computer-generated labels (except for one-time or nonrecurring medications, there is no hand transcription onto the MAR).
- Expanded roles for pharmacy technicians. The pharmacy technical support staff perform many functions performed by pharmacists in other institutions (e.g., order entry). This gives the pharmacists more time to complete clinical activities.
- Advanced clinical reference information readily available on the hospital intranet (e.g., Micromedex, Stat-Ref, full-text electronic journals).
- Advanced electronic repository with a substantial amount of patient information that is readily available on personal computers throughout the health system. (It should be emphasized that UWHC does not have a complete electronic medical record.)

Lucian Leape and colleagues identified drug knowledge dissemination and patient information availability as two of the most common system failures that lead to medication errors and preventable ADEs.[27] The last two items on this list address these areas.

Although the UWHC health system already has many key safety components incorporated into the medication use system, it is recognized that there still is significant room for improvement for UWHC to strive to achieve a zero-defect rate in its medication use process. To further enhance medication safety at UWHC, the pharmacy department has developed six guiding principles:

1. Improve organizational awareness about medication safety by providing education to healthcare professionals and hospital administrators.
2. Improve medication error reporting and root cause analysis.
3. Foster and promote a nonpunitive culture regarding medication errors within the organization.
4. Maximize the appropriate use of new technologies by standardizing systems and incorporating best demonstrated practices for safety.
5. Enhance collaboration across all disciplines.
6. Continue to leverage and maximize the use of decentralized clinical pharmacists.

Medication Safety Committee

The Medication Safety Committee is a multidisciplinary subcommittee of the Pharmacy and Therapeutics (P&T) Committee. Initially called the Medication Error Committee, the committee's name was changed and its membership expanded shortly after the release of the 1999 IOM report. The membership expansion and the name change were intended to reflect an expanded systems approach to medication safety. In August 2000, an afternoon-long retreat was organized to provide sufficient time to develop a strategic plan and mission statement that would help define the expanded scope and focus of the committee. The committee accomplished three objectives during its retreat:

1. A summary of key medication use safety principles, literature, and national recommendations was presented to the group.
2. A mission statement was developed (Table 33.5).
3. An extensive list of potential system improvements that could maximize patient safety was identified.

TABLE 33.5 Mission Statement of the UWHC Medication Safety Committee

Medication Safety

- Oversee and maximize the safety of the medication use process throughout the UWHC continuum of care by incorporating fail-safe procedures and safety surveillance systems.
- Ensure systems are in place to conduct and review root cause analysis and trends for reported medication errors and preventable adverse drug events. Facilitate implementation and monitoring of system changes to help prevent similar events in the future.

Medication Error Reporting

- Maintain simple, consistent reporting procedures for both actual and potential medication errors in all UWHC care areas.
- Ensure that a nonpunitive system exists so that fear of retribution is not a barrier to medication error reporting.

Awareness

- Increase healthcare practitioner and administrator awareness about medication safety.
- Ensure that employees know how the medication error reporting process works at UWHC.
- Increase consumer/patient awareness about medication safety.

The final objective, to identify medication safety initiatives that could be the focus of the committee during the subsequent year, was identified after the retreat. Each committee member ranked the possible system improvements identified during the retreat according to their potential impact and feasibility (i.e., time and resources necessary). The four highest-impact system improvements were (1) developing safety criteria for an ideal ambulatory and inpatient CPOE system to help guide the selection and implementation of this technology, (2) improving the medication error and ADE reporting form, (3) developing an electronic MAR using point-of-care technology, and (4) developing computerized maximum dosing alerts for high-alert drugs. The four most feasible system improvements were (1) having a clinical pharmacist in the emergency department (ED), (2) including a space on the medication error and ADE reporting form for employees to provide ideas for improving medication safety, (3) working with public affairs to promote medication safety initiatives to patients and the public, and (4) improving the dissemination of information included in the biweekly *Institute of Safe Medication Practices (ISMP) Medication Safety Alerts*.

These eight system improvements served as the focus of the committee for the subsequent year. The Medication Safety Committee now holds an annual afternoon-long retreat to review new published best practices, review occurrence trends, and develop annual committee goals based on impact and feasibility.

UWHC Medication Error Reporting Process Task Force

Improving the medication error and ADE reporting process was one of the high-impact initiatives identified during the Medication Safety Committee retreat. A multidisciplinary task force was formed with volunteers from the Medication Safety Committee to improve the medication error reporting process by redesigning the reporting form; developing a new hospital-wide, nonpunitive medication error/preventable ADE policy and procedure; and improving the tracking, trending, and analysis of medication error data.

The group began by redesigning the form used to report medication errors and other medication-related occurrences. The previous process for reporting medication-related incidents involved the use of a general Occurrence

Screen form that was also used to report a variety of non-drug-related incidents such as slips and falls, equipment malfunction, and incorrect blood administration. Some of the problems that were identified with the previous form included the following:

- The form lacked space for healthcare professionals to suggest ways to improve the medication use system.
- No mechanism was provided to distinguish actual from potential errors.
- Too much narrative and time were needed to complete the form.
- The form was not scannable.
- Very few reports were generated in the emergency department, operating room/recovery room, and ambulatory clinics.
- Attributable and root cause assessments were not incorporated into the form.

The process for following up on error reports was also not standardized, and the path for routing the form to the appropriate disciplines often was very convoluted. Consequently, follow-up on medication errors and report processing were often severely delayed.

The redesigned Medication Occurrence (Error) Report is now used for reporting actual and potential medication occurrences. A section has been incorporated into the form for suggesting system changes that could improve medication safety. A check box format exists throughout the form to minimize the time necessary to complete the form. The form prompts healthcare professionals to report the following characteristics of the occurrence: whether it is an actual or potential occurrence; the location; the practitioner(s)/staff involved; the timing; the suspected type of occurrence (e.g., incorrect dose, incorrect drug); the name, dose, and route of medication ordered compared to that given; the age of the patient; the source of the medication (e.g., automated dispensing device, patient's medication drawer); and the name and discipline of the person completing the report.

The revised reporting process also consists of a follow-up form that is completed by pharmacy managers. The sections on this form include assessment of the attributable system factors that contributed to the occurrence, assessment of the patient outcome (utilizing the NCCMERP scale), an assessment of any additional costs incurred, the category of medication(s) involved in the occurrence, and a section to record the follow-up actions taken. The follow-up section also utilizes a check box format and is completed for all reported occurrences and near misses.

The revised UWHC medication error occurrence policy and procedure incorporates many of the points already described. In addition, the policy also emphasizes that "the focus of the program is quality improvement, not punishment. UWHC assumes that practitioners are doing their very best and that occurrences are not the result of incompetence or misconduct." These statements reflect the organization's evolving nonpunitive systems approach to reporting errors. In the past, there have been instances in which medication errors have been used in the performance review of employees. However, using medication errors in employee performance reviews undermines efforts to encourage reporting. The task force realized that creating a nonpunitive organizational culture is an ongoing process that is not as simple as adding a statement to a policy. Unfortunately, all of the hard work invested to create the culture change can be undone by one instance in which an employee is disciplined or terminated for committing an error. Even one instance is enough to change employees' perceptions about the policy and suggests that the organization is not as committed to a nonpunitive culture as the policy implies.

Development of a database to facilitate the trending and analysis of medication occurrences is ongoing. UWHC participated as an alpha site with University HealthSystem Consortium to develop and test an anonymous online occurrence-reporting program. The goal of using the database to run queries and generate reports is to easily identify areas for potential system improvements and to communicate meaningful feedback to healthcare professionals. Preliminary experience with the system indicates that it makes reporting more convenient and efficient for staff, electronically prompts managers via an email message that follow-up is needed, prevents the need for data entry into a trending database, and automates the generation of useful trending reports. This program is now being utilized by 15 other academic medical centers who actively share data and learning about errors and error reduction.

Medication Ordering Performance Improvement Project

A multidisciplinary team was commissioned to develop and implement a standardized system for medication order initiation and implementation for all patient care areas at UWHC.* The original impetus for the project was to improve efficiency and minimize the time from when medication orders are written to the time that medication orders are entered into the pharmacy computer system.

The team approached the problem by flowcharting the existing ordering systems, in which orders could be stored, initiated, and implemented in one of three ways. Having three nonstandardized systems was one of over 30 problems identified with the UWHC medication ordering system. As the group began to explore strategies for improving the efficiency of the system, it quickly became clear that many of the system changes that would improve efficiency would also improve medication safety. For instance, standardizing systems, eliminating handoffs and unnecessary steps, improving training about the system, and improving interdisciplinary communication are all efficiency enhancers that are also best practices for improving medication safety.

*Please note that the new medication ordering system is not a CPOE system. It is a manual system with improved processes for flagging and processing orders.

One of the most valuable components of the new medication ordering system has been the requirement that all healthcare professionals attend a 30-minute training presentation and complete a competency examination on the new system before it is implemented on a given unit. The training describes the specifics of the new program and includes 10 minutes on safe order-writing practices (Table 33.6 lists some of the safe order-writing practices covered in the training program). The classes, especially the component of the class describing safe order-writing practices, have been very well received. A training video has also been developed to facilitate participation by healthcare professionals who primarily work on the third shift. The system was implemented housewide over a 12-month period. A Web-based medication ordering system training course and safe order-writing training course and accompanying competency test will be incorporated into new employee orientation for all clinical disciplines via the hospital's intranet.

High-Alert Medication Policy

High-alert drugs are broadly defined as those drugs that have a heightened potential for causing patient harm when misused. The UWHC P&T Committee has approved a policy and procedure identifying specific medications that will be considered high risk (e.g., neuromuscular blocking agents, dobutamine, dopamine, heparin, and insulin). The safety procedures incorporated into the high-alert policy and procedure are designed to minimize the potential for patient harm. These safety procedures include the following:

- Double-checking with another licensed professional occurs when the medication is being prepared from a multidose vial.
- Nurses complete a competency examination for appropriate high-alert medication administration procedures. The competency program is incorporated into new nurse orientation.

TABLE 33.6 Safe Order-Writing Practices

All orders are handwritten in ballpoint pen. Orders are never written in felt tip pen or pencil.

All the required elements of an order are included: patient name (or addressograph), generic name of medication, drug strength, dosage form, amount to be dispensed, complete directions for use, and signature/title. An optimal order would also include indication, duration of therapy (when applicable), and the prescriber's pager number.

Appropriate policies and procedures exist for verbal orders:

> Numbers should be communicated by pronouncing each numerical digit separately (e.g., "one three" instead of "thirteen").
>
> The healthcare professional (HCP) receiving the order should confirm the indication with the prescriber to verify that the medication makes sense for the patient.
>
> The HCP receiving the order should repeat the order back to the prescriber for verification.
>
> The HCP should record the order directly onto an order sheet in the patient's chart immediately.
>
> The HCP should time, date, and sign the orders per institution policy.
>
> The physician countersigns all verbal orders in a timely manner per institution policy.
>
> The use of verbal orders is minimized by limiting verbal orders to situations when the prescriber is with another patient and cannot leave (e.g., surgery) or when the prescriber is not in the hospital and direct physical assessment of the patient is not necessary.

Unfamiliar drug names should be verified by spelling out the name.

Verbal orders for chemotherapy are never accepted.

For institutions that utilize a duplicate or triplicate order form, orders must never be written on order forms when the duplicate and/or triplicate order form has already been pulled.

Indications are provided.

Leading zeros are used for any decimal expression of dosage less than 1 (e.g., 0.3 mg *not* .3 mg).

Medication orders are complete and contain no ambiguity. Examples of ambiguous orders include "continue previous medications," "take as directed," or "resume all pre-op medications."

Potentially dangerous abbreviations and medication abbreviations are prohibited.

Specify infusion rate when ordering IV solutions (TKO is not acceptable).

Specify the exact dosage strength rather than the dosage form unit when writing medication orders. (Do not use terms such as *one vial*, *one ampule*, *one tablet*, or *one bottle*. Many drugs have multiple strengths.)

Specify the salt when ordering electrolytes (e.g., calcium chloride vs. calcium gluconate).

Terminal zeros are never used when expressing doses (e.g., write 2 mg *not* 2.0 mg).

Weights, volumes, and units are expressed with the metric system. The apothecary system is not used.

- Nurses complete an annual competency examination for administering high-alert medications.
- At the end of each shift, on admission and transfer, the off-going and oncoming nurses check intravenous infusions of high-alert medications to ensure appropriateness (e.g., right medication, right patient, right infusion rate, and right medication concentration). The amount infused is also reset each shift.
- Infusion pumps are labeled with the name of the medication being infused by placing a label or piece of tape across the door of the pump.
- High-alert medications are specially labeled when they are dispensed from the pharmacy.
- The pockets of the automated dispensing cabinet that contain high-alert medications and the MAR for each high-alert medication are specially labeled to call attention to their high-alert status.

Chemotherapy medications are one group of high-alert medications. Within UWHC, a multidisciplinary chemotherapy quality improvement team standardized the chemotherapy administration process among all settings and populations (e.g., inpatients, outpatients, adults, pediatrics). This team also revised all UWHC chemotherapy policies, developed a new process for annual review of preprinted orders and order sets for investigational protocols, and developed a new chemotherapy order function that incorporated fields to help stimulate the provider to include all the required elements of a chemotherapy order.

Recheck Campaign

In response to several high-profile reports of healthcare professionals overrelying on automated dispensing systems, a campaign was designed to provide healthcare professionals with simple strategies to maximize medication administration accuracy and patient safety. Because of the multiple-check system required to ensure safe medication administration, the initiative is called the "Re-✓" campaign (Figure 33.2). The campaign was launched in the summer of 2001 as part of a hospital-wide medication safety awareness program. Laminated stop signs with the "Stop and Re-✓" phrase have been placed throughout the hospital in certain strategic areas (e.g., on the automated dispensing cabinet and other conspicuous locations in patient care areas). A Web-based training program is currently under development for all clinical disciplines to complete during new employee orientation via the hospital's intranet.

Abbreviations

One of the recommendations made by the Institute of Medicine was to "standardize prescription writing and prescribing rules." Minimizing the use of problem-prone abbreviations is one way to standardize prescription writing. As part of a citywide patient safety collaborative (please see the section "Citywide and Statewide Approach," later in this chapter), UWHC and the other hospitals in Madison are targeting the elimination of error-prone abbreviations (Table 33.7). UWHC collected baseline data and found the use of problem-prone abbreviations to be very prevalent.

To educate healthcare professionals about problem-prone abbreviations, an interactive educational session was developed for all UWHC healthcare professionals to complete on the hospital intranet. The training program is now mandatory and is included in the new nurse orientation, new pharmacist training, and the orientation for new house staff. Incorporating a safe prescription-writing course into the medical school curriculum is also being explored. In addition to the training programs, educational pocket cards were distributed to all clinicians to highlight the problem-prone abbreviations. Pharmacists provide timely feedback on actual error-prone abbreviation use directly to prescribers via an audit form. A duplicate of these forms is maintained in the quality improvement office for trending

FIGURE 33.2 A portion of the recheck campaign (*Continued*)

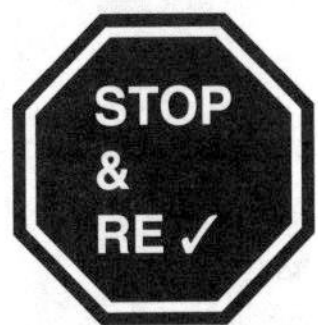

Check and re-check
Practice the "3-time check." First compare the medication label with the original order or patient kardex, second when preparing the medication for administration, and third just before giving the patient the medication. Keep drugs in their labeled packages until you are ready to administer them at the patient's bedside. Read all labels very carefully. Realize that two completely different medications may have very similar packages and even similar sounding names. Always check back with the physician or pharmacist if you cannot clearly read the order.

Engage the patient
Remind patients about the importance of proper identification before drug administration, and suggest that they actively participate by stating their name and holding out their name bracelet. Always verify patient identity via the patient's wristband (inpatient setting) and/or verbally by verifying the patient's name (ambulatory setting) before administering a medication. Additionally, one should verbally verify the drug name and purpose with the patient before administering the medication. Take the patient's concerns seriously. If a patient says a pill looks different than what he or she usually takes, double-check the medication identity and/or indication for that drug prior to administration. Additionally, perform all necessary monitoring before administering select medications (e.g., heart rate and blood pressure for beta blockers, blood sugar for antidiabetics, etc.).

Do not take automation for granted
Do not assume that the medication in the AcuDose™ cabinet is exactly the medication that has been ordered for the patient. Incorrect medications may be placed in the wrong location within the AcuDose™ cabinets or they may become dislodged from their correct storage pockets. Additionally, matrix drawer configurations allow for the wrong medication to be retrieved and dispensed if one is not careful. Except in emergency situations, first doses of medications stored in AcuDose™ cabinets should not be administered to patients until the pharmacist has reviewed and signed off on the medication order.

First do no harm
It is easy to be tempted to take shortcuts when one is busy. For instance, one may be tempted to not be as rigorous in performing the 3-check process. However, being busy is never an excuse for taking shortcuts that may jeopardize patient safety. Additionally, never administer a medication with which you are unfamiliar.

You are part of a team
Every person working in the medication use process provides an opportunity to assure that the appropriate medication is administered to the patient. Asking co-workers to verify one's work when handling complex or powerful medications, or whenever there is ambiguity, is a best practice. It also is best practice to perform this double check when drawing a dose from a multiple-dose vial. This means double-checking the order, the label on the medication, as well as the dose that is drawn up. Remember, too, that there are several double checks provided by pharmacists on the inpatient units. One of the checks provided by pharmacists is verification of all the medications that are sent to the floor. Because pharmacists provide this double check, medications should never be removed from the pharmacy delivery bins by anyone other than a pharmacist. While it is important to start drug therapy as soon as possible, often the clinical need for quick administration does not outweigh the safety of having the pharmacist review the order first.

(*continues*)

FIGURE 33.2 A portion of the recheck campaign (*Continued*)

Write all verbal orders immediately after they are received
Verbal orders are one of the most common causes of medication errors. Best practice is to completely eliminate such orders. However, this may not always be feasible. Strategies to make the verbal order process more safe include immediately repeating the order back to the prescriber to ensure that you clearly understood the order, as well as documenting the order in writing and having it reviewed by another healthcare professional prior to administering the first dose of medication. In the inpatient setting, if urgency necessitates administration of a scheduled medication before it is reviewed by a pharmacist, the nurse should check the medication label against the original order to verify accuracy prior to administration of the medication. Medications may only be administered pursuant to an order from an authorized prescriber.

Forgive yourself, report all errors, and make suggestions to improve the system
No one is perfect. Most healthcare professionals have had at least one experience with an error. If you are involved with an error, immediately report the facts to your supervisor and fill out a medication variance reporting form. It is only through insightful information from those who have made errors that we learn about their system-based causes and remedies.

purposes. Follow-up data on the use of problem-prone abbreviations are being collected at periodic intervals to assess the impact of the program after the educational sessions are complete.

Medication Safety Week

To help improve organizational awareness about medication safety, a dedicated UWHC Medication Safety Week is held. UWHC hosted several nationally renowned speakers who provided Grand Rounds lectures for all interested Madison-area healthcare professionals. Other presentations and posters were offered that week to launch new safety programs (e.g., the "Re-✓" campaign and the new reporting process) and to present existing UWHC initiatives that maximize medication safety.

UWHC Technology Model

The vision at the University of Wisconsin Hospital and Clinics is to develop an integrated information system that follows medication orders and medications from the physician's electronic prescription pad to the pharmacy and then to the patient. It is believed that such a system, when integrated with appropriate automation, will maximize patient safety and the efficiency of the medication use process. Figure 33.3 illustrates the UW Hospital vision for the acute care medication use process, whereby a CPOE system is coupled with heavy use of automated dispensing systems that rely on the use of bar codes. Every drug product is bar coded at each phase of the medication use process, from the point of purchasing through documentation of medication administration to the patient.

The department currently uses a single integrated pharmacy computer system for processing all inpatient and ambulatory medication orders and prescriptions at all sites. To maximize patient safety and minimize costs, a hybrid approach to medication distribution has been implemented throughout the organization using centralized robotics. Decentralized automated dispensing cabinets are used to dispense controlled substances and as-needed medications. Matrix drawers are used only to store drugs with low potential for harm, abuse, or misuse. A handheld wireless point-of-care system for verifying and documenting medication administration is currently implemented on a 27-bed inpatient hematology/oncology unit. The system is used by all nurses on the unit and employs bar code technology to provide a three-way link between the patient, medication, and nurse

TABLE 33.7 Problem-Prone Abbreviations (*Continued*)

Abbreviation	Intended Meaning	Error	Recommendation
U	Units	Misread as 0, 4, or cc (e.g., an order for 10 U of insulin can be misread as 100)	Write out "units."
BIW, TIW	Two times a week, three times a week	Misread as two or three times a day	Specifically write out "two" or "three times a week," or write out specific days medication is to be administered (e.g., q Mon, Wed, Sat).
µg	mcg	Misread as mg, or µ misread as 0 and units read as grams	Use "mcg" instead.
AU, AS, AD	Both ears, left ear, right ear	Misread as OU, OS, OD	Specifically write out intended route of administration.
OU, OS, OD	Both eyes, left eye, right eye	Misread as AU, AS, AD	Specifically write out intended route of administration.
cc	Cubic centimeters (milliliters)	Misread as "U" (units)	Use "mL" instead.
QD, QID, and QOD	Every day, four times daily, and every other day	Each can be mistaken for one of the others	Write "daily," q am or q pm; write "four times daily" or "4x daily"; write "every other day."
Trailing zero (e.g., 1.0 mg)	1 mg	Misread as 10 mg	*Do not use* trailing zeros after a decimal point.
No leading zero (e.g., .1 mg)	0.1 mg	Misread as 1 mg or 11 mg	Always use a zero before a decimal point.
X3d	For three days	Misread as for three doses	Write out "for 3 days."
Apothecary symbols (e.g., 10 gr)	10 grains	Misread as 10 grams	*Do not use* apothecary symbols.

(*continues*)

TABLE 33.7 Problem-Prone Abbreviations (*Continued*)

Abbreviation	Intended Meaning	Error	Recommendation
IU	International units	Misread as intravenous	In most cases, eliminating the word "international" and fully writing "units" will suffice.
Medication Abbreviations*			
Nitro	Nitroglycerin or nitroprusside	Misread as the unintended agent	Never abbreviate medication names. Always use the full generic name of drugs.
PIT	Pitocin (oxytocin) or Pitressin (vasopressin)	Misread as the unintended agent	
Levo	Levofloxacin, levothyroxine, levodopa, others	Misread as the unintended agent	
MSO_4	Morphine sulfate	Magnesium sulfate	
$MgSO_4$	Magnesium sulfate	Morphine sulfate	
ARA-A	Vidarabine	ARA-C (Cytarabine)	

*These are just a few of the many medication abbreviations that exist. Because of their error potential, *all* medication abbreviations should be avoided.

to help ensure accuracy. All drugs as well as patients' and healthcare professionals' name badges are bar coded. This system receives real-time patient information and medication profiles from the pharmacy computer system.

A multidisciplinary team is in the early stages of planning the use of an inpatient CPOE system. UWHC has developed extensive safety criteria for an ideal CPOE system to help guide the implementation of this technology from a patient safety perspective. An implementation team has recently been created, and a physician champion has been identified. The resources and technological infrastructure are being developed to meet a target CPOE implementation date of 2003. A centralized pharmacy data repository has been established that ties together data from all pharmacy, billing, and admit/discharge/transfer (ADT) information systems, as well as automated dispensing technologies. Responsibility for developing an integrated patient medical record rests with the hospital's information systems department, but the organization's goal is to provide caregivers rapid access to patient information and electronic documentation of care by integrating all hospital information systems, including pharmacy, laboratory, billing, ADT, and nursing.

Citywide and Statewide Approach

UWHC has taken an active role in several Madison-area and Wisconsin-wide medication and patient safety initiatives. The Madison Patient Safety Collaborative is a group of Madison-area hospitals that have been meeting since the middle of 2000 to help design strategies to minimize medical errors. The first strategies being worked on by the group include the elimination of error-prone abbreviations, initiatives to reduce falls, and the distribution

FIGURE 33.3 Vision of the UWHC medication use process

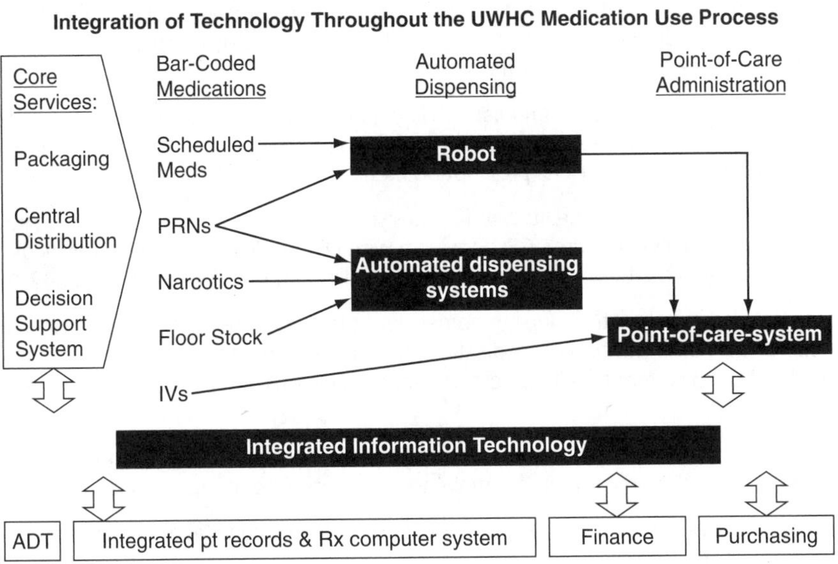

of consistent consumer information on how to avoid medication errors throughout the community.

UWHC has also been involved at a state level to improve medication safety. In May 2000, representatives from a diverse group of Wisconsin organizations (e.g., healthcare purchasers, state professional societies, healthcare organizations, consumer groups) assembled to discuss ways to improve patient safety and reduce medical errors in the state of Wisconsin. The group endorsed the concept that patient safety must be a priority in every healthcare setting. A subgroup of that original panel developed 10 recommendations designed to improve medication safety, which were ultimately presented at the Patient Safety Forum in November 2000 (Table 33.8).

These 10 recommendations were the first steps that the group made toward improving patient safety in Wisconsin. The group has since been incorporated into a funded nonprofit entity called the Wisconsin Patient Safety Institute (WPSI). The mission of the WPSI is to enhance and promote patient safety by advocating the adoption of safe practices in healthcare organizations throughout Wisconsin. The Institute encourages research leading to improvements in patient safety, the improvement of public and professional awareness of patient safety issues, implementation of effective safety initiatives, and partnerships among healthcare providers, consumers, purchasers, educators, researchers, and leaders in government. Future efforts of the group will also involve developing practices to assist healthcare purchasers and patients; ensuring appropriate medication administration procedures, including the use of infusion devices; and expanding the scope of the group beyond medication errors to include fall prevention, blood transfusion errors, wrong-site surgeries, and other medical errors.

The authors of this chapter have been involved at a state level with the Pharmacy Society of Wisconsin (PSW). They have helped to develop the *PSW Medication Use Practice Standards to Maximize Patient Safety*. This resource has been distributed to healthcare professionals and other interested parties (e.g., healthcare purchasers, legislators, media, and

TABLE 33.8 Medication Safety Recommendations for Wisconsin Health Providers

1. Hospitals, extended care facilities, nursing homes, and other healthcare facilities need to provide 24-hour pharmacy coverage either on-site or on-call (by telephone access to a staff pharmacist or contracted through a community pharmacist).
2. Hospitals, community pharmacies, ambulatory clinics, and other healthcare facilities that dispense medication should utilize available computer software to provide clinical screening to maximize patient safety in the dispensing of all prescription medications.
3. Hospitals and other appropriate healthcare facilities should conduct an evaluation of an integrated computerized prescriber order entry (CPOE) system with clinical decision support for medications and other ordered services by January 1, 2002, with implementation by January 1, 2004.
4. Hospitals, extended care facilities, nursing homes, and other appropriate healthcare facilities responsible for the administration of medications to patients should implement an oral and inhalant unit-dose distribution system for all non-emergency medications administered within the facility by January 1, 2002.
5. Hospitals and ambulatory healthcare centers should utilize a pharmacy-based and pharmacist-managed process for the preparation of intravenous admixture solutions.
6. Pharmacies and physicians should include the generic name on the label of prescription medications dispensed to patients.
7. Hospitals and other appropriate healthcare facilities should investigate and evaluate the use of bar-coding systems for packing and administration of medications by January 1, 2002.
8. Hospitals and other appropriate healthcare facilities should prepare and maintain written policies and procedures for the use of select high-risk medications within the facility.
9. Prescribers should institute actions to eliminate the use of symbols and phrases that are commonly misinterpreted by pharmacists and other healthcare providers.
10. Prescribers and pharmacists should include the intended use on all prescription orders and prescription drug labels and packages for consumers.

Developed by the Wisconsin Patient Safety Institute

patients) within the state of Wisconsin as well as nationally. It is available for free on the PSW Web site (www.pswi.org). The document is an effort by PSW to identify minimum practice standards and best demonstrated practices that maximize consumer safety and safe medication use; provide consumers with practical strategies to make safe use of their medications and protect themselves from errors inside and outside the hospital; and recommend criteria that healthcare purchasers should consider when selecting a healthcare organization, health system, or pharmacy to care for their members. This resource was later reviewed and revised by a multidisciplinary team. PSW has subsequently published *Maximizing Patient Safety in the Medication Use Process: Practice Guidelines and Best Demonstrated Practices*.

GENERAL CONSIDERATIONS FOR HEALTH SYSTEMS

Given the complexity and the multitude of steps in the medication use process, designing safe systems that prevent and eliminate medication errors can seem like a daunting task. However, it is critical that institutions begin to address the problem. For some organizations that are struggling to find their way, it may be best to pick the low-hanging fruit by choosing projects that are the most feasible.

This strategy of considering both the impact and the feasibility of potential projects has worked well at UWHC. After all, it does not make sense for an organization to begin with a project that is not very feasible and has low potential for making a significant difference in improving medication use safety.

The following 10 items are key principles that organizations can use to help guide them as they strive to improve the safety of the medication use process.

1. Collaboration is essential. Various departments need to interact. Avoid the "silo approach" that historically has been prevalent in many hospitals and healthcare institutions. Improving medication safety should be a multidisciplinary process because the processes that create medication errors span many disciplines.
2. Secure buy-in from key leadership. Support and leadership from upper administration is essential to accomplishing meaningful change.
3. Learn from other organizations. In other words, interhospital collaboration is needed in addition to intrahospital collaboration.
4. Seek to have better reporting of actual *and* potential errors. System improvements can only be made if there is a good understanding of existing problems.
5. Embrace a nonpunitive culture for medication errors by adopting a systems approach. Punishing healthcare professionals for mistakes does little to fix the underlying problem and will hamper reporting efforts and identification of system problems. Medication errors often result from a complex interplay of multiple factors and are rarely caused by the carelessness or misconduct of single individuals.
6. Technology is helpful, but it is not a cure-all. Existing systems need to be sound before technology is implemented. Remedy process problems within the existing system before implementing technology. Do not place sole emphasis, resources, or reliance on automation at the expense of sacrificing other safety initiatives.
7. Understand the existing system (consider flowcharting it). Conduct prospective analyses to understand where errors can occur in the process. (This is a process known as failure mode effects analysis. More information has been published elsewhere.[28,29]) Seek to simplify the existing system by standardizing, reducing the number of steps and handoffs (e.g., transfer of orders from one person to another), using forcing functions and constraints, avoiding reliance on memory, using protocols and checklists, and improving access to information.
8. Include front-line personnel in efforts designed to improve medication safety. Healthcare professionals who are on the sharp end of active failures possess unique insight into the importance and feasibility of any initiative designed to improve the safe use of medications.
9. Leverage clinical pharmacists. Pharmacists are critical to the safety of the medication use process. Make sure that pharmacists are deployed in patient care areas and are able to provide clinical services and are not just relegated to a strictly dispensing role.
10. Perform a safety self-assessment. Organizations should compare their medication use system with the best practices advocated in the Institute of Medicine report and other literature on safe medication use processes (e.g., the Advisory Board's *Prescription for Change I* and the Medication Safety Self Assessment from the Institute of Safe Medication Practices).

CONCLUSION

Healthcare organizations should strive for a zero defect rate in the medication use process. Although many of the examples described in this chapter are from an academic medical center, many of the concepts and strategies can be applied across a variety of practice settings. It is hoped that this chapter has helped to further stimulate ideas for improving the safety of the medication use process. Creativity and ingenuity will be necessary to achieve a zero defect rate because as Albert Einstein once said, "We should not try to solve problems with the same ideas that created them in the first place."

Acknowledgments

The authors would like to acknowledge the following members of the UWHC Medication Safety Committee for their contributions to many of the projects described in this chapter:

Bonnie Albaugh, RN
Sarah Bland, RPh
Jan Brassington
Myra Enloe, RN
Robert Judd, MD
Jim Klauck, RPh
Sue Lehnherr, RN
Diana Renken, PharmD
Ian Robins, MD
Mark Schroeder, MD
Carl Selbo
Kathy Speck, RN
Deb Tinker, RN

References

1. Kohn, L. T., Corrigan, J. M., Donaldson, M. S., ed. *To err is human: Building a safer health system*. Washington DC: National Academy Press, 1999.
2. Committee on Quality of Health Care in America. *Crossing the quality chasm: A new health system for the 21st century*. Washington DC: National Academy Press, 2001.
3. Business Roundtable. Press release: The Business Roundtable launches effort to help reduce medical errors through purchasing clout. Available at: http://www.brtable.org/press.cfm/464. Accessed November 16, 2000.
4. Joint Commission on Accreditation of Healthcare Organizations. Revisions to Joint Commission standards in support of patient safety and medical/health care error reduction. Available at: http://www.jcaho.org/standard/fr_ptsafety.html. Accessed January 21, 2001.
5. Kaiser Family Foundation and the Agency for Healthcare Research and Quality. *Americans as health care consumers: An update on the role of quality information*. Available at: http://www.ahrq.gov/qual/kffhigh00. htm. Accessed December 12, 2000.
6. National Coordinating Council for Medication Error Reporting and Prevention. http://www.nccmerp.org. Accessed August 1, 2000.
7. Bates, D. W., Boyle, D. L., Vander Vliet, M. B., Schneider, J., and Leape, L. Relationship between medication errors and adverse drug events. *J Gen Intern Med* 1995;10:199–205.
8. World Health Organization Technical Report, Series 425, 1969.
9. Brennan, T. A., Leape, L. L., Laird, N. M., Hebert, L., Localio, A. R., Lawthers, A. G., et al. Incidence of adverse events and negligence in hospitalized patients: Results of the Harvard Medical Practice Study I. *N Engl J Med* 1991;324:370–6.
10. Leape, L. L., Brennan, T. A., Laird, N., Lawthers, A. G., Localio, A. R., Barnes, B. A., et al. The nature of adverse events in hospitalized patients: Results of the Harvard Medical Practice Study II. *N Engl J Med* 1991;324:377–84.
11. Cullen, D. J., Bates, D. W., Small, S. D., Cooper, J. B., Nemeskal, A. R., and Leape, L. L. The incident reporting system does not detect adverse drug events: A problem for quality improvement. *Jt Comm J Qual Improv* 1995;10:541–8.

12. Classsen, D. C., Pestotnik, S. L., Evans, R. S., and Burke, J. P. Computerized surveillance of adverse drug events in hospitalized patients. *JAMA* 1991;366:2847–51.
13. Bates, D. W., Cullen, D. J., Laird, N., Petersen, L. A., Small, S. D., Servi, D., et al. Incidence of adverse drug events and potential adverse drug events. *JAMA* 1995;274:29–34.
14. Jha, A. K., Kuperman, G. J., Teich, J. M., Leape, L., Shea, B., Rittenberg, E., et al. Identifying adverse drug events: Development of a computer-based monitor and comparison with chart review and stimulated voluntary report. *J Am Med Informatics Assoc* 1998;5:305–14.
15. Johnson, J. A., and Bootman, J. L. Drug-related morbidity and mortality: A cost-of-illness model. *Arch Intern Med* 1995;155:1949–56.
16. Johnson, J. A., and Bootman, J. L. Drug-related morbidity and mortality and the economic impact of pharmaceutical care. *Am J Health-Syst Pharm* 1997;54:554–8.
17. Classen, D. C., Pestotnik, S. L., Evans, R. S., Lloyd, J. F., and Burke, J. P. Adverse drug events in hospitalized patients: Excess length of stay, extra costs, and attributable mortality. *JAMA* 1997;277:301–6.
18. Bates, D. W., Spell, N., Cullen, D. J., Burdick, E., Laird, N., and Petersen, L. A. The costs of adverse drug events in hospitalized patients. *JAMA* 1997;277:307–11.
19. Reason, J. Human error: models and management. *BMJ* 2000;320:768–70.
20. Vincent, C., Stanhope, N., and Murphy, M. C. Reasons for not reporting adverse incidents: An empirical study. *J Eval Clin Prac* 1999;5:13–21.
21. Rough, S. The pharmacist-technology interface: Current and future implications for the practice of pharmacy. In: Mueller, B., Bertch, K., Dunsworth, T., et al., eds. *The pharmacotherapy self-assessment program*, 4th ed. Kansas City, MO: ACCP, 2001.
22. Sutter, T. L., Wellman, G. S., Mott, D. A., Schommer, J. C., and Sherrin, T. P. Discrepancies with automated drug storage and distribution cabinets. *Am J Health-Syst Pharm* 1998;55:1924–6.
23. Barker, K. N. Ensuring safety in the use of automated medication dispensing systems. *Am J Health-Syst Pharm* 1995;52:2445–7.
24. Borel, J. M., and Rascati, K. L. Effect of an automated, nursing unit-based drug-dispensing device on medication errors. *Am J Health-Syst Pharm* 1995;52:1875–9.
25. Weaver, P. E., Perini, V. J., and Pierce, D. Random sampling process for quality assurance of the $R_x$obot dispensing system. *ASHP Midyear Clinical Meeting* 1998;33:289E.
26. Bates, D. W., Leape, L. L., Cullen, D. J., Laird, N., Petersen, L. A., Teich, J. M., et al. Effect of computerized physician order entry and a team intervention on prevention of serious medication errors. *JAMA* 1998;280:1311–6.
27. Bates, D. W., Teich, J. M., Lee, J., Seger, D., Kuperman, G. J., Ma'Luf, N., et al. The impact of computerized prescriber order entry on medication error prevention. *J Am Med Informatics Assoc* 1999;6:313–21.
28. Leape, L. L., Bates, D. W., Cullen, D. J., Cooper, J., Demonaco, H. J., Gallivan, T., et al. Systems analysis of adverse drug events. *JAMA* 1995;274:35–43.
29. Cohen, M. R., Senders, J., and Davis, N. M. Failure mode and effects analysis: A novel approach to avoiding dangerous medication errors and accidents. *Hosp Pharm* 1994;29:319–30.
30. American Society of Health-System Pharmacists. Suggested definitions and relationships among medication misadventures, medication errors, and adverse drug reactions. http://www.ashp.org/public/proad/mederror/draftdefin.html. Accessed August 31, 2000.

34

Using Simulation to Advance Patient Safety

Keshia Carswell

INTRODUCTION

The safety and quality of healthcare delivery is dependent on a number of multifaceted interactions between healthcare professionals and administrators, healthcare facilities, and regulatory governing bodies. The individuals in these categories are highly educated and trained, and for the most part experienced in delivering (or in the case of regulatory bodies, providing for the delivery of) such care. However, despite the education and experience of those providing medical care, safety and quality issues continue to plague the U.S. health delivery system. In fact, the Agency for Healthcare and Quality Research (AHQR) recently reported that the average rate of improvement in health outcomes for a variety of conditions has risen a mere 1.6% per year since the Institute of Medicine (IOM) released its report on the alarmingly high occurrence of preventable medical errors over 10 years ago.[1] In that time, several unsuccessful efforts have been made to enhance patient safety and quality.[2] However, one method seems to be yielding promising results: simulation.[3]

BACKGROUND

Generally speaking, simulation is a technique or device that attempts to create or recreate real-world scenarios.[4] In health care, simulation refers to a wide variety of these techniques and scenarios in the clinical setting.[4] They are designed to promote clinical thought processes and decision making and critical thinking, and to demonstrate clinical procedures.[4] Simulation allows students or practicing medical professionals to participate in interactive learning experiences and provides them an opportunity to develop, refine, and apply knowledge and skills in realistic clinical situations. Simulation is used regularly in medical education settings but is often used to improve the training and education of practicing clinicians as well.[5] Simulation techniques allow an educator to control and adapt the learning environment to create clinical scenarios of all kinds.[4] Thus, the educator can mimic the reality of the clinical environment by introducing distractions or complications that would occur in a particular clinical setting.[4] As such, it is not surprising that simulation techniques come in many forms ranging from relatively simple to highly complex.[4] Simulation modalities range from role-playing to interactive human–patient simulators to complete virtual reality.[5]

Part Task Trainers

Part task trainers, also known as static task trainers, are designed to replicate a specific area of the body or clinical environment.[4] They range in complexity from food items—such as oranges to teach injection techniques[4]—to devices that simulate laparoscopic surgery.[5] These task trainers generally represent portions of the human body selected to teach basic psychomotor skills and procedures.[4] The advantage to part task trainers is that they are, more or less, inexpensive, and oftentimes they are widely available for use within the same organization, which allows for larger amounts of people to learn.[4]

Standardized Patients or Actors

Standardized patients are actors commonly used in nursing and medical education.[6] They are laypersons specially trained to play the role of a patient in a clinical encounter.[6] They are given a medical history and symptoms to complain of, and they understand enough about the condition to improvise in response to questions asked by clinicians or learners.[5] Standardized patients are useful in teaching physical assessment skills, history taking, and communication skills.[4] Oftentimes, they are used to practice sensitive topics and exam skills, such as "breaking bad news" and performing gynecological examinations.[6] Standardized patients provide real benefits to medical and nursing education because students can refine and improve their techniques for certain examinations, such as prostate or breast exams, because the actors are able to provide live feedback as the exam is being performed.[4] In fact, simulated patients have been so successful in the education arena that medical students are required to take a "simulated patient exam" as part of the United States Medical Licensing Examination Step 2.[6] However, this type of simulation can be expensive and also presents scheduling challenges.[4] Additionally, standardized patient exercises are limited by the absence of genuine pathologic findings in actors, such as heart murmurs or abnormal lung sounds.[6]

Screen-Based Computer Simulators

Screen-based simulators are designed to model different aspects of human physiology.[4] Users interact with computer programs by using information provided by the program to make clinical decisions.[4] These simulators are often aimed at single users who play the role of a clinician, while the computer plays the role of the patient.[5] The advantage to these systems is that they are relatively inexpensive and can be reused.[4]

Complex Task Trainers

Complex task trainers engage the learner with virtual reality and haptic technology.[4] Haptic technology is technology that employs sensors that sense touch and measure the amount of pressure applied by the touch.[4] This kind of technology is particularly useful where the educator cannot accurately gauge the learner's technique, such as in pelvic examinations.[4] Complex task trainers are often combined with part task trainers so that physical interactions can be mimicked in a virtual environment.[4] While complex task trainers can be reused, they can be costly.[4]

Mannequin Simulators

Mannequins are human patient simulators capable of realistic physiological responses, such as respiration, heart sounds, urinary output, and pupil reaction.[4] Mannequins are the most technologically advanced simulators[6] and are capable of simulating entire biological processes, such as childbirth.[7] They allow trainees across several disciplines to interact with one another, as well as with the mannequin, and to manage problems of varying complexity.[6] The mannequin is programmed with computer software that can be manipulated by educators to change the scenario in real time.[6] Generally, after a simulation exercise with a mannequin, the trainees or learners will meet with the educator for a debriefing session.[6] Advantages to mannequin simulators are the realistic physiological reactions to the mannequin and the ability of educators to change the scenario without disrupting the learning experience. However, because these mannequins represent the most advanced types of simulation, they can be extremely expensive to purchase and maintain.

Hybrid Simulators

Because simulations come in so many forms and levels of complexity, different types of simulators are often combined with one another into hybrid forms. For example, standardized patient actors are mixed with part task trainers,[5] and suturing skills can be performed on an actual person fixed with plastic suture model arms.[6] These kinds of hybrid simulations allow institutions to adapt simulation techniques to their needs and employ simulation modalities within their means financially.

SIMULATION AND PATIENT SAFETY

There is widespread recognition, largely due to the publication of *To Err Is Human* that harm posed to patients by preventable medical errors is unacceptably high. Despite the fact that medical education and training in the United States is among the best in the world, many have come to the conclusion that this very education and training is the root cause of preventable errors that pose such great harm to the patient population.[6] Healthcare training and practice are notorious for a plethora of tensions between different groups of clinicians (nurses, medical students and residents, and physicians), which together have created a system that produces widespread preventable medical injury on a daily basis. Because this education and training is a contributing factor at the root of these issues, efforts such as simulation have been incorporated into nursing, medical student, and clinician education and training to teach (or refine) skills and to address communication breakdowns that lead to patient harm. In fact, the IOM recognized that simulation could be used to enhance patient safety and prevent medical errors stating: "[H]ealth care organizations and teaching institutions should participate in the development and use of simulation for training novice practitioners, problem solving, and crisis management."[8] The use of simulation as an educational tool can contribute to patient safety and quality by providing students and practitioners with opportunities to gain experience in clinical scenarios and to act in those scenarios without posing a risk to the patient. I will address the role of simulation and its benefits to patient safety in each category of clinician groupings mentioned previously.

Nursing Education

Nursing education has used simulation in some form for many years to teach principles and skills of nursing care.[4] As such, there are several aspects of nursing care that have been able to, or have the potential to, benefit from the use of simulation. These areas include prevention of medication errors, critical thinking and clinical decision-making skills, effective communication, and teamwork. These are areas that significantly affect patient safety and that can easily incorporate the use of simulation in educating and training nurses.

Preventing Medication Errors

In 2006, the IOM released a report that concluded at least 1.5 million preventable medication errors occur each year in the United

States, and this figure does not take into account errors of omission.[9] The report goes on to say that, on average, a patient in a hospital is subjected to more than one medication error each day.[9] Research has shown that medication errors, which are also known as adverse drug events (ADEs), are most likely to occur during the prescribing and administration stages, and most commonly occur at transition points during hospitalization.[4] Because the administration of medication is a task almost always performed by nurses,[4] medication errors are directly related to the nursing sector. Medication errors usually involve dosage issues, overlooked allergies, administration of the wrong drug entirely, and incorrect administration sites.[4] All of these errors are affected by environmental factors in the hospital such as distractions during administration, miscommunication, and drug labeling issues.

Because medication administration is such an important part of nursing practice, teaching nursing students practices to safely administer drugs should be a primary concern in nursing schools. In doing so, it is important to recognize that educating students is multifaceted and encompasses more than mathematical skills, but critical thinking and decision making as well. Students must be able to manage side effects and educate the patient about the appropriate treatment regimen.[4] It is here where simulation can come into play.

Patient simulators, such as mannequins, can provide a realistic setting to practice administering medication without any accompanying patient safety risks. For example, bar code systems that match patients to their appropriate medications are commonplace in many hospitals.[4] This could easily be applied and practiced in nursing education using simulation, without any risk of harming a patient. For instance, in advanced human patient simulators such as mannequins, specific medications can be scanned to activate physiologic responses that are consequences of incorrect dosages or administration sites, or incorrect medication.[4] Another opportunity for simulation use in nursing care is in crisis situations. In these scenarios, students are exposed to the reality of medication administration in emergent situations and can use simulation as a technique to learn procedural methods to avoid ADEs. Additionally, effective patient handoffs and patient family education can be practiced using role-play simulation techniques.[4]

Incorporating medication administration into simulation exercises provides numerous and valuable learning experiences to nursing students. Using simulation in medication administration education can assist students in identifying high-risk areas for ADE occurrence, such as patient handoffs and shift reports and transitions.

Critical Thinking and Clinical Decision-Making Skills

A large part of nursing education and training deals with developing critical thinking and decision-making skills. Nursing educators have to teach their students to go beyond memorization to learn how to synthesize and apply their knowledge when planning and evaluating nursing care.[4] Simulation techniques allow students to experience situations that they may not encounter during their clinical practicum. Simulators enable educators to provide scenarios that engage the students and require critical thinking and clinical decision making instead of attempting to find a "rare patient" care opportunity in the hospital setting.[4] As students analyze the symptoms and medical history of a simulated patient, they can use critical thinking skills to make clinical determinations. More importantly, in simulation scenarios, the student can think and decide without the pressure of potentially harming the patient.

Effective Communication

Effective communication in the healthcare setting is integral to promoting and maintaining patient safety. The Joint Commission identifies deficient communication as the root cause of approximately 70% of all sentinel events.[10] In its report, The Joint Commission went on to say, "[P]atient safety is improved when communication is clear, accurate, complete, and timely."[4]

Currently, interdisciplinary communication is the focus of healthcare curriculum, and each discipline has its own terminology and idiosyncrasies.[4] This presents significant barriers to effective communication among various disciplines within the nursing sector and across other healthcare disciplines as well. SBAR—situation (a statement of what is happening at the present time that has triggered the SBAR), background (background information that puts the situation into context and explains the circumstances that have led to the situation), assessment (a statement of the communicator's thoughts regarding the problem), and recommendation (a statement of what should be done to correct the problem, when and by whom)—is a proposed model of interdisciplinary communication that has gained increased consideration.[4] Simulation techniques provide methods to teach nursing students to use standardized, such as SBAR, communication effectively. With little effort, SBAR can be incorporated into all of a given institution's simulation modalities and used to develop and refine communication techniques to practitioners at all levels. This would be particularly useful in the educational setting because students across all disciplines could work together in simulations to practice communication techniques that are representative of a realistic healthcare setting.

Teamwork

Nursing schools, as well as medical schools, train nurses as individuals despite the fact that, in practice, they are most often required to work as teams.[4] In practice, nurses, physicians, and other medical staff interact on a regular basis as part of their daily job functions. Thus, it follows that improving teamwork by sharing information among team members can improve patient safety and quality. In fact, research has shown that the risk of serious adverse events is reduced when team training has been implemented within an institution.[4] In 2000, the IOM report urged healthcare organizations to develop strategies to improve team function in an effort to increase quality of care for patients.[4]

Simulation techniques are excellent methods to educate and train nurses (and other healthcare professionals) to operate effectively in team settings. Simulation scenarios can be created to emphasize group work by assigning students specific roles such as "primary nurse, secondary nurse, medication nurse, communicator, or recorder."[4] In this example, students learn to delegate tasks, follow directions, and communicate effectively with other nurses and clinicians. This simulation technique allows students to refine communication skills by presenting them with an opportunity to assess the patient and situation, to identify information that must be communicated to other health providers, and to then practice that communication.

Medical Student Education

Like nursing education, the primary advantage of using simulation as an educational tool in medical education is that it provides realistic learning experiences without any risk of harm to an actual patient. Medical schools have traditionally relied on training with real patients to educate students.[11] However, in this kind of experiential learning, making mistakes is inevitable, and those mistakes pose a serious threat of harm to patients. Consequently, as technology advances and public policy efforts demanded better quality care for patients, simulation has begun to play an important role in medical education.

In an interview about simulation, Bannis, a third-year medical student said, "I like simulations because [they] give . . . me an opportunity to practice my skills without the added pressure of a human being's health being at stake."[12] Simulation allows students to learn, practice, and repeat procedures as often as necessary to correct mistakes and fine-tune their skills—all without compromising the safety of real patients. Additionally, simulation is useful in that it provides a bridge between the theory of medicine and clinical practice. Furthermore, learning experiences with simulation allow medical students to identify gaps in their knowledge, can boost self-confidence, and help to reduce students' anxiety in actual patient care settings.

One setting where simulation training can be particularly important and beneficial is in the emergency department. Medical students (or residents) can gain experience with various types of emergency conditions that they may not encounter in their rotations or shifts. Patients with volatile conditions may not get second chances. Thus, when medical students are confronted with emergency situations, prior experience handling that situation from simulation training could make the difference between life and death.

Studies have shown that medical students who have undergone simulations perform better on subsequent simulated tasks.[6] For example, a cohort study studied medical students at five academic medical centers where cohorts were differentiated by simulation training experience.[6] One group underwent two weeks of cardiac bedside skills simulation followed by two weeks of traditional ward work.[6] The second group was not exposed to any simulation training and engaged in four weeks of traditional ward work.[6] The simulation group performed at twice the level of the ward group in half the amount of training time.[6]

In another study, researchers showed residents with simulation training were more likely to adhere to professional medical association patient care guidelines than those with no simulation training.[6] In this study, residents who were simulator trained in resuscitation were more likely to adhere to American Heart Association guidelines for such resuscitation in real patients.[6] Notably, *second*-year residents with simulation training adhered to guidelines 68% of the time compared to *third*-year residents, without simulation training, who adhered to guidelines 44% of the time.[6] Additionally, in a random, double-blind study of gall bladder surgery, specifically laparoscopic cholecystectomy, residents trained using virtual reality simulation techniques significantly outperformed their counterparts who were not simulation trained.[6] Virtual reality trained residents made six times fewer intraoperative errors in addition to performing the procedure 29% faster.[6]

The Best Evidence Medical Education Collaborative (BEME), a group of individuals and institutions committed to promoting medical education, issued a report about the benefits of simulation in medical education.[6] BEME concluded that the characteristics of simulation that best facilitate learning include the ability to provide feedback, repetitive practice, curriculum integration, and the ability to create a range of difficulty levels.[6] BEME summarized the educational benefits of simulation as deliberate practice with feedback, exposure to uncommon scenarios, reproducibility, and the opportunity to assess students.[6] Despite these benefits, BEME determined that the rigor and quality of research in educational simulation could use improvement.[6] However, overall, BEME concluded that medical simulations are effective in the educational area and simulations complement training of practicing clinicians in patient care settings.[6]

All of the aforementioned studies, in addition to studies being performed at present, support the notion that simulation in medical education is extremely beneficial to patient safety and that simulation has a well-warranted, if not essential, role in medical education.

Practicing Clinicians

It is problematic that care is given by a variety of clinicians in different disciplines who work closely together under stressful conditions yet the training of each of these players is separate and distinct. Because of this, each group of clinicians develops individual cultures and norms, and when they are brought together to deliver care, these cultures often clash. Unfortunately, oftentimes it is the patient who suffers as a result. In addition to communication and cultural divides among providers, clinicians who have been practicing for many years may encounter rare or uncommon scenarios, such as malignant hypothermia, for the first time with little to no knowledge of what to do in that situation. For both communication and deficient knowledge issues, simulation provides a model for training and continued education that can complement traditional training for existing practitioners.

For certain procedures, it has been established that volume of experience decreases patient complication rates.[6] Thus, by incorporating simulation exercises into clinician practice, these clinicians will develop such experience prior to working with real patients, and complications in actual patients will be reduced. Although data regarding improvements in patient outcome is minimal to date, as discussed previously, there is significant evidence of the benefits of simulation training in educational outcomes.[6] Furthermore, several insurers providing medical malpractice insurance offer discounts for institutions whose faculty participate in simulation training.[6] Additionally, in 2004, the Food and Drug Administration (FDA) took on simulation as a measure of competency assessment for procedure performance.[6] As a result, the FDA will certify the competency of practicing clinicians to perform certain procedures, such as carotid stenting, only if competency is first demonstrated in simulation.[6]

With respect to cultural issues among different groups of clinicians, cultural clashes and communication breakdowns pose a significant threat to patient safety. Louisiana State University (LSU) performed an internal study using simulation to assess and improve the impact of teamwork effectiveness on operating room (OR) culture.[13] LSU identified a culture of safety that was lacking in its hospitals and was least present in emergency departments and ORs.[13] Ineffective teamwork was found to be at the center of the culture of safety issue.[13] LSU identified role confusion, poor communication, and disruptive behavior as leading contributors to these problems and employed simulation training as a solution.[13] The institution set up a mock OR and conducted half-day sessions with interdisciplinary teams to address role clarity, flatten the hierarchy, practice situational mental rehearsal, and increase situation awareness.[13] LSU concluded that while cultural change is a very slow process, simulation at the point of care can be used to promote and facilitate cultural change, particularly relating to their culture of safety concerns.[13] LSU also noted that behavior changes must precede any cultural change that is to take place and that organizational support is essential to successfully implement change processes.[13]

It is easy to see the impact that simulation can have in addressing numerous factors that affect patient safety, such as cultural, communication, and experience issues. Accordingly, the section below discusses various institutions that have utilized simulation techniques and how those institutions have benefited from their use of simulation.

INSTITUTIONAL SIMULATION PROGRAMS

Since the IOM reported on the prevalence of preventable medical errors over 10 years ago, several academic medical institutions and hospital systems have employed or developed existing simulation modalities.[4] One such institution is HealthPartners, a healthcare system in Minnesota, which in collaboration with the University of Minnesota's School of Medicine, designed and built a fully functioning simulation center.[11] The simulation center was built after HealthPartners received a grant from the Robert Wood Johnson Foundation and Institute for Healthcare Improvement in 2001.[11] The purpose of the grant was to increase effectiveness and safety in patient care delivery.[11] Thus, the simulation center was designed to educate and train nursing students, medical students, and residents in the health system.[11]

The simulation center offers five kinds of training for its learners: human patient simulators, simulated clinical environments (which is a fully equipped mock hospital setting including a mock ICU, ED, OR, and exam rooms), virtual procedure stations (a computer-controlled simulation device available to teach bronchoscopies, colonoscopies, and flexible sigmoidoscopies), an electronic medical record (EMR) system, and performance recording (so observers can watch simulation activities in nearby conference rooms and simulation participants can watch their simulation exercise after the fact for feedback).[11] Each type of simulation offers a variety of clinical scenarios, and HealthPartners plans to continue to invest in simulation technology and equipment.[11]

In addition to its role in educating University of Minnesota medical students and nurses, the HealthPartners simulation center plays a large role in training existing clinicians within the HealthPartners network.[11] Emergency medicine residents at Regions hospital are required to spend a significant amount of time in the simulation center as part of their training. Residents spend anywhere from 30 to 40 hours in the simulation center each year of their three-year residency.[11] This is equivalent to five emergency room shifts annually.[11] According to Felix Ankel, the assistant professor of emergency medicine and residency director, "[E]xperiential learning is essential, and simulation enhances this aspect of the [emergency medicine] program."[11]

According to educators at the HealthPartners simulation center, the students and residents utilizing the services "value [the] opportunit[y] to make mistakes and learn from them in a safe educational environment."[11] Ankel goes on to say that the residents "appreciate the chance to simulate cases that they may not see in their emergency room shifts as opposed to just reading about them in textbooks and hearing about them in lectures."[11]

Simulation has also made its way into the continuing education arena.[11] The HealthPartners simulation center hosts continuing medical education (CME) courses as well.[11] Carson Harris, the director of emergency medicine toxicology education at Regions, teaches fundamentals of critical care to groups of intensive care unit (ICU) and critical care unit (CCU) nurses using the simulation center.[11] Similarly, Duke University's Human Simulation and Patient Safety Center offers one-day simulation training courses in anesthesia and crisis management.[14] Duke simulation courses are endorsed by the American Society of Anesthesiology and meet the simulation course-training requirement for part of the Maintenance of Certification in Anesthesiology (MOCA).[14] As such, it is clear that the importance and benefits that simulation has with respect to patient safety are widely recognized by educators, regulators, and clinicians alike.

CONCLUSION

The safety and quality of patient care is highly dependent on successful teamwork and interactions of multiple healthcare professionals. However, for many reasons, including lack of experience, cultural clashes, ineffective teamwork, and miscommunication, safety and quality issues continue to plague the U.S. health delivery system. Since the Institute of Medicine released its report, *To Err Is Human*, regarding the prevalence of preventable medical errors over 10 years ago, several efforts have been made to enhance patient safety and quality including a number of simulation techniques. These simulation techniques range from role-playing, to standardized patient actors, to complete virtual clinical realities.

Over time, there have been significant advancements in simulation modalities, likely due to the shock and unwillingness of the U.S. public to accept the astounding amount of preventable medical errors that occur on a daily basis. Many have come to the conclusion that, despite the fact that U.S. medical training is among the best in the world, this very education is the root cause of preventable medical errors. Healthcare practice is notorious for tensions between different groups of clinicians, including nurses, medical students and residents, and physicians. Together, those tensions have created a system that causes significant (numbers of preventable) medical injuries.

To address these issues, simulation techniques have been incorporated into nursing, medical student, and clinician education and training to teach (or refine) skills and to address communication breakdowns that lead to patient harm. To date, most (if not all) nursing and medical schools use these simulation techniques to educate and train students without posing any actual harm to patients. The use of simulation as an educational tool contributes to patient safety and quality by allowing students to gain experience in clinical scenarios and to develop critical thinking and decision-making skills without posing a risk of harm to the patient population.

In addition to the use of simulation in the educational arena, simulation has been useful in refining or practicing skills for existing practioners. With existing practitioners, simulation techniques have been particularly useful in improving teamwork and communication. Thus, whether it is to practice or refine clinical skills, learn new skills, improve communication and teamwork, or resolve cultural bounds, simulation provides a model for training and continued education that has the power to significantly improve patient safety and affect the delivery of health care for the better.

References

1. Holmboe, E., Rizzolo, M. A., Sachdeva, A. K., Rosenberg, M., & Ziv, A. (2011). Simulation-based assessment and the regulation of healthcare professionals. *Simulation in Healthcare, 6*(7), S58–S62. doi:10.1097/SIH.0b013e3182283bd7.
2. Beresford, L. (2009 November). Medical mistakes, 10 years post-op. The Hospitalist. Retrieved from http://www.the-hospitalist.org/details/article/423625/Medical_Mistakes_10_Years_Post-Op.html.
3. U.S. Department of Health and Human Services, Agency for Healthcare Research and Quality. Realistic simulations improve teamwork and care processes in the operating room. Retrieved August 2005 from http://www.innovations.ahrq.gov/content.aspx?id=2209.
4. Hughes, R. G. (Ed.). (2008). Patient safety and quality: An evidence-based handbook for nurses. AHRQ. Retrieved from http://www.ahrq.gov/qual/nurseshdbk/.
5. Youngberg, B. J. (2011). *Principles of risk management and patient safety* (p. 353). Sudbury, MA: Jones & Bartlett.
6. Diane Sliwka, Simulation in Medicine, Retrieved May 25, 2012 from https://simdoc.wordpress.com/2009/01/02/simulation-in-medicine-a-knol-by-diane-sliwka/.
7. Gynecological models, obstetrical models & childbirth model. Retrieved from http://www.buyamag.com/gynecological_models.php.
8. Kohn, L. T., Corrigan, J. M., & Donaldson, M. S. (Eds.). (1999). *To err is human: Building a safer health system*. Washington, DC: National Academies Press.
9. Institute of Medicine. (2006). Preventing medication errors: Quality chasm series. Retrieved from http://www.iom.edu/Reports/2006/Preventing-Medication-Errors-Quality-Chasm-Series.aspx.
10. Joint Commission on Accreditation of Healthcare Organizations. (2006). Sentinal event statistics. Retrieved May 25, 2012 from http://www.jointcommission.org/sentinel_event_statistics_quarterly/.
11. Patow, C. A. (2005). Advancing medical education and patient safety through simulation learning. Retrieved from http://www.psqh.com/marapr05/simulation.html.
12. Interview with Dillon Bannis, medical student at University of Miami Miller School of Medicine. (2011 December).
13. Paige, J., Kozmenko, V., Gururaja, R. P., Yang, T., & Chauvin, S. (2007). Impact of the system for teamwork effectiveness and patient safety (STEPS) on operating room culture. Retrieved from http://internationalforum.bmj.com/forum-resources/presentation-files/C5%20paige.pdf.
14. Simulation Training for Maintenance of Certification in Anesthesiology® (MOCA®). Retrieved from http://simcenter.duke.edu/moca.html.

35

Moving from Traditional Informed Consent to Shared Patient–Provider Decision Making

Shannon Flaherty

INTRODUCTION

The informed consent doctrine has evolved from medical, legal, and ethical principles as a protection of a patient's right to self-determination.[1] This doctrine formalizes a patient's fundamental right to personal autonomy by requiring that a provider discuss all necessary information so that the patient may make informed choices about his or her medical care.[1,2] However, as experienced by many patients in the contemporary clinical setting, informed consent can take the form of a transaction rather than a discussion. This transaction may consist of a provider or administrative staff member presenting a legally defensive, standardized form to the patient to sign.[3] This style of implementation has led some providers to refer to the process as "consenting" patients, not "informing" them.[4]

The legal doctrine developed, in part, as a reaction to the historically paternalistic medical culture, in which the provider had no formal obligation to communicate treatment information to patients. Given this starting point, even rote disclosures to patients are preferable to no disclosures. Yet the legal mandate implies an exchange of information and a minimum amount of discussion between providers and patients. Unfortunately, the legal doctrine places a heavy emphasis on the active role of the provider to communicate medical information, while the patient retains the right to consent or refuse the proposed treatment, establishing an almost adversarial dynamic.[2] The provider, as the holder of all medical information, carries all the risks associated with failed or insufficient communication.[2] The patient is granted legal recourse for an unclear, unwanted, or undesirable outcome if the provider failed to garner the patient's informed consent.[1] The looming threat of litigation and the one-sided emphasis on the provider's duty to disclose distract focus from the ultimate goal of patient understanding.

The legal doctrine of informed consent has not generated the level of change required to increase patient understanding. There is evidence that traditional efforts to inform patients are inadequate. In a review of 540 informed consent documents from 157 randomly selected U.S. hospitals, the documents were shown to have limited educational value.[4] In a study of surgical patients, almost 70% did not read the informed consent form.[5] As a result, many patients misunderstood the benefits and risks of their procedure.[6] When informed consent is applied in the clinical setting, studies of primary care physicians and surgeons have shown that the discussion of treatment alternatives occurred in only 5.5 to 29.5% of patient–provider interactions, of pros and cons in 2.3 to 26.3% of interactions, and of uncertainties associated with the decision in 1.1 to 16.6% of interactions.[7] In all scenarios studied, the providers rarely explored whether patients understood the proposed treatment (0.9–6.9% of interactions).[8]

Nevertheless, the foundational doctrine endures, both as an ethical ideal and as a litigation threat.[3] Certain aspects of the traditional informed doctrine are important and necessary to set boundaries and to provide a consequence for noncompliance; however, the medical and legal communities have shifted the focus toward increasing patient–provider communication as an ethically sound and legally preventative method of achieving informed consent.[3] The movement toward patient understanding has demanded that new mechanisms and models for effective patient–provider communication be developed. Proponents of the leading model, shared decision making, emphasize the importance of patient involvement as partners in the decision-making process. Medical research of the shared decision-making model has shown promising results including improved patient adherence to prescribed treatment and health outcomes. Implementing the shared decision-making model presents challenges; however, many organizations believe that the benefits of this model outweigh the risks.

THE MEDICAL AND LEGAL ORIGINS OF INFORMED CONSENT

Standards for the patient–provider relationship have changed drastically over the course of the 20th century. However, it can be helpful to understand the historical context of patient–provider relationships. Elements of this early, paternalistic model have a lingering influence in contemporary medical practice and in the application of informed consent.

The Paternalistic Model for Patient–Provider Relationships

The historical dynamic of the patient-provider relationship has accurately been described as paternalistic. The paternalistic model explicitly assumes a passive role for the patient, dependent on the physician's expert role to make treatment decisions.[9] In the most extreme scenario, a physician would authoritatively inform a patient of when and what type of medical intervention would be initiated.[9] In a less extreme scenario, the patient may view the provider as dominating the medical encounter even if the provider unintentionally established this dynamic.[9] The patient's decision-making power would be limited to consent or nonconsent to what the provider considers best.[9] Additionally, there was no formal requirement or mechanism for the provider to elicit the patient's preferences for treatment alternatives.[9]

The American Medical Association (AMA) Code of Ethics codifies the values to which AMA physicians and leadership have committed themselves.[9] The AMA Code of Ethics has evolved over time, paralleling changes in health care and the medical profession's values in clinical practice.[9] The AMA promulgated the first edition of its Code of Ethics in 1847; the most recent edition was published in 2010.[10] The code has evolved markedly from edition to edition; however, the first edition is notable in several ways. First, it was unanimously adopted by AMA as the world's first national code of professional medical ethics.[10] Second, the first edition of the AMA Code of Ethics advised the provider to not engage the patient in discussions of expected outcomes or risks:

> [Physicians] should study in their deportment, so to unite tenderness

> with firmness, and condescension with authority, as to inspire the minds of their patients with gratitude, respect and confidence.
>
> A physician should not be forward to make gloomy prognostications, because they savor of empiricism, by magnifying the importance of his services in the treatment or cure of the disease. But he should not fail, on proper occasions, to give to the friends of the patient timely notice of danger when it really occurs; and even to the patient himself, if absolutely necessary.
>
> It is a sacred duty to guard himself carefully in this respect and to avoid all things which have a tendency to discourage the patient and to depress his spirits.[11]

Though this text may seem anomalous or comical in the world of modern medicine, as recently as the 1970s, only 25% of physicians reported that they always disclosed the details of the patient's diagnosis to the patient.[1] The shift away from this model was greatly influenced by external societal and legal movements.

Informed Consent as a Response to Medical Paternalism

The legal doctrine of informed consent developed, in part, as a response to medical paternalism and is predicated on two basic principles of law.[12] The first is the fundamental legal principle that a competent individual has a right to determine what will be done with his or her body, and the second is the fiduciary nature of the provider–patient relationship.[12] The right to personal autonomy is protected by numerous criminal laws. Additionally, the tort of battery provides a civil cause of action to protect this right. A tort is a civil wrong for which the law provides a remedy, and the person who committed the tort may be liable to pay damages to the person injured.[13] The U.S. legal system has recognized the tort of battery since at least the 1800s, and the judicial roots of this tort in the British legal system date back to the 1400s.[14] Battery is defined as intentional conduct that directly or indirectly results in harmful or offensive contact with another person.[15] The element of intent does not require that the actor desire to do harm, only that the actor intentionally invaded another's personal autonomy in a way that the law forbids.[16] The U.S. legal system began to recognize the provider's liability under the tort of battery in the late 1800s.[17] As applied in the medical context, even if the patient outcome is beneficial, the provider's contact can be considered offensive if the patient did not consent to treatment.[18]

As the number of cases in this area grew, courts began to recognize a need for providers to disclose relevant information regarding treatment risks, benefits, and alternatives so that a patient could grant the provider "informed consent."[19] The need to fully inform patients of a recommended treatment was incorporated into providers' standard of professional care. Judicial recognition that a reasonable provider had a duty to inform patients created another cause of action under the legal principle of negligence. Liability under the principle of negligence is premised on unintentional, careless action or an omission (i.e., a failure to disclose is an omission that breaches this duty).[2] A breach of this duty that causes injury to a patient can make the provider liable to the patient for damages.

While nearly all jurisdictions have adopted informed consent into a provider's standard of care, they have struggled with how to define the provider's duty. The first articulation was a provider-based standard, in other words, what a reasonable provider would disclose with regard to treatment.[19] When applying this standard, judges sought to protect patient autonomy but deferred to the discretion of medical professionals.[19] To prove a breach of the provider's duty to disclose, a patient needed a medical expert to testify that the provider neglected to share information that another, reasonable provider would have.

In 1960, the well-known case of *Natanson v. Kline* articulated a provider's duty to disclose under this standard as "primarily a question of medical judgment."[19]

Subsequent to the *Natanson* decision, other jurisdictions adopted a more patient-centered standard. An objective, patient-based standard, often referred to as the reasonable patient standard, was described in the seminal case of *Canterbury v. Spence*. This highly influential judicial opinion by the Court of Appeals for the District of Columbia influenced courts nationally on the issue of informed consent. The court in *Canterbury* frames a violation of informed consent as a provider's failure to inform a patient of risks and undesirable consequences:

> The root premise is the concept . . . that [e]very human being of adult years and sound mind has a right to determine what shall be done with his own body. . . . True consent to what happens to one's self is the informed exercise of a choice, and that entails an opportunity to evaluate knowledgeably the options available and the risks attendant upon each.
>
> We hold that the standard measuring performance of that duty [to disclose] by physicians, as by others, is conduct which is reasonable under the circumstances.

In our view, the patient's right of self-decision shapes the boundaries of the duty to reveal. That right can be effectively exercised only if the patient possesses enough information to enable an intelligent choice [regarding] [a]ll risks relevant to the decision by patient.[20]

The shift away from battery toward negligence as a theory of liability has created challenges in the practical application of informed doctrine in the clinical setting. All jurisdictions recognize exceptions to informed consent in the cases of emergency, incompetency, patient waiver, and therapeutic privilege.[21] While all jurisdictions seem to recognize the duty to disclose particular treatment risks and alternatives, including the alternative of no further treatment, the method of determining which risks should be disclosed varies by jurisdiction. Twenty-five states have defined the standard of care as what a reasonable provider would disclose with regard to treatment.[19] However, 23 states have defined the standard in terms of what a reasonable patient faced with a treatment decision would want to know.[19] A few jurisdictions have further personalized the patient-based standard beyond the *Canterbury* opinion, defining the standard as what this particular idiosyncratic patient needed to know under the circumstances.

Practical application of all three standards of informed consent has been difficult. The provider-based standard presupposes that all reasonable providers would agree on a standard of disclosure; however, research has shown that there are significant differences in disclosure standards based on a provider's locality and expertise.[22] This research has demonstrated consistency between what individual providers view as essential versus nonessential information; however, it also demonstrates that providers have significantly different opinions on what information is important to communicate to patients. Similarly, the objective patient-based standard assumes that there is one appropriate standard of care for most treatments regardless of individual patient preferences.[19] While acknowledging patient preferences, the subjective patient standard places providers in a vulnerable position of being held liable based on a patient's hindsight that he or she would have declined treatment if he or she had known of a risk before treatment.[19] Such statements are inherently suspect because the risk of the poor health outcome has typically materialized and is the cause of litigation. Few patients would testify that they would have knowingly accepted such risk after the resulting harm occurred. In summary, all three standards presume that the provider is aware of the information that the patient needs or wants to know, a fundamental flaw.

Recognition of the Legal Doctrine of Informed Consent in Medical Practice

Due in part to the development of the legal doctrine of informed consent, the traditional, paternalistic model of a provider as the medical expert and unilateral decision maker has been questioned within the medical community. This shift mirrored, and was potentially influenced by, larger societal movements, such as the consumer rights movement.[9] The perspective shift included an increased focus on patient autonomy in addition to patient challenge of physician authority, narrowing the disparity of information and control between providers and patients. From the late 1970s to the early 1990s, informed consent gained recognition and influence in the medical profession, as reflected in the 1980 AMA Principles of Medical Ethics: "A physician shall be dedicated to providing competent medical service with compassion and respect for human dignity. A physician shall deal honestly with patients. . . . A physician shall respect the law . . . and shall respect the rights of patients."[23]

Developments in Medical Research and Practice: Shifting Toward Patient Involvement

Medical research began to explore the patient's perspective on illness and the patient–provider relationship in the 1950s, as well as the effects of social and psychological factors on illness.[24] The results of this research indicated that psychosocial factors and the patient's personal experiences during treatment should be considered during medical decision making.[25] Additionally, clinical practice demonstrated a varying tolerance of side effects and risks associated with a particular treatment from patient to patient.[26] Recognition of these variables prompted the development of a more patient-centered view of health care within the medical community.

This shift coincided with changes to the nature of medical practice as it moved away from acute care to chronic care. Caregivers and providers spent more time managing long-term illnesses rather than focusing on an immediate cure, translating to longer term provider–patient relationships.[9] Effective management of ongoing and chronic illness necessitates shared responsibility. The patient has responsibility for implementing his or her regimen outside of the clinical setting (e.g., by taking prescription pharmaceuticals or supplements, following a prescribed diet, or checking blood sugar).[27] To effectively manage a chronic illness, a patient must accept a certain amount of responsibility.[28] Research has shown that patient participation in healthcare decisions increases the patient's engagement, knowledge, confidence, skills, and commitment to making an optimal treatment.[29]

An example highlighted by several commentators has been an early-stage diagnosis of breast cancer.[30] Patients with an early diagnosis have numerous treatment options that were historically unavailable. More specific, certain mastectomy procedures do not have higher cure rates for early-diagnosed breast cancer than do lumpectomy procedures.[31] Therefore, a patient's values can be instrumental in distinguishing and determining the treatment option that would be preferable from both the patient's and the provider's perspectives. Some women would elect to have a mastectomy to reduce anxiety about recurrence, whereas other women may find the associated change in body image to be overwhelming.[31] In this situation of curative equivalence, each woman should be able to express the decision that best meets her emotional and situational needs.[31] Cost, convenience, and recovery time can be important factors in selecting the appropriate treatment in this case, as well as in many others.

NEW PATIENT DECISION-MAKING MODELS TO ACHIEVE INFORMED CONSENT

The movement toward patient involvement necessitated new patient decision-making models for obtaining informed consent, shared decision making being one of them.[9] All of the models attempted to correct the imbalance of information between patient and provider. However, patients and providers play different roles in each of the models.

The Informed Decision-Making Model

In the informed decision-making model, the balance of knowledge shifts toward the patient.[9] The provider is responsible for increasing the patient's knowledge of the possible risks of alternative therapeutic options and their clinical effectiveness so that the patient can make a decision that reflects both his or her preferences and medical knowledge.[9] This is not typically a shared decision because the patient then possesses information regarding his or her own preferences and all relevant medical information.[9] This leaves the provider outside of the decision in many respects, limiting the role of the provider to information transfer.[9] Although this model increases patient autonomy, it can be imperfect for many situations and patients.[9] Studies have shown that although patients want information about their medical condition and treatment options, they do not necessarily want to be the ultimate decision maker.[9] Rather, the majority of patients would prefer to choose their level of involvement in the decision-making process.[26]

The Professional-as-Agent Model

In the professional-as-agent model, the patient's involvement in the decision-making process is very limited. This model addresses the imbalance of information between patient and provider by shifting the information toward the provider.[26] The provider elicits the patient's preferences for future health states, lifestyle, etc.[26] Once the information and preferences are clear to the provider, the provider becomes the sole decision maker.[26] When applying this model to clinical practice, there is a strong risk that providers would assume the patient's preference, without verification, equating to a much higher risk of litigation based on lack of informed consent.[9]

The Shared Decision-Making Model

Both the informed decision-making model and the professional-as-agent model address the imbalance of information between patient and provider, providing alternatives to strictly provider-based models.[9] However, these models represent two distinct extremes as to who owns the ultimate decision. Studies have shown that individual patients vary in their desire to influence the ultimate decision regarding treatment (even that a patient's preference can change over the course of lengthy treatment).[9]

Shared decision making has been described as the only model that requires providers and patients to be actively involved in the decision-making process.[9] Shared decision making "denotes an interactive process in which patients and providers collaborate to make healthcare decisions."[26] It assumes that both patient and provider have important information to contribute to the process. While providers have expertise as to benefits and risks associated with relevant medical interventions, patients are the experts of their own values, preferences, and ideal outcomes.[9] There is no one, definitive way to implement shared decision making. However, several criteria are required for truly shared decision making that have been noted by commentators. Those criteria, and methods for achieving each criterion, are discussed following:[9]

At Least Two Parties in the Treatment Discussion

Shared decision making requires at least two parties in the discussion of medical treatment, the patient and the provider.[9] However, additional parties may be involved without affecting the integrity of the model.[9] Additional parties may include a relative, friend, another provider, or a decision coach. Third parties can act on behalf of the patient as information gatherers, advisors, negotiators, or caretakers. In particular, a trained decision coach can work with a patient to identify impact of treatment options to the patient's values and goals so that the patient can have a more effective conversation with his or her provider.[19] In some situations, the addition of a third party confidante or advocate may be necessary to achieve full patient understanding, particularly for patients with low health literacy.[9]

Active Participation by Parties Involved

The model further requires that both providers and patients take steps to actively participate in the decision-making process.[9] To ensure active and appropriate participation, complementary role expectations and behaviors between provider and patient must be established. Much of the responsibility to establish role expectations lies with the provider.[9] Perhaps due to paternalistic origins, many patients look to set the norms of interaction in the medical encounter. If the provider is not motivated to share decision making, it is difficult, if not impossible, for the patient to force the interaction.[9]

Effective Communication

Shared decision making shifts the focus from adequate, perfunctory disclosures toward the goal of effective communication.[2] Providers should not rely on a patient's questions as the sole basis for communication. If a provider perceives value in the involvement of the patient as a partner, the discussion can begin with simple questions such as "What do you think?" If the patient responds, "You're the doctor," the provider could respond with a comment such as "Yes, and I will provide you with information and my expert opinion, but I really do want to include your thoughts and wishes in our planning together."[2]

Similarly, basic disclosures should not be discontinued but should be used to initiate a more involved, bilateral discussion.[2] Because a patient will not know what to ask all of the time, the provider's opinions can be very useful to a patient's consideration of treatment options.[8] Effective communication encompasses facts that the provider should provide, questions the provider should ask, and how the provider should interact with the patient. Providers should facilitate communication by inviting active participation by patients in the context of an informational exchange and encouraging questions.

Providers can utilize verbal and nonverbal skills to more effectively elicit and respond to patients' concerns.[32] One technique to improve communication is to have either party repeat back, in his or her own words, the ideas he or she has heard so that the other party knows that mutual understanding has been established.[2,8] Another simple but effective strategy is to have the patient prepare a written list of questions before the appointment.[2] There is not one single method for implementing a shared decision-making model; however, some of these examples can be leveraged to achieve more effective communication.

Patient Understanding

Advocates of shared decision making have suggested criteria to achieve patient understanding including acknowledgment by the patient that he or she is giving permission for a specific treatment and articulation of definite and possible consequences of that treatment, as well as the patient's own remaining responsibilities.[2]

Studies have shown that the use of decision aids and guidelines can be effective as means of structuring the decision-making process and ensuring that patients receive accurate, unbiased information on treatment options.[9,19] Decision aids can take many forms: videos, decision boards, interactive computer programs, or a combination of these. They can be used by the patient individually or as a discussion tool for the patient and the provider.[26] Ideally, these aids would be created by clinical staff and researchers and regularly reviewed by the same group for accuracy.[19]

An effectively designed decision aid has been shown to clarify a patient's values regarding what is at stake and what it is that he or she is trying to achieve as a result of treatment.[9] Study results show that these aids help patients feel as though they were offered a treatment choice.[9] Additionally, studies have shown that a patient's communication with his or her provider noticeably improved after the patient had time to review and understand a decision aid.[19] Evaluations of decision aids have shown that patients that use them are more informed, make decisions with their doctor that are more consistent with their expressed preferences, and are more likely to follow through with treatment decisions.[33]

Confirmation of Patient Understanding

A provider can never be completely certain that a patient has an adequate understanding to make substantially autonomous choice. However, a provider can use assessment techniques to gauge a patient's understanding and elicit any remaining doubts or questions:[2]

- *Improved consent materials:* Presenting easy-to-read and understandable written consent materials to patients after a decision has been reached.
- *Recognition test:* Asking patients to complete a brief, multiple-choice or true-false test at the end of a shared decision-making discussion.
- *Feedback loop:* Asking patients to restate in their own words what has been disclosed, followed by professional feedback as to correctness.

CHALLENGES AND BENEFITS OF IMPLEMENTING A SHARED DECISION-MAKING MODEL

Shared decision making has been implemented in several organizations. One of the leaders in this area has been the Dartmouth-Hitchcock Medical Center, which created a Center for Shared Decision-Making. Studies conducted by Dartmouth and other medical researchers have noted numerous challenges associated with the implementation of shared decision making, which appear to be significantly outweighed by the benefits. This section outlines some of the common challenges, the overriding benefits, and areas for continual improvement.

Challenges Implementing the Shared Decision-Making Model

There are several challenges associated with the implementation of the shared decision-making model. Implementation of this model may create challenges related to (1) changes in patient–provider relationship and communication, (2) provider concerns regarding additional time required with patients, and (3) resources needed to develop communication tools such as decision aids.

Challenges Related to Communication: The Patient–Provider Relationship

Even providers who advocate for shared decision making have difficulty effectively communicating with patients.[34] Many providers find it challenging to convey the treatment risks, benefits, and associated probabilities in a way that patients can understand.[19] Furthermore, the historically paternalistic medical culture has led some providers to withhold treatment information.[35] Additionally, patient–provider relationships are usually complicated by inherent imbalances in power and knowledge.

Research has shown that providers are not often able to anticipate the patient's preference without a well-developed discussion.[19] These providers may ask questions and elicit emotions from their patients but find it hard to acknowledge and incorporate patients' opinions that do not coincide with their views of medical treatment.[36] As a result, providers should be careful not to withhold relevant information in an effort to ensure that a patient makes the "correct" medical choice.[19]

To further complicate matters, many patients who desire an active, participatory role in the decision-making process can often remain passive while interacting with providers.[26] Empirical research has shown that patient preference for information does not necessarily translate into information-seeking behavior while interacting with a provider, creating a danger that the provider's values will influence the patient, even unintentionally. In one study, only 10% of patients took an active role in decision making, while another study found that 90% of patients indicated that they would like to have an active role in the decision before the visit.[26] Patients, particularly older generations, have been socialized to think that the provider knows best and agreeing with the provider will result in better or more personal care.[26] The traditional paradigm of the provider–patient relationship and the resulting barriers to effective communication need to be acknowledged and addressed if an organization implements shared decision making.

Provider Concerns Regarding Additional Time with Patients

Even under traditional informed consent models, providers have complained that limited time with a patient presents a barrier to completing consent discussions.[26] This has translated to a fear that shared decision making will only amplify the burden on already precious time with the patient. In the clinical setting, additional time with a patient equates to lost revenue from another patient visit, with no additional financial reimbursement for any extra time spent having a meaningful discussion with the first patient. However, there has been little research illustrating how much additional time it would actually take to conduct a shared decision-making discussion. Though it seems logical that more time would be needed, some studies have indicated that doctors trained in communications skills do not take significantly longer to conduct patient interviews.[37] Although an initial patient encounter involving informed shared decision making may take longer, there is evidence that shared decision making may improve a patient's health outcome, netting overall efficiency gains.[37] Furthermore, any financial loss associated with longer patient visits could be counterbalanced by fewer malpractice claims based on a lack of informed consent though further research is needed here. Nevertheless, any organization that considers implementation of shared decision making should acknowledge the potential need for longer patient encounters.

Resources Needed to Implement Communication Tools

Implementing informed decision making requires additional resources not limited to increased provider time spent with patients. For example, it can be expensive and time consuming to create new decision aids that are clear, complete, and unbiased.[19] Decision aids are not available or easily accessible for all major medical decisions. While decision aids are not essential to implement the shared decision-making model, they can be a very helpful method to increase patient understanding. The use of additional resources, such as trained decision coaches, can be very beneficial to effectuate patient communication; however, organizations would need to train and/or hire decision coaches for that role.[19]

Benefits of Implementing a Shared Decision-Making Model

There are significant benefits associated with the implementation of the shared decision-making model, particularly for the patient. Implementation of a shared decision-making model allows provider's to better (1) address an individual patient's need for information and involvement, (2) improve patient well-being and health outcomes, and (3) improve patient recall of risk discussions.

Address an Individual Patient's Need for Information and Involvement

Shared decision making allows patients to control their role in the decision-making dialogue.[19] Most contemporary medical procedures are performed to improve the quality of a patient's daily life; therefore, it is important to consider patient preference about treatment choices.[19] Patients have a strong desire for medical information. In some studies, over 90% of participating patients expressed a strong desire for information on illnesses, treatments, and side effects.[26] In contrast, observational studies suggest that patient's preferences to be better informed are rarely reflected in medical encounters with their providers.[26] The implementation of a shared decision-making model provides medical professionals with an effective toolset to better understand a patient's values.[26]

Improve Patient Well-Being and Health Outcomes

While overall results are mixed, there is a growing body of research demonstrating that shared decision making has a positive impact on a patient's well-being and health outcomes. Outcomes of care and adherence to treatment regimens improve when patients are more involved.[38]

Several studies have shown that patient-centered communication is associated with reduced patient psychological distress and improved functional status.[26] Specific provider behaviors associated with these benefits include asking more questions to understand the patient's problems, expectations, and perspectives; encouraging the patient to ask more questions; giving clear information; showing support and empathy; and allowing the patient to share in decisions.[26] Patients who felt they had expressed themselves fully and received all the information they wanted had better functional outcomes.

In general, patients who perceive that they are actively involved in treatment decisions generally have better physical health outcomes, whereas a low sense of control has been associated with less behavioral involvement in care, poorer self-rated health, and increased illness burden.[26] Patients surveyed expressed less discomfort, greater reduction of symptoms and improvement in general medical conditions if they were more involved in decision making.[26] One surgical study showed that patients who were active in treatment decisions experienced improved short-term recovery, which researchers attributed to lower postsurgery anxiety.[26] Interestingly, there was no resulting, longer term health benefit six months postsurgery.

Another study of hypertensive patients on a chronic care plan demonstrated a correlation between improved treatment outcomes and increased patient involvement. Patients in that study were also more likely to comply with treatment regimens as a result of being invested in the treatment decision.[26] Patient adherence was sometimes related to communication variables, though it is unclear which communication variable influenced this result. The effect of decision making on patient outcomes is a relatively new area of research; however, the research to date has indicated many potential benefits.

Improve Patient Recall of Risk Discussions

Clinical research has associated the use of individualized consent forms with patient-specific risks with improved participation in the consent process, reduced anxiety, and better risk recall.[39] In one study, all patients underwent a nonemergent cardiac catheterization procedure.[39] Patients who received the personalized consent form reported higher rates of reading the consent form, increased perception of shared decision, and decreased anxiety about the procedure compared to patients who received the original consent form.[39] Although there were no differences between groups in patients' ability to name specific complications, more patients in the group who received individualized consent forms recalled being informed of their estimated risk of likely complications.[39]

SUGGESTIONS FOR IMPROVED IMPLEMENTATION OF SHARED DECISION MAKING

There are several proposals and suggestions for the improvement of the shared decision-making model. Three areas of improvement with the potential to greatly benefit patients are (1) improving provider education, (2) improving patient education, and (3) personalizing patient consent forms.

Improving Provider Education

Provider–patient communication is a "central clinical function."[40] However, it is markedly underrepresented in medical school curricula and continuing professional education.[8] Most medical curricula limit the discussion of communication skills to gathering patient diagnostics and social history, breaking bad news, and general health promotion.[37] Based on the potential benefits of improved communication with patients, curriculum development in this area at all levels of medical education may be appropriate. Although there is no prescriptive checklist of questions that would enable an effective decision-making discussion, research by Angela Towle and William Godolphin has suggested that provider education should focus on the following core competencies:[37]

1. Develop a partnership with the patient;
2. Establish or review the patient's preferences for information (such as amount or format);
3. Establish or review the patient's preferences for role in decision making (such as risk taking and degree of involvement of self and others) and the existence and nature of any uncertainty about the course of action to take;
4. Ascertain and respond to the patient's ideas, concerns, and expectations (such as about disease management options);
5. Identify choices (including ideas and information that the patient may have) and evaluate the research evidence in relation to the individual patient;
6. Present (or direct patient to) evidence, taking into account competencies 2 and 3, framing effects (how presentation of the information may influence decision making), etc. Help the patient to reflect on and assess the impact of alternative decisions with regard to his or her values and lifestyle;
7. Make or negotiate a decision in partnership with the patient and resolve conflict;
8. Agree on an action plan and complete arrangements for follow-up.

Improving Patient Education

Patient education has been shown to be an effective method of improving patient–provider communication skills in clinical settings.[40] For example, studies have successfully educated patients on communication skills through distribution of information packages and through waiting-room training sessions.[40] Further research by Angela Towle and William Godolphin has suggested that developing the following core competencies in patients could improve the decision-making process:[40]

1. Define (for oneself) the preferred patient–provider relationship;
2. Find a physician and establish, develop, and adapt a partnership;
3. Articulate (for oneself) health problems, feelings, beliefs, and expectations in an objective and systematic manner;
4. Communicate with the physician to understand and share relevant information (such as from competency 3) clearly and at the appropriate time in the medical interview;
5. Access information;

6. Evaluate information;
7. Negotiate decisions, give feedback, resolve conflict, and agree on an action plan.

Personalizing Patient Consent Forms

Another possible area for improvement is format of patient consent forms, particularly in the context of elective procedures.[6] Harlan Krumholz has proposed the use of a standardized format with personalized content to the patient's characteristics and treatment.[6] The standardized format would contain treatment information in five key areas: risks, benefits, alternatives, costs, and provider experience.[6] The estimate of the risks and anticipated benefits would consider each patient's unique characteristics. If a potential treatment benefit is uncertain, the patient should be so informed, which would also facilitate meaningful discussion with his or her provider. Ideally, the cost would reflect the patient's individual insurance coverage.[6] The standardized format should be easy to read and relatively concise, avoiding the cumbersome nature of existing consent forms.

Krumholz also suggests including information regarding the provider's experience, an additional aspect of consent not previously discussed in this paper.[6] This would include information about experience with this treatment and number of times performed.[6] Additionally, it could include information about provider and institutional performance, focusing on outcomes and benchmark comparison.[6] If this information was not known by the institution, the lack of knowledge could be disclosed to the patient.[6]

Krumholz advocates for the use of such a form as a tool to facilitate informed consent discussions, not to replace them.[6] Use of improved, yet standardized, informed consent documents should not preclude personalized discussions of medical treatment. If patients are given adequate time to read the forms before scheduling procedures, the forms could be useful tools to enhance the discussion. See Figure 35.1 for an example of a consent form.

THE FUTURE OF INFORMED CONSENT AND SHARED DECISION MAKING

The legal doctrine of informed consent, even in its earliest form, was a progressive step toward patient involvement in medical decision making. Over the past 50 years, there has been growing momentum within the medical community for more patient-centered care and patient involvement.[6] Recently, the Institute of Medicine (IOM) named patient-centered care as one of its six core attributes of a high-quality healthcare system.[41] The IOM defined patient centeredness as "providing care that is respectful of and responsive to individual patient preferences, needs, and values, and ensuring that patient values guide all clinical decisions." Shared decision making fits nicely within the IOM's objective by facilitating dialogue between providers and patients in the decision-making process.[6]

Some members of the medical and legal community have called for a different way of viewing and structuring the process of soliciting patient consent that would expand current legal and regulatory disclosure requirements to include new models of decision making.[1,26] One proposal is that a patient could be asked to sign an informed consent form acknowledging that he or she has engaged in shared decision making with the provider and that he or she has no remaining questions that would deter him or her from a specific course of treatment.[26] Such a proposal has not yet been adopted by the courts, and more time is needed to determine whether the concept of shared decision making will be adopted into the legal doctrine of informed consent.[26] Regardless of judicial adoption, shared decision making appears to have great potential in medical practice to foster more complete patient understanding, address a patient's personal needs, and improve a patient's health outcome.

FIGURE 35.1 Example of a consent form[6]

- **Background**

Lay-person description of physical symptoms and cause.

- **Procedure**

Brief, high-level description of procedure, perhaps providing print material for patient to take home and read and discuss with significant others.

- **Potential Benefits***

Likely benefit: __ of every 100 patients who have this procedure have less __, and __ of every 100 no longer have it.

**Benefits that will not be achieved, but could be easily confused with benefits of this treatment, could also be included.*

- **Potential Risks**

This treatment has a small risk of causing __ :

(1) the chances of you experiencing this risk are __ in 1000;

This treatment has a large risk of causing __ :

(2) the chances of you experiencing this risk are __ in 100.

- **Other Available Treatments**

Brief description of other treatment options, including the option of no treatment.

- **Experience of Your Healthcare Team**

Your doctor has performed __ number of procedures in the past year. Standards suggest that doctors should perform at least __ each year. Your hospital has performed __ procedures in the past year. Standards suggest that hospitals should perform at least __ procedures each year.

- **Cost**

Taking your health insurance into account, the procedure will cost you about $__ if things go as planned. The doctor will cost you $__. Taking ongoing prescriptions for __ months will cost about $__ per month, totaling $__ for the year.

References

1. Switankowsky, I. S. (1998). *A new paradigm for informed consent*. Lanham, MD: University Press of America.
2. Faden, R. R., Beauchamp, T. L., & King, N. M. P. (1986). *A history and theory of informed consent*. Oxford: Oxford University Press.
3. Krause, J. H. (2010). Can health law truly become patient-centered? *Wake Forest Law Review, 45*, 1489–1503.
4. Krause, J. H. (2010). Can health law truly become patient-centered? *Wake Forest Law Review, 45*, 1489–1503, referencing Berg, J. W., Appelbaum, P. S., Parker, L. S., & Lidz, C. W. (2001). *Informed consent: Legal theory and clinical practice* (2nd ed.). New York, NY: Oxford University Press.
5. Krumholz, H. (2010). Informed consent to promote patient-centered care. *JAMA, 303*,

1190–1191, referencing research by Holmboe, E. S., Fiellin, D. A., Cusanelli, E., Remetz, M., & Krumholz, H. M. (2000). Perceptions of benefit and risk of patients undergoing first-time elective percutaneous coronary revascularization. *Journal of General Internal Medicine, 15*, 632–637.

6. Krumholz, H. (2010). Informed consent to promote patient-centered care. *JAMA, 303*, 1190–1191.
7. Weston, W. W. (2001). Informed and shared decision-making: The crux of patient-centered care. *Canadian Medical Association Journal, 165*(4), 438–439, referencing Braddock, C. H., Edwards, K. A., Hasenberg, N. M., Laidley, T. L., & Levinson, W. (1999). Informed decision making in outpatient practice: Time to get back to basics. *JAMA, 282*(24), 2313–2320.
8. Weston, W. W. (2001). Informed and shared decision-making: The crux of patient-centered care. *Canadian Medical Association Journal, 165*(4), 438–439.
9. Charles, C., Gafni, A., & Whelan, T. (1997). Shared decision-making in the medical encounter: What does it mean? (or it takes at least two to tango). *Social Science & Medicine, 44*(681), 681–692.
10. American Medical Association (AMA) Ethics Group. *History of AMA ethics*. Retrieved from http://www.ama-assn.org/ama/pub/physician-resources/medical-ethics/code-medical-ethics/history-ama-ethics.page?
11. Code of Ethics of the American Medical Association (adopted May 1847), as cited in Katz, J. (1984). *The silent world of doctor and patient*. Mankato, MN: The Free Press.
12. 70 C.J.S. *Physicians and Surgeons* § 115.
13. Prosser, W. L., Wade, J. W., Schwartz, V. E., Kelly, K., & Partlett, D. F. (2010). *Torts: Cases and materials* (12th ed.), 1. Note that breach of contract is a separate area of civil law, excluded from tort law.
14. See references in historical British case law dating back to at least 1466 in *Hulle v. Orynge*, Y.B.M. 6 Edw. IV, folio 7, placitum 18 (1466), in which the right to personal autonomy and to be free from injury is recognized.
15. *Restatement (Second) of Torts* § 13 (1965).
16. See *Wallace v. Rosen*, 765 N.E. 2d 192; see also American Law Institute. (2010). *A concise restatement of torts* (2nd ed.), §16.
17. See *Schloendorff v. Society of New York Hospitals*, 105 N.E. 92, 93 (1914); *Bang v. Charles T. Miller Hospital*, 251 Minn. 427 (1958); and *Berkey v. Anderson*, 1 Cal.App.3d 790 (1969).
18. See *Mohr v. Williams*, 104 N.W. 12 (Minn. 1905), where patient consulted an ear specialist, complaining of issues with her right her. Upon examination, the physician found the right ear to be diseased. Patient consented to surgery on the right ear. While patient was anesthetized, the physician deemed that the condition of the right ear did not require surgery; however, he found a serious condition in the left ear, which he proceeded to operate on. Although the operation was performed skillfully and successfully, the physician was held liable to the patient under the tort of battery and paid moderate damages to the patient.
19. King, J. S., & Moulton, B. (2006). Rethinking informed consent: The case for shared medical decision-making. *American Journal of Law & Medicine, 32*, 429–501.
20. *Canterbury v. Spence*, 464 F.2d 772, 784-86 (D.C. Cir. 1972).
21. Flinn, J. L. (2009). Personalizing informed consent: The challenge of health literacy. *Saint Louis University Journal of Law & Policy, 2*(2), 379–412.
22. King, J. S., & Moulton, B. (2006). Rethinking informed consent: The case for shared medical decision-making. *American Journal of Law & Medicine, 32*, 429–501, referencing research by Wennberg, J. E., & Peters, P. G. (2002). Unwanted variations in the quality of health care: Can the law help medicine provide a remedy/remedies? *Wake Forest Law Review, 37*, 925–941; and research by Feldman-Stewart, D., Brundage, M. D., McConnell, B. A., & MacKillop, W. J. (2000). Practical issues in assisting shared decision-making. *Health Expectations, 3*, 46–54.
23. American Medical Association principles of medical ethics (1980), as cited in Katz, J. (1984). *The silent world of doctor and patient*. Mankato, MN: The Free Press.
24. Adams, J. R., & Drake, R. E. (2006). Shared decision-making and evidence-based practice. *Community Mental Health Journal, 42*, 87–105, referencing research by Balint, M. (1957). *The doctor, the patient, and his illness*. London: Tavistock; and Engel, G.

(1960). A unified concept of health and disease. *Perspectives in Biology and Medicine, 3*, 459–485.

25. Adams, J. R., & Drake, R. E. (2006). Shared decision-making and evidence-based practice. *Community Mental Health Journal, 42*, 87–105, referencing research by Ellwood, P. (1988). A technology of patient experience. *New England Journal of Medicine, 318*, 1549–1556.
26. Adams, J. R., & Drake, R. E. (2006). Shared decision-making and evidence-based practice. *Community Mental Health Journal, 42*, 87–105.
27. Adams, J. R., & Drake, R. E. (2006). Shared decision-making and evidence-based practice. *Community Mental Health Journal, 42*, 87–105, referencing research by Anderson, R. M. (1995). Patient empowerment and the traditional medical model. A case of irreconcilable differences? *Diabetes Care, 18*, 412–415.
28. Adams, J. R., & Drake, R. E. (2006). Shared decision-making and evidence-based practice. *Community Mental Health Journal, 42*, 87–105, referencing research by W.A. MacColl Institute for Healthcare Innovation. (1998). *A model of practice and system supports for effective chronic illness care*. Group Health Cooperative of Puget Sound.
29. Adams, J. R., & Drake, R. E. (2006). Shared decision-making and evidence-based practice. *Community Mental Health Journal, 42*, 87–105, referencing research by Auerbach, S. M. (2001). Do patients want control over their own health care? A review of measures, findings, and research issues. *Journal of Health Psychology, 6*, 191–203.
30. Adams, J. R., & Drake, R. E. (2006). Shared decision-making and evidence-based practice. *Community Mental Health Journal, 42*, 87–105. See also Whitney S. N., McGuire, A. L., & McCullough, L. B. (2003). A typology of shared decision making, informed consent, and simple consent. *Annals of Internal Medicine, 140*, 54–59; and King, J. S., & Moulton, B. (2006). Rethinking informed consent: The case for shared medical decision-making. *American Journal of Law & Medicine, 32*, 429–501.
31. Whitney, S. N., McGuire, A. L., & McCullough, L. B. (2003). A typology of shared decision making, informed consent, and simple consent. *Annals of Internal Medicine, 140*, 54–59.
32. Adams, J. R., & Drake, R. E. (2006). Shared decision-making and evidence-based practice. *Community Mental Health Journal, 42*, 87–105. Joos, S. K., Hickam, D. H., Gordon, G. H., & Baker, L. H. (1996). Effects of a physician communication intervention on patient care outcomes. *Journal of General Internal Medicine, 11*, 147–155.
33. Estabrooks, C., Goel, V., Thiel, E., Pinfold, P., Sawka, C., & Williams, I. (2001). Decision aids: Are they worth it? A systematic review. *Journal of Health Services Research and Policy, 6*(3), 6170–6182.
34. Roter, D. L., Stewart, M., Putnam, S. M., Lipkin, M. Jr., Stiles, W., & Inui, T. S. (1997). Communication patterns of primary care physicians. *JAMA, 277*(4), 350–356. (1997).
35. Katz, J. (1984). *The silent world of doctor and patient*. Mankato, MN: The Free Press.
36. Gwyn, R., & Elwyn, G. (1999). When is a shared decision not (quite) a shared decision? Negotiating preferences in a general practice encounter. *Social Science & Medicine, 49*, 437–447.
37. Towle, A., & Godolphin, W. (1999). Framework for teaching and learning informed shared decision-making. *BMJ, 319*, 766–771.
38. King, J. S., & Moulton, B. (2006). Rethinking informed consent: The case for shared medical decision-making. *American Journal of Law & Medicine, 32*, 429–501, referencing research by Keating, N., Guadagnoli, E., Landrum, M., Borbas, C., & Weeks, J. (2002). Treatment decision making in early-stage breast cancer: Should surgeons match patients' desired level of involvement? *Journal of Clinical Oncology, 20*, 1473—1479. See Towle, A., & Godolphin, W. (1999). Framework for teaching and learning informed shared decision-making. *BMJ, 319*, 766–771.
39. Arnold, S. V., Decker, C., Ahmad, H., Olabiyi, O., Mundluru, S., Reid, K. J., . . . Spertus, J. A. (2008). Converting the informed consent from a perfunctory process to an evidence-based foundation for patient decision making. *Circulation. Cardiovascular Quality and Outcomes, 1*(1), 21–28.
40. Stewart, M. A. (1995). Effective physician-patient communication and health outcomes:

A review. *Canadian Medical Association Journal, 152*, 1423–1432.
41. IOM Report, Institute of Medicine Committee on Quality of Health Care in America. (2001). *Crossing the quality chasm: A new health system for the 21st century*. Washington, DC: National Academies Press.

36

Trust, Disclosure, Apology: How We Act When Things Go Wrong Has an Impact on Patient Safety

Keith Siddel

Trust: reliance on the integrity, strength, ability, surety, etc., of a person or thing; confidence.[1]

Disclose: to make known; reveal or uncover.[2]

Apology: a written or spoken expression of one's regret, remorse, or sorrow for having insulted, failed, injured, or wronged another.[3]

Many industries have given high reliability concepts top priority for more than 20 years, but healthcare institutions have only recently embraced these concepts. I believe that trust, disclosure, and apologies when appropriate are essential components of achieving high reliability, particularly in healthcare organizations. The five key characteristics of high reliability are trust and transparency, reporting, flexibility in hierarchy, organizations perceived to be just and accountable, and engagement and dedication in terms of continual learning.[4] There are many things a healthcare institution can do to become a high-reliability organization, but this chapter will focus on those things they can do when things go wrong. With scrutiny from a growing number of external stakeholders, healthcare institutions must seek the path of change now or face an uncertain future.

In the past, healthcare providers have allowed the fear of litigation to pervade all aspects of their operation. Concern about liability erodes professional integrity and destroys the relation of trust that health care is built on. It is no wonder that many healthcare providers now view each patient as a potential litigant.[5] "To err is human; to forgive, divine."[6] This quote demonstrates that there are two parts to an error: the error itself and what comes next. We spend enormous amounts of resources focusing on preventing errors, as we should. Yet, in high-reliability organizations, the work that occurs after the error is equally important.

TRUST

The concept of trust incorporates a number of the high-reliability characteristics including transparency, justness, accountability, and reporting. The physician–patient relationship, and by extension the hospital–patient relationship, is built on the foundation of trust. In spite of the plethora of developments in the last century, the provider–patient relationship has been the one unchanging principle in medicine. Once the trust begins to fade, the relationship can no longer be effective.[7] When an error occurs, there is a violation of this trust. The provider compounds the injury when he or she fails to disclose the error and to apologize. We expect that someone worthy of our trust will behave ethically by taking responsibility for harming us. The state of Colorado realized this, and made it the basis for one of the most far-reaching "I'm sorry" laws in the United States.[8] The stated legislative intent of Colorado's law was to promote a continued open and trusting relationship between physicians and patients following a medical error.[7]

Trust is not just a two-way street; rather it is a complex highway interchange involving many parties. Healthcare providers at all levels involved in patient care need to be included in the process. Patients' immediate and extended families, who play a role in support, should be taken into account. Maintaining the balance of trust is difficult when things go wrong or when errors happen, but it is essential to a successful program. The patient-centered ethic underscores the provider's obligation to inform the patient of potential adverse outcomes.[9]

DISCLOSURE

The concept of disclosure incorporates a number of the high-reliability characteristics including transparency, accountability, and reporting. A sizable gap exists between patients' desire to be told about medical errors and the current level of information which is shared.[10] Physicians generally agree that the information they disclose to a patient widely varies. A 2002 survey found that disclosure of errors occurred in less than one-third of cases, falling short of patient expectations.[11] In a 2006 study of physicians, when asked what they would disclose, 42% said they would use the word *error*, while 56% mentioned the adverse event but not the error; 50% would disclose specific information about what the error was, while 13% would not volunteer any details unless asked by the patient.[12] Similarly, 52% would disclose specific information about why the error happened, but 19% would volunteer no such information. Overall, 94% would apologize, with 61% offering an expression of regret ("I am sorry about what happened"), and 33% choosing an explicit apology ("I am so sorry that you were harmed by this error").[12] Regarding error prevention, 9% would provide no information unless asked, 54% chose a general pledge to prevent recurrences, and 37% would discuss detailed plans for preventing recurrences.[12]

There is wide disparity between what various organizations and providers believe should be disclosed to the patient. Some believe that what should drive the decision is the outcome of the error, while others look to the potential for harm to the patient. For example, should the provider disclose a medication error when it occurs but there is no adverse effect on the patient? Is the patient owed an apology in this situation? When the term *never event* was coined in 2001, the focus was on outcomes. Likewise, when The Joint Commission required that hospitals report sentinel events in 1995, they defined them as "an unexpected occurrence involving death or serious physiological or psychological injury, or the risk thereof."[13] Under the National Quality Forum definition of never events, 15 of the 28 events require death or serious disability before the error is considered a true never event.[14]

Health care often looks to other high-risk industries when modeling its safety plans. Yet none of these industries has a disclosure policy close to health care. It is true that industries such as commercial aviation, nuclear power, and hydrocarbon have extensive reporting processes for near misses; however, none of these processes suggest that those involved receive an apology for the near miss. (I wonder what would happen if during a transatlantic flight the pilot came on the overhead and reported a near miss to the passengers?) The healthcare industry is divided on the position of apologizing for near misses, and only time will show whether disclosure requirements will be expanded to include them, as well as those errors with serious or fatal outcomes.

The practice of nondisclosure arose out of the fear of litigation and a desire to preserve the organization's and the provider's reputation. Providers drove medical mistakes underground, believing that admitting errors would damage their reputations and lead to lawsuits. If the mistake could not be hidden, the institutions stalled all inquiries, but were these actions justified?

A recent study of over 5,800 physicians found that more than 60% of physicians older than 55 had been sued at some point in their careers.[15] Over 20% of the physicians were defendants in lawsuits more than once. Some specialties such as surgery had a litigation rate as high as 90%. Over 50% of OB-GYN physicians under the age of 40 years old have already been sued. The question is what is behind all this litigation? Is it that physicians and healthcare providers make that many mistakes, or is there possibly another reason that patients turn to the legal process for answers?

This same study found that 65% of the legal claims filed resulted in withdrawal or dismissal. Looking at this number one might conclude that there are many frivolous lawsuits,[16] but perhaps there is another answer. It is possible that the patients file lawsuits simply to force the provider to disclose information that the patient seeks about a perceived error. Do patients feel that a lawsuit is the only way to get answers when the outcome is unexpected?

In 1990, Harvard University conducted a study that suggested fewer than one in eight victims of medical negligence actually filed a claim.[17] Some would argue that in many of these cases the patient might not have known that an error occurred and that is why the patient does not file a claim. This belief has certainly been the basis for the argument that physicians should keep quiet when errors occur. In this study, of those people who did sue, two-thirds of the plaintiffs walked away with no money because 61% of the cases resulted in dismissal or withdrawal.[17] (This result compares closely to the result of the first study quoted at 65%.) While the outcomes will vary as much as the claims, it is possible that once patients found out the information they sought, they had no reason to continue with the suit. Of note, 32% of the cases that did settle had an average payout of $300,000.[17] Of the 7% of the cases that go to trial, plaintiffs prevail in approximately 20% (only one in five) cases.[17] This is a very small fraction of the total number of medical malpractice claims actually filed—representing a mere 1.3%.[17] Eighteen years later, another study produced similar results and indicated that of the cases that went to trial, the plaintiff prevailed on only 10%.[15]

Responding to these situations, lawmakers in most states considered a variety of legislative reforms. Some reforms focused on reducing providers' liabilities, while others sought to make it easier for patients to get information about what happened during their care. One such reform that has gained widespread support, albeit in different forms, is what is commonly called apology or disclosure laws.

Some have argued that if the physician could apologize for an error or unexpected outcome without fear of the apology being used against him or her, he or she would.[18] The other side of this same issue is the belief that patients often sue their physicians out of anger and frustration from lack of information and accountability. Patients who experience adverse medical events almost inevitably desire to know what happened. If the medical provider does not offer that information, some patients or their families will file a lawsuit to get it.[19] One study reported that patients offered the following reasons for deciding to file a medical malpractice case: (1) families believed that physicians would not listen (13%), (2) would not talk openly (32%), (3) attempted to mislead them (48%), or (4) did not warn about long-term problems (70%).[20] As these results indicate, the lack of clear, open, honest communication is at the center of the conflict between patients and their physicians.[21] Researchers have found that after a medical error the factors that put physicians at risk of a lawsuit are not the quality of medical care,[23] not chart documentation,[23] and not technical negligence[24] but rather ineffective communication with patients.[25]

Both the American College of Physicians and the American Medical Association state that ethics requires physicians to disclose medical errors to patients. As the AMA has explained:

> It is a fundamental ethical requirement that a physician should at all times deal honestly and openly with patients. Patients have a right to know their past and present medical status and to be free of any mistaken beliefs concerning their conditions. Situations occasionally occur in which a patient suffers significant medical complications that may have resulted from the physician's mistake or judgment. In these situations, the physician is ethically required to inform the patient of all the facts necessary to ensure understanding of what has occurred. Only through full disclosure is a patient able to make informed decisions regarding future medical care.[26]
>
> While most physicians would agree with this principle in theory, full disclosure has not always been the norm.[27]

The elements of a successful disclosures program should be an explanation, an open investigation, involvement of the patient and perhaps the family, an apology, compensation, and an acknowledgment of harm. For those who remain concerned that a program of this nature would increase litigation and damage their reputations, the following study offers the response.[28] This study indicated that, after full disclosure and an apology, patients felt that they trusted their providers more, were more satisfied, and were less likely to change physicians than when they received incomplete and evasive explanations. The study also indicated that the form of disclosure did not reduce the likelihood that the patient would consult a lawyer, at least in the case of serious harm. Seeking that sort of expertise did not inevitably mean that it would result in adversarial litigation.

APOLOGY

An apology is typically defined as "a written or spoken expression of one's regret, remorse, or sorrow for having wronged another," but that may be an oversimplification of a very complex type of communication. One study divides apologies into three broad categories: (1) those that are full, personal, and sincere and that are accompanied by an acknowledgment of responsibility; (2) those that are impersonal or nonspecific; and (3) those that accept responsibility on behalf of the institution or a third party. It is easy to conclude that from the patient's perspective (1) would be most effective, but it also presents the most legal risk to the person apologizing. Apologies (2) and (3) would be less effective but would appear to lessen the legal liability for the person giving the apology.

Many people believe that a partial apology is always preferable to saying nothing. However, research in the context of a nonmedical tort suggests that where fault is clear a partial apology may have a worse effect than saying nothing. If an individual who was clearly responsible for an injury fails to take responsibility, the injured party is less likely to accept a settlement. In that situation, no apology may be preferable to a partial apology. This leads me to conclude that, if a provider cannot or will not give an apology as defined in (1), it is better to not give the type of apology defined in (2) and (3).

Many physicians and healthcare providers would agree with the principle of apologizing for errors in theory, but few actually practice it. The healthcare industry has seen medical malpractice premiums skyrocket over the years, primarily in specific specialties such as obstetrics-gynecology and neurosurgery, which is reflective in the litigation patterns previously discussed. Because of increased risk and the increased premiums that accompany the risk, many physicians view each patient as a potential litigant. This attitude is reflected in two surveys designed to assess attitudes toward disclosure. The studies revealed that fear of litigation was the primary reason for both physicians' and hospitals' reluctance to disclose errors, unanticipated outcomes, or to apologize.

Under existing U.S. law, fault-admitting apologies are ordinarily admissible to prove liability. Rule 801(d)(2) of the Federal Rules of Evidence (FRE) and analogous state provisions provide that an admission by a party-opponent is not considered hearsay and therefore not excluded from admissibility by the hearsay rule(s). The rule states that an admission by a party-opponent is the party's own statement, in either an individual or a representative capacity. Therefore, even though you might at first consider the statement to be hearsay, as an out-of-court statement, it will not be considered so under the FRE. The key here is to note it is not necessarily the fault-admitting part of the apology that creates the risk but rather that it is a statement. Thus, when you consider the three types of apologies as defined previously they all carry the same risk.

Many state laws prevent apologies from admission when they occur during mediation or settlement negotiations. When viewed in this same light, medical apologies could likewise be excluded, but few courts have taken this position. One case where the court did take this position is in *Deese v. Carroll City County Hosp*. In this case, the Court of Appeals of Georgia concluded that "activity constituting a voluntary offer of assistance made on the impulse of benevolence or sympathy should not be considered as an admission of liability."[29]

OUTCOMES

One example of a high-reliable risk program that incorporates these concepts is at the University of Michigan health system. In 2002, the university began a program in which physicians report errors after review by risk management, disclose the error, and apologize to the patient. The impact on the health system's rate of litigation has been quite dramatic. In June 2001, the average number of open claims against the system was 250 to 260, and it took an average of 1,100 days to dispose of cases.[30] In December 2004, Rick Boothman, the Chief Risk Officer at the University of Michigan, reported that the number of open claims had fallen to the 120 to 130 range and that claims were resolved in 320 days.[30] He also reported that the annual cost of handling claims had declined from approximately $3 million to $1 million.[31]

Studies at other hospitals have found the same results.[32,33] While not conclusive that the increased use of disclosure and apology was the sole factor in the impact at these hospitals, it is clear that it did play some part. A number of other studies took another approach. They provided participants with hypothetical situations, and they found that apologies may reduce the subjects' likelihood to litigate.[28,34–36]

Apology and disclosure laws are not without their critics. The critics argue that, by disclosing the error and offering an apology, the providers will actually be placed in a worse situation because the majority of patients in the adverse medical event are unaware of medical errors and unsolicited apologies could possibly induce more malpractice claims.[37] In this study,

65 experts completed the survey (response rate: 83%) and predicted that, among patients who experienced severe injury as a result of negligence, disclosure would on average deter 32% from suing and prompt claims by 31% of patients who would not otherwise have sued.[37]

Perhaps one of the most robust studies performed to date was completed in September 2010 and relied on National Practitioner's Data Bank (NPDB).[38] Since 1991, all malpractice payments, either as part of a settlement or as part of a court judgment, made by or on behalf of a licensed healthcare provider are reported to NPDB within 30 days. This database has a robust data set and is comprehensive in nature. Using this data, researchers compared state claims data to compare those with disclosure and apology laws to those that do not have these laws. The results are striking. There is a consistent 14 to 15% increase in closed claims after the adoption of the apology law.[38] Furthermore, as expected, the total compensation also shows an increase of 20 to 27%.[38] These results may be surprising to some, but to those critics of the apology laws, this is the proof that their conclusions are correct. The researchers were surprised at the result as well and decided to further break the data down by medical severity. (This also limited the data set to claims since 2002 since that is when medical severity was initially added as an element to the database.) They reasoned that insignificant injuries would most often benefit from the apology laws, and the results supported this conclusion. There was a net reduction of 17.7 to 18.5% in the number of cases that did not involve major permanent injury or death.[38] Further analysis supports the conclusion that, after the disclosure and apology laws pass in a state, the number of claims rise for a short period of time for those cases that take years to resolve. However, there is an overall decline in those cases involving insignificant injuries. Perhaps the best news for the providers is that the study indicated that after the law is adopted claim severity is reduced by 17% for severe cases and 20% for the most severe cases.[38]

As previously identified, Colorado has one of the most extensive disclosure and apology laws of any state. In 2000 a large, private physician-directed medical malpractice insurance carrier in Colorado, COPIC Insurance Company (COPIC), instituted its 3Rs program. This program is one of the more commonly cited programs by apology advocates, but a careful examination of this program will show it has both advantages and disadvantages. First, a little background on COPIC. COPIC is the primary liability insurer for Colorado, insuring 6,000 physicians and 120 facilities.[39] The 3Rs program stands for recognize (unanticipated event), respond (soon after event), and resolve (related issues). 3Rs is a nonfault-based program designed to prevent medical injuries from entering the ineffective, inefficient, and adversarial legal system. Under the program, once a physician has reported an incident to COPIC and COPIC determines that the incident qualifies for its 3Rs program, the physician has a frank discussion with the patient, including an apology if warranted. The key is that although the patient still retains his or her right to sue the physician, he or she cannot use the apology as evidence of liability even if fault is admitted under Colorado's broadly protective apology statute. Apology advocates will tell you that only a few lawsuits have ever been filed following a 3Rs claim, but that is only half of the story. The advocates will tell you there are few lawsuits because of the apology, but there is more to the story. The key is to remember that the 3Rs is a no-fault program. There are a number of exclusions where if COPIC believes there may be obvious negligence, such as a never event, then the claim will not qualify for the 3Rs program. Other exclusions include patient deaths, formal written demands for compensation, summons/complaint, attorney involvement, request for action from a state licensing board, and incidents involving certain nationally recognized unacceptable outcomes (never events).[39] The advantage of the program is that if the error meets the 3Rs criteria the patient is eligible to receive reimbursement of related out-of-pocket medical expenses up to $25,000 and $100 per day up to 50 days to recognize extended loss of time from normal activities, and reimbursement is received in a timely fashion.

During the first five years of the program, COPIC reported that its malpractice claims against COPIC physicians dropped by 50% and settlement costs dropped by 23%.[30] Since the program has begun, COPIC has reviewed 13,053 incidents and concluded that 8,496 met the 3Rs criteria (65%).[39] The program has reimbursed 1,829 patients (21% of incidents that met the 3Rs criteria and 14% of all incidents), and the average amount paid per incident was $4,977.[39]

The disadvantage to this program is that it would be a mistake to conclude that it is anything more than a limited program designed to handle outcomes that are unlikely to involve serious negligence or injury. The focus is on minor errors and near misses, which limits its effectiveness.

CONCLUSION

Disclosure and apology are not only the ethical thing to do but also maintain the trust that is the bedrock of the healthcare relationship. If providers needed another reason to incorporate these concepts in their risk management and patient safety programs, studies show it ultimately is good for the bottom line. In the end, what more can providers ask for but a financial reward for doing what's right!

References

1. Trust. (n.d.). In *Dictionary.com*. Retrieved from http://dictionary.reference.com/browse/trust?s=t.
2. Disclose. (n.d.). In *Dictionary.com*. Retrieved from http://dictionary.reference.com/browse/disclose?s=t.
3. Apology. (n.d.). In *Dictionary.com*. Retrieved from http://dictionary.reference.com/browse/apology?s=t.
4. Youngberg, B. J. (2011). *Principles of Risk Management and Patient Safety*. Sudbury, MA: Jones & Bartlett.
5. Wojcieszak, D. *Doctors, insurers, lawyers, hospital administrators, patients, and researchers joining together to provide a "middle ground" solution to the medical malpractice crisis*. The Sorry Works! Coalition. Retrieved from http://www.sorryworks.net.
6. Alexander Pope, *An Essay on Criticism*, Part II (written in 1709, first published in 1711). Retrieved May 26, 2012 from http://www.quotecounterquote.com/2010/12/to-err-is-human-to-forgive-divine.html.
7. Cohen, J. R. (2004). Toward candor after medical error: The first apology law. *Harvard Health Policy Review, 5*, 21–24. Retrieved May 27, 2012 from http://www.hcs.harvard.edu/~hhpr/publications/previous/04s/Cohen.pdf.
8. Evidence of admissions—civil proceedings—unanticipated outcomes—medical care. Colo Rev Stat sec 13-25-135 (2003). Retrieved from http://www.state.co.us/gov_dir/leg_dir/olls/sl2003a/sl_126.pdf.
9. Youngberg, B. J., & Hatlie, M. J. (Eds.). (2004). *The Patient Safety Handbook*. Sudbury, MA: Jones & Barlett.
10. Gallagher, T. H., Garbutt, J. M., Waterman, A. D., Flum, D. R., Larson, E. B., Waterman, B. M., . . . Levinson, W. (2006). Choosing your words carefully: How physicians would disclose harmful medical errors to patients. *Archives of Internal Medicine, 166*(15), 1585–1593.
11. Blendon, R. J., DesRoches, C. M., Brodie, M., Benson, J. M., Rosen, A. B., Schneider, E., . . . Steffenson, A. E. (2002). Views of practicing physicians and the public on medical errors. *New England Journal of Medicine, 347*, 1933–1940.
12. Gallagher, T. H., Garbutt, J. M., Waterman, A. D., Flum, D. R., Larson, E. B., Waterman, B. M., . . . Levinson W. (2006). Choosing your words carefully. *Archives of Internal Medicine, 166*, 1585–1593.

13. The Joint Commission. *Facts about the sentinel event policy*. Retrieved from http://www.jointcommission.org/assets/1/18/Sentinel_Event_Policy_3_2011.pdf.
14. National Quality Forum. *Serious reportable events*. (2008). Retrieved from http://www.qualityforum.org/Publications/2008/10/Serious_Reportable_Events.aspx.
15. Kane, C. K. (2010). *Medical liability claim frequency: A 2007–2008 snapshot of physicians*. Retrieved from http://www.ama-assn.org/resources/doc/health-policy/prp-201001-claim-freq.pdf.
16. American Medical Association. (2005). *Medical liability reform now!* http://www.legalreforminthenews.com/Reports/Medical-LiabilityReformNow-AMA-142005.pdf.
17. Houk, C., & Moidel, B. (2003). Integrated conflict management systems in health care: A practical innovation whose time has come. *ACResolution, 2*, 30–31.
18. Novack, D. H., Detering, B. J., Arnold, R., Forrow, L., Ladinsky, M., & Pezzullo, J. C. (1989). Physicians attitudes towards using deception to resolve difficult ethical problems. *JAMA, 261*(2), 2980–2985.
19. Gilbert, S. (1997). *Wrongful death: A medical tragedy*. New York, NY: W.W. Norton.
20. Hickson, G. B., Wright Clayton, E., Githens, P. B., & Sloan, F. A. (1992). Factors that prompted families to file medical malpractice claims following perinatal injuries. *JAMA, 267*, 1359–1363.
21. Kielhorn, T. M. (1997). Reducing risk by improving communication. *The Permanente Journal, 1*(1), 69–70. Retrieved from http://xnet.kp.org/permanentejournal/sum97pj/risk.pdf.
22. Litman, R. S. (2009). Physician communication skills decrease malpractice claims. *ASA Newsletter, 73*(12), 20–21. Retrieved from http://depts.washington.edu/asaccp/prof/asa73_12_20_21.pdf.
23. Entman, S. S., Glass, C. A., Hickson, G. B., Githens, P. B., Whetten-Goldstein, K., & Sloan, F. A. (1994). The relationship between malpractice claims history and subsequent obstetric care. *JAMA, 272*, 1588–1591.
24. Harvard Medical Practice Study. (1990). *Patients, doctors, and lawyers: Medical injury, malpractice litigation, and patient compensation in New York*. A report by the Harvard Medical Practice Study to the State of New York. Retrieved May 26, 2012 from http://www.oshmanlaw.com/Harvard-Medical-Practice-Study.pdf.
25. Lester, G. W., & Smith, S. G. (1993). Listening and talking to patients: A remedy for malpractice suits? *Western Journal of Medicine, 158*, 268–272.
26. Retrieved May 26, 2012 from http://www.ama-assn.org/ama1/pub/upload/mm/-1/positionprescribing.pdf.
27. Bender, F. F. (2007). "I'm sorry" laws and medical liability. *Virtual Mentor, 9*(4), 300–304. Retrieved from http://virtualmentor.ama-assn.org/2007/04/hlaw1-0704.html.
28. Mazor, K. M., Simon, S. R., & Gurwitz, J. H. (2004). Communicating with patients about medical errors: A review of the literature. *Archives of Internal Medicine, 164*, 1690–1697.
29. *Deese v. Carroll City County Hosp.*, 203 Ga. App. 148 (1992), Court of Appeals of Georgia.
30. Simon, S. (Producer). (2004, December 18). *Hospitals: 'Sorry' reduces malpractice cases*. [Audio podcast]. Retrieved from http://www.npr.org/templates/story/story.php?storyId = 4234901.
31. Berg, M. (2004). Hospitals implement programs that encourage clinicians to apologize for mistakes. *Nursing Executive Watch, 5* (December 10).
32. Liebman, C. B., & Hyman, C. S. (2005). *Medical error disclosure, mediation skills, and malpractice litigation: A demonstration project in Pennsylvania*. Retrieved from http://www.pewtrusts.org/uploadedFiles/wwwpewtrusts-org/Reports/Medical_liability/LiebmanReport.pdf.
33. Kraman, S. S., & Hamm, G. (1999). Risk management: Extreme honesty may be the best policy. *Annals of Internal Medicine, 131*(12), 963–967.
34. Gallagher, T. (2003). Patients' and physicians' attitudes regarding the disclosure of medical errors. *JAMA, 289*, 1001–1007.
35. Witman, A. B., Park, D. M., & Hardin, S. B. (1996). How do patients want physicians to handle mistakes? A survey of internal medicine patients in an academic setting. *Archives of Internal Medicine, 156*, 2565–2569.
36. Wu, A. W., Huang, I. C., Stokes, S., & Pronovost, P. J. (2009). Disclosing medical errors to patients: It's not what you say, it's what they

hear. *Journal of General Internal Medicine, 24,* 1012–1017.

37. Studdert, D. M., Mello, M. M., Gawande, A. A., Brennan, T. A., & Wang, Y. C. (2007). Disclosure of medical injury to patients: An improbable risk management strategy. *Health Affairs (Millwood), 26*(1), 215–226.
38. Ho, B., & Liu, E. (2010). *What's an apology worth? Estimating the effects of apology laws in medical malpractice.* Retrieved from http://www.socialsciences.cornell.edu/0912/Ho.pdf.
39. Tarrant, C. A. *Recognize, respond to and resolve patient injury.* CAPSAC Annual Convening, April 30, 2010. Sacramento, CA. Retrieved from http://www.capsac.org/wp-content/uploads/2012/03/COPICs-3Rs-Program Recognize-Respond-to-and-Resolve-Patient-Injury.pdf.

37

Why, What, and How Ought Harmed Parties Be Told? The Art, Mechanics, and Ambiguities of Error Disclosure

John D. Banja, PhD

Although the law bases the patient–health provider relationship on the latter's "reasonable and prudent" behavior, ethics understands that relationship as grounded in beneficence, wherein the professional subordinates his or her self-serving interests to furthering and advancing the welfare of his or her patients.[1–3] Virtually all ethical codes of physician behavior require that health providers elevate their patients' welfare above their own, and state licensing laws and regulations generally begin by noting that their primary purpose is to protect the interests of citizens and consumers of the professional service.[3–5]

Using the language of ethics, then, we might translate the question of "What ought persons who have been harmed from medical error be told?" into the following questions:

- What does ethics say persons are "owed" by way of informational disclosure when they have experienced adverse consequences from medical error?
- Assuming the existence of a moral obligation requiring disclosure of harm-causing medical error to affected parties, what ought the content and scope of that disclosure be?
- How ought the persons involved in the error understand and communicate it—in a purely factual way, as a breach of trust, as sorrow and regret, or as legally owing a compensation?
- How ought healthcare training programs and institutional attitudes be configured according to the ways these questions are answered?

This chapter addresses these questions and offers a series of suggestions as to how to conduct what is not only a bad-news conversation, but one wherein the error operators expose themselves to the possibility of adverse litigation as a consequence of their disclosure. Also, a number of ambiguities surrounding certain facets of the disclosure process that require further discussion and even research will be identified as the chapter proceeds. As a prelude to all of this, however, I will offer a fundamental ethical argument as to why the disclosure of serious harm-causing medical error *must* occur because without such a conceptual foundation, harm-causing error operators might not admit a need to learn and implement the mechanics of an error disclosure conversation.

WHY ERROR DISCLOSURE IS A MORAL IMPERATIVE

A considerable amount of literature appeared during the 1990s attesting to the utility of error disclosure. Commentators noted that the policy and practice of error disclosure can result in a diminished incidence of malpractice litigation or its associated costs, improve quality of care and diminish future risk of error, alleviate guilt and relieve stress among error operators, heighten the public trust, improve health professional–patient relationships, and abolish counterproductive myths (e.g., physician omniscience and perfectionism) that are slow to leave institutional cultures.[6–8]

Besides the benefits that derive from disclosure, however, we ought to note a substantive moral reason for disclosure whose merit and persuasiveness does not derive from its positive or materially useful consequences. This reason has been alluded to earlier by way of the primacy of the patient's welfare. A fundamental concentration on the patient's good not only derives from our traditional and historical understanding of the health provider's obligation to patients and the ideal formation of his or her character, but from the very meaning of normative ethics itself. That is, to be ethical or act ethically *means* to be other-regarding. The ethical act is ordinarily understood to be the one that furthers the interest of the other for his or her own sake, not for the sake of the moral agent's.[9] Whether one adopts a Kantian ethic of duty or a utilitarian ethic of realizing the greatest good for the greatest number, both moral theories are unequivocal in requiring the decision maker to be other-regarding.[10] It is simply counterintuitive—indeed, it runs contrary to the way we talk about and understand professional ethical behavior—to call an act ethical that primarily promotes the actor's self-interest.

The unassailability of this simple observation—that professional ethics is grounded in other-regarding sensibilities—explains why the discovery of an intentional act of concealment of harm-causing error is so shocking, embarrassing, and shameful. The guilty parties have no argument that is morally acceptable with which to justify their concealment because no publicly acceptable justification for their behavior exists.[6] Rather, their motivation for concealment is as obvious as their guilt: Their refusal to disclose derives from placing their own interests (in the form of averting harm to themselves, usually in the form of malpractice litigation) over those of the very party whose welfare they had promised to protect. Not only did they fail the patient once by delivering care that fell below a professional standard, they failed a second time by placing their own interests above the patient's, thereby depriving him or her of some recourse based in justice.

The idea of a "recourse based in justice" deserves some elaboration. Simply put, when a patient places his or her welfare into the hands of a health provider, not only does that patient have the right not to be maltreated, he or she has a fundamental right to know how his or her welfare is being affected by the ministrations of the health provider.[1,6] The contractual as well as fiduciary dimensions of the professional–patient relationship obligate the professional to inform the patient about how his or her care program is faring, given the fact that the health professional is morally responsible for whatever outcomes are reasonably connected with or result from that care. Consequently, whether the care program is succeeding or failing, the patient has a categorical right to know "What is causing this?" when that information is reasonably available because of the trust and honesty that must prevail in their relationship. (In the alternative, how many patients would enter into such a relationship if the understanding was that the physician will only tell you why you are feeling better, not why you are feeling worse?)

Now, this does not imply that patients have the right to be free from harm when they enter into a healthcare relationship, since a patient's condition might deteriorate despite the most technically sophisticated and skillfully delivered care. Patients do have the right, however, to understand how their health is a function of the care they are receiving, as well as to be free from behavior that fails to accommodate how a reasonable and prudent health provider ought to act.[2] A patient who experiences a harm-causing error, then, not only has a right to know about it, but also has a justice-based right to determine whether and how his or her harm (or loss) should be managed or remedied.

Section 8.12 of the American Medical Association's *Current Opinions on the Code of Medical Ethics* nicely underlines the trust and honesty that are at the basis of this "right to know," especially in the event of error:

> It is a fundamental ethical requirement that a physician should at all times deal honestly and openly with patients. Patients have a right to know their past and present medical status and to be free of any mistaken beliefs concerning their conditions. Situations occasionally occur in which a patient suffers significant medical complications that may have resulted from the physician's mistake or judgment. In these situations, the physician is ethically required to inform the patient of all the facts necessary to ensure understanding of what has occurred. Only through full disclosure is a patient able to make informed decisions regarding future medical care . . . . Concern regarding legal liability that might result following truthful disclosure should not affect the physician's honesty with a patient.[4, pp. 141–142]

Dispatching that duty, of course, might require enormous courage. Besides the way an individual's interest in professional self-preservation can be threatened by error disclosure, error operators might feel so wretched that exposing themselves to scrutiny via disclosure would be intolerably painful. Indeed, perhaps an emphasis on the way moral argument requires disclosure entirely misses certain broader and more powerful psychological forces that militate against it. Enormous fear of professional and public censure coupled with shame, guilt, and humiliation can easily persuade the professional whose error caused harm to numb himself or herself to recollections of the event, to "misremember" certain details or forget the incident altogether, to blame but then excuse someone else, or to reinterpret the error or its gravity (e.g., "the patient was desperately ill anyway," "these things happen—we can't always be perfect," "perhaps the error wasn't the harm-causing event after all").[7,11–13]

To the extent these factors play an influential role in error concealment, this chapter ends with some comments on how healthcare institutions, practicing professionals, and programs of medical education must commit themselves to changing the *character* of healthcare delivery and education in responding to medical error. Otherwise, it is unlikely that the following recommendations and strategies on how best to communicate harm-causing error will be taken seriously.

HOW TO COMMUNICATE HARM-CAUSING ERROR

The following suggestions are inspired by and frequently taken directly from Robert Buchman's and Yvonne Kason's classic treatise *How to Break Bad News*.[14] For any number of reasons—but perhaps most important, because professional training programs often do not sufficiently teach and maintain the skills associated with bad-news conversations—this book ought to be required reading for health professionals. Because the disclosure of medical error is a species of bad-news conversation, this text's numerous suggestions and insights are immensely valuable in conducting error disclosure conversations.

Assuming, then, that risk management and whatever other parties involved in error analysis have determined that a harm-causing error has indeed occurred and that the requisite professional courage has been secured to disclose it, the following considerations are offered with the hope that their implementation will reduce the occurrence of additional harm resulting from a poorly or ineptly conducted error disclosure conversation.

Consideration 1: The Initial Contact

If the harmed individual is of legal age and able to tolerate and engage in an error disclosure conversation, then he or she ought to be the first individual contacted. Because he or she sustained the harm, the institution's first obligation is to respect his or her right not only to know what happened but to determine what redress, if any, should be considered. If the harmed individual is not able to engage in the conversation, then his or her legally authorized surrogate, proxy, guardian, or nearest next of kin ought to be contacted and told.

If the individual who has suffered the harm-causing error is no longer receiving care at the facility—which may often be the case—then the patient or the patient's legally authorized representative or both will need to be contacted, probably telephonically, which raises the issue of framing that conversation. I shall assume in most of what follows that the harm-causing error was at least moderately serious and that, in all likelihood, the harmed party or his or her representatives will desire to schedule a face-to-face meeting after an initial telephonic contact. Whether the harm was serious or not, however—which, after all, is for the harmed party to decide—I suggest the telephone caller should be prepared at the outset to clarify the reason for the contact. Although some professionals might prefer that the caller say, "Mr. Jones, we'd like to discuss some issues with you that came up while your father was receiving care here some weeks ago. What date and time might fit your schedule for a meeting here at the hospital?" and then hedge or obfuscate if Mr. Jones asks for details, a better strategy, I believe, is for the caller to say, "Mr. Jones, the reason I'm calling is to discuss with you or whomever you'd like something we've learned that transpired with X's care while he was here. Would you like me to go into any details right now, or would you prefer to wait until we can set up a face-to-face meeting here at the hospital?" If Mr. Jones asks for details, then he should receive them—as discussed later—since they might assist him in deciding whether a face-to-face meeting is warranted and, if so, who else he might want to invite, such as an attorney. Also, if Mr. Jones does opt for a formal meeting, it might be wise to suggest to him that he might regard the information to be discussed at that meeting as confidential and so should choose his invitees according to their sensitivity toward maintaining confidentiality.

The identity of the telephonic caller is a significant issue for consideration and, perhaps, debate. One report in the literature has the initial contact to the harmed party made by the hospital's chief of staff.[8] Another strong candidate would be the harmed party's attending physician. Yet another might be someone from risk management or administration. Still another might be the health provider with whom the patient had the most favorable rapport, which might be a night nurse. In any case, the telephonic caller should anticipate that many if not most persons will want some detail about X's care, and that if the caller admits that an error was committed, many if not most persons will request considerable detail. Proceeding with such detail, however, will not only require a deep familiarity with the harm-causing error but might well cause considerable psychological pain to the listener. Indeed, the situation is not unlike a telephonic death disclosure to a family member.

Buckman and Kason's suggestions for handling that situation seem relevant to the error disclosure conversation as well. That is, if the caller is asked to go into some detail about the harm scenario, he or she might preface his or her remarks by saying something like, "Mr. Jones, what I'm going to say might be difficult for you to hear. Is there someone with you right now in the event you might want or need some company? [pause and wait for answer] Would you like me to contact someone to be with you? [pause and wait for answer] Do you believe you'll be all right until we can arrange a meeting?"

Although many health professionals will object to my suggestion that the telephonic caller be prepared to discuss the harm-causing error because they believe it would be too traumatic for the listener, the ability of persons to withstand the disclosure of painful news is usually much better than healthcare providers have traditionally supposed. Decades of experience with providing risk disclosure information in informed consent scenarios—which was once repudiated as unnecessarily upsetting for the "average" patient—show that most persons can handle bad news at least tolerably well.[15,16] Indeed, the healthcare provider who argues that it would be cruel for patients or family members to learn telephonically about harm-causing error may well be transferring his or her own anxiety about disclosing the information to the listener. Nevertheless, a very small number of persons likely exist for whom such telephonic disclosure would have devastating and perhaps even disabling impact. Further research and commentary is needed to provide confident procedures for discerning who this population might be and determining how best to proceed.

Should a face-to-face meeting be requested, which is likely, its scheduling should obviously respect the harmed parties' schedules because it is for their benefit. Indeed, consideration should be given to holding the meeting at the harmed party's dwelling. The purpose of the meeting, after all, is for the harmed party's sake so that the institution can fulfill its ethical duty to provide whatever benefits might culminate from disclosure. Consequently, as soon as a facility confirms that a harm-causing error has occurred, it should notify the involved parties and prepare for the meeting. The more time that elapses between the error discovery and the error disclosure, the more the harmed parties might feel they have been ignored or deprived of their right to know and of whatever time is necessary to heal from the event.

Consideration 2: The Meeting Setting

Buckman and Kason point out that bad news is frequently communicated in noisy, public environments (hospital hallways, waiting rooms, in front of elevators, at the bedside within earshot of strangers, etc.) that disrespect and can even heighten the emotional discomfort the news might precipitate. Consequently, a first order of business is to schedule the conversation in a private and quiet space that is free from background disturbances (e.g., conversations among other staff, phones or faxes ringing) and that promotes a calm atmosphere.

Communicators ought further to eliminate any artifacts that suggest institutional superiority or power. Buckman and Kason urge that when bad news is about to be communicated, not only ought the communicator(s) sit down, but that there be no desk between the conversants because a desk creates a geographical space that demarcates one zone of power—that is, where the doctor or administrator sits—from another, considerably disempowered one. The psychological context of an error disclosure conversation ought to be one wherein institutional authorities refrain from striking a politically superior position to the harmed parties.

Individuals disclosing the bad news must recognize that their communicational style ought to convey concern and profound regret. Once the harmed parties realize what has happened, they might feel enormously angry and betrayed and convey their emotions to the staff. Thus, communicators who are used to managing angry patients or family members by getting angry back or by assuming a bodily posture such as a stiffened spine, an icy or disapproving stare, a jutting, defiant chin, or an aloof communicational style (e.g., haughty, sermonizing, condescending, authoritative) should realize that these behaviors will be interpreted as arrogant and will probably arouse the anger of the patient or the family all the more.

Consequently, not only should the physical environment convey respect for the emotional gravity of the occasion, but extreme consideration should be paid to the tone of one's voice and even one's bodily posture. Buckman and Kason even suggest that bad-news communicators consider sitting lower in their chairs, because it is psychologically more difficult to have sadistic feelings toward someone positioned beneath your eye level than someone at or above it. Casual body language such as sitting back with one's legs crossed should be forgone in favor, perhaps, of a slightly forward-leaning sitting posture that communicates concern. The communicator's voice should be soft and gentle, and words should be expressed slowly. The communicator should speak in plain English, not medicalese. As will be noted later, the communicator should pause frequently so as to give the listeners an opportunity to ask questions. A box of tissues should be available if someone begins to cry.

Consideration 3: Who Should Be Present?

Root cause analysis overwhelmingly suggests that errors more often occur from systemic breakdowns than from a single individual making a terrible blunder with no one to blame but himself or herself. Indeed, analysis shows that in most cases, the error operator's mistake may simply have been the last in a mistake event chain that enables or facilitates the harm's occurrence.[17,18] If most harm-causing errors are the result of a systemic breakdown, then one might argue that key representatives of that systemic breakdown ought to be present.

I believe that the professional members attending a disclosure meeting should minimally include the patient's attending physician, a representative from hospital administration, and probably a representative from hospital risk management. It might also be a good idea to invite someone with experience in managing emotionally painful or traumatic conversations, such as a psychiatrist, psychologist, or social worker. Kraman and Hamm note that when such meetings occurred at their facility, the institutional representatives included "the chief of staff, the facility attorney, the quality manager, the quality management nurse, and sometimes the facility director."[8]

Additional commentary and study seem warranted here on how to achieve the best chemistry among and representation of institutional staff so as to enable an artful conveyance of harm-causing error. For example, should the facility's legal counsel be present, especially if the harmed party has announced that he or she will be accompanied and represented by counsel? Can the facility's legal counsel be expected to foster the objectives of a truthful and "healing" disclosure of information, or would his or her advocacy role for the facility cause a situation that might result in the attorney's guiding the conversation toward something less than a comprehensive disclosure of information?

Another area where serious disagreement might occur is over whether any of the error operators should be present. There are a number of reasons suggesting they should be. Consider that the error operator was an eyewitness to the error, might best know what happened (assuming his or her psychological stability and veracity), and represents the physical embodiment of the institution's intention to deal truthfully, directly, and honestly with the situation. Consider, too, how this individual might use the meeting to gain some sense of guilt relief over what has happened.[12] Also consider how the absence of the error perpetrator from the discussion (e.g., "Please forgive

Dr. or Nurse X for not being here; he or she was simply too shaken to attend our meeting.") might aggravate a patient's or family's desire for revenge. After all, the harmed parties are present and are experiencing the anguish of the disclosure. Why should the error operators be spared? A patient or family who has been harmed and is feeling terribly angry is unlikely at first blush to pity the error operator or, for that matter, pity anyone directly involved in the error's commission. Sadly but understandably, during the early moments of error disclosure, certain harmed parties might experience intense feelings of hatred or sadism. This invites yet a third suggestion on impaneling the meeting participants. That is, so as not to make it appear that the error operator is being offered up as a sacrificial lamb to the harmed party, the facility might consider inviting as many staff involved in the error as possible. The psychological effect of inviting a large number of professionals is not only to show in a most dramatic fashion how each person might admit a role in the error's occurrence, but to redirect the patient's or family's anger from one or a few persons to many persons, who might more effectively absorb that anger.

Many aggrieved parties might be impressed by such a generous admission and demonstration of concern, culpability, and regret, but certain harmed parties might feel suffocated by a large number of institutional representatives, not to mention how such a large group would need to be prepared in advance for comporting themselves during what might be an emotionally wrenching discussion. (Indeed, suppose the principal error operator is a particularly inept communicator or is psychologically fragile. What, when, and how much ought he or she be prepared to discuss?) Moreover, regardless of how many or how few persons represent the institution at the disclosure conference, care must be taken to ensure that they substantially agree on what happened. Again, it seems that more research and reflection is needed. How to determine the best mix and number of institutional persons is an important issue that deserves future study and insight.

Consideration 4: Framing the Disclosure

Buckman and Kason suggest that the following considerations guide the form and content of a bad-news conversation:

- Be guided by the patient's or family's agenda (i.e., their questions, considerations, concerns, speculations, accusations, and anxieties).
- Speak slowly, pause often, and refrain from medical jargon.
- Deliver the bad news gently but truthfully and straightforwardly.
- Don't assume how the bad news will be received.
- Use empathic listening skills (e.g., "This must be awful [dreadful, astonishing] for you to hear").
- Respect and use the therapeutic power of silence.

In bad-news conversations such as delivering a dreadful diagnosis, Buckman and Kason strongly recommend finding out how much the patient or family already knows about the situation, which can be elicited by asking, "Mr. Jones, what is your understanding of what has happened to you thus far?" Or, "Mr. Jones, tell me what your doctors have told you thus far." The point of these questions is to determine the extent and accuracy of Mr. Jones's information as well as to gauge the level of informational complexity the patient or family can handle.

Error disclosure is a different case, however, wherein these questions seem inappropriate because the harmed party's knowledge of what has occurred up to that point will largely be irrelevant to the actual purpose of the meeting. Therefore, after introducing the persons attending the meeting, it would be best for the principal communicator—who might well be either the attending physician or chief of staff—to begin by saying, "Mr. Jones, the reason for having this meeting today is to discuss with you a very serious situation that we have learned occurred with X's care. This is very difficult for me to tell you, but an error occurred that probably contributed to or outright caused Y to happen. [pause] Now, the individuals gathered in this room are prepared to talk about this with you and answer any of your questions. So, I'd like for you to tell me how to proceed. Would you like me to go into considerable detail, or would you like to know just in general what occurred? Or if you'd prefer for me to discuss this information at length with someone else whom you'd appoint, I'd be perfectly willing to do that." At this point, the communicator should stop and allow Mr. Jones to speak.

Consideration 5: How to Talk

One of the most challenging aspects of the conversation for the communicator, especially if he or she is a physician, will be to *remain silent and listen* to the harmed party or his or her representative while they speak or display emotions. Medical curricula generally pay insufficient attention to teaching empathic listening skills, and many physicians complain they don't have time to listen to patients. Furthermore, the institutional representative who communicates the error disclosure may feel frightened or anxious and be unable to resist his or her own psychological defenses insinuating themselves into the conversation. Thus, the communicator might be tempted to downplay the gravity of the harm committed, use humor inappropriately, anxiously and continually interrupt the harmed individual, or even, as has been reported on at least one occasion, lecture the harmed party at length on the theological merits and value of forgiveness.[19] The point of the conversation, however, is not for the communicator to protect his or her feelings but to inform the harmed party in a compassionate way about the error and allow that individual to express his or her feelings. The artful communicator, then, will know how to manage his or her feelings, not only in the midst of what might be a very emotionally charged discussion, but in a way that enables the harmed party to discharge his or her feelings in a nonharmful manner. In effect, once the communicator discloses the error, he or she ought to be led by the questions, concerns, and expressions of feeling of the harmed party, not the feelings and concerns of the institution (even though they will be powerfully present and always wanting to intrude).

Furthermore, communicators ought not to sugar-coat the bad news. For example, physicians sometimes communicate a diagnosis of cancer obscurely with words like *irregularity* or *shadow*, but this language primarily serves to lessen the discomfort of the communicator, not the patient. (And often the patient finds out anyway and becomes angry at the physician's reluctance to be more truthful.) While it is as simple to say as it is difficult to do, the best delivery of bad news ought to be done straightforwardly, concisely, truthfully and, of course, respectfully: "Mr. Jones, just before your father's surgery, he received twice the dosage of a drug that was ordered. This probably caused his heart to stop during the operation and contributed to his eventual death [pause, wait for response]." The communicator should look at the harmed party while saying this, not down at the floor or away. If direct eye contact is too painful for the communicator, he or she should pick out a spot on the harmed party's forehead and direct his or her gaze there.

Although arguments may occur over the precise content of the error disclosure, institutions might give serious consideration to including the following in an error disclosure conversation: an apology; a description of the nature of the harm-causing error and the time, place, and circumstances of the harm occurrence; the likely consequences of the harm-causing error for the patient; actions taken to treat or diminish the harmful consequences of the error on the patient; institutional measures taken to prevent recurrence of the accident; names of persons who will manage ongoing care of the patient; a description of the error analysis so far; names and phone numbers of persons who will manage ongoing communication with the patient or family; information on obtaining support and counseling regarding the error; and that charges and expenses directly related to the harm-causing error will be removed from the patient's account.[20]

Interestingly and importantly, Buckman and Kason urge that the communicator anticipate nothing as to how the news will be received. The intent of this rule is not to denigrate the psychological astuteness or insight of the communicator, but rather to encourage him or her to adopt a mind-set that enables an honest and straightforward informational disclosure. The communicator who, during the disclosure of error, cannot get his or her mind off imagining some dreadful scene erupting just moments away risks delivering a distracted, fragmented, fitful, and incoherent account of what occurred. By not anticipating how the news will be received, the communicator is in a better psychological position to articulate the error disclosure articulately and efficiently.

Consideration 6: Empathizing

Although a common definition of empathy is "feeling what another feels," a more correct characterization of empathy is understanding or imagining what the other is feeling and then exploring the roots of that feeling.[19] An empathic communicator not only does not dismiss or ignore a person's displaying his or her emotions, but realizes that they represent that person's being at that moment. How I *feel* is a manifest expression of what, at that moment, I *am*. Consequently, the communicator's saying, "Mr. Jones, I realize this is difficult but please try to get control of yourself" is in effect saying, "Mr. Jones, I'm uncomfortable with the 'Mr. Jones' I'm observing right now, so please present me with a different 'Mr. Jones' whose behavior I find more acceptable." If Mr. Jones is beside himself with anger or grief, what he really wants is an indication that his emotional pain is recognized and respected. The best response to Mr. Jones is either to be silent—because silence communicates respect—or to say, "This must be unimaginably difficult for you to bear."

A guiding consideration for the communicator is that he or she should mightily resist his or her own defensive behaviors. Whereas the purpose of activating our psychological defenses is so they protect us, the purpose of the error disclosure conversation is to inform and support the harmed party. The communicator, therefore, must be prepared to feel vulnerable and even to absorb the harmed party's rage, grief, bewilderment, and so on. The more the communicator expresses respect for and permission to the harmed party to say or express his or her feelings, the better. These facilitations best occur through empathic techniques such as reframing the other's statements or questions, for example, "What I hear you saying, Mr. Jones, is. . . ." Or "Let me see if I understand your question, Mr. Jones. You're asking me whether. . . ." The communicator might also simply reflect back the harmed party's feelings: "I realize you're feeling awful, Mr. Jones. This is utterly dreadful."

Many harmed parties might try, without realizing it, to provoke the communicator's rage by projecting their own rage onto the communicator. Thus, the harmed party might cry out, "How can you sit there and tell me this? I don't believe this. Is this some kind of joke? Are you sitting there telling me you killed my father? My God, then you're the ones who should be dead, not him." The most unproductive thing for the communicator to do at this moment would be to get angry or testy because doing so would only aggravate the harmed party's pain. Nor would it be particularly prudent for the communicator to argue or try to convince the harmed party how sorry everyone on the staff is: "But Mr. Jones, don't you see how sorry we are? Look at all we went through to set up this meeting and the courage it takes to sit down and tell you this. We could have kept the error a secret, you know, but we chose not to. Surely, you must give us credit for that." Although this might seem a perfectly logical response, an emotionally traumatized person might not be thinking logically or might not be inclined to sympathize with how rotten the error operators are feeling. An enraged harmed party might rather focus exclusively on his or her own grief, anger, or sense of betrayal. Consequently, the best response to the harmed party's provocations will be either to say nothing or say, "I am so sorry."

All of this will likely be extremely difficult for individuals not trained in empathic skills. Health care providers are accustomed to talking a lot, which is understandable. After all, persons come to them requesting their expertise and clinical knowledge. Consequently, when health providers feel uncomfortable in a professional situation, it is natural for them to preserve their self-esteem by calling upon what they know best and are most comfortable with: namely, reaching into their knowledge banks and talking. But in a bad-news situation such as error disclosure, elaborate explanations or justifications may be nontherapeutic unless the patient or harmed party requests them. Again, the rule is to be guided by the harmed party—who might indeed request lengthy and repeated descriptions of what went wrong or, instead, express a desire to terminate the present meeting and schedule another one. Consequently, delivering bad news requires the health professional to tolerate what will occasionally be deafening and heart-wrenchingly uncomfortable periods of questions, accusations, threats, and silence.

Consideration 7: Follow-up

When an individual hears emotionally devastating news, a common reaction is for that person to feel terribly isolated and alone.[21] One of the objectives of a bad-news conversation, therefore, is to convey to the patient or family that he or she will not be abandoned in the days, weeks, and months ahead. Thus, in a typical bad-news communication, Buckman and Kason suggest the communicator say something like, "Mr. Jones, I wonder if you might want to consider the following [treatments, self-help groups, other professionals, information, etc.]." In the context of an error disclosure conversation, a variant might be: "Mr. Jones, please know that despite what has happened, we're here to answer any questions or schedule any future meetings with you that you'd like. Although you may not desire it, please know we sincerely want to support you in any way we can. We'll give you contact information for certain members of our staff whom you can call anytime, day or night. And should you wish to secure an attorney, please know that our staff will accommodate his or her questions or requests." Although an interest in a continuing relationship might sound odd in an error disclosure conversation, it implies the possibility of a nonhostile, supportive, and continuing relationship that can be extremely therapeutic (not unlike airline staff who assist family members whose loved ones died or were injured in airplane disasters with shopping, laundry, housecleaning, and so forth).

Error disclosure communicators must realize that many individuals who have been harmed by medical error can come to admire an institution's effort to disclose. If done artfully, disclosure will impress many harmed parties that their welfare remains a significant concern among the error operators and institutional representatives. Consider, in the alternative, how the relationship between the harmed and harming parties might transpire if institutional representatives intentionally engage in a conspiracy of error concealment and the harmed parties find out.

Error communicators ought to develop a list of suggestions or considerations for the harmed parties. Institutional authorities ought to suggest their availability for future meetings to work with harmed parties and their representatives to bring emotional closure. Harmed parties might especially want precise and elaborate information as to how the error-causing chain of events played out. A need to know in great detail everything that happened helps certain types of persons by providing a sense of calm, as it not only takes the individual's mind off of his or her pain by focusing it on the facts associated with the harm-causing event, but also allows a harmed party to feel a vicarious sense of empowerment (i.e., "Well, even though I couldn't prevent what happened, at least I know what happened"). Indeed, institutions might want to include broaching the issue of a financial settlement early on in conversations with the harmed party. This might prove very wise in instances where the resultant harm has reached significant proportions because a settlement, if skillfully negotiated, might turn out to be considerably less than what an elaborate malpractice trial culminating in a jury verdict would cost.[8]

WHAT IS REQUIRED FOR A PATIENT-CENTERED POLICY ON ERROR DISCLOSURE?

Carrying out these steps of error disclosure calls for organizational, psychological, communicational, and ethical sensibilities and skills that are missing in many, if not most, of today's healthcare institutions. I believe that if something like the steps in error disclosure discussed here become commonplace in America's healthcare facilities, it will primarily be due to profound changes in the training, attitudinal formation, and core beliefs of healthcare providers and institutional representatives that incorporate some of the following suggestions.

First, unnecessarily oppressive elements of medical training need to be eliminated in undergraduate and graduate medical education programs. These include not only the common practice of having students and residents go for long periods without food or sleep, but also the elimination of various unethical practices that trainees not only frequently observe but in which they are asked to participate. Considerable literature on third-year medical students' experiences, for example, describes how they are privy to conversations wherein certain patients are called derogatory names ("dirtball" or "stool"), are asked to secure consents from patients for procedures with which the medical student is thoroughly unfamiliar, are expected to conspire in subterfuge or outright lying to patients and even to attending physicians, forge interns' signatures at their request, and knowingly expose patients to nonsterile procedures.[22–24] If we wonder how it comes about that healthcare providers can subordinate the ethic of patient-centered care to protecting their own self-interests by concealing harm-causing error, the ubiquity of unethical practices occurring in training programs might provide part of the explanation. Because actual behaviors and practices usually win out over moral rhetoric or exhortation, it is extremely tempting to believe that exposure to unethical practices early on—such as in the third year of undergraduate medical training—lays the groundwork for concealing harm-causing error. As such, training programs must operationally insist that disrespecting the rights and dignity of patients in any form is absolutely forbidden.

Second, institutions must recognize that healthcare providers who are brutally intolerant of performance that is less than perfect and who teach or instruct by embarrassment or humiliation are probably troubled souls in need of lengthy counseling or psychotherapy. Also, these persons might respond maladaptively when error occurs because their reaction will likely issue from painful, probably childhood, experiences that derive from problematic rather than caring relationships.[25] Consequently, hospitals should not only routinely maintain counseling programs for their staff but should also recognize that those services might be especially valuable for error operators who are terribly disturbed over the harm their error has caused.

Third, institutions need to operationalize an understanding of what root cause analysis has shown for some time, namely, that healthcare institutions are complex systems, that complex systems are hazardous, and that where hazard and complexity exist, error is inevitable.[26] Risk management strategy, therefore, ought to reject the myth of error-free care, but should design clinical systems with a keen eye to the probability of their malfunctioning. In other words, at every step of system design, the architect should ask himself or herself, "How might this system, as it incorporates elements A, B, C, and so forth, break down?" and then build in appropriate fail-safe elements.[18] Accordingly, error disclosure will be facilitated as more and more institutions become convinced of what errorologists such as James Reason have been observing for over a decade: that serious errors are more often the result of system flaws such as poor monitoring or supervision, faulty technological design, or unreasonably high levels of psychological stress than they are the result of a single individual doing something inexplicably inept.[27]

Last but hardly least, more research is needed on the economic value of error disclosure. At first blush, the idea that comprehensive error disclosure does not increase but might actually decrease the associated cost of malpractice litigation seems counterintuitive, although some early data seem to indicate precisely that.[8] However, if this counterintuition is consistently supported by data and the data are widely and conspicuously disseminated, such efforts should ultimately have a positive effect on encouraging error disclosure.

A Final Point

There is some literature that suggests that individuals choose health care as a career because of deep, unconscious insecurities about the threat of sickness and their own mortality.[28] On this account, their vocational choice of health care turns out to be an unconscious defense mechanism or derives from a psychological formation that mollifies their deepest worries and insecurities. Interestingly and fortunately, these unconscious insecurities become consciously expressed by a disposition toward altruism, wherein health providers feel good by advancing the welfare of others. Perhaps, though, these psychodynamic phenomena offer another explanation as to why error disclosure is as difficult as it is infrequent: Error disclosure powerfully threatens the deepest and most profound insecurities of healthcare providers. As James Reason has pointed out, an error operator may often manifest "a desire to escape from the evidence of one's own inadequacy."[27, p. 93] Thus, those healthcare providers and their institutional representatives who have decided to disclose error truthfully and comprehensively, as painful as it might have been, have successfully managed their insecurities with a sense of right and a sense of self that is, I believe, punctuated by a healthy regard for their own dignity, self-respect, and, indeed, self-love. That is, the individual who has a healthy regard for himself or herself—a healthy narcissism—will be better poised to care for patients and do the right thing when error occurs than those who may be supremely technically skilled but whose singular concentration on the development of those skills occurred at the expense of dismissing the patient who is presumably the beneficiary of those skills. It has been said that, "Great physicians are great human beings first, and great clinicians second." To the extent that healthcare training programs and institutions can operationalize that idea and concentrate on developing narcissistically healthy human beings who are also skillful clinicians, the practice of truthful and comprehensive error disclosure should witness substantial improvement.[25]

References

1. Beauchamp, T., and Childress, J. F. *Principles of Biomedical Ethics*, 4th ed. New York: Oxford University Press, 1994, pp. 259–325.
2. King, J. H. *The Law of Medical Malpractice in a Nutshell*, 2nd ed. St. Paul, MN: West Publishing Company, 1986, pp. 9–82.

3. Rodwin, M. A. *Medicine, Money & Morals.* New York: Oxford University Press, 1993.
4. Council on Ethical and Judicial Affairs, American Medical Association. *Code of Medical Ethics, Current Opinions with Annotations, 1998–1999 Edition.* Chicago, IL: American Medical Association, 1999.
5. Gorlin, R. A. (ed.). *Codes of Professional Responsibility,* 2nd ed. Washington, DC: The Bureau of National Affairs, 1991.
6. Smith, M. L., and Forster, H. P. Morally managing medical mistakes. *Cambridge Quarterly of Healthcare Ethics* 2000;9:38–53.
7. Joint Commission on Accreditation of Healthcare Organizations. *What Every Hospital Should Know About Sentinel Events.* Oakbrook Terrace, IL: Author, 2000, pp. 89–106.
8. Kraman, S. S., and Hamm, G. Risk management: Extreme honesty may be the best policy. *Annals of Internal Medicine* 1999;131:963–967.
9. Bayles, M. *Professional Ethics.* Belmont, CA: Wadsworth Publishing, 1989.
10. Munson, R. (ed). *Intervention and Reflection: Basic Issues in Medical Ethics,* 4th ed. Belmont, CA: Wadsworth Publishing, 1992, pp. 1–45.
11. Christensen, J. F., Levinson, W., and Dunn, P. M. The heart of darkness: The impact of perceived mistakes on physicians. *Journal of General Internal Medicine* 1992;7(July/August):424–431.
12. Wu, A. W., Folkman, S., McPhee, S. J., and Lo, B. How house officers cope with their mistakes. *Western Journal of Medicine* 1993;159:565–569.
13. Wu, A. W., Folkman, S., McPhee, S. J., and Lo, B. Do house officers learn from their mistakes? *JAMA* 1991;265:2089–2094.
14. Buckman, R., and Kason, Y. *How to Break Bad News.* Baltimore, MD: Johns Hopkins University Press, 1992.
15. Gillick, M. Talking with patients about risk. *J Gen Intern Med* 1988;3(Mar–Apr):166–170.
16. Meisel, A., and Kuczewski, M. Legal and ethical myths about informed consent. *Arch Intern Med* 1996;156:2521–2526.
17. Leape, L. L. Error in medicine. *JAMA* 1994;272:1851–1857.
18. Joint Commission on Accreditation of Healthcare Organizations. *Root Cause Analysis in Health Care: Tools and Techniques.* Oakbrook Terrace, IL: Author, 2000.
19. Platt, F. W., and Gordon, G. H. *Field Guide to the Difficult Patient Interview.* Philadelphia: Lippincott Williams & Wilkins, 1999, p. 81.
20. Adapted from the Disclosure of Patient Safety Events policy of Licking Memorial Health Systems. Available from Legal Services, Licking Memorial Health Systems, 1320 West Main Street, Newark, Ohio 43055.
21. Gunther, M. Countertransference issues in staff caregivers who work to rehabilitate catastrophic-injury survivors. *Am J Psychother* 1994;48:208–220.
22. Feudtner, C., Christakis, D. A., and Christakis, N. A. Do clinical clerks suffer ethical erosion? Students' perceptions of their ethical environment and personal development. *Academic Med* 1994;69:670–679.
23. Novack, D. H., Epstein, R. M., and Paulsen, R. H. Toward creating physician-healers: Fostering medical students' self-awareness, personal growth, and well-being. *Academic Med* 1999;74:516–520.
24. Branch, W. T. Supporting the moral development of medical students. *J Gen Intern Med* 2000;15:503–508.
25. Miller, A. *The Drama of the Gifted Child,* 3rd ed. Translated by Ruth Ward. New York: Basic Books, 1997.
26. Cook, R. I., Render, M., and Woods, D. D. Gaps in the continuity of care and progress on patient safety. *BMJ* 2000;320:791–794.
27. Reason, J. *Human Error.* Cambridge, UK: Cambridge University Press, 1990.
28. Graber, G. The role of compulsiveness in the normal physician. *JAMA* 1985;254:2926–2929.

38

Moving Beyond Blame to Create an Environment That Rewards Reporting

Doni Hass

The story related in this chapter describes the coordination of one hospital's response to a sentinel event that ultimately took the life of 7-year-old Ben Kolb. Woven throughout the story of Ben's fatal journey are the actions of many on the hospital staff that supported risk management efforts in the coordination of the response to and investigation of an unusual event.

The control of risk and promotion of patient safety had always been at the forefront of Martin Memorial's corporate objectives. Every employee was evaluated annually on specific risk and safety measurements. Each manager had specific goals, and the bar was always rising. Because of the emphasis on and support for risk management, unfortunate events were approached by a team seeking solutions, not micromanagers seeking to place blame. The following story is not about people making mistakes, it is about a failed system that allowed humans to err. The case also illustrates how Ben's family responded when the event, its investigation, and the disclosure were handled with diligence, integrity, and compassion. It is a story of tragedy and of trust. This is Ben's story.

December 15, 1995, was the first day of Christmas vacation. It was a good day for Ben Kolb to have some routine ear surgery in plenty of time to be able to enjoy the Christmas holidays with his 12-year-old sister Margaret and their parents. Ben was scared, but he had known his surgeon since he was a baby. They were "buddies." Mom and the nurses joked with him to ease his fear. Like many Moms before and since, she gave her only son a kiss and he was wheeled off to the operating room.

Twenty minutes into the operation, the surgeon injected the local anesthetic into the four quadrants surrounding Ben's ear. The scrub technician felt the child's chest "pounding" through the surgical drapes as the Certified Registered Nurse Anesthetist (CRNA) saw precipitous changes in the blood pressure and pulse. The supervising anesthesiologist was summoned to lead the management of the hypertension and tachycardia. The child responded immediately to the treatment and stabilized within minutes. The anesthesiologist, recognizing the timing of the event, instructed the scrub technician to save the syringes, intending to follow up on the cause of this unusual reaction to lidocaine 1 % with epinephrine 1:100,000.

Nine minutes later, the child experienced a cardiac arrest. The chaplain was summoned for family support and the risk manager for coordinating the response to and investigation of an unusual event. It was weeks later that the error that caused the reaction was identified.

When Ben left the operating room 2 hours later, he was in a profound coma and on a ventilator. A pacemaker had been inserted during the resuscitative efforts. Meanwhile, in the surgical waiting room, Tammy Kolb had been anxiously wondering what was taking so long when the volunteer quietly told a visitor, "I'm sorry sir, they have asked me to hold all visitors to intensive care. They are getting ready for a critical child from OR." Tammy rose to her feet.

The surgeon and anesthesiologist, after meeting briefly with the risk manager, came to tell Tammy Kolb. In a private room, they gently gave a thorough explanation of how Ben's heart had stopped and how difficult it was to restart. The chaplain joined them to support Tammy, who insisted "I know he'll get better, I've seen this on TV." Again, the physicians tried to help her begin to cope with the seriousness of his condition. "Ben is in a deep coma, he may not be able to wake up . . . we'll do everything we can."

Usually, operating rooms (ORs) are cleaned and readied for the next operation rapidly. This room was left undisturbed as the director of surgical services met with the risk manager to review details of the event with the staff. The risk manager focused on the timing of the event and selected the syringes of lidocaine with epinephrine, the original vial, and the bottle of topical adrenalin. The vials had been discarded in the "red box." There was one other vial of each in the box. The two syringes and four vials were handed directly to the risk manager.

Thinking she was dealing with a product problem, the risk manager took the items directly to the pharmacist, who initiated the product recall procedure, removing all solutions with the same lot numbers. An alert was faxed to the U.S. Pharmacopoeia. A portion of the contents of one syringe was drawn into a third syringe and prepared for shipment with a vial of adrenalin and lidocaine with epinephrine to a lab capable of analysis. The pharmacist searched for the lab. The risk manager went to the intensive care unit and met with Ben's mom, who was holding her son's limp hand and calling softly to awaken him. Tammy wanted to know what happened. The risk manager replied, "We honestly do not know, but it is my job to try to find out what happened. I will exhaust my resources to find you an answer. I will let you know as soon as I find out." She then met with the CEO and marketing director, outlining the event and her plan for response. Returning to the pharmacy, she and the pharmacist selected the lab at the University of Georgia. The items were sent by overnight mail.

Ben died the following day, after being transferred to a tertiary care center. The risk manager called the defense counsel and insurer to alert them to the event, review the planned response, and obtain advice on the proposed investigation. The board and senior management were called in to a special meeting. The coroner was contacted and told of the analysis under way in Georgia.

Individual meetings were held with every person who entered the OR suite during the procedure. Each one made drawings detailing the location of all equipment and people. The anesthesia team had been positioned at the child's feet to allow room for the microscope to be wheeled into position over Ben's head. Each person's role was outlined, step by step, on poster paper. Everyone seemed to know the proper procedure and appeared to be very competent. After each interview, the risk manager taped the drawings and procedural detail to the walls in an empty office. Procedurally, the only variation was a failure to label the syringes of lidocaine. A pharmacist was relieved of her usual duties by the CEO and assigned to the investigation. She and the risk manager pored over the posters, the procedure, and Ben's previous medical records. Both investigators, to learn how others handled medications in the operating room, called colleagues across the country. They searched the literature for similar cases. One was identified in London. The article described a cardiac arrest in a small boy during ear surgery. The child did not respond to treatment. Efforts to identify the site failed.

The lab notified them that two substances had been isolated in the product test. Further tests were under way to match the substances with the vial contents.

During this time, the risk manager called the Kolb family to express sympathy and renew her pledge to seek an answer. "Please, don't let this happen to another child. Please don't stop, don't ever, ever stop. Please find an answer," was Ben's mother's plea. The anesthesiologist attended the funeral home viewing. The surgeon attended the funeral.

During a routine sentinel event meeting, the details of the event were described by the CRNA, anesthesiologist, and surgeon. The chief of anesthesia, chief of surgery, vice president of medical affairs, physician chair of the quality committee, the president of the medical staff, and the risk manager brainstormed a root cause. At this meeting, the chief of anesthesia said, "I'll bet I know what happened; we saw the same thing in Miami years ago. Someone had mixed up the two medicines. The child died from receiving an injection of the concentrated adrenalin." Everyone agreed that scenario would explain the resultant symptoms. The risk manager focused the discussion on the medical management because she was getting the product analyzed. "If that happened, we will know it," she reminded the group of concerned physicians.

After the meeting, the risk manager met with the director of surgical services to question her on the possibility of a drug mixup. "That's impossible," insisted the nurse. "We followed procedure. It simply cannot happen—we used the same procedure everyone else does. It simply cannot happen, period." In a later meeting with the medical center administrator, a group of circulating nurses and scrub techs in the OR were assigned to a process improvement task force to examine the procedures used in the OR when handling medications.

On December 19, the University of Georgia called to say they were unable to identify the contents. They would continue to try if an additional sample was available. That afternoon, the coroner called to see if the lab results were in. He said he was ruling the death an idiosyncratic reaction to lidocaine with epinephrine. The story could have ended here with a resultant lawsuit and no answers, no truth for Ben's parents.

An additional sample was sent. January 2 brought a chilling call from Georgia. The sample did not match the control of lidocaine with epinephrine. They were running tests for the topical adrenalin properties.

During this time, the director of surgical services, working closely with risk management and the task force, identified an unnecessary step in the commonly accepted process for transferring medications to the sterile operating room environment. This step was also identified as an opportunity for error that could be eliminated. That step was the use of intermediate containers. Using sterile technique, pharmaceuticals were transferred to small plastic and stainless containers on the operating room table by pouring or by use of a syringe. The circulating nurse and scrub technician would verify visually and audibly the contents and expiration dates. The intermediate containers had been labeled by the scrub tech during set-up. The scrub tech would then finish the preparation by withdrawing the injectable pharmaceutical into a syringe. The syringe should have been labeled. The investigation found that it was not uncommon for this step to be skipped when only one injectable was used. The topical solution was poured on cotton pellets to dab on bleeders during the procedure. As the tech finished, the circulating nurse would finish the room set-up and bring the patient to the OR. The task force recommended the use of a filter straw or spike for the scrub tech to attach a labeled syringe to. Intermediate containers were eliminated.

The risk manager, pharmacist, vice president of medical affairs, and the president decided to engage a crisis management firm and locate a second lab with different testing methods in order to confirm the findings.

A quarter of a cubic centimeter of the substance remained in the syringe that had actually been used on Ben. All of the pharmaceuticals had been sealed in wax on December 15 to protect their integrity. That syringe was hand-carried along with control vials to National Medical Services in Willow Grove, Pennsylvania. The pharmacist accompanied the specimen throughout the testing processes. The following day, she called to tell the risk manager the findings, which confirmed what had been learned at the University of Georgia. The syringes of lidocaine 1:100,000 actually contained topical adrenalin. There had indeed been a tragic, fatal error.

As soon as the written reports were received, the risk manager called the Kolb family. Arrangements were made to meet them the following day at their attorney's office. The surgeon and anesthesiologist were notified. A copy of the lab reports was taken to the coroner. He informed the hospital that he would have to change his ruling, but agreed not to do so until after the family was informed.

The following day, the risk manager, accompanied by the anesthesiologist, went to the Kolbs' attorney's office. There, in the presence of many attorneys, the Kolb family, and a court reporter, the risk manager sat near the Kolbs and focused directly on them. They were told how and why the two medicines were used in the surgery, how the risk manager had saved the pharmaceuticals and sent them for testing, and what the tests found. She told them on behalf of the hospital that Martin Memorial accepted full responsibility. This was their error, and it was no one else's. The staff somehow had made a mistake in the transfer process. They are working diligently to make the process safer so that this event never occurred again. She told them sincerely that they were very, very sorry. The attorney escorted them out to another office. It was a very emotional time for everyone. The attorney said he did not know how to respond: The law firm had never had this happen, but they had an obligation to their client. The risk manager, having worked closely with her defense counsel and the insurer, was prepared to respond: "Our defense counsel and insurer are fully informed and are willing to meet with the Kolb family today or as soon as you specify, to try to bring this part of the tragedy to closure. We feel a settlement would be in their best interest."

That evening the Kolb family, their attorney, the risk manager, and the hospital attorney reached a confidential settlement and approved a mutually acceptable press release. The story again could have ended here. Martin Memorial, using the new procedure, would have eliminated one system problem that placed caring, competent professionals in an environment where error occurred. They could try to put this event, their darkest hour, behind them. They could hope as time passed that the OR staff members, manager, and physicians would no longer awaken in the night, no longer doubt their competence, no longer feel that others did not trust them.

"Please don't let this happen to another family. Don't stop, don't ever stop!" These were the words that haunted the risk manager. The picture of Ben's smiling face, bright eyes, and blond hair was a constant reminder that this was not about Martin Memorial, this was about health care as an international industry. This industry had accepted the use of intermediate containers; untold numbers of patients were at risk. Any surgical staff member, given the right circumstances, could make the same error. The risk manager therefore wrote an article for an OR management journal, describing the error and the procedural changes that were developed to keep this type of error from occurring. Copies of the new procedure were offered. Many requests were received.

During 1996, in the months following the error, the American Medical Association was planning what eventually became the first Annenberg Conference on Medical Error, where the National Patient Safety Foundation was officially announced. The insurer of Martin Memorial was on the committee planning the conference. When the committee needed a case study, Ben's story was considered.

In October 1996, Ben's story was told to a hushed audience of 300-plus researchers, clinicians, and concerned citizens. Several other journal articles followed. Lectures were given 12 times a year. Ben's story began a journey of many years as the face of health care and the mystique of medical error went through radical changes.

The calls began. Five calls were received in which risk managers, insurers, and attorneys who had heard about Ben were inquiring to see if their cases, all children having ear surgery, were similar to Ben's experience. Four were. They were from all over the country, the children ranging from 4 to 7 years of age. They did not survive. The fifth call was about a young girl having ear surgery. Her pulse and blood pressure rose. Her nurses called the risk manager, who called Martin Memorial's risk manager for guidance. She was reminded what the investigation had found. In real time, the team was told and was able to realize it had made the same mistake. Now they knew the treatment had to be different. The child lived.

Ben's family supported continued reference to their tragedy. In return they have witnessed a sea change in operating room procedures and patient safety. They are grateful that other families have been spared their loss. That is Ben's story.

Ben's legacy will serve as an inspiring example of the value of system analysis and the futility of a culture that places blame. Safety is being redefined for patients. The environment of health care delivery is in the international spotlight. Error is no longer the other person's problem or the other institution's problem: Error is everywhere. The discovery, reporting, and proper management of error have great value. All must learn to embrace error and hold it up for the world to see. Hold it up, and the world will change.

39

The Role of Ethics and Ethics Services in Patient Safety

Erin A. Egan, MD, JD

Clinical medical ethics has existed since the time of Hippocrates and Aristotle.[1] Currently many hospitals offer clinical ethical services, and The Joint Commission now mandates that hospitals have a process in place for dealing with ethical issues.[2] Clinical ethics services are important tools in patient protection and in development of an institutional ethic that emphasizes patient safety. Hospitals and other institutional providers of health care must foster an atmosphere that values patient safety in order to improve patient safety. Offering competent and clinically relevant ethics services is a key element of this atmosphere.

Medical ethics is grounded in traditional Western philosophy and has always been a fundamental aspect of healthcare provision. The oath taken by physicians as they become doctors, the Hippocratic oath, and similar oaths taken by many healthcare providers, provide a framework for professionalism and ethical provision of care. These philosophical underpinnings reflect the inherent moral obligations assumed by healthcare providers. The moral obligations create a series of duties incumbent on providers. Central among these duties is the responsibility to guard the safety of the patient. Medical ethics is therefore fundamentally tied to patient safety.

Several well-respected medical ethicists have considered patient safety as a fundamental aspect of clinical medical ethics. Patients are in a position of particular vulnerability and need as a result of their illness, and medical ethics places the patient's specific vulnerabilities and needs at the center of the ethical analysis.[3] This is particularly important as the healthcare environment becomes increasingly subject to a variety of economic and administrative interests that are not inherently patient oriented. Ethics consultation services, whether provided by an individual, a team, or a committee, should be guided by the following goals:

- To maximize benefit and minimize harm to patients, families, healthcare professionals, and institutions by fostering a fair and inclusive decision-making process that honors patients'/proxies' preferences and individual and cultural value differences among all parties to the consultation.

- To facilitate resolution of conflicts in a respectful atmosphere with attention to the interests, rights, and responsibilities of those involved.
- To inform institutional efforts at policy development, quality improvement, and appropriate utilization of resources by identifying the causes of ethical problems and promoting practices consistent with ethical norms and standards.
- To assist individuals in handling current and future ethical problems by providing education in healthcare ethics.[4]

Any ethics committee that makes an effort to live by these goals can play a vital role in patient safety initiatives.

PRINCIPLES OF CLINICAL MEDICAL ETHICS: BENEFICENCE, PATERNALISM, NONMALEFICENCE, JUSTICE, AND FIDUCIARY DUTIES

Clinical medical ethics is a field grounded in the practical application of the duties physicians and other healthcare providers have to patients. These duties serve as starting points for analyses of ethical behavior. All these duties involve an understanding of the patient's experience and the patient's needs in obtaining care. These principles, when adhered to for the patient's best interest, promote a focus on patient safety. The basic foundation of these duties is the legal and moral obligation of providers to act in their patients' best interest. The ethical implication of these duties can be applied to solve problems, make policy decisions, and guide behavior on issues of patient safety.

Beneficence is the principle of acting for the benefit of others and contributing to their welfare. Rules of beneficence, as articulated by Beauchamp and Childress, include protecting the rights of others, preventing harm, rectifying conditions that may cause harm, and aiding those in need of rescue. Adherence to principles of beneficence lays an excellent foundation for a safety-oriented environment. Practical application of this principle seeks a course of action, policy, or solution that is of maximal benefit and most likely to prevent or reduce harm. In analyzing patient safety problems and issues, identifying beneficent principles can help reach a plan that emphasizes benefit and patient welfare.[5]

Paternalism is a subtype of beneficence where someone with more knowledge, experience, or authority determines what actions would be in another's best interest. The intent in paternalism is beneficent, but it generally involves the imposition of one set of values on another. The typical, healthy manifestation of this type of beneficence is, as the name suggests, parenting. Parents use their superior judgment and experience to make decisions for their children, at times against the child's wishes, until the child has the maturity to assume responsibility for his or her own best interest. Health care often involves a similar paternalism, which can facilitate a healthy doctor–patient relationship and promote safety or can act to undermine those things. A patient seeks out health care to utilize the knowledge, experience, and skills of healthcare professionals. Trust in the provider allows the patient to rely on the beneficence of the caregiver and accept some level of paternalism in the interest of preventing or treating diseases. Paternalism is a fundamental part of the relationship because the patient must rely on the knowledge, judgment, and skill of the provider to do what is best for the patient. However, paternalism has a limited role in health care, and the failure of providers to curb their own paternalism can compromise patient safety. The balancing principle, respect for the patient's autonomy, is discussed next. A proper balance between paternalism and respect for patient autonomy is the cornerstone of quality health care and safe health care.

Autonomy is respect for the patient's ability and right to determine what happens to his or her own body. The Greek roots of the word mean "self-governance."[6] Autonomy in health care requires that certain conditions be met. The patient must be competent—capable of understanding and making healthcare decisions. The decision itself and the process of making the decision must be voluntary. Respect for a patient's autonomy requires full disclosure, with adequate explanation to facilitate decision making.[7] Autonomy is the interest that balances paternalism. To respect patients' autonomy and to facilitate their autonomous decision making, the provider or providers must limit their own paternalism. Some patients may demand that the healthcare team limit its feelings of paternalism by insisting on autonomy. Other patients may not do so, but are entitled to a similar limitation, self-imposed by the provider. Respect for a patient's autonomy is still important outside the decision-making context. Disclosure of mistakes respects patients' right to know the truth about their care and their body. There may not be any decisions, or at least healthcare decisions, that need to be made or are affected by a mistake, but the patient has the right to know about errors as an autonomous entity. Less than full disclosure may be premised on the belief that it will only hurt the patient or family more to know the truth, but this belief is an expression of paternalism and ignores the patient's or the family's autonomous rights.

The principle of *nonmaleficence* is embodied by the phrase "first, do no harm." Patient safety concerns are firmly rooted in this principle. Before a provider or institution undertakes the effort to improve a patient's health, each should be very sure that the patient wouldn't be injured and in worse condition as a result of the care received. Patient safety is not a movement aimed at creating new and better cures or treatments. It is aimed at ensuring that no preventable harm is done to patients. It is important to note that patient safety is not completely devoted to nonmaleficence. Patient safety focuses on eliminating preventable harm, but not eliminating all harm. Some genuinely indicated and competently performed healthcare services cause harm. The nonmaleficence embraced in the patient safety movement is not that no risks are justified for better health, because the decision of what is acceptable risk lies with the competent patient. Nonmalificence does not always override autonomy. Our respect for patients' abilities and right to make their own decisions means that we will allow them to experience risk. Patient safety emphasizes eliminating preventable, unnecessary injury. The role of nonmaleficence in patient safety is immense but requires proper limitation in its application.

Justice is a principle based on rights and fairness. Something is unjust if it denies rights or distributes benefits and burdens unfairly.[8] Typically, the rights of individuals and what is fair or unfair distribution are concepts defined by a society. Some are common to most societies, such as the injustice of killing. Others vary widely, such as the injustice of modes of access to health care. In medical ethics, justice can be a troubling consideration. Societal considerations of fairness and scarcity issues may have a very limited role in bedside decision making. In the area of patient safety, however, justice is usually a proper consideration. Justice enters into issues of disclosure, as well as issues of policy and institutional ethics. Allocation of resources is important in patient safety, both as a cause of medical error and as a solution. How an institution distributes its efforts to improve patient safety will have implications for what is accomplished and how successfully. Throughout this discussion, justice is an underlying concern, even if it is not expressly mentioned.

Fiduciary duties are legal duties, which, in health care, consider the relative vulnerability of the patient relative to the provider. The legal concept of a fiduciary responsibility attempts to enforce some professional ethical principles by creating legal consequences for violating them. A *fiduciary* is a person who voluntarily agrees to act primarily for the benefit of another.[9] Generally, a fiduciary relationship involves "good faith, trust, special confidence, and candor."[10] Breaching a fiduciary duty has legal and professional consequences. Physicians, and often other healthcare providers, have a fiduciary duty to patients and are required to act in the best interest of the patient. This duty is somewhat paternalistic, but it recognizes that patients seek health care for knowledge that they don't have and to receive services they can't perform. Sometimes the patient must rely on the healthcare provider's perception of what is good for him or her under the circumstances. However, fiduciary duties include candor and trust. Therefore, disclosure is a fiduciary, as well as a moral and ethical, duty. Similarly, ensuring the safety of the patient, especially in a hospital setting where the individual has little control over his or her own environment, is a fiduciary duty because it is undertaken in the patient's best interest. In many ways the fiduciary relationship between a patient and a healthcare provider is merely a formal, legal recognition of the ethical obligations the provider has to the patient.

ETHICS COMMITTEES AND CONSULTATION SERVICES

Although medical ethics began thousands of years ago, ethics committees and ethics services are relatively new concepts. Ethics committees, ethics consultation teams, and individual ethics consultants allow ethics to be an active clinical service. Ethical analysis is useful to proactively prevent problems through education and formation of policies, and is important for retrospective review to learn from mistakes and identify weak areas. The strength of providing ethics consultation services is that ethical considerations need to guide decision-making processes and pervade clinical care. Clinical medical ethics focuses on the role of ethics in the active clinical environment. The American Medical Association *Code of Medical Ethics* recommends that ethics committees or services be educational and advisory, and that they be available to healthcare professionals, families, and patients to provide information and assistance when asked.[11] Ethics committees typically espouse three primary goals: case consultation, education, and policy development.

The idea of hospitals providing ethical assistance in active cases through ethics services was the result of a suggestion by the judge charged with deciding the case of Karen Ann Quinlan.[12] *Quinlan* was one of the first cases to look at the possibility of discontinuing a ventilator in a patient who was in a persistent vegetative state but with no immediately terminal conditions.[13] The court in *Quinlan* suggested that situations such as the one faced by the Quinlan family would be best addressed by medical personnel with some training and ability to deal with complicated and emotionally charged dilemmas and disagreements.[14]

Ethics committees are often composed of members with diverse backgrounds, including physicians, nurses, attorneys, patient advocates, and religious leaders. Ethics committees can consider active cases by allowing medical personnel to attend the meeting and present a case, or by offering consultation services and later discussing the case with the committee. The consultant is able to respond quickly to a request, gather information, and talk to providers and families. The consultant is more experienced in ethical consultation than a typical medical team and is therefore able to collect information quickly and sort out relevant information. If the medical team needs to make an immediate clinical decision, the consultant is available for an immediate recommendation. However, whenever possible, the consultant will meet with the full ethics committee and present the case prior to making a recommendation. If there is not time to present the case prior to offering a recommendation, a recommendation is made to the team, and the committee reviews the case and gives feedback at the next meeting. This mixed committee/consultant structure allows for immediate clinical ethics involvement in active cases, providing the capability of responding to the pace of clinical medicine, while maintaining the benefit of a group process and the input of people with varied backgrounds whenever possible.[15] This interaction between a consultant and the larger committee has been analogized to the interaction between a trial court and a court of appeals.[16]

There are many variations in the way ethics services are offered by hospitals or other institutions. Services may be limited to an ethics committee without consultation services, or may involve a consultation service without an ethics committee. Many institutions have a single person, often with formal or informal training in ethics, available for ethics consultation. Whichever structure an institution uses, it is important that the ethics consultant or committee make a distinct effort to provide education and policy assistance in addition to clinical case consultation.

The role of clinical ethics consultants or committees in patient safety involves all three facets of clinical ethical services. Any active case where there is any type of patient safety concern warrants an ethics consultation. The role of the ethicist in specific situations is discussed in depth later in this chapter. However, the ethicist can provide a framework for determining which obligations are most important to meet the patient's needs and improve the outcome. An ethics committee can provide an opportunity for discussion of the issues and the conflicts involved in a nonthreatening, patient-focused environment. It is important that the ethics committee be a forum for discussion and not a penalty tribunal.

The educational and policy roles of ethics are important in developing a safe patient environment. The ethicist can assist in making ethical, patient-oriented, outcome-improving policies that help prevent problems and conflict. Developing an ethically sound institutional policy on issues of provider incompetence, medical mistakes, and informed consent helps ensure patient safety as a preventive measure and facilitates rapid action in the face of problems. Educating all members of the healthcare team on their duties and responsibilities to patients as a result of their moral, ethical, and legal obligations assists team members in understanding their role in patient safety and emphasizes the importance of a patient safety commitment. Educational interventions should be provided both case by case, educating the team members as consults arise, and in broader efforts that target groups, including lectures, journal clubs, case conferences, and lunch seminars.

Ethics consultation services are frequently consulted on issues of withdrawing or withholding therapy, more than any other single issue and constituting 49% to 65% of consultations in one study.[17] An additional 37% of consultations in the same study involved end-of-life decision making and how to approach resuscitation.[18] Making sure these decisions are made competently and ethically, with maximum participation by the patient and family, is both a quality of care issue and a patient safety issue. Other ethical issues of particular importance for patient safety are medical mistakes and disclosure, impaired or incompetent providers, issues of informed consent, and disagreements between professionals or between patients, families, and providers. Finally, the ethical atmosphere of the institution, the way the institution values ethical and safe healthcare provision, and emphasis on candid and critical discussions about patient safety and quality improvement are all within the scope of ethics services and are the basis for long-term improvement in patient safety.

PATIENT SAFETY AS AN ETHICAL ISSUE

The previous section focused on ethical principles and the nature of clinical ethics services. This section discusses patient safety as a clinical medical ethical issue. The principles discussed earlier provide the philosophical framework for analyzing patient safety issues in a clinical ethical context. The next section focuses on application of ethical principles in specific types of patient safety–related problems. Medical ethics, to be relevant, must move beyond the philosophical roots of ethics and become clinically relevant. Clinical relevance requires a meaningful contribution to the process of providing care to patients and improving the outcomes for individual patients. Ethics in this context becomes a dynamic application of principles to improve care and assist the healthcare team in resolving the issues they face daily.

The common ground of ethics, health care, and the patient safety movement is that all emphasize improving outcomes. This common ground is all that is necessary for these fields to interact synergistically for the benefit of the patient. All three areas begin with nonmaleficence, the desire to do no harm, and strive for maximal beneficence, the opportunity to do the most possible good. Providers seek these goals through their technical knowledge and the healing quality of their interactions with patients. Ethicists seek these goals through "improving the process and outcomes of patients' care by helping identify, analyze, and resolve ethical problems."[19] Patient safety becomes involved because the patient's well-being is the goal of health care, and safety is essential to well-being. Patient safety concerns are in a realm where the philosophical, technical, and personal aspects of medicine overlap.

A further basis for patient safety issues as an ethical concern is that the focus on patient safety needs to be pervasive and requires a paradigm shift in the way professionals deal with mistakes and problems. Creating a paradigm shift in a field such as health care requires constant vigilance to ethical principles in order to avoid creating a system that is ethically flawed.[20] This paradigm shift requires the development of an institutional ethic, a pervasive policy of commitment to ethical principles that is reflected in how the institution as a whole prevents and responds to patient safety concerns. The institutional ethic should be something that goes far beyond a policy governing certain situations to be a general atmosphere of commitment to patient safety that is as apparent in unpredictable occurrences as in established policies. An institutional ethic that focuses on complete internal consistency in protecting the patient's interest will inherently promote patient safety, because safety is clearly in the patient's best interest. The institution must accept and enhance the fiduciary duties of providers to protect the patient's interest. The principles of beneficence, nonmaleficence, and fiduciary responsibility must be apparent in every policy and action endorsed by the institution.

As a result of framing patient safety concerns as ethical issues, additional benefits arise from the central involvement of the ethicist or committee in patient safety promotion. Ethics services frequently assist teams and patients when the primary problem is one of disagreement. As many as 24% to 45% of an ethics service's consultations involve dispute resolution.[21] Formal clinical medical ethics training usually includes some dispute resolution training.[22] Dealing with the aftermath of a medical mistake can foster hostility and disagreement, and because ethicists are experienced in dispute resolution, they can provide valuable guidance.

Finally, ethical concerns and ethical services can play an important role in quality improvement efforts. Improving patient safety is inherently quality improvement, and these fields can go hand in hand. Especially when quality improvement and utilization review are closely linked in the hospital's administrative structure, ethical principles and quality improvement initiatives help create boundaries to the effort to control costs so that patient safety is not compromised by cost control. Ethics and quality improvement are similar in that they promote a goal of ideal behavior and policy, which although never perfectly achieved should always be sought.[23]

SPECIFIC APPLICATIONS OF ETHICS IN PARTICULAR SITUATIONS

Medical Mistakes

The first and foremost issue in patient safety is medical mistakes. Since the publication of the Institute of Medicine's report indicating that medical error is a severe problem in U.S. health care, this issue has properly received a lot of attention both from patients and providers.[24] Medical error, and the aftermath of errors, has always been an area of focus for clinical medical ethics. Most legal, professional, and ethical guidelines agree that disclosure and the duty to report are fundamental issues.

Disclosure is often the hardest aspect of mistakes for healthcare professionals. Disclosure refers to being honest with the patient or the family or both about the mistake and the consequences of the mistake. Despite the difficulty providers have with disclosure, it is the cornerstone of the relationship between patients and providers. Disclosure is a fundamental manifestation of respect for autonomy. The American Medical Association's Principles of Medical Ethics require a physician to "deal honestly with patients."[25] The legal fiduciary duty requires trust and candor, and candor requires honest disclosure. In 1999 the *British Medical Journal* published the Tavistock Group's statement of "shared ethical principles for everybody in health care."[26] These principles include cooperation and leadership by healthcare professionals, and an approach of personal responsibility for errors.[27] Ethics education and prioritization of ethical behaviors facilitate this personal responsibility. In addition to being traditionally considered the ethical response, disclosure may decrease the likelihood of litigation.[28] Providers and institutions must realize that disclosure and honesty are important parts of the healthcare process. Understanding autonomy and its implications facilitates this realization.

Another issue, one that precedes the issue of disclosure, is the duty to report. Medical errors may go unreported 50% to 96% of the time.[29] For obvious reasons, there can be little improvement without accurate information about the nature and frequency of medical mistakes. Ethics education can provide the basis for each provider believing that the importance of reporting outweighs the possible negative effects to the provider who is the reporter. Justice and respect for autonomy demand reporting. Conversely, the immediate unpleasant consequences, real or imagined, of reporting the errors of colleagues or one's self can create a compulsion to keep things quiet. However, if providers and those around them are constantly encouraged to place the patient's interests above all others, and are rewarded for doing so, reporting mistakes will be easier for providers to undertake.

Provider Impairment and Incompetence

All healthcare providers are aware of the potential and actual danger of incompetent and impaired providers. However, this is an area where healthcare professionals have extreme difficulty. In contrast to medical mistakes, which are a fact of being human, incompetence or impairment is limited to a group of providers and is not a common experience. The one element of commonality, which influences providers to be forgiving and supportive, is that most providers have had to practice in an impaired condition from lack of sleep. However, persistent impairment from drugs or other problems, or persistent incompetence, is an intolerable danger in health care. No one wants to be the snitch. Providers may feel that reporting will do little good and make their own lives intolerable. Every provider accepts the principle that he or she has a duty to report problems with colleagues, but often the practical barriers to doing so seem insurmountable.

This is an area where ethics education and an institutional ethic are crucial. Every provider must feel a personal responsibility to ensure the safety of every patient. Every provider must be willing to take all possible steps to prevent unnecessary harm. If providers value their ethical and legal duties, they are more likely to act on those principles in spite of barriers. Reminding providers of the moral underpinning of their responsibilities will cause providers to reflect on these duties and prioritize adherence to them. The institution must create an environment that encourages reporting. Whistle blowers should be given genuine protection. If the whistle blower requests, he or she should be transferred to avoid retribution. However, immediate intervention with all members of a department or area where there has been a report to review and emphasize the obligatory nature of reporting may help other providers realize the value of reporting. Because this is a particularly threatening area for providers, change will be slow and institutions and ethics services must commit to long-term education and support.

Informed Consent

Informed consent is one of the areas most traditionally considered "ethical." Informed consent issues can be complicated, and ethics services are well positioned to assist in complex cases. More important, ethics services can emphasize the importance of proper informed consent in every routine instance. Proper informed consent can prevent a variety of problems and misunderstandings. The institution must insist that providers make a concerted effort to have a detailed personal conversation with each patient on issues of consent. Obtaining consent for a procedure may fall to the lowest person on the totem pole and may be viewed as one more paperwork requirement. Institutions need to require the provider performing the procedure to obtain the consent. Providers need to be reminded of the importance of the consent process, including preventing misunderstandings or disappointment after a procedure. Providers should be trained in giving consent, and quality management or utilization review should ensure that the consent form was signed by a provider who was appropriate to obtain the consent. The principles of informed consent and the reasons for it are topics of education. Enforcing proper informed consent procedures is administrative.

CONCLUSION

This overview of ethical principles and applications has attempted to integrate clinical medical ethics services into a coordinated patient safety initiative. Acting alone, ethics service providers may have little material impact on improving patient safety. Ethics education and clinical ethical consultations will have an effect on improving patient safety, but require an organized effort for maximal effectiveness. As institutions evaluate mechanisms to improve patient safety, diverse groups should be involved. Ethicists and ethics committees have a unique role, and their potential contribution to patient safety is critical. Even without a designated ethicist or ethics service, these principles can and should be incorporated into any patient safety initiative. In institutions that have the advantage of having designated ethicists or ethics committees, those people should be given a central role in developing a comprehensive patient safety agenda.

References

1. Aristotle, *The Nichomachean Ethics*, and the writings of Hippocrates in general.
2. Joint Commission on Accreditation of Healthcare Organizations, *1995 Comprehensive Accreditation Manual for Hospitals* (Oakbrook Terrace, IL: JCAHO, 1994).
3. Edmund Pellegrino, "Allocation of Resources at the Bedside: The Intersection of Econom-

ics, Law and Ethics," *Kennedy Institute of Ethics Journal*, vol. 4 (1994), 309.
4. John C. Fletcher and Mark Siegler, "What Are the Goals of Ethics Consultation? A Consensus Statement," *J Clin Ethics*, vol. 122 (Summer 1996), 125.
5. Tom L. Beauchamp, and James F. Childress, *Principles of Biomedical Ethics* (New York: Oxford University Press, 1994), 277–318.
6. Ibid., 120.
7. Ibid., 146.
8. Kathleen Mitchell et al., "The Synergistic Relationship Between Ethics and Quality Improvement: Thriving in Managed Care," *J Nursing Care Quality*, vol. 1 (Oct. 1996), 9.
9. *Black's Law Dictionary*, abridged 6th ed. (St. Paul, MN: West Publishing, 1991), 431.
10. Ibid.
11. American Medical Association, *Code of Medical Ethics* (Chicago: AMA, 1997), 151. Although this citation is to an older edition of the code, the substance of this reference has not changed in later editions.
12. *In re Quinlan*, 70 N.J. 10, 355 A.2d 647 (1976).
13. Ibid.
14. Ibid.
15. Peter A. Singer, Edmund D. Pellegrino, and Mark Siegler, "Ethics Committees and Consultants," *J Clin Ethics*, vol. 1 (Winter 1990), 263.
16. Mark Siegler, Edmund D. Pellegrino, and Peter A. Singer, "Clinical Medical Ethics," *J Clin Ethics*, vol. 1 (Spring 1990), 5.
17. John LaPuma et al., "An Ethics Consultation Service in a Teaching Hospital: Utilization and Evaluation," *JAMA*, vol. 260 (Aug. 12, 1988), 808.
18. Ibid.
19. Fletcher and Siegler, "What Are the Goals of Ethics Consultation?" 124.
20. Cheryl A. Anderson, "Ethics Committees and Quality Improvement: A Necessary Link," *J Nursing Care Quality*, vol. 11 (Oct. 1996), 17–25.
21. LaPuma et al., "Ethics Consultation Service," 809.
22. For example, the postdoctoral fellowship in clinical medical ethics offered through the MacLean Center for Clinical Medical Ethics at the University of Chicago Hospitals includes formal and informal training in dispute resolution.
23. Anderson, "Ethics Committees and Quality Improvement."
24. Institute of Medicine, *To Err Is Human: Building a Safer Health System* (Washington, DC: National Academy Press, 1999), 1.
25. American Medical Association, *Code of Medical Ethics*, xvii.
26. R. Smith et al., "Shared Ethical Principles for Everybody in Health Care: A Working Draft of the Tavistock Group," *BMJ*, vol. 318 (1999), 248.
27. Peter A. Singer, "Medical Ethics: Clinical Review," *BMJ*, vol. 321 (July 29, 2000), 282.
28. Robert L. Lowes, "Made a Bonehead Mistake? Apologize," *Med Econ*, vol. 74 (May 12, 1997), 94.
29. Paul Barach and Stephen D. Small, "Reporting and Preventing Medical Mishaps: Lessons from Non-medical Near Miss Reporting Systems," *BMJ*, vol. 320 (March 18, 2000), 759.

40

TELEMEDICINE—RISK MANAGEMENT AND PATIENT SAFETY

John Blum, JD, MHS and Doni McCoy, JD, LLM

Telemedicine lies at the intersection of several major phenomena, namely the explosion in telecommunications, the rapid expansion of information technologies, the related developments in software design, the evolution of user-friendly PC applications, and mobile phones. It is the intersection of these noted elements that has led to the growth and development of telemedicine, often broadly cast as e-health, which encompasses an array of technologies that link health providers to patients across distances. E-health raises challenges for both risk management and patient safety because it alters the traditional physical environment and moves diagnosis and treatment into two or more settings outside the confines of a single, controlled environment. This chapter provides an overview of telemedicine for the patient safety officer. Specifically the chapter will explore the definitions of telemedicine, liability concerns and standards, privacy/security matters, and federal regulatory compliance considerations, as well as state law licensure and credentialing policies.

DEFINITIONS

It is difficult to provide an exact definition of telemedicine because it is not a unitary technology. But for purposes of this chapter, a good generic definition can be taken from the American Telemedicine Association (ATA). The ATA defines telemedicine "is the delivery of any healthcare service or transmission of wellness information using telecommunications technology" (ATA).[1] Such a definition is wide in that it encompasses an array of communication technologies and a range of applications such as specialist referral services, patient consultations, remote patient monitoring, medical education, and provision of consumer medical and health information. Traditional telemedical delivery modes as identified by the ATA include various ways of linking providers, such as networks and point-to-point connections, and patient connections, such as primary/specialty care to homes, homes to monitoring centers, and Web-based patient e-health service sites.

The applications of telemedicine are expanding with clearer visual resolution, reliability of use, and acceptance of appropriateness of these treatment modalities, making future definitional accuracy challenging. Robotics and virtual reality, once the realms of science fiction, are now part of the armaments of medicine and are moving rapidly into various e-health applications. Thus even the broad parameters of the ATA definition of telemedicine—electronic communication and movement of data from one site to another—will be subject to regular reanalysis. As healthcare entities reorganize themselves around shifting inpatient and ambulatory models, telemedicine will not only link patients from remote sites but will routinely be used to connect sick individuals to providers within the given distances in a particular organization, such as from a doctor's office to the patient bedside, and will serve as key elements of infrastructure for emerging entities such as accountable care organizations.[2] On the other hand, the likely growth and increased capacity of small, easy-to-use computers and cell phones will provide greater ability to link individuals from afar to medical personnel for a widening array of informational and clinical applications.[3]

Clearly telemedicine is poised for growth as a result of major changes in related technologies, as well as a growing awareness of the need to address severe shortages in primary care and specialty medical services in too many parts of the country. There are several policy challenges raised by telemedicine, starting with reimbursement and accompanying regulatory barriers, which, in large part, have posed more serious problems in the growth of this area than have those of a technical or medical nature. For the patient safety officer, the challenges of telemedicine occur at the micro level and are anecdotal to the organization and nature of service in question. Still, resolution of broad policy questions will have a profound impact on the adoption of telemedical services, and in turn, those matters of adoption will frame the nature of how a given risk management and patient program deals with this area of practice.

MAJOR VARIABLES FOR RISK MANAGEMENT/PATIENT SAFETY

In the risk context, telemedicine raises a number of broad issues that warrant exploration and policy development. Key variables that must be explored include medical liability and the development of practice standards and guidelines, privacy and security, and regulatory compliance. No doubt many other factors could be added to the patient safety officer's list of relevant e-health matters, but those variables noted provide a good jumping off point for consideration of patient safety/risk management in established and emerging areas related to cyber medicine.

Medical Liability

Picture a scenario where a patient at an originating site is separated from a physician at a distant site and via telecommunications technologies the patient and physician are transported across miles. A high resolution of the patient on a large screen enables the distant clinician specialist to direct care at the originating site where a physician extender is following his or her directions, and the encounter is a successful way to treat the sick party, who can only receive specialized care in this manner. Another scenario that can be drawn in telemedicine is in the area of diagnostics, where radiological tests are batched and eventually electronically forwarded to a radiologist who provides diagnostic interpretations of the digitized images from quite literally anywhere in the world. Envision the intensivist who, from the comfort of home, is using his or her PC to examine a patient in an ICU who is being electronically monitored by a robot. Or the patient who suffers from chronic health conditions monitors vital signs via a smartphone and transmits that information to his or her clinician. These are but four possible scenarios that can be identified in telemedicine, each of which can be viewed from a liability and patient safety standpoint, illustrating the types of encounters that can go amiss and as such form a basis for consideration of possible legal liabilities.

In considering liability in any of the scenarios noted, three factors must be considered. First, telemedicine is merely a format for health delivery so that, in and of itself, it does not alter established principles of either liability or patient safety. Policies and procedures that have been developed in inpatient and outpatient settings for risk prevention should be extended to telemedical services. Second, like with most of risk management, the key challenge is to understand and control the environment to prevent and contain risks, and to assure patient safety. The e-health environment is odd because it introduces risk management and patient safety into two, and possibily more, venues, as well as into the new dimension of cyberspace. But such oddities need to be accounted for in the context of traditional policies. In the typical example of electronic treatment linking originating and remote sites, the patient safety officer in the tertiary remote site must develop practices and procedures for the consultation site, and develop mechanisms to create assurance that the originating site of patient care is being properly managed. In addition, safety considerations must take into account any potential problems that could arise as a result of using electronic technology as the medium for linking patient and physician. The third factor to be appreciated in addressing liability matters in telemedicine is an awareness of the lack of specific common law guidance. At this stage in telemedicine, there is no body of case law to draw on for reference. Undoubtedly, although considerable discussion on liability in cyberspace has occurred, the courts have yet to address the area directly, so liability analyses need to draw on the general principles of malpractice law developed in more traditional contexts.

Medical liability, regardless of jurisdiction, follows a fairly set format including the existence of a duty, a breach of that duty that entails a violation of the relevant standards of practice, establishing a causation link between the breach of duty and the injury in question, and a showing of the damages the injured party was exposed to.[4] In the first scenario referred to above—the traditional link between an originating site and a distant tertiary center—the question can be addressed as to whether a doctor–patient relationship is established via this electronic medical encounter. For such a relationship to be created there needs to be an agreement, explicit or implied, on the part of the key parties—physician and patient—that treatment is being sought and provided. Largely the circumstances dictate the existence of the physician–patient relationship and in turn that sparks a duty on the part of the treating doctor. One avenue of inquiry is whether telemedicine fits within the definition of medical practice or constitutes a service outside the definitions of a state medical practice act. A view that telemedicine is not medical practice is largely an unsustainable position that would have credibility only in the area of the Internet where a user avails himself or herself of information on a medical Web site and has no interaction with the given health professional or institutional site sponsor. Certainly if a physician–patient relationship can be sparked on the telephone without physicality being necessary, an encounter where direct treatment is provided triggers all the action verbs of medical practice acts (i.e., diagnose, treat, etc.) and would undoubtedly result in the creation of a duty relationship between the patient and the telemedicine doctor.[5] Even in the case of diagnostic evaluation, as in the above example, the consultant radiologist would be hard pressed to argue that he or she has no duty to the patient because such consultation has a direct impact on the individual's medical care even if it occurs via electronic medicine practiced over distance.

An interesting concern in the duty area involves the second classic element of duty, namely the scope of the obligation.[4] This question is particularly germane in reference to the consulting physician in the distant site. Specifically, what is the scope of the consultant's duty for care that he or she provides at the originating site? Such a question would be dealt with using the traditional test of foreseeability, namely, is it foreseeable that if the consultant makes an error that such error would be compounded by those professionals in attendance at the originating site? Here, courts may want to recognize the physicality of the bifurcated care and place limitations on the scope of duty of the consultant; but, of course, there is no guarantee that such narrowing of obligation will occur. Rather, in the agreement struck between consultants and the originating site, scope of liability will need to be covered by contract. For example, the originating site may want to specify in contractual language that the consulting doctor is not an agent and thus bears no corporate liability for his or her conduct.

The second element of medical liability, the breach of duty, concerns the matter of practice standards. Here, there is a twofold inquiry. On one hand, the standards of practice that govern the conduct of health professionals in traditional settings would apply to telemedicine. Thus, the specialist consultant cannot argue that the world of electronic medicine allows for a diminished practice standard, but the level of service, regardless of the novelty of the medium, must be akin to professional performance in traditional settings. The more interesting question that arises in the e-health context concerns whether the nature of telemedicine is such that it warrants the development and application of different practice standards. With the exception of radiology, we do not see the emergence of evidence-based medical standards that are unique to telemedicine, although broader trends in diagnosis and treatment that push practice standards in conventional environments certainly spill over into telemedicine. In the future, it is conceivable that telemedicine practice may be facilitated by means of technologies that will require distinct skills such as the use of virtual reality. Perhaps robotics used in diagnostics will necessitate special training on the part of the specialist, who will need to be able to understand the distinct capabilities and limitations of such technologies, as well as possess requisite skills to use such technology. And of course, robotics may actually raise the standards of practice for medicine generally by introducing levels of precision in procedures that have not previously existed in an all-human environment.

An interesting question in the standards area concerns whether the presence of telemedicine will raise the level of responsibility for an individual clinician or institution by virtue of its presence. If a given health professional or facility has the capacity to provide diagnosis or treatment via telemedicine and fails to use that capacity, will the courts find negligence in such failing? It is certainly reasonable that the individual physician who has access to specialized services via telemedicine should bear the same responsibility he or she would have for failure to seek on-site, traditional consultation. In turn, the institution that voluntarily chooses to expand its diagnostic and treatment capabilities would have a responsibility to use such services. For example, if a small hospital or clinic holds itself out as a stroke care center, poses the technology to treat via electronic medium, and fails to do so, it would bear liability. Clearly in the stroke center example, telemedicine becomes a type of core technology that is integral to the operation of the facility, and failure to use it would be no different from malfeasance in use of any other, more traditional diagnostic and treatment resources. Where telemedicine expands possibilities of care, there may be more room for argument that the individual clinician should not be expected to use an unfamiliar technology, but such an argument seems to be one that is short lived as this technology is increasingly becoming more mainstreamed.

The causation element of medical liability opens up a variety of legal considerations that touch on both matters of fact and details of legal proof.[4] For purposes of patient safety, the key factor in causation is the determination, based on a given factual scenario, as to which party (parties) in a telemedical encounter is responsible for an ensuing medical error. While causation in a conventional setting is not always easily determined, when the care at issue occurs in different sites, the factual determination of who is at fault, or more appropriately, discerning the comparative fault of the parties, is a challenging matter. There is also an issue as to whether individuals at the site of the treatment could have intervened to prevent an error that stemmed from following the distant consultant's advice. Determination of the originating site professional duty quickly moves causation into the realms of legal causation. Under the doctrine of legal causation, the matter at issue becomes one for the courts to determine whether given conduct will be viewed under law as inappropriate. Telemedicine is a novel area for the common law, so it would be reasonable to expect that courts must grapple with matters of how much liability they want to attribute to the involved parties.

The fourth element of medical liability concerns damages.[4] In fact, the damage element is the single most critical factor in this arena, and though lawyers may argue that equity drives malpractice actions, reality is lodged in financial assessments. It is very difficult to speculate on how telemedicine gone amiss may affect immediate damages in the abstract, but certainly the availability of telemedicine may impact future medical costs. The more immediate concerns over damages relate directly to questions of liability insurance coverage. Certainly all involved individual parties and organizations in telemedicine need to be aware of whether their respective liability insurance coverage includes telemedicine. Existing policies may need to be amended to include this area, and in some cases, special liability insurance must be purchased. In institutional cases in which entities self-insure, risks for telemedicine must be factored into reserve adequacy, and secondary carriers must agree to provide necessary reinsurance. Calculation concerning telemedicine liability insurance will not be easy because there is no claims history in this area. Insurers will need to consider matters of medical quality and the adequacy of the technology and professional training, and even assess the levels of confidence clinicians exhibit in given e-health diagnostics and treatment applications. An interesting challenge that applies to insurance coverage and liability actions generally involves determination of the jurisdictional question raised by interstate telemedicine. Which law applies to a given telemedicine action—the law of the originating site where the patient is located or the law of the remote site where the e-health professional is located? Largely, legal experts have concluded that the jurisdiction in which the patient is treated would be the controlling one, and as such it is the doctor who travels electronically to the sick party. As such, the law of patient residence would serve as the basis for framing and resolving a dispute, and insurance would reflect the realities of risk in the originating site.[6] It has been argued that the telemedicine scenario should be seen as moving patient to physician, and interestingly enough, this small change in perspective holds a significant implication for liability and regulation in this sector.

Of special note in the liability area is the doctrine of informed consent.[6] Generally, the law underpinning informed consent in all states requires that patients be provided with material information about their treatment including details concerning risks, benefits, alternatives, and ramifications of not being treated. The refinement of what materiality is in a given situation is impacted by how the law of a particular state has characterized the disclosure duty. Jurisdictions measure the information disclosure responsibility in three ways—from what the reasonably prudent physician would disclose in similar circumstances, to those states that evaluate the doctrine from the standpoint of the reasonable patient, to a minority that measure informed consent from the particular patient perspective. Thus, the manner in which telemedicine informed consent is worded must first reflect the disclosure duty in a given state. The challenge is, however, deciphering what elements of electronic medicine fit into the three streams of duty noted. Generally, it would seem appropriate to disclose that the particular treatment is being provided over distance, the nature of the technology involved, the parties who will be participating in the treatment, and the potential for any material risks to occur. The fact that telemedicine is remote and that originating sites may be the only option for care should not minimize the nature of the disclosure made by the treating parties.

Practice Standards and Guidelines

It may be obvious to any patient safety officer that specific uses of telemedicine will require that the organizations in question develop policies and standards that guide the applications of these technologies. Such standards and guidelines must be tailored to the diverse settings where telemedicine occurs, as well as to the array of diagnostic and clinical uses for such care. As will be discussed, there are points of reference in developing clinical guidelines and procedures for e-health that can be drawn on, but certainly the idiosyncrasies of a given program must be factored into any standard setting process. The goal for patient safety is to treat telemedicine as any other medical service and to regularize these processes at the requisite level of professional service that would be expected generally. Standardization underpins quality and from the safety standpoint becomes a core element in minimizing potential liability, as well as in the promotion of a safer environment.

In searching for models of best practices in telemedicine, there are developed standards and guidelines that can be referenced. The American Telemedicine Association (ATA) has issued several practice guidelines in the area that can serve as valuable resources for individual programs.[7] For example, the ATA has issued practice guidelines for videoconferencing (VTC)-based telemental health, which provides a very helpful template for this growing e-health application.[7] The ATA telemental health standards are accommodating enough to cover clinical applications such as physician consultations, emergency evaluations, case management, and clinical supervision, as well as nonclinical applications such as distance learning, research, and administration. Concerning operations, the ATA guidelines cover staffing, privacy/confidentiality protections and patient rights, billing and coding, documentation and record keeping, and administrative matters. In addition, the ATA telemental health guidelines delineate necessary general practices in patient encounters, from criteria covering particular types of examinations, to specific patient safety details in areas such as developing patient reports and psychotherapy and pharmacotherapy management. Special considerations for children, elderly, and rural populations are noted, together with ethical standards. Particularly unique to telemedicine are necessary technical specifications for VTC that are addressed in the guidelines, such as concerns over the adequacy of picture resolutions, data transmission issues, information security and encryption, and physicality elements such as room setup, lighting, and ergonomic considerations. Even a cursory examination of the ATA telemental health guidelines reveals the high level of sophistication and understanding that the patient safety officer must bring to this area, as well as the need for a safe environment to be elemental in the development of these services.

Privacy/Security Considerations

There are numerous privacy and security concerns in telemedicine. The employment of telemedicine technology means that protected health information can be sent anywhere in the world in a matter of seconds. The vast reaches of e-health provide a panoply of positive uses, as well as potential opportunities for abuse. In general the law requires the consent of the individual prior to the disclosure of protected health information, a baseline patient right.

At both the state and federal levels, personal health information receives a heightened level of privacy protection compared to other types of personal information due to the particularly sensitive nature of such information, and such protections are highly germane to telemedicine.[8] The fear in allowing more lax protections for this type of information is the fact that possession of personally identifiable health data could be powerful and damaging if accessed by those with malicious intentions.[9] There are generally three principles dealing with the protection of health information. The first principle is that typically, the government will set a standard of privacy across the spectrum of information. Once the default standard is set, carve outs, or exceptions to the rule, are allowed. Typically, the exceptions are allowed for the public good. As a general rule, health data that has been de-identified and aggregated is not required to be protected. This type of data is typically used for benchmarking and research purposes.

The second principle entails establishing trust with the patient populations. This is achieved through development of practices to foster openness and transparency in the process. In essence, the patient has a right to know what information is being kept by his or her healthcare providers and with whom it is being shared. Transparency requires that the patient know the key pieces of information concerning his or her care. The patient must give consent to the process. The patient also has a right to view his or her own records and correct erroneous information, as well as to remove information that is not timely, accurate, and relevant or complete. The third generic health data principle requires that privacy protections be integrated into all systems. This would include any information system that is accessed regarding a given patient's care. These systems would include records kept by a physician, ancillary providers, and health institutions, and even records maintained by a payer organization. Implementation of safeguards will include protection against loss, unauthorized access, destruction, use and modification, and disclosure.

In 1996 the Health Insurance Portability and Accountability Act (HIPAA) was enacted.[10] HIPAA's Administrative Simplification section serves as the primary focal point for privacy law in the United States at the federal level and is the touchstone for understanding the legal mandates for law in this area.[11] While safety officers dealing with patient data must be aware of state laws in their respective jurisdictions, HIPAA is the basis on which specific institutional patient privacy policies should be crafted. Under HIPAA, the standards for collecting, sharing, and storing individuals' personal health information (PHI) are established. PHI refers to four categories of information: information concerning past, present, or future physical or mental health conditions; information concerning payments or provisions of care; data that identifies an individual or serves as a basis to do so; and patient information held by a covered entity under the law (health plan, provider, clearinghouse). The Department of Health and Human Services (DHHS) has published two major rules dealing with standards for electronic transactions and information privacy.[12] These are commonly known as the Administrative Simplification Rules, and they deal with two main issues. The first issue addressed by the rules is reducing the amount of administrative overhead costs. The idea is that healthcare entities can streamline processes and vastly reduce overhead costs by reducing paper and operating in the realm of technology. The second issue addressed by these rules is protecting individually identifiable health information in the electronic world.

This HIPAA rule covers health plans, healthcare clearing houses, and healthcare providers that transmit protected health information in paper or electronic form. Using outside providers to maintain and manage the covered data cannot circumvent the rule. Outside providers become what are known as business associates, and pursuant to the rule, business associates are covered by HIPAA and must sign an agreement with the primary entity with whom they are contracting.[13] Individual information that falls under this rule is a person's name and address, date of birth, social security number, payment history, account number, and name and address of healthcare provider and/or health plan. The rule also requires a patient to give consent prior to the release of this information. In the use of electronically stored, used, or transmitted data, HIPAA requires that the data be encrypted and that video sessions be secured to the greatest practical extent, all factors highly germane to telemedicine.

It has been suggested by commentators that all health information networks must be fortified against unauthorized access.[14] Stringent security features should include encrypted email communications, facial recognition to clearly identify patients on the network, a digital identity card issued after identity has been authenticated, verification of access to all point-of-service computers, and a network that is protected by a continuously monitored firewall. Most of these security features reach beyond what is currently mandated by law and for some providers would be cost prohibitive.

There are several scenarios that have yet to be anticipated by HIPAA and other legislation in the realm of e-health. According to health researchers Chiang and Starren, because legal advances have failed to keep pace with technological progress, there are gaps, which could result in information being wrongfully disclosed or misused if these gaps remain.[15] For example, one such scenario raising uncertainty is seen with differences in the stringency of safeguards from state to state and between the federal and state levels. Also, HIPAA preempts state law unless the state law is more stringent. This presents a unique compliance issue. If a practitioner in one state performs a telemedicine consult in another state with different local privacy laws, there could be situations in which there is conflict in determining whether the laws of state one or state two are controlling or whether federal law controls. This jurisdictional disparity is not addressed by HIPAA but needs to be dealt with by patient safety officers.

Another telehealth scenario that isn't covered under HIPAA is one in which an argument could be made that telemedicine is a healthcare operation and therefore falls under *treatment, payment, or healthcare operations* (TPO), a zone specified in the law. If categorized as such, the use and disclosure of patient's protected information can be made without the patient's consent. DHHS rules have not addressed this issue. Another unaddressed scenario outlined by Chiang and Starren is the situation in which a telemedical consultation may, by necessity, need to include additional nonclinical personnel, such as technicians and camera operators, who are not traditional providers in the healthcare arena. These individuals will need to comply with HIPAA. While this situation has not been specifically addressed, it appears that these "outsiders" to the traditional process could be covered through the use of business associate agreements.

Undoubtedly as noted, the cyber environment raises high levels of concern over individual privacy because it compounds points of vulnerability in the context of a virtual world in which safeguards are still evolving, and complacency can yield a high price. For the patient safety officer, the challenges of insuring privacy and developing adequate security protections are constant as telecommunications technologies and their applications are continually progressing. No area is more illustrative of these challenges than the explosion in the use of wireless technologies in health care, so-called mobile health or m-health.[16] Wireless devices, such as cell phones, tablets, and PDAs, are an increasing presence in medical delivery as a dizzying array of new appliances are being proliferated to provide a unique range of information and monitoring services. For example, in various settings, patient monitoring is being conducted via smartphones, which track various patient biometrics.[17]

While not every m-health application has HIPAA implications, those that involve the use of protected health information by covered entities must adhere to privacy and security laws.[18] Email serves as a good example of the types of policies that need adoption in m-health. Under HIPAA security requirements, email security requires unique user identifications, emergency access procedures, automatic log off, and use of encryption and decryption, as well as special hardware and software.[19] While email regulation is a helpful example, each m-health application may have unique privacy/security mandates and will need careful independent assessment for purposes of risk management and patient safety. It is also important to note that m-health and other telemedicine products (both hardware and software) are subjected to regulation by the U.S. Food and Drug Administration (FDA). In 2011, the FDA issued a regulation covering medical device data systems (MDDS), those that passively transfer or communicate health data without modification, interpretation, or any value addition.[20] The MDDS regulation applies to anyone who manufactures an MDDS and may even extend to healthcare facilities. Draft guidelines have been issued by FDA that apply to mobile medical applications, including software, for use in diagnosis, treatment, or disease.[3] For example, the use of a smartphone to perform telehealth assessments could conceivably be regulated as a mobile medical application (app).

Key Federal and State Regulatory Concerns

There are many issues that arise when various states and agencies of the federal government attempt to regulate the practice of telemedicine. These can complicate how the practice actually is implemented, particularly when telemedical practices cross state lines. Practitioners often fail to optimize their telemedicine activities out of fear of being found out of compliance with the state and federal licensing, billing and reimbursement laws.

Billing Issues and Telemedicine

Uncertainty about legal, regulatory, and billing issues surrounding telemedicine is the reason that many practitioners are reluctant to use it. Research has shown that the major barrier to telemedicine is the absence of consistent and comprehensive reimbursement policies.[21] With the current cost of health care and the poor payment histories of both Medicare and Medicaid programs, providers are reluctant to use technology that does not enjoy widespread acceptance for fear that their efforts will go unreimbursed. This lack of comprehensive reimbursement, together with specialist shortages, poses a particular challenge for the delivery of health care in rural areas. One such example of serious rural access issues can be seen in the area of stroke care. Each year in the United States, 795,000 strokes occur, but only four neurologists are available per 100,000 patients.[22] Patients who are able to make it to a medical facility may be misdiagnosed because up to 30% of nonspecialists may misdiagnose an acute ischemic stroke.[22]

Improvement of stroke care through timely intervention and access to specialty care is a distinct benefit that can be offered by telemedicine. So-called telestroke care is an excellent example wherein advanced technology has been employed to address the critical need in one area for health care. The American Heart Association and the American Stroke Association recommendations support the use of telestroke as a means for providing stroke care in rural, remote, and underserved areas.[23] There are two telestroke models that provide a microcosm in which to analyze reimbursement and billing issues present in telemedicine.[22] The first model is the hub and spoke arrangement. In this model, hub hospitals are certified by The Joint

Commission (TJC) as primary stroke centers with advanced care capacities including the availability of neurologists and neurosurgery capabilities 24/7.[24] The spoke hospitals are typically smaller and do not possess neurosurgery support. These hospitals may be community (critical access) hospitals that are located in underserved rural or suburban areas, and may or may not have a stroke center certification. The second telestroke arrangement is the third-party consult model. In this model, the third-party provider, also known as the remote provider, employs neurologists to provide telestroke services. The spoke hospitals have ICU capabilities for treating nonsurgery patients, and more complicated patients are stabilized and transported to tertiary hospitals. This treatment mechanism is referred to as "drip and ship," meaning that an I.V. of some antithrombolytic medication is administered and then the patient is transported to a better-equipped facility. The challenges in building a telestroke infrastructure are the same challenges that are faced by building most telemedicine infrastructures. These challenges include funding, legislative and regulatory changes, methods for reimbursement that include clarity in the system, when it will occur, and dealing with drip and ship patients. Other issues that need to be faced concern licensure and credentialing, hardware and software legal issues, and certainly patient safety and medical error prevention.

All telemedicine services face reimbursement issues from Medicare, Medicaid, and private health insurance payers.[6,25] The Balanced Budget Act (BBA) of 1997 authorized partial Medicare reform for telehealth services.[26] Unfortunately, because technology in 1997 was not as advanced as it is today, these reforms did not go far enough in anticipating the issues now being faced. The Benefits Improvements and Protection Act (BIPA) of 2000 included an amendment to the Social Security Act (SSA), which removed some prior constraints but maintained substantial limitation relating to geographic locations, originating sites, and eligibility for telehealth services.[27] While support is often voiced for telemedicine by various health officials, the Patient Protection and Affordable Care Act fails to address expansion of reimbursement in this area.

Presently, Medicare reimbursement for telemedicine or telehealth services is divided into three basic areas: (1) remote patient face-to-face services seen via live videoconference, (2) non-face-to-face services that can be conducted through live videoconference or via store and forward telecommunication services, and (3) home health services.[6,28] Medicare requires that the originating site must be either in a rural health professional shortage area or in a county not included in a metropolitan statistical area (MSA). The service must be provided by an interactive telecommunications system that includes, at minimum, audio and video equipment permitting interactive, two-way real-time communication between a distant site practitioner and patient. Telephone conferences do not qualify for reimbursement. The reimbursement for telemedicine services provided by the physician or other practitioner at the remote site is the same as if the service were provided without the use of telecommunication equipment. Medicare pays a flat facility fee to the facilitating site. Reimbursement for telemedicine is separate from Medicare Severity–Diagnosis Related Group (MS-DRG) payment.

Medicaid also reimburses for some telemedicine uses.[6,29] Most states' Medicaid programs provide for the reimbursement of some transportation to and from healthcare service providers. Many of these states have decided to cover telemedical services, reasoning that this could greatly diminish covered transportation expenses. Currently, the majority of states allow for the reimbursement of some telehealth services, and there has been a rapid expansion in Medicaid reimbursement for behavioral health services. Other states have indicated amenability to the idea of establishing or enhancing telemedicine reimbursement policies. The barriers to this, however, are serious budgetary constraints and the requirement that new coverage must be based on solid cost-benefit data.

While still evolving, reimbursement trends in telemedicine are evident in the development of billing codes in this area. For example, the American Medical Association (AMA) has developed current procedural terminology (CPT) codes for the reimbursement of telemedicine services. The AMA approved two new Category III CPT codes that may be used to report critical care provided by physicians via telemedicine, not limited to stroke care. CPT Code 0188T is for remote, real-time interactive videoconferenced critical care, evaluation, and management of critically ill or critically injured patients. This code is to be used for the first 30 to 74 minutes of medical care. CPT Code 0189T is to be used for each additional 30 minutes and should be listed separately from the code for primary service. These codes became effective on July 1, 2008.[30]

Federal Fraud and Abuse Regulation

A significant consideration in the Medicare and Medicaid reimbursement area for participating providers, including those billing for telemedicine services, is compliance with federal and state fraud and abuse laws.[6] Over time, a series of statutes have been enacted as amendments to the federal Medicare law, or in tandem with the law, which have added significant compliance requirements to those involved in delivering health services under program auspices. While there is an array of laws in this area, three statutes dominate the fraud and abuse field, and become points of initial focus for participating providers. They include the so-called Antikickback Statute, the Stark Law, and the Federal False Claims Act.[31] Risk managers and patient safety officers who oversee telemedicine services must pay careful attention to Medicare fraud and abuse compliance requirements that are outlined in the law and thus be cognizant of current and evolving complexities presented herein.

The Antikickback Statute

The Antikickback Statute is designed to prevent financial and other types of remuneration being provided to a Medicare provider in return for patient referrals.[32] The statute has both civil and criminal implications, but with a strong criminal law basis, it requires proof of intent as a core element of a violation. The statute prohibits the knowing and willful payment, direct or indirect, that results in referrals or the purchase of items covered under the Medicare program. The Antikickback Statute is so broad in its construction that Congress had to enact safe harbors that exempt certain types of actions from criminal prosecution. While behavior that falls outside a safe harbor is not necessarily illegal, conduct within the safe harbor allows for providers to assure that reimbursement will be forthcoming for legitimate activities that could on their face be construed as a violation of law.

For purposes of telemedicine, there are three long-standing safe harbors that are significant: payments to bona fide employees, discounts or price reductions disclosed in cost reports, and rebates paid under specified circumstances to group purchasing agents.[33] Qualification for the safe harbors noted is not automatic, but parties seeking to find shelter therein must meet a series of regulatory requirements to qualify. More recently, in 2006, two new safe harbors were created by the Office of the Inspector General (OIG) under the Anti kickback Statute related to electronic prescribing, as well as to electronic medical records.[34] The electronic prescribing/medical records safe harbors allow designated health service providers to donate electronic health record software, IT, and training services to physicians, and for hospitals to provide physicians with such items as noted. These newer safe harbors were forged not so much in recognition of business practices but rather to overcome regulatory barriers to the implementation of new technology.

In addition to statutory safe harbors, the OIG, on request, may issue opinions that interpret specific safe harbors, which provide greater guidance on how these exceptions are interpreted by the regulator. In one case, the safe harbor for rental equipment was at issue in a situation where an eye care generalist leased equipment from an eye specialist that was used for both diagnostics and telemedicine. The OIG concluded that the arrangement even if it had potential antikickback implications did not violate the law if the eye care generalist did not market or charge a fee for telemedicine consultations and the patients were free to go to any specialist for consultation.[35] In another advisory opinion, the OIG confronted the issue of a relationship between a hub tertiary center and a number of small, rural facilities in which the rural facilities had been given telemedicine technology by the hub center under the auspices of a federal grant. When the grant terminated, the relationship continued between the involved provider entities, and on its face constituted a violation of the Antikickback Statute because the donated telemedicine equipment was resulting in patient referrals to the hub. In this case, the OIG felt that the benefits of the arrangement in expanding access in a rural setting, containing costs, and overcoming physician isolation were factors that offset the application of the statute.[36] While the hub-spoke advisory opinion can't be generalized to the point where it can be argued that a regulation can be trumped by circumstance, it does, at least, demonstrate that potential violations of this law must be seen in the context of the delivery environment in which they occur.

Stark Law Issues

The Stark Law is a multifaceted and complex piece of legislation that has expanded over time since its initial provisions against physician self-referrals were enacted in the Omnibus Budget Reconciliation Act of 1989.[37] Simply stated, Stark prohibits referrals by physicians treating Medicaid and Medicare patients to a provider of designated health services if the referring physician or an immediate family member of the physician has a financial relationship with the entity receiving the referral unless the referral falls within an exception. Because the Stark Law is a strict liability statute, it does not require proof of intent to induce referrals. There are no criminal penalties for a Stark violation, but the civil penalties can be severe. These penalties include the denial of a payment to the provider, a requirement for the provider to refund a payment made in violation of the law, a $15,000 penalty per service violation of the law, and a $100,000 penalty for each arrangement that is found to be part of any scheme designed to circumvent the law.

Proponents of the Stark Law find support in the idea of conflict-of-interests concerns. They argue that if such referrals are allowed, they could lead to overutilization of services, thereby driving up the costs of health care. They also argue that such a system of referral would create a closed or captive referral system, which could result in limits on competition. Those who argue against the Stark prohibitions claim that it is an unlimited intrusion into the practice of medicine and that the law is too complex. They also argue that the prohibitions found in Stark impede a physician's ability to practice in managed care networks.

Stark poses some unique challenges in the area of telemedicine. One such challenge may be the difficulty in figuring out exactly if and when the physician–patient relationship attaches. A physician at a distant sight may claim that the law does not apply in certain circumstances if there is no actual physician–patient relationship. Another challenge may arise if the referring physician at the originating site has some financial interest in either the telemedicine operation or the equipment used to facilitate the process. Another example of an unintended Stark violation could arise in situations where a large originating hospital provides telemedicine equipment to a small community or rural facility for the purpose of facilitating a telemedicine relationship between the two facilities. Because the relationships between physicians and facilities in the telemedicine arena are not always clear cut, all proposed relationships should be reviewed with legal counsel to assure compliance with the Stark Law.

False Claims

The False Claims Act prohibits knowingly submitting false claims for government funds.[38] Those who do so can be liable for three times the government's damages plus civil penalties of $5,500 to $11,000 per false claim. Because physicians, hospitals, and other medical providers receive government funding through Medicare and Medicaid, the False Claims Act is directly applicable to the practice of medicine. As applied to medicine, the Act prohibits providers from billing Medicare or Medicaid for services that were either not performed or were performed unnecessarily.[6]

Because the government has such limited resources to pursue these claims and millions of dollars of federal funds are paid as a result of these claims, the Act contains qui tam, or whistleblower, provisions in an effort to reduce these claims or recover funds that were paid as a result of them. This provision allows citizens with evidence of fraud against the government to sue on behalf of the government to recover the funds. In exchange for their willingness to bring the action, they can be awarded a percentage of funds recovered, usually between 15 and 25%.

The False Claims Act requires that all bills for services from healthcare providers appropriately document that services were performed and were necessary. As with Stark, compliance with the False Claims Act can pose unique issues for telemedicine practitioners. One specific area where practitioners will need to be fully cognizant of the requirements of the Act is in the emerging telestroke practices. Providers in these and other telemedical practices will need to fully document the necessity of the services when billing for these services. Further, precaution will need to be taken to document what, exactly, was provided via telemedical consultation.

Licensure

Because telemedicine enables physicians licensed in one state to, in essence, practice in another state via remote technology, state licensing has been a long-standing concern that has been followed and reviewed by several medical groups over the years. The issue of licensing for the practice of medicine is rooted in the traditional exercise of police power in which states, pursuant to their 10th Amendment authority, endeavor to protect the public from practitioners without requisite education and experience. Every state has a designated Board of Medical Practice, which operates under the auspices of enabling legislation and a regulatory code.[39] Licensure is a type of regulatory floor that establishes entry requirements into the profession. It is also a process that exercises continuing oversights during the duration of the license. Licensing sets the standard of rights, responsibilities, discipline, and continuing competence of physicians. Until now, licensure was an issue largely left within the purview of state regulation. Major issues, however, are encountered as this process faces the realities of electronic medicine that cuts across borders in the new reality of cyberspace.

Licensing, like any other regulatory process, is composed of a series of variables that may make grappling with this area challenging. First, there is a strong federalism tradition in the area of licensing. The states, not the federal government, have retained considerable authority for a range of public health regulations of which licensure is a critical function. In addition to medical licensing, individual professional licensure has expanded to cover an array of health professionals who function in an expanding set of roles that are independent of physicians or as physician extenders. These include nurses, nurse practitioners, physicians' assistants, and others. Any issue concerning telemedicine must be viewed in the context of broader health professional licensing generally. Additionally, states also license medical facilities. States also wield a great deal of power over the licensure of entities and are often locked into established regulatory patterns that may beg the question of effectiveness. In essence, because of the deeply rooted regulatory traditions, it often appears that form is chosen over substance. A preemption of licensing authority from the state to the national level would require changes in the law at both the state and federal levels, as well as a willingness on the part of state regulators to walk away from this traditional function. This concept sounds simple. When one considers, however, the power structures built on the state level and the bureaucratic deliberation that takes place on the federal level, this is a process that will not be accomplished quickly.

A related reality in licensure is the political and structural nature of this process. Licensure, as it currently exists, is supported by the majority of organized medicine. There is, at present, no groundswell to alter the existing process. The most significant organization in the licensing arena is the Federation of State Medical Boards, and the Federation has developed a reformed licensure model that is under revision.[40] This model may support a type of mutual recognition, but it does not support the abandonment of medical licensing at the state level. The fact is that, if telemedicine levers a national license, there is a very compelling case for further broadening the licensing laws to allow for a general medical practice license, which is really the heart of the political concern. From a structural standpoint, licensing cannot be seen independent of undergraduate and postgraduate medical education. While there is a great deal of national uniformity in medical education, it is tightly linked to state-based regulatory systems.

There is also a state concern about public protection that reaches the licensing process. In an era when the federal authority is assuming a massive new role in oversight and following healthcare reform, questions emerge about the regulatory capacity of the federal government to take on the role of a national licensing authority for telemedicine. Clearly, a new regulatory structure would need to be developed. The growth and evolution of telehealth technologies could pose considerable challenges. Related to this concern are questions regarding federalizing liability issues, risk management, and patient safety. Additionally, practical economic concerns arise in licensure, namely, the revenue received by the states for these processes.

None of this is to suggest that the world will remain totally flat forever and that changes in licensing that affect telemedicine cannot occur. Given the fact that states are not brilliant regulators and that many are in dire financial straits, alternative regulation may be an attractive prospect. Further, the realities of shortages in rural health, manpower challenges in primary care, and the lack of geographic balance in specialty care make a strong case for eliminating barriers to telehealth. There are several approaches to simplifying cross-border medicine, none of which are novel. As noted earlier, states can choose to provide mutual recognition or reciprocity to physicians with comparable training. Some jurisdictions have used special telehealth licenses that have distinct entry requirements and place providers under the jurisdiction of a given medical board. One frequent exception is taken from consultation provisions in licensing laws, which consider the telemedicine physician in a secondary role providing advice to the on-site, licensed treating doctor.[41]

Rather than create a national license that is dependent on oversight, the American Telemedicine Association or a comparable group could create a national specialty board for telemedicine. This specialty board would be much closer to developments in telehealth and be in a position to respond to the needs for practice standard development that will arise as technology evolves. Dependence on a federal scheme may ease concerns about barriers but, at the end of the day, would not necessarily address what should be the foundation of licensure, namely, the enhancement of quality.

Credentialing, Federal Rules Change

Credentialing is a process of formal recognition and attestation that a physician is competent and qualified. This process verifies that a doctor meets certain standards set by an organization.[42] During the credentialing process, a physician's education, training, experience, license, certification, character, professional judgment, malpractice, and adverse clinical occurrences are reviewed by way of investigation and observation. Credentialing is an ongoing process throughout the professional life of the physician. It is not enough for a physician (or other healthcare professional) to hold the required license in a given jurisdiction, but he or she must also obtain privileges in both the originating and distant hospitals. The most typical dilemma in credentialing concerns the specialist who, at the distant site, is not credentialed in the originating location. The process is highly bureaucratic, time consuming, and costly. This requires small facilities, and often rural hospitals, to meet a high bar.

Medicare hospitals' conditions of participation are explicit in the credentialing area.[43] The general Medicare rule was that no physician should be permitted to bill for services in a facility in which he or she is not credentialed. This is of particular importance when one considers that nearly every hospital in the United States receives some Medicare funding. Credentialing across jurisdictional boundaries for the purpose of practicing in the telemedicine arena stood out as a major impediment to growth of this technology.

Several years ago, TJC attempted to strike a compromise position that allowed diagnostic services to be provided by individuals who are not credentialed in originating facilities. This proxy credentialing, however, was determined by the Centers for Medicare & Medicaid Services (CMS) not to meet the Medicare conditions of participation. In 2011, CMS amended the Medicare Conditions of Participation (COP) to allow for a more flexible credentialing and privileging process for telemedicine.[43] To recognize distant-site credentialing/privileging, four conditions must be met. The distant site must be a Medicare participating hospital, the physician or other practitioner must hold privileges at the distant site for the service in question, the physician/practitioner is licensed in the state where the originating site is located, and the distant-site clinician undergoes peer review in the areas relevant to telemedicine.

CONCLUSION

Telemedicine as it evolves into multiple applications holds great promise for improving access to care and empowering consumers. Like many areas of technology, the law trails behind the innovations in electronic medicine. Adherence to current legal mandates and anticipation of future requirements are essential to the successful diffusion of telemedicine at macro and micro levels. Safety officers and risk managers on the front lines will be challenged by the unique environments of cyber medicine but must work to assure that the same principles that apply to brick-and-mortar healthcare facilities are translated to the world of virtual medicine. The issues visited in this chapter—liability, privacy/security, reimbursement, fraud and abuse, licensing, and credentialing—provide a general framework of matters that need to be considered but is only an initial template of law that will inevitably be expanded into a broader arena as e-health develops and grows.

References

1. Retrieved June 9, 2012 from http://www.americantelemed.org/i4a/pages/index.cfm?pageID=3308.
2. Wood, D. (2011). The move to accountable care organization includes telemedicine. *Telemedicine Journal and E-Health, 17*(4), 237–240.
3. Dolan B. (2010, December 17). *Report: 70 percent want access to mhealth.* Mobihealthnews. Retrieved from http://mobihealthnews.com/9789/report-70-percent-want-access-to-mhealth.
4. Heydemann, H. W., Macdonald, M. G., & Neely, E. J. (2011). Medical malpractice (chapter 12). In M. G. Macdonald, R. M. Kaufman, A. M. Capron, & I. M. Birnbaum (Eds.), *Treatise on health care law*. New York, NY: Matthew Bender.
5. Blum, J. D. (2003). Internet medicine and the evolving legal status of the physician-patient relationship. *The Journal of Legal Medicine, 24*, 413–455.
6. Fleisher, L. D., & Dechene, J. C. (2004). *Telemedicine and e-health law*. New York, NY: Law Journal Press.
7. American Telemedicine Association. *Telemedicine standards & guidelines*. Retrieved June 10, 2012 from http://www.americantelemed.org/i4a/pages/index.cfm?pageid=3311.
8. For example, see Sharp HealthCare's 2011 Compliance Education Module 1: Safeguarding Privacy. Retrieved from http://www.sharp.com/b2b/students/upload/pp2011-Safeguarding-Privacy-2-18-11-Final.pdf.
9. U.S. Department of Health & Human Services, Office of the National Coordinator for Information Technology. *Advancing privacy and security in health information exchange*. Retrieved June 10, 2012 from http://healthit.hhs.gov/portal/server.pt/community/healthit_hhs_gov__privacy_and_security/1147.
10. 42 USC 1301 et seq.
11. U.S. Department of Health & Human Services. *HIPAA administrative simplification statute and rules*. Retrieved from http://www.hhs.gov/ocr/privacy/hipaa/administrative/index.html.
12. 45 CFR Parts 160, 162, and 164.
13. 45CFR164.502(e), 164.504(e), and 164.532(d) &(e).
14. Gaya, J. (2010, March 18). *Telemedicine–Enhancing network security to achieve hipaa compliance*. Retrieved from http://ezinearticles.com/?Telemedicine---Enhancing-Network-Security-to-Achieve-HIPAA-Compliance&id=3950233.
15. Chiang, M., & Starren, J. Data Confidentiality and HIPAA. chapter, Home Telemedicine for Health Care Provider, Informatics for Diabetes Education and Telemedicine (IDEAtel) pilot project. Retrieved from http://www.ideatel.org/syllabus.hipaa.html.
16. Stross, R. (2011, September 3). Tracking vital signs, without wires. *The New York Times*. Retrieved from http://www.nytimes.com/2011/09/04/technology/wireless-medical-monitoring-might-untether-patients.html.
17. Sarasohn-Kahn, J. (2010). *How smartphones are changing healthcare for consumers and providers*. Prepared for California HealthCare Foundation. Retrieved from http://www.chcf.org/~/media/MEDIA%20LIBRARY%20Files/PDF/H/PDF%20HowSmartphonesChanging-HealthCare.pdf.
18. Scher, D. L. (2011, October 28). *Mhealth and HIPAA*. The Digital Health Corner. Retrieved from http://davidleescher.com/2011/10/28/mhealth-and-hipaa/. For a helpful summary of regulatory law impacting Mhealth, see Brooke, M. J., Kendall, L. R., & Stout, D. Apps and accessories. *EPC*, 22–27. Retrieved from http://www.ebglaw.com/files/45619_EPC%20June%202011%20-%20%28Jason%20Brooke,%20Leah%20Kendall%29%20%282%29.PDF.
19. 45 CFR sec.164.312(a),312 (c)(1),312 (e)(1).
20. 21 CFR 880.6310.
21. Advani, P. (2009, November 6). Telemedicine: Good innovation hampered by outdated policies. iHealthBeat. Retrieved from http://www.ihealthbeat.org/perspectives/2009/telemedicine-good-innovation-hampered-by-outdated-policies.aspx.
22. Activase. *Telestroke allows for specialized stroke care in underserved areas*. Retrieved from http://www.activase.com/telestroke/telestroke_networks.jsp.
23. Jeffrey, S. (2009, May 11). *New AHA/ASA guidelines on TIA management and telemedi-*

cine in acute stroke released. theheart.org. Retrieved from http://www.theheart.org/article/968715.do.

24. The Joint Commission. *Advanced certification for primary stroke centers.* Retrieved from http://www.jointcommission.org/certification/primary_stroke_centers.aspx.
25. Medicare Carriers Manual Part 3-Claims, Chapter XV, Section 15516, Medicare Payment for Telehealth Services. Retrieved from http://www.cms.gov/Regulations-and-Guidance/Guidance/Transmittals/downloads//R1798B3.pdf.
26. 42 USC 13951.
27. 42 CFR 410.78.
28. *Telehealth services fact sheet.* (2009, July). Retrieved from http://www.telemedicine.com/pdfs/TelehealthSrvcsfctsht.pdf.
29. Medicaid.gov. *Telemedicine.* Retrieved from http://www.medicaid.gov/Medicaid-CHIP-Program-Information/By-Topics/Delivery-Systems/Telemedicine.html.
30. Department of Health and Human Services, CMS Manual System Pub. 100-04 Medicare Claims Processing, Transmittal 997.
31. 42 USC 1320, 42 USC 1395m, and 31 USC 3729. In addition to the three laws noted, the other important legal consideration in this area is civil monetary penalties that require those submitting bills to certify that services were provided in accordance with all applicable federal and state laws, 42 CFR sec. 410.12. It is also important to be aware of the fact that there are state fraud and abuse laws and, in some cases, special telemedicine fraud and abuse provisions (e.g., see 22 Tex. Admin.Code sec.174.3).
32. 42 USC 1320.
33. 42 USC 1320(a)-7b(b).
34. 70 FR 59015 (Oct. 11, 2005).
35. See Waxman, J. M. (2011, September 16). *OIG issues new telemedicine advisory opinion.* Retrieved from http://www.foley.com/publications/pub_detail.aspx?pubid = 8505. There have been four major advisory opinions on telemedicine issues by the Office of Inspector General. The advisory opinion concerning eye care, the first OIG opinion in the telemedicine area, is OIG Advisory Opinion 98-18.
36. OIG Advisory Opinion 99-14.
37. 42 USC 1395m.
38. 31 USC 3729.
39. For example, see the Texas Medical Practice Act, Chapter 153. Or more generally, Federation of State Medical Boards. (2003). *A guide to the essentials of a modern medical practice act* (10 ed.).
40. Federation of State Medical Boards. Public Policy Compendium, 2011, 140.005. Telemedicine Model Policy.
41. Jacobson, P. D., & Selvin, E. (2000). Licensing telemedicine: The need for a national system. *Telemedicine Journal & e-Health, 6*(4), 429–439. Retrieved from http://deepblue.lib.umich.edu/bitstream/2027.42/63348/1/15305620050503915.pdf.
42. Becker, S., & Macdonald, M. G. (1998). *Health care law: A practical guide.* New York, NY: Mathew Bender.
43. 42 CFR 482.22 (2003).
44. 42 CFR 488.12 and 483.22. For a more detailed discussion of this rule change, see 76 Federal Register, Credentialing and Privileging of Telemedicine Physicians and Practitioners, 25550-25565, May 5, 2011.

41

The Criminalization of Medical Malpractice from Past to Present and the Implications on Patient Safety and Voluntary Error Reporting

Laverne Largie, JD, LLM

INTRODUCTION

This chapter will explore the concept of criminalization of medical malpractice from the past to the present and its implications on patient safety and voluntary error reporting. Committing medical malpractice used to not be regarded as a criminal matter and was historically handled primarily in the civil tort system. In more recent times, however, society has been holding negligent healthcare practitioners criminally responsible for their harmful acts. This paper will explore some of the more recent cases involving the criminal treatment of medically negligent acts by practitioners including an analysis of the circumstances surrounding the celebrity deaths of Michael Jackson and Anna Nicole Smith and how their physicians were treated in this context.

HISTORY OF CRIMINALIZING MEDICAL MALPRACTICE

Criminalizing medical errors of physicians and other healthcare professionals is a recent phenomenon.

> Criminal prosecution of healthcare negligence was historically reserved for intentionally ending a person's life through euthanasia, or in angel-of-death cases, where a provider decided to play God, or in cases where the provider would benefit from the death through personal gain (doctor killing his wife for the life-insurance money). A surgeon who operates on an individual while intoxicated similarly resulted in criminal charges, as this act demonstrated intentional disregard for human life. (p. 272)[1]

There is a recent push for such acts to be thought of as so reckless that in addition to tort liability they also warrant criminal punishment. Additionally, the criminal pursuit of healthcare professionals is not limited to just physicians. Nurses, pharmacists, and other medical professionals are also being pursued in this regard.

Currently, states across the country are prosecuting nurses, pharmacists, and nursing assistants for negligent care of patients in any setting where they are providing care.[2] Negligence is not just limited to nursing homes but, in a relatively recent case in Wisconsin, involved a hospital and an OB patient. In the 2006 Wisconsin Board of Nursing disciplinary proceedings case, a nurse was charged with criminal neglect of a patient by causing great bodily harm in the medication error–related death of a young woman during childbirth.[1] "The criminal complaint alleged that the nurse failed to follow the 'five rights' of medication administration (right drug, right patient, right route, right time, and right dosage), and that she did not use an available bedside bar-coding system (p. 273)."[1] The unusual thing that happened in this case is that she was charged with a felony for an unintended healthcare error by an overzealous prosecutor.[1] The normal course of proceedings should have only involved her being sued civilly and the Department of Regulation and Licensure (DRL) being the only entity involved in the handling of this infraction.[1] Fatigue and a number of other contributing factors contributed to this unintentional error and led to the tragic occurrence for which she cooperated fully, leading her to make incriminating statements that were disclosed in an incident report that was used against her in the criminal case.[1] Furthermore, because the nurse was being accused of a criminal act, she was fired from her job. Because the hospital's malpractice insurance carrier did not cover her, she had to hire an attorney on her own.[1] The charges against this nurse were eventually dropped from felonies to misdemeanor pleas for two counts of illegally administering prescription medications.[1] The Wisconsin Board of Nursing was at the same time looking into disciplining the nurse as well, and a day before her court appearance had even suspended her license for nine months and found that her conduct violated the minimum standards of the nursing profession necessary for the protection of the health, safety, and welfare of a patient or the public, which also included unprofessional conduct.[1] The criminal charges brought against this nurse evidences the problems associated with criminalizing medical errors. Clearly, this was not the case of a nurse who intended to harm the patient, and it was a result of clear unintended error. Other factors contributed to this error such as fatigue, persistent staffing shortages, and systemic failures.

Another example of a medical professional being criminally prosecuted involves the 2005 Hurricane Katrina disaster, when a physician and two nurses in New Orleans were arrested and criminally prosecuted for causing the deaths of critically ill hospitalized patients who died while in their care.[1] The charges against them were eventually dropped when a New Orleans grand jury refused to indict them for the alleged mercy killings after a yearlong prosecutorial ordeal.[1] What was scary was the fact that, if those healthcare providers were found guilty, the ramifications could have been far reaching and may still have led to unanticipated negative impacts in response planning for future disasters where the need to elicit the assistance of medical professionals in these efforts would be futile.[1] The general public could not find enough faults with these practitioners to punish them for their mercy killings. Perhaps these grand jury members thought that criminal punishment was too severe for the type of acts alleged.

"These recent examples demonstrate that prosecution of criminal medical negligence is a growing trend. With these increasing numbers, there is a greater concern regarding how medical negligence is applied in the criminal system and the difficulties that are associated with applying those standards in a criminal setting."[2] This leads us to the following question:

> What medical acts transform tort negligence into criminal negligence remains anybody's guess. Courts and common law have not been helpful in clarifying how criminal negligence applies to the practice of

> medicine. However, current definitions do not seem to contemplate that criminal negligence is more than a mistake in judgment. That notion can be found in the following definitions: that degree of negligence or carelessness which is denominated as gross, and which constitutes such a departure from what would be the conduct of an ordinarily careful and prudent man . . . as to furnish evidence of that indifference to consequences which in some offenses takes the place of criminal intent.[3]

This definition clarifies what can be thought of as warranting criminal prosecution. It is such a high degree of carelessness that a healthcare practitioner utilizes that leads to this result, which warrants a healthcare practitioner being punished in this manner. For example, a Supreme Court case involved a 1994 incident in which Dr. Suresh Gupta, a plastic surgeon, operated on his patient to remove a nasal deformity and made an incorrect incision that resulted in blood seeping into the patient's respiratory passage leading to his death. This incident also did not rise to the level of an offense that could take the place of criminal intent.[4] The court concluded:

> To fix criminal liability on a doctor or surgeon, the standard of negligence required to be proved should be so high that it can be described as gross negligence or recklessness and not merely lack of necessary care, attention, and skill. Every careless act of a medical person cannot be termed "criminal" only when doctors exhibit gross lack of competence or inaction, and wanton indifference to their patients' safety, as a result of gross ignorance or gross negligence. When a patient's death results merely from an error of judgment or an accident, no criminal liability should be attached to it. Mere inadvertence or some degree of want of adequate care and caution might create civil liability but not criminal liability. It was held that but for this approach, the hazards in the medical profession which include civil liability would also unreasonably extend to criminal liability, and doctors would then be at risk of landing up in prison, a result that would shake the mutual confidence between doctors and patient.[4]

This is a very powerful phrase in that it explains the problems with criminalizing medical errors in judgment. Surely, Dr. Gupta's actions in this scenario did not meet that level, and he should not have been criminally prosecuted for the same. The court reached the right conclusion in this scenario, and he was acquitted without a trial.[4]

In the past, there have not been many instances of physicians being held criminally responsible for their negligent behavior. For example, in the United States for the period from 1809 to 1981, there were only 15 reported appellate cases involving the criminal prosecution of physicians for medical malpractice.[5] Then for the period from 1981 to 2001, there were approximately two dozen cases of this sort, and from 2001 to 2011, there were approximately 37 cases, or about three times the rate for the prior two decades.[5] Though still small in number, these figures represent the growing trend of prosecutors taking on these types of cases. Perhaps it's how society has evolved in viewing gross negligence that has led to the increase in prosecutions. There is a parallel surge in prosecutions for negligence by healthcare practitioners who negligently prescribed addictive medication for their patients, which contributed to drug abuse.[5] In 2003, there were about 15 reported physician arrests that resulted in convictions, while in 2008 this figure had increased to 43.[5]

The AMA's Position on Criminal Prosecution May Limit Appropriate Accountability

The American Medical Association (AMA) has concluded that the criminalization of medical malpractice interferes with the practice of medicine.[5] In 1995, they adopted a resolution that opposes criminalizing medical negligence by physicians and have reasoned that healthcare decision making should not be penalized, which now is the current trend.[5] The AMA does not think that physicians' errors can rise to the level of a criminal nature.[5] Erroneous healthcare decision making is just a decision that should be penalized in the civil tort system.[5]

> The cost of defending a criminal case can be significant. In civil suits, doctor's legal bills are usually covered by their malpractice insurance plans, which don't extend to criminal charges. The AMA has argued that the civil tort system is sufficient for holding doctors accountable for negligent or incompetent actions.[5]

(Interesting, however, since the AMA also constantly criticizes the tort system.) The AMA feels that the financial exposure is enough of a deterrent because most physicians caught in this situation will have to pay restitution from their own pockets. The threat of paying out these oftentimes very large awards should be enough of a deterrent in their own right.

For advocates of patient safety, this aggressive, punitive, and often unwarranted prosecution can also lead to providers who are less willing to come forward and openly discuss and acknowledge error. The culture of silence described in the Institute of Medicine's (IOM) report, which was ascribed to a fear of malpractice litigation, will only be fueled in providers who are under a threat of criminal prosecution. This is even the case in a culture where criminal prosecution was not the threat, but only civil prosecution. The widespread tendency of physicians to avoid disclosing the commission of errors is not merely the result of commonly felt pressures; it is entrenched in the culture of medicine to the extent that physicians are taught to strive for the unrealistic ideal of an error-free practice.[1] These are unrealistic goals, as is echoed throughout the IOM report.[1]

> Recognition of medical malpractice is the longest-standing social-incentive structure that attempts to promote safety in health care delivery and represents an ethos of individual responsibility; however, recent criticisms by physicians allege that not only does this system fail to promote safety, it may even prevent them from reporting errors and making health safer. (p. 104)[1]

The IOM report further finds that, ironically, the medical malpractice system has encouraged physicians to practice defensive medicine to reduce the risk of liability, even by ordering tests and procedures that are of marginal or no medical benefit.[1] The culture of health care being punitive has hampered our ability to learn from our mistakes.[1] By continuing to criminalize medical errors, all of the successes already obtained in the IOM report might be impeded. This is because the criminal system is something that not even the medical arena can control and the effects of being punished are so grave that no practitioner wants to take the risk of being prosecuted in this area, thus engendering a culture of silence.

Society also feels different about how egregious cases of medical malpractice should be handled. As previously discussed,

> Criminal cases involving physicians have increased by about 33 percent between 1981 and 2011, prompting the AMA to emphatically reject criminal prosecution. Attempted criminalization of malpractice interferes with medical decision-

> making, making the argument that malpractice cases should only stay in the civil court. Most criminal cases brought against physicians involve prescription drug abuse or other egregious behavior. AMA officials don't get that the vast majority of medical malpractice cases don't wind up in the criminal courts. Only those cases where the doctor's misconduct crosses the line show up in criminal courts and in order to preserve the integrity of the profession they too should be interested in identifying those individuals and having them held accountable in a manner consistent with other professionals. Many egregious malpractice cases, that either injure or maim patients, end up in arbitration, usually in the hands of skillful mediators.[6]

Therefore, they don't even go through the entire channels of the legal system which could possibly expose them to more scrutiny. This growing trend has indicated that society wants to hold the most egregious acts as criminal so that they won't happen again.

HOW SEVERE CASES OF MEDICAL MALPRACTICE ARE HANDLED TODAY: AN ANALYSIS SURROUNDING THE MEDICAL CARE RESULTING IN THE DEATHS OF MICHAEL JACKSON AND ANNA NICOLE SMITH

A very good recent example of a case where society has criminalized acts by a physician involves the Dr. Conrad Murray case. He was the live-in physician of acclaimed pop star Michael Jackson. When Dr. Murray was accused and charged with involuntary manslaughter for his ongoing administration of the powerful anesthetic Propofol (which is generally used only in an operating room where continuous monitoring is available) to treat insomnia, objections were raised in the medical community because such acts that fell beneath the standard of care or gross negligence typically were handled by the civil courts.[6] Murray's case involves a doctor who didn't practice medicine but instead practiced experimentation without any medical precedent.[6] Murray concocted his own way of treating insomnia by anesthetizing Jackson with a fast-acting operating room anesthetic.[6] AMA officials can't possibly believe that such behavior should not invoke the severest of punishment or that physicians should be treated in a manner different from the manner in which the lay public is treated.[6] When the world looked on in horror at Nazi medical experiments after WWII, no one defended the actions as medical practice.[6] They saw it for what it was—pure sadism, controlled violence perpetrated on innocent victims.[6] This is how society viewed Dr. Murray's actions of giving Propofol to Michael Jackson while he was at home outside of a hospital setting. The public did not have a problem with the charges that were brought against him because they wanted someone to blame for causing Jackson's untimely death. They were relying on facts surrounding his senseless death that would call into question Dr. Murray's professional conduct. Dr. Murray's lack of experience in treating insomnia or in using anesthesia to induce sleep fell closely in line with the standard "outside the usual course of professional practice" and not for some "legitimate medical purpose," which falls within the strict medical definitions of gross negligence.[6] Dr. Murray will be held to have acted grossly negligent by his experiments on Michael Jackson even though in a sense he was only trying to help him get some sleep.

"Even experts at the AMA or any other professional organization must confess that Murray's Propofol drip breached every known rule of practicing medicine. He concocted his own anesthesia machine for which he had no experience, training or expertise to treat an equally unfamiliar condition to him called insomnia."[6] Furthermore,

> there is no clearly definable point at which a health care provider's negligence results in criminal culpability. To cross the line from civil to criminal negligence, there must be a gross or flagrant deviation. Using Dr. Conrad Murray as an example, the prosecution only needed to prove that he should have been aware of the risks associated with administering Propofol outside of a hospital setting, and not whether he had actual knowledge of those risks.[2]

Clearly, the jury hearing this case found there was not only a deviation from the standard of care, which is attributable to Michael Jackson's untimely death, that warranted attention but also reckless conduct committed by Dr. Murray, which directly contributed to Mr. Jackson's death. The question remains whether it warrants criminal culpability. "It's one thing to get sued for malpractice and quite another to go to jail for doing your job and becoming a victim ('second victim') of a healthcare delivery system that allowed you, the healthcare provider, to make an unintended mistake (p. 272)."[1] The burning question is, was it enough of a deviation in this case to warrant Dr. Murray spending up to four years in prison? Is it enough that a medical error exposes a healthcare practitioner to jail time for a judgment call seems to be the inquiry that affects us all.

The Difference Between Civil and Criminal Prosecution

The legal standards for prosecuting criminal versus negligent behavior differ with respect to medical malpractice cases.

> Criminal litigation applies different legal standards. Charges are brought by a state prosecutor against the Defendant and evidence is controlled by the prosecutor's office. There is a higher burden of proof than in a civil case, and findings must go beyond a reasonable doubt before the Defendant is found guilty of the charges. If the Defendant is found to be guilty of the charges, he or she faces monetary fines, prison time, and often probation. Only the Defendant has the right to appeal the verdict in criminal cases. No insurance policy covers these types of monetary fines and criminal-defense fees are usually excluded from professional-liability policies. (p. 270)[1]

Thus, as one can see it is very hard to defend these cases, and it can also be very costly since insurance companies won't cover these types of offenses. Whether it is worth it will next need to be explored since in a criminal prosecution the main goal is to deter performance of a criminal act with retribution by punishment.[1]

In a civil case of healthcare negligence the culpable Defendant (or their insurance provider) has to pay the Plaintiff for the negligent performance of a medical act or omission and the question becomes whether the criminal prosecution would have the desired effect as a deterrent for his passing.

> This case is only about whether or not Dr. Murray caused his death. . . . His guilt or innocence should not be a symbol of anything, his indictment should not be in order for prosecutors to make a statement about deterrence, but rather this should be a statement that our legal system is based on justice and nothing else.[7]

Perhaps this highly publicized case was taken out of context because of the fame of the victim. There are some scholars who are looking for new or interesting legal frameworks with respect to affirmative defenses for physicians administering medications that can result in death.[7] They feel that it is unfair for the physicians to be treated as criminals for this type of mistake.

Another interesting case with a different outcome is the Anna Nicole Smith case, where physician Dr. Sandkeep Kapoor was charged with illegally providing Smith with several prescription drugs that ultimately led to her death.[5] This case was based on a controlled substance law and hinged on whether Dr. Kapoor believed in good faith that there was a medical purpose for all of the prescriptions to be prescribed for Smith.[5]

> Kapoor, 42, who was Smith's internist, wrote numerous prescriptions for opiates and sedatives during the period he treated her. He followed a drug regimen originated by Smith's previous doctor who sold his practice to Kapoor. Prosecutors Renee Rose and David Barkhurst argued that Kapoor blurred the line between patient and doctor when he was photographed kissing her at a party. . . . pointed to a diary in which Kapoor discussed the "mesmerizing" experience of riding with her in a gay pride parade when he wondered: "Can she ruin me?"[8]

These factors raised questions about the validity behind Smith requiring these prescription drugs for valid medical purposes. However, the standard that needed to be scrutinized was whether a physician has a good-faith belief that a patient is in pain, and then he or she is not guilty of a crime for prescribing the controlled substance to relieve suffering.[8] For a physician to violate the law, he or she would need to knowingly and willfully prescribe, dispense, or administer a controlled substance to an addict for a nontherapeutic purpose.[8] Although Kapoor administered drugs to Smith, he claimed he did not know that she was an addict.

The jury ultimately dismissed the charges against Dr. Kapoor.[5] It was probable that the jury did not believe Dr. Kapoor thought Smith was an addict and that he knowingly and willfully prescribed her drugs anyway. The medication he prescribed was not uncommon or deadly, but it was the dangerous mix of drugs and the overdose that contributed to Smith's death. On the other hand, the difference in the Michael Jackson case was that prosecutors were not charging Dr. Murray with violating a controlled substance law.[5]

> That's because Propofol, the anesthetic Murray is accused of giving to Jackson, is not a controlled substance. The drug administered intravenously is used to induce anesthesia and has rarely been abused as a narcotic. Prosecutors instead alleged Murray breached the medical standard of care when he administered the anesthetic to Jackson at home, and that his gross negligence caused the singer's death at age 50.[5]

Although this seems similar to breaching a prescription drug law that Dr. Kapoor was charged with, the distinction is the type of drug that was involved in the allegations. Also there was a great deal made of the lack of appropriate monitoring that should have been done since Dr. Murray was physically present. Propofol is much stronger than a drug per se because it is used as an anesthesia and is not a controlled substance that is inherently subject to stronger controls. Whether this distinction is enough to subject Dr. Murray to jail time while Dr. Kapoor gets off scot free is yet to be seen. It is more likely than not that Dr. Kapoor had some inclination that Smith had a history of drug abuse.

The Wisconsin, Hurricane Katrina, and Dr. Gupta cases incorporate a very important distinction from the Jackson and Smith cases regarding criminal culpability, which is really more common than these other high-profile celebrity cases. The distinction lies in the level of culpability that the practitioners in the Wisconsin, Hurricane Katrina, and Dr. Gupta cases had versus those in the Jackson and Smith cases. The physicians in the foregoing cases appeared to make honest, unintentional medical errors, which could have easily been made by anyone else put in similar situations. These situations are exactly like the types of events described in the IOM report, where a conflagration of system problems sets these individuals up for failure. On the other hand, the physicians in the Jackson and Smith cases had a little more control over their decisions, unhampered by medical emergencies, systemic failures, and fatigue. As a result of the lack of an emergency situation surrounding Dr. Jackson and Smith's decision making process included many poor choices and few system problems. Thus, it appears that they are probably really more culpable than the first set of physicians described above. The physicians for Jackson and Smith had the time and resources to make sound medical decisions regarding the care of their celebrity patients, and they still did not do so. Their professional judgment came into play because they lacked reasonable judgment when formulating their decision making in regard to their patients, while in the Wisconsin, Hurricane Katrina, and Dr. Gupta cases, one could see that it was only a result of unintended medical error that tragedy resulted. Even though Smith's physician was eventually acquitted, reasonable minds could still have inferred that he knew or should have known of Smith's drug use. The lines are considerably more blurry in the Wisconsin, Hurricane Katrina, and Dr. Gupta cases. The AMA is more concerned about these types of cases garnering criminal culpability. These types of cases are more in line with what exemplifies which actions should be exonerated from criminal culpability.

The Impact That Criminalizing Medical Malpractice Has on Patient Safety and Voluntary Error Reporting

There is an impact that is felt in the areas of patient safety and voluntary error reporting as a result of criminalizing medical malpractice. Some feel that criminalizing the decisions that healthcare providers make puts more pressure on them to strive for perfection. They, therefore, do not wish to report errors that they make for fear of the consequences, especially if they risk going to jail for these errors. For example, if a risk manager is working for a hospital or healthcare system that is governed by an accrediting body's standards, they know that event analysis and disclosure are mandated.[1] "The balancing act of doing the investigation and event analysis while protecting the organization and the healthcare provider involved in the incident from having statements and facts used against them in the criminal matter can be challenging (p.275)."[1] There must be an ability to distinguish between the systemic failures of a system that often predisposes a provider to act in a manner that harms others and the personal and often reckless conduct of a professional that directly leads to harm. Personal accountability has to be part of the analysis. This can be extremely difficult to achieve since a balancing act has to occur within the organization and the required system of disclosure. Each case must be individually evaluated to determine what the best advice will be for those involved.[1]

There are some things that a risk manager can do to cut down on the impact of criminalizing medical negligence including the following: 1) educating all staff on the differences between civil and criminal liability and the types of behavior that can give rise to criminal charges, 2) adding a criminal defense extension endorsement to the entity's professional-liability policy that includes defense costs incurred in defending against a criminal proceeding, 3) developing a second-victim support program so that when healthcare providers are involved in a tragic error they are treated with respect, compassion, and understanding, 4) limiting organizational use of overtime to assure patient and provider safety including educating all employees and physicians that they are responsible for knowing when fatigue could impact personal performance, 5) if a significant event occurs that could appear in the media, the risk manager should recommend notifying the public affairs department and the governing board, 6) preparing the organization for a regulatory visit, which could very likely follow a significant event, 7) developing a safe healthcare delivery system and analyzing the near-miss events (as time allows) to continually strive for system improvements, 8) setting clear expectations for staff performance and emphasizing the need to understand why, not just what, to encourage the development of the critical thinking skills, 9) performing failure mode and effects analysis; prior to introducing new programs, procedures or technology, 10) utilizing error-reduction toolboxes and other strategies that should be utilized whenever possible to reduce the likelihood of human-error occurrence, and 11) utilizing the just culture checklist-tips to assist the organization in becoming a fair, accusation-free environment (276–277)[1] Implementation of these procedures should minimize the effect of potential devastating criminal prosecutions.

Should More Acts of Negligence Be Considered Criminal?

The next question that needs to be explored is whether this new phenomenon of criminalizing health professional's negligent behavior and thereby exposing them to criminal penalties and jail time is effective in improving the healthcare system. The preferable option is for actions of medical negligence to remain strictly a matter of civil liability unless the behavior is so reckless that even a reasonably prudent person would be shocked by it and there was an intention to harm.[2]

> Civil liability for medical negligence is itself not a perfect system, but it provides redress for civil wrongs that have been committed. A civil claim for medical negligence provides the Plaintiff patient with the opportunity to receive compensation for injuries, and it gives the health care provider a chance to reform conduct without the unnecessary punishment of prison.[2]

The civil system used in this regard still accomplishes the mission of providing redress for the injured victim while punishing the negligent healthcare provider financially and professionally for the harm he or she has caused. Plaintiffs can potentially receive both economic and noneconomic damages.[2] Economic damages enable the plaintiff to be able to recover for objective monetary losses such as medical expenses and lost wages, while noneconomic damages such as pain and suffering, loss of enjoyment of life, and loss of consortium can be recovered.[2] These types of awards to the injured plaintiff serve to make him or her whole again and will be attributable to the negligent health professional's conduct and pocket.

There are also other things that can be done to the health professional to punish him or her besides a prison sentence.[2]

> These punishments are imposed by medical and nursing boards. Each state maintains its own medical board, which is tasked with monitoring physician conduct and investigating complaints received from the public. State nursing boards carry the equivalent duty of protecting the public from the negligent conduct of licensed nurses. Investigations from these boards can lead to punishments that include reprimands, suspension or revocation of licenses, or probation. Alternatively, the medical or nursing board can also choose to focus its attention on re-educating and retraining the health care provider, a remedy not feasible within the confines of a prison cell . . . and the focus should be on providing these professionals with the opportunity to learn from their mistakes, not to punish them with criminal sanctions.[2]

Thus, one can see the variety of mechanisms that can be used as effective deterrents—not only the threat of compensation being paid to the victim but also of possibly losing one's license, which can mean the end of livelihood for the negligent professional. These two factors alone can be effective deterrents and should make the entire system safer. Thus, the need for criminal prosecutions should not be great since the punishments are just as effective. The result would be that society does not need to criminalize medical negligence.

CONCLUSION

Whether we are going down the correct path by criminalizing negligent behavior by healthcare professionals is yet to be seen. The arguments for continued criminalization of medical negligence are strong since those advocating for criminalization want to deter those who are in a position to know best and who are skilled in the art of providing care from harming unknowing patients who have given them control of their lives. This theory lies on the premise that,

> Proponents of criminal prosecution rely on utilitarian and retributive theories of justice to rationalize their position. Utilitarians believe criminal sanctions are appropriate when punishing negligent conduct because prosecution encourages all individuals to conduct themselves with more caution. Utilitarian theory applied to health care supports the notion that the threat of criminal sanctions would force physicians to monitor their own practices. Retributive justice, a theory centered on the notion that punishment is justified on the grounds that the criminal has created an imbalance in the social order, also supports criminal sanctions for medical acts. A physician's inadvertent risk taking may be viewed as a fault in social interaction that should be punished through criminal sanctions.[3]

The public wants to punish those who are reckless and careless in this regard, as can be evidenced by the Dr. Conrad Murray trial and Michael Jackson's untimely death. As stated:

> Criminal punishment for medical negligent conduct is a growing trend. Studies of these cases indicate that the triers of fact tend to place a greater emphasis on the defendant's subjective state of mind. The concern is that a jury may render a "guilty" judgment without considering whether the health care provider's conduct fell within the objective standard of care. Moreover, the criminalization of medical negligence fails to serve the true goals of criminal law. Criminal culpability for health care providers should be limited to instances of recklessness. Providers who are reckless will be criminally punished for undertaking actions in which they were aware of the risks.[3]

On the other hand, there are those who say criminalization of medical health practitioners' negligent acts is not the best way to go. They reason that

> ultimately civil liability is the preferred method for settling issues for negligent conduct. It provides the patient with the opportunity to recover for his or her injuries and medical expenses. Additionally, medical and nursing boards already have existing procedures for punishment and reform, all of which supersede the necessity of a prison sentence. With these existing civil liabilities and sanctions, the focus should be on rehabilitating these health care providers to prevent them from repeating the same mistakes, and not imprisoning them for unintentional error.[2]

Furthermore, the sentiment is that

> [t]hose who oppose criminally punishing negligent medical conduct argue that a just criminal system should only punish those who have voluntarily committed a wrong. Based on this theory, it would be unjust to punish an actor for risk taking that is inadvertent or when the actor is unaware that the conduct creates a risk of danger. In addition, a negligent actor who fails to identify her dangerous conduct would also fail to comprehend the potential threat of sanctions for such conduct. Therefore, it would be unjust for such a defendant to lose her liberty and be stigmatized. Medical associations and physician specialty groups add that criminal prosecution for clinical errors would set a dangerous precedent. They argue such a precedent will drive physicians away from taking hard cases or experimenting in new areas. Others argue that such a precedent will encourage the practice of defensive medicine and further drive up the cost of health care. There may come a day when only the bravest or most foolhardy clinician will opt for anything but the least controversial option.[3]

As one can see, there are several implications on patient safety and voluntary error reporting as a result of criminalizing this behavior. As was seen in the Wisconsin, Hurricane Katrina, and Dr. Gupta cases, it did more harm than good to attempt to criminally prosecute these healthcare practitioners for clear medical errors. It further disincentivized the goals set out to reform the profession as a result of learning from one's mistakes. If criminalization of medical malpractice is left for only the most egregious of circumstances, then this will fare better overall on the healthcare community. This concept will also foster the growth of more openness about error in the medical community. Thus, the new philosophy is that less severe punishment will contribute more to voluntary error reporting and patient safety. If this pattern is followed, what needs to be emphasized in regard to learning from one's mistake will still be taken care of, and for everyone involved it will be a win-win situation.

References

1. Youngberg, B. J. (2011). *Principles of risk management and patient safety*. Sudbury, MA: Jones & Bartlett.
2. Barcus, H. A., & Shen, E. (2010). *When does medical negligence become criminal?* Retrieved from http://www.latlaw.com/index.php/firm-news-articles/articles-2010/88-when-does-medical-negligence-become-criminal.
3. Monico, E., Kulkarni, R., Calise A., & Calabro, J. (2007). The criminal prosecution of medical negligence. *The Internet Journal of Law, Healthcare and Ethics, 5*(1).
4. Hariharan Nair, M. R. (2004). Criminal liability for medical negligence: A drastic change? *Indian Journal of Medical Ethics, 1*(4). Retrieved from http://www.issuesinmedicalethics.org/124hl126.html.
5. Baynes, T. (2011, September 12). Michael Jackson's doc represents rise in criminal prosecutions. *Thomson Reuters News & Insight*. Retrieved from http://newsandinsight.thomsonreuters.com/California/News/2011/09_-_September/Michael_Jackson_s_doc_represents_rise_in_criminal_prosecutions/.
6. Curtis, J. M. (2011, September 12). AMA defends Dr. Murray against criminal acts. *LA City Buzz Examiner*. Retrieved from http://www.examiner.com/article/ama-defends-dr-murray-against-criminal-acts.

7. Wood, D. B. (2011, February 8). Case against Michael Jackson's doctor centers on gross negligence. *The Christian Science Monitor*. Retrieved from http://www.csmonitor.com/USA/Society/2010/0208/Case-against-Michael-Jackson-s-doctor-centers-on-gross-negligence.

8. Associated Press. (2010, October 28). Anna Nicole Smith's doctor acquitted in drug case, psychiatrist and boyfriend convicted. *FoxNews.com*. Retrieved from http://www.foxnews.com/entertainment/2010/10/28/anna-nicole-smiths-doctor-acquitted-drug-case/.

42

Aligning Patients, Payers, and Providers: Bringing Quality and Safety into the Reimbursement Equation

Caitlin Podbielski, JD

INTRODUCTION

Traditionally, many of the decisions made within healthcare organizations have been financially rooted. The effectiveness technologies, supplies, and even procedural protocols are frequently evaluated for cost effectiveness rather than for quality effectiveness. Patient safety has suffered as a result. Reimbursement reform is a unique mechanism through which cost and quality can be simultaneously achieved. The current fee-for-service reimbursement mechanism juxtaposes cost efficiency against clinical efficiency by rewarding volume and ignoring outcomes. Because reimbursement is the means through which providers recognize financial gain, it is the most appropriate venue to align financial and clinical incentives. Changing the current payment mechanism to recognize quality, clinical efficiency, which in turn generates cost efficiency, will better align patients', providers', and payers' interests. The inclination to compromise patient safety in favor of financial gain is eliminated because quality health care is necessarily safe care.

This chapter will begin by developing a plan for reimbursement reform, which requires both defining the relevant terms and formulating a set of objectives to guide implementation. Next, this chapter will cover how basic principles of a pay-for-performance reimbursement system will recognize quality, and this chapter will evaluate three pay-for-performance programs that each approach the concept in a different manner. Last, this chapter will advocate for hybrid models, which can protect patients against unintended consequences and account for geographic, demographic, and infrastructure variances. Ultimately, this chapter will conclude that reimbursement reform is not a one-size-fits-all solution but can be an effective mechanism for extracting quality, safety, and value out of the American healthcare system if stakeholder objectives are aligned.

IDENTIFYING THE VARIABLES AND CONSTANTS

To formulate a plan to improve the current system, it is important to recognize the ways in which the current system fails patients, providers, and payers. To illustrate the inadequacies, the Institute of Medicine offered the following example to demonstrate how payment policies work against quality initiatives:

> A physician group paid primarily on a fee-for-service basis instituted a new program to improve blood sugar control for diabetic patients. Specifically, pilot studies suggested that tighter diabetic management could decrease hemoglobin A1c levels 2 percentage points for about 40 percent of all diabetic patients managed by the physician group. Data from two randomized controlled trials demonstrated that better sugar controls should translate into lower rates of retinopathy, nephropathy, peripheral neurological damage, and heart disease. The savings in direct healthcare costs (i.e., reduced visits and hospital episodes) from avoided complications have been estimated to generate a net savings of about $2,000 per patient per year, on average, over 15 years. Across the more than 13,000 diabetic patients managed by the physicians group, the project had the potential to generate over $10 million in net savings each year. The project was costly to the medical group in two ways. First, expenses to conduct the project, including extra clinical time for tighter management, fell to the physician group. Second, over time, as diabetic complication rates fell, the project would reduce patient visits, thus, revenues as well. But the savings from the avoided complications would accrue to the insurer or a self-funded purchaser.[1]

This example illustrates that the current system does not reward innovation because value is not created for the innovator. Clinically efficient providers suffer economically for such achievements because the savings accrue only to the payer. While providers certainly want to see their patients healthy, the current system forces them to choose between their patients and their financial well-being. It would be naive to believe that altruistic motives will prevail at this crossroad; instead, tying economic benefit to improved patient care eliminates the choice.

Hopefully, changing the way in which providers are paid will change the way in which providers interact with patients, the way in which organizations operate, and the way in which patients engage providers. However, to assure such changes produce positive results, any plans for reform must have clear objectives, and implementation should be a manifestation of those objectives. Fundamentally, the primary objective of reimbursement reform should be to achieve more quality and value. The current system rewards only volume; thus patients are reduced to a commodity, or a means to a financial end. When the payment is tied to the patient in a more meaningful way, providers are held accountable for the care they deliver and the patient's response. Similarly, a system that incentivizes patients to participate in their own health produces quality and value. Thus, the first step in developing feasible objectives for reform is to define the relevant terms.

Defining the Relevant Terms

If the overarching objective is to create more quality and value in the healthcare system, then quality and value must be defined. Henceforth, quality means clinical, evidence-based practices employed to yield a typical result. Patient safety is a clinical input essential to produce quality. Furthermore, when value recognizes clinical outcomes, quality and patient safety are inherent by-products. Accordingly, value must next be defined. Superficially, value implies a return on investment, but the substance of that return differs depending on the investor. Accordingly, value must be defined for all stakeholders: patients, providers, and payers.

Turning first to patients, value is defined as obtaining a benefit, measured in better health or best possible outcomes, in return for financial investments and opportunity costs. Patients' financial contributions in insurance premiums, copays, and out-of-pocket costs come at the sacrifice of using those dollars for other purposes, such as for children's needs, food, and shelter, among other important or desired expenditures. With medical debt accounting for two-thirds of bankruptcies in the United States, it is difficult to dispel the premise that the healthcare system asks for a substantial financial investment from patients.[2] In return, patients expect to derive benefit from the services and products purchased with their hard-earned income. Currently, the healthcare system is not accountable for producing such value. Reformed reimbursement mechanisms should give patients more for their money in better health care on an individual level and, globally, more efficient use of resources to lower overall costs.

Turning next to providers, there are several avenues through which providers invest in the healthcare system and seek value in return. As an initial investment, the average physician incurs $150,000 in debt throughout his or her medical education.[3] Additionally, many providers take on substantial financial risk establishing and operating medical practices, which require expensive overhead and expose the physician to immense liability. Providers, like any other working professional, are asked to sacrifice time with their families for the sake of their work. Certainly, providers are financially compensated for their service, which provides economic benefit for their families; however, if the system in which providers operate is riddled with waste at the expense of time at home, there is arguably little value generated to justify the personal sacrifice. Providers, as businesspersons and breadwinners, are motivated by economic benefits to an extent. But as medial professionals bound by an oath to do no harm, providers are also driven to heal by treating patients to the best of their ability. Thus, value for providers is adequate compensation, professional recognition, and successful patient outcomes.

Payers, defined as insurers, obtain value when patients and providers receive value because money is used efficiently and beneficiaries are healthier. For example, lowering patient readmissions or managing chronic diseases creates value for the payer by reducing costs and lowering risk, but both are equally valuable to patients and providers. True to the principles of risk distribution governing insurance products, a healthier pool of beneficiaries reduces direct financial costs for the insurer. Tangentially, satisfied participants can also translate into increased participation and disburse risk even further. Similarly, efficient providers reduce utilization costs for payers. Alternatively, payers can be defined as employers, for whom value is mainly derived from healthier employees. Further, employers with self-funded insurance products directly benefit from lower costs in the way insurers do. Ultimately, value for either type of payer is the net effect of creating value for patients and providers.

Formulating Reform Objectives

After establishing that creating value for all stakeholders will safeguard quality and patient safety, the next step is to formulate objectives by which to evaluate possible reimbursement mechanisms. To assure that all stakeholders recognize value from the new system, it is important to consider the objectives of each stakeholder. Accordingly, Table 42.1 details those objectives.

All three groups fundamentally agree that a healthcare system that emphasizes quality and creates value is possible. The Institute of Medicine, advocating objectives favoring patient interest in quality health care, set forth six principles to govern payment reform. Ideally, the dollar amount of payment should be adequate to promote reengineering and process design, yet providers should not gain or lose because of patients' severity of illness. Further, when the payment is based on quality measures, it

TABLE 42.1 Stakeholders' Objectives for Reimbursement Reform

Patients: Institute of Medicine[1]	Providers: American Board of Internal Medicine Foundation 2009 Stakeholders Meeting[4]	Payors: CEO Council[21]
• Avoid adverse selection	• Collaboration	• Change delivery incentives
• Data transparency for providers	• Cost-effective resource use	• Make data transparent
• Empower the consumer	• Information sharing and improvement	• Best preventative-care practices
• Evidence-based reimbursement	• Innovation and flexibility	• Engage and empower employers
• Reduce fragmentation of care		• Tort reform

Data from the Institute of Medicine (2001). Crossing the Quality Chasm: A New Health System for the 21st Century, 18. National Academies Press. http://www.nap.edu/catalog.php?record_id=10027. Accessed March 1 2012; and Cara S. Lesser et al (2010). Physician Payment Reform: Principles That Should Shape It, 29 Health Affairs, no. 5 at 948, 949; and Laura Landro, Health Care: Change the Incentives, Wall Street Journal CEO Council (NOV. 22, 2010). http://online.wsj.com/article/SB10001424052748703688704575620850148494216.html. Accessed March 1 2012.

should produce valuable data, which can be used to develop processes of care. In turn, such data should be equally available to providers to enable widespread implementation and to consumers to make educated decisions about where to receive care.

Alternatively, the American Board of Internal Medicine Foundation brought together physicians, nurses, patient and consumer advocates, policy researchers, health system leaders, and payers to develop 10 principles for payment reform, which fall into four areas of focus. To promote collaboration, payment must incentivize team-based care in two respects. First, payment per service devalues the contributions of other members of the caregiving team. Instead, providers should be incentivized to coordinate care across settings, over time. Second, the emphasis on volume in the current system deters providers from engaging with patients as active partners in their health. Alternatively, payment should incentivize shared decision making, which has been shown to lead to better outcomes and lower costs.[4]

Finally, *The Wall Street Journal* sponsored a task force discussion on health care wherein the participants concluded that the solution was not to repeal federal health reform but, instead, to charge the industry and government with working together to revolutionize the way care is delivered by changing the incentives for employers, physicians, and consumers. The task force offered five recommendations. First, reimbursement should recognize outcomes, team-based care, and appropriateness of setting. Second, employers and consumers alike should have readily available data on provider performance compared to nationally accepted standards. Similarly, providers should be incentivized to use that data to formulate and disseminate best practices. Third, a focus on disease management and prevention programs is an important part of data aggregation and the proliferation of best practices. Fourth, granting employers more flexibility in developing benefits plans and offering workplace wellness programs can provide both the carrot and the stick for patient–employees to take control of their own health outside of the provider setting. Last, physicians utilizing evidence-based medicine should be protected, requiring an overhaul of liability laws in favor of alternative dispute resolution mechanisms.

TABLE 42.2 "Five Guiding Principles" for Reimbursement Reform

1. Data Sharing and transparency
2. Allocating responsibility between patient and provider
3. Coordination of caregivers
4. Dissemination of evidence-based medicine
5. Greater flexibility in delivery of care models

From these three perspectives emerge common themes that can be developed into a comprehensive set of objectives. Table 42.2 sets forth five objectives cumulatively representative of all stakeholders (henceforth referred to as the Five Guiding Principles), against which proposed pilot programs for reimbursement will be evaluated.

PAYING FOR PERFORMANCE INSTEAD OF VOLUME

With principles by which to evaluate reimbursement innovations, the next step requires determining what reimbursement will reward. It is well established that the current system rewards volume, and the consequences of such incentives are readily apparent. If the reformed system is to effectuate the Five Guiding Principles, it should reward performance. The pay-for-performance concept can generally characterize the pilot programs evaluated below. This concept has been employed in several other industries with much success, but it is important recognize the appropriate standards for "performance" in the healthcare setting that the new reimbursement scheme should reward.

Pay-for-performance programs in healthcare seek to pay providers to deliver quality. The "pay" aspect will be defined by the reimbursement mechanism, examples of which will be discussed in the following part. On the other hand, "performance" can be defined in several respects. Performance can be evaluated from several perspectives, including payment system, provider group, and individual physician levels. The effect of rewarding certain aspects of performance at each level is varied, and the definition of performance must be tailored to address the unique perspective. Studies indicate the way in which performance is defined impacts the effectiveness of the payment mechanism for quality, generally referred to as the financial incentive. Additionally, performance can pertain to the process of care or patient outcomes, focusing on provider behaviors or the results thereof. For example, confining performance to process of care ignores outcome, and improved quality may be the result of improved documentation rather than actual improvement in patient care.[5] Alternatively, performance confined to outcome can induce adverse selection, where providers choose to treat only healthier patients with the greatest chance of achieving the desired outcome.[5] Thus, the design of the incentive is important to avoid unintended consequences and to produce meaningful results. The pilot programs discussed below illustrate the variety of ways in which performance can be measured and defined. The benefits and drawbacks of each will be discussed, and recommendations for hybrid models to account for unintended consequences follow.

Bundled Payment

Much of federal health reform has been in response to the exorbitant cost of the healthcare system. Accordingly, an attractive option for reimbursement reform is the bundled payment model, which combines payment for all services associated with an episode of care. In some respects, the bundled payment is capitation, allocating a set dollar amount for a defined scope of services for a specific diagnosis rather than a per-patient payment. Section 3023 of the Patient Protection and Affordable Care Act, as amended by the Health Care and Education Reconciliation Act, authorizes the Centers for Medicare & Medicaid Services (CMS) to implement the bundled payment pilot program, slated to begin January 1, 2013. Alternatively, The Center for Medicare & Medicaid Innovation has launched the Bundled Payments for Care Improvement, which offers four models that will cover a variety of services and provider settings.[6] The hope is that this predictive cost model will force providers to evaluate the allocation of resources; the effect will be increased efficiency and quality through mandatory reporting on certain quality measures. Preliminary data from several pilot programs have seen cost reductions and quality improvement as a result of the adherence to guidelines, elimination of waste and utilization reduction, and physician–hospital alignment.[7]

There is currently flexibility in how the bundled payment rate is set. For episodes of care that involve a small number of providers, payers are able to negotiate the rates much the same as the current contracting process. Regardless of the process, there are three main valuation methods that can serve as the basis for the payment rate. First, historical costs and reimbursement data can set the initial rate. Second, standard guidelines dictating appropriate levels of care could determine which services will be bundled. Last, evidence-based case rates, representative of required care in accordance with established clinical guidelines, can incorporate quality measurement into the payment rate. In addition to the base rate, bundled payments can be risk adjusted to provide for variations in the severity of illness among patients.[7]

Turning to the Five Guiding Principles, the bundled payment model fairly obviously fosters coordination of care and flexibility in the delivery of care. Alternatively, little accountability is shifted to the patient under this model. In fact, the patient is arguably confined to the same passive role as the recipient of services rather than as an engaged decision maker. Similarly, the only mechanism with the potential to disseminate evidence-based medicine is the payment calculation. If payers decide to base the rate on historical cost and claims data, no meaningful examination of best practices and necessary processes is performed or communicated. Further, there is little incentive to communicate best practices among providers without a comparative component to encourage transparency. Reliable data on patient diagnoses and comorbidities is essential for basing rates on historical episodes, but current programs have been utilizing data designed only for fee-for-services payments, which lacks the necessary detail for meaningful clinical evaluations.[7] Ultimately, the adequacy of the bundled payment model depends on the payer–provider relationship and the extent to which each seeks to keep costs stagnant or to revolutionize the delivery of care in favor of quality and efficiency.

Value-Based Purchasing

A more data-intensive approach to extracting quality from the healthcare system is the value-based purchasing model. The theory of value-based purchasing is to hold providers accountable to buyers through the compilation of information on healthcare quality, such as outcomes and processes of care.[8] The idea is based on five key elements: (1) contracts, (2) information, (3) quality management, (4) incentives, and (5) education. Contracting is the process through which the responsibilities of providers as suppliers and employers or insurers as purchasers are memorialized. Information is used for quality management purposes and to influence purchasing decisions. Incentives encourage and reward providers for executing desired practices developed as part of quality management. Last, education refers to the process of empowering healthcare consumers with quality data and comparisons. Results from the largest Medicare hospital demonstration project show promising indicators of quality and patient outcomes improvements. Over six years, the participants improved quality scores by almost 19% on average, saved approximately 8,500 heart attack patients, and received $60 million in Medicare awards.[9]

The Medicare Value-Based Purchasing (VBP) program[10] for hospital inpatient services is an example of how this model can be effectuated. In 2013, VBP will begin reimbursing on performance scores based on patient satisfaction and clinical process of care measures found in Table 42.3. In 2014, outcome measures, detailed in Table 42.4, and efficiency measures will be added to the equation. Efficiency is measured by spending per beneficiary based on claims data and episodes of care. CMS has already begun to measure cost-efficiency and quality measures to set the baselines by which performance and improvement will be evaluated in relation to thresholds (50th percentile of national performance) and benchmarks (mean value for the top 10 %). To fund the program, Medicare diagnosis related group (DRG) payments will be reduced by 1 % in 2013.

TABLE 42.3 Final FY2013 Clinical Process of Care and Patient Experience Measures for VBP

Acute Myocardial Infarction
• Fibrinolytic therapy received within 30 minutes of hospital arrival • Primary PCI received within 90 minutes of hospital arrival
Heart Failure
• Discharge instructions
Pneumonia
• Blood cultures performed in ED prior to initial antibiotic received in hospital • Initial antibiotic selection for CAP in immunocompetent patient
Healthcare-Associated Infections
• Prophylactic antibiotic received within one hour prior to surgical incision • Prophylactic antibiotic selection for surgical patients • Prophylactic antibiotic discontinued within 24 hours after surgery end time • Cardiac surgery patients with controlled 6 a.m. postoperative serum glucose
Surgeries
• Surgery patients on a beta blocker prior to arrival that received a beta blocker during the perioperative period • Surgery patients with recommended venous thromboembolism prophylaxis ordered • Surgery patients who received appropriate venous thromboembolism prophylaxis within 24 hours prior to surgery to 24 hours after surgery
Patient Experience of Care Measures
• Hospital consumer assessment of healthcare providers and systems survey

Data from the Centers for Medicare & Medicaid Services: Medicare Program; Hospital Inpatient Value-Based Purchasing Program, 76 Fed. Reg. 26490, 26510 (to be codified at 42 C.F.R. pts. 422 & 480).

TABLE 42.4 Final FY2014 Outcome Measures for VBP[10]

Mortality Measures (30-day rates)	AHRQ Patient Safety/ Inpatient Quality Indicators	Hospital-Acquired Condition Measures
• Acute myocardial infarction • Heart failure • Pneumonia	• Complications/patient safety for selected indicators • Mortality for selected medical conditions	• Foreign object retained after surgery • Air embolism • Blood incompatibility • Pressure ulcer stages III and IV • Falls and trauma • Vascular catheter-associated infection • Catheter-associated urinary tract infection • Manifestations of poor glycemic control

Data from the Centers for Medicare & Medicaid Services: Medicare Program; Hospital Inpatient Value-Based Purchasing Program, 76 Fed. Reg. 26490, 26511 (to be codified at 42 C.F.R. pts. 422 & 480).

Operationally, providers will still receive the traditional fee-for-services payment, but performance and improvement scores will be combined to produce an achievement score that may entitle the provider to an additional bonus payment. Even though the fee-for-service model is still employed, the incentive to define performance by volume is mitigated by the way in which the bonus payment is calculated. In the VBP program, providers can be paid more without increasing volume. To illustrate, the current model incentivizes more patient visits per day by physicians regardless of what occurs or the results from those visits. Alternatively, under the VBP model, two physicians seeing the same number of patients could be reimbursed differently *because of* what happens during and after those visits. Consequently, the incentive is not to maximize the volume of patient encounters but to maximize the value of patient encounters irrespective of quantity.

Specifically, the hospital's DRG payments will be reduced for lower scoring hospitals or increased for higher scoring hospitals. Where hospitals fall on the continuum is based on achievement, in comparison to national performance, and improvement, in comparison to the hospital's own baseline. The achievement score is the composite of 0–10 scores per measure. Hospitals receive a score of 10 for measures at or above the benchmark, a score of 0 for scores below the threshold, and a score of 1–9 for performance in between. The improvement score is the composite of 0–9 scores per measure. The hospital receives a score of 1–9 for performance improvements since the baseline period but still between the threshold and benchmark. Further, the four domains are weighted differently for each calculation, ranging from 20 to 30%. For the year 2012, providers receive the full DRG for reporting the already required hospital inpatient and outpatient reporting measures.

In general, value-based purchasing programs achieve several of the Five Guiding Principles. Such detailed performance tracking necessitates data sharing. Although not specifically part of the VBP program, the reported performance measures include those available to the public on the Medicare Hospital Compare[11] Web site and will be publicly available on the Physician Compare site on January 1, 2013.[12] Further, since the clinical process of care measures evaluate adherence to well-established principles of care, the dissemination of evidence-based medicine is an inherent part of establishing and evolving the program. Accordingly, there is minimal flexibility in delivery of care models because of the emphasis on standardization rather than on innovation. Value-based purchasing programs do not specifically address patient responsibility, but the inclusion of a patient experience domain (and the substantial weight it is in given in the payment calculation) keeps the patient relevant to the equation. As illustrated above, providers cannot improve clinical processes at the expense of the patients' experience. Similarly, coordination of caregivers is not explicitly rewarded, but collaboration could prove to be an effective means of improving clinical processes and engaging patients, much in the same way the bundled payment envisions.

Medical Home

The patient-centered medical home (PCMH) combines reimbursement reform with health IT and the five pillars of patient care, as outlined in Table 42.5. The PCMH model strives to engage the patient on three levels: (1) sharing in decision making in their own care, (2) improving quality in the primary care practice, and (3) implementing policy and research development. Shared decision making refers to a formal process wherein the patient is provided with evidence-based decision aids to understand the risks and benefits of various treatment options, after which the patient communicates personal concerns regarding the risks and benefits to the provider and the provider and patient dialogue to decide how to proceed with treatment. Informal shared decision-making processes still involve the

TABLE 42.5 "Five Pillars" of the Patient-Centered Medical Home Model[13]

1. Comprehensive care
2. Patient centered
3. Coordinated care
4. Accessible services
5. Quality and safety

Data from the Agency for Health Research and Quality (2011). Patient-Centered Medical Home Decisionmaker Brief: Strategies to Put Patients at the Center of Primary Care. http://pcmh.ahrq.gov/portal/server.pt/community/pcmh__home/1483/PCMH_Home_Papers%20Briefs%20and%20Othe%20Resources_v2 (link to downloadable PDF); and Defining the PCMH, pcmh.ahrq.gov, http://pcmh.ahrq.gov/portal/server.pt/community/pcmh__home/1483/pcmh_defining_the_pcmh_v2. Accessed Dec. 11, 2011.

patient by soliciting patient preferences and providing evidence-based information to help the patient understand treatment options. An important aim of empowering the patient is to improve patient safety in the areas of safe medication use, infection control initiatives, and reporting complications or errors. Similarly, patients can participate in quality improvement efforts in a general sense by contributing feedback on surveys, patient/family advisory councils, or participating in quality improvement activities such as pilot programs.[13] Holistically, policy makers should assure patients are involved in the design and study of medical home demonstrations to assure that programs are actually *patient centered* rather than system or provider centered.

There are several ways in which PCMHs can be reimbursed, ranging in the level of necessary administrative transformation from the current model.[14] Building on the current fee-for-service structure, providers could receive enhanced payments for service evaluation or management, or additional codes could be added for medical home activities. Further, a per-patient-per-month payment could supplement fee-for-services payments for medical home providers. Alternatively, this model favors a capitation scheme, such as a risk-adjusted comprehensive per-patient monthly payment. Drawing on lessons learned from the health maintenance organization era, capitation payments do not provide the service-level data necessary to derive utilization and quality data. However, if the medical home is able to employ health IT in a meaningful way, such concerns may be appeased.

The five pillars of PCMHs demonstrate the ways in which this model achieves or fails to achieve the Five Guiding Principles. First, data transparency is achieved at the practice level through the emphasis on health IT. A core goal for the PCMH model is to employ practice-based population health, which utilizes functionalities of information management in five domains. Practice information technology should enable providers to target subpopulations of patients, examine detailed characteristics of subpopulations, create reminders for patients and providers, track performance measures, and make data available in multiple formats, such as graphical representation.[15] Second, engaging patients in the process of shared decision making achieves the principle of allocating responsibility between the patient and provider in a meaningful way. Third, coordinated care is one of the five pillars of PCMHs and particularly emphasizes transition processes among care settings, such as discharge from the hospital. Fourth, the production of evidence-based decision-making aids for patients necessarily implicates the dissemination of evidence-based processes and best practices. Last, the PCMH allows for a variety of delivery of care models such as alternative methods of communication, including email and telephone care, electronic access to personal medical records, and an enhanced experience when the patients visit the provider in person. At the practice level, the PCMH model achieves the Five Guiding Principles to incorporate all stakeholder objectives. However, this model fails to emphasize data sharing and the dissemination of information in a meaningful way beyond the patient's immediate caregivers. This model can be improved on by an emphasis on sharing the quality improvement studies and policy research discussed above as opportunities for patient engagement.

RECOGNIZING OPPORTUNITIES FOR HYBRID MODELS

None of the above-described models are necessarily exclusive of another. The current model stresses uniformity, without recognizing important geographic, demographic, and structural differences among care settings and patient populations. Certain adaptations are made for rural versus urban settings or among providers of different payer mixes, such as critical access hospitals. However, these accommodations confine these providers mainly to the traditional delivery of care models and instead provide supplemental financial support rather than allowing for an infrastructure change to better adapt to that particular patient population's needs or environments. Because patients and environments are not uniform, reimbursement mechanisms do not have to be standardized. Inadequate mechanisms in favor of ease of administration have already proven insufficient. Instead, reform should evaluate the experiences of pilot programs and determine in which setting and where each is appropriate. Further, there may be instances in which a hybrid model is more appropriate because of specific clinical or infrastructure variances.

Consolidating Stakeholders: The Emerging Trend of Payer–Provider Entities

The role of the payer in the PCMH is passive, and initiatives for active involvement could interfere with the clinical decision making of providers and patients. For example, the reigning insurance product model could restrict the shared decision-making process when patients choose a provider or course of treatment outside the scope of coverage, implicating a higher out-of-pocket cost. Alternatively, the PCMH model may be an excellent structure in instances where the payer is financially responsible for the providers, such as with Highmark's ownership of West Penn Allegheny Health System in Pittsburgh, Pennsylvania.[16] Where the provider is part of the payer organization, the provider's decisions regarding care may be given more weight than those of an external provider; yet, the risk of payer interference with clinical decision making is still prevalent if the payer's aim is not consistent with the Five Guiding Principles to produce cost-effective, quality care. Notably, this type of infrastructure could be particularly effective in rural settings, where the number of providers is limited and there is generally limited competition among payers for the finite beneficiary population.

Combining Payment Mechanisms: Enhancing Capitation with Incentive Payments

One limitation on the bundled payment model is that the diagnosis dictates the payment rather than the patient dictates the payment, thus the payment is best suited for conditions with a defined timeframe from diagnosis to recovery. To the end, the payment assumes that the patient's condition upon presentation to the hospital can be viewed and treated in isolation, when more commonly patients present with manifestations of several untreated or mismanaged comorbidities. A relevant example of how episode-of-care reimbursement fails to recognize the related but distinct nature of diseases can be found in persuasive criticism of the new, final three-day DRG rule—requiring the bundling of preadmission diagnostic and nondiagnostic services "clinically related" to the hospital admission. Critics posture that if a patient received outpatient treatments for depression, a comorbidity, within the three-day window of a leg amputation because of diabetes, those services could be viewed as clinically related; yet each diagnosis and treatment is distinct.[17] Though extreme, that example illustrates the reasons patients and conditions cannot be viewed in isolation. This also raises patient safety concerns because there is a substantial risk that the patient is rendered a constant rather than a variable in this equation.

The bundled payment also presumes perfect diagnosis on the part of providers, precluding flexibility for the differential diagnosis process and requiring a level of diagnostic precision that may not exist for all conditions. The pressure on providers to reduce unnecessary utilization under this model also risks deterring providers from administering necessary care. The current system is criticized for fostering defensive medicine, but the bundled payment forces the provider to choose between economic gain and liability mitigation because the assignment of responsibility is difficult in some instances. For example, a hip replacement has more predictable care assignments than a heart attack, thus the delineation of responsibility for the heart attack may be confusing and infeasible with a bundled payment.[7] Accordingly, the bundled payment incentivizes adverse selection.

To address these concerns, the bundled payment can be coupled with performance incentives, much like the Geisinger Health System's ProvenCare program. The revolutionary program initially offered coronary artery bypass surgery for a flat fee, including all related charges for 90 days after discharge, nicknamed the "90-day warranty."[18] The surgeries are governed by 40 specific clinical measures, which require surgeons to "explicitly assure the surgery is appropriate, document a shared decision-making process with the patient, and initiate postdischarge follow-up to assure compliance with medication and rehabilitation recommendations."[19] After the first year, Geisinger experienced a 10% reduction in readmissions, shorter average length of stay, and reduced hospital charges.[19] Eighteen months later, readmissions decreased 44%. This particular hybrid of payment mechanisms is best suited for a provider that is already clinically integrated, with the infrastructure to support systemwide processes. A stand-alone hospital and individual physician groups will likely not have the infrastructure, such as compatible electronic health records, to manage patients' treatment to this level of particularity.

Alternatively, a global payment in lieu of a bundled payment could be coupled with performance measures to address some of the patient-centered concerns about bundled payments. A global payment is a capitation mechanism paid per enrollee for a defined scope of services irrespective of care provided. One such example of this hybrid is the alternative quality contract (AQC) implemented by Blue Cross Blue Shield Massachusetts. Medical groups in the program agree to manage spending for designated beneficiaries in return for a risk-adjusted global budget.[20] The participating medical groups range in size, specialty, and experience with the capitation model. The program was launched in 2009 but has since expanded to 12 medical groups, accounting for 11 % of Massachusetts's insured population.[20]

The five strategies employed by AQC participants to implement and maximize the benefits of the program closely align to the Five Guiding Principles. First, improving quality scores enables primary care physicians to increase compensation by 50 % above the existing Blue Cross fee schedule.[20] The medical group determines how quality bonuses are allocated, which can create flexibility in the delivery of care by providing payment from the bonuses for traditionally uncompensated services. Second, changing referral patterns to less expensive sites of care is a strategy that allows medical practices to coordinate care by monitoring where patients are receiving care and evaluating whether a different setting is more appropriate. Third, coordinating care for high-risk enrollees is mainly patient-safety driven, focused on case management to avoid hospital admissions, readmissions, and emergency department visits.[20] Fourth, linking physician compensation to performance is a mechanism for holding practice members accountable, but thus far such linkage has not been established because incentive payments were necessary for capital investments in the infrastructure to administer the program. Last, redesigning care processes for delivery system reform directly speaks to flexibility in this area, as well as to coordination of care. Most of the practices do not have the infrastructure to implement reform in a meaningful way, but a favored possibility is the medical home model.[20]

Based on the experiences of these medical groups in Massachusetts, the enhanced global payment model is best suited for the managed care setting, where the payer has a greater degree of control over how and where beneficiaries receive care. Currently the AQC applies only to members of HMOs who are required to select a primary care provider, through whom the beneficiary can obtain referrals for specialty care. The AQC requires the provider to share in 50 to 100 % of the financial risk for meeting budget targets. However, the fact that the incentive payments have allowed the medical practices to improve the infrastructure during the program indicates that the AQC model may be feasible for a broad array of providers.

CONCLUSION

There are benefits and drawbacks to all reimbursement mechanisms. However, the effectiveness of any model at recognizing value and quality in the healthcare system is whether all stakeholders have been represented in developing the model. Clear objectives, such as the Five Guiding Principles set forth herein, are critical to ensuring that the underlying goal is not compromised. Patient safety should never be sacrificed for financial gain, but quality medical services cannot be rendered without significant financial investment. This paradox does not preclude one in favor of the other because reimbursement can address both.

Furthermore, reimbursement reform is not necessarily onefold. Hybrid models can recognize variances in care settings and patient needs. Effectively, fragmentation of care is exchanged for fragmentation of payment, but if lives are saved, providers offer quality in addition to care, and payers contain costs, then all stakeholders should agree it is worth the administrative burden. In summary, reimbursement reform may the solution to solving the U.S. healthcare problem, but this equation has more than one correct answer.

References

1. Institute of Medicine. (2001). *Crossing the quality chasm: A new health system for the 21st century*. Washington, DC: National Academies Press. Retrieved from http://www.nap.edu/catalog.php?record_id=10027.
2. Himmelstein, D. U., Thorne, D., Warren, E., & Woolhandler, S. (2009). Medical bankruptcy in the United States, 2007: Results of a national study. *American Journal of Medicine, 122*(8), 741–746. Retrieved from http://www.pnhp.org/new_bankruptcy_study/Bankruptcy-2009.pdf.
3. Sanchez, C. (Producer). (2010, March 9). *Cost of medical school rises in recession* [Audio podcast]. Retrieved from http://www.npr.org/templates/story/story.php?storyId=124501284.
4. Lesser, C. S., Fineberg, H. V., & Cassel, C. K. (2010). Physician payment reform: Principles that should shape it. *Health Affairs, 29*(5), 948–952.
5. Petersen, L. A., Woodard, L. D., Urech, T., Daw, C., & Sookanan, S. (2006). Does pay-for-performance improve the quality of health care? *Annals of Internal Medicine, 145*(4), 265–272.
6. For more information, see Centers for Medicare & Medicaid Innovation Center, *Bundled payments for care improvement initiative frequently asked questions*. (2011). Retrieved from http://innovations.cms.gov/Files/x/BundledPaymentsFAQ_2_29_12.pdf.
7. American Hospital Association. (2010, May). *Bundled payment: An AHA research synthesis report*. Retrieved from http://www.aha.org/research/cor/bundled-payment/index.shtml.
8. U.S. Department of Health and Human Services, Agency for Healthcare Research and Quality. *Theory and reality of value-based purchasing: Lessons from the pioneers*. Retrieved from http://www.ahrq.gov/qual/meyerrpt.htm.
9. BusinessWire.com. (2011, November 8). *Nation's largest hospital value-based purchasing demonstration achieves continued improvements in quality and patient outcomes*. Retrieved from http://www.businesswire.com/news/home/20111108005935/en/Nation's-Largest-Hospital-Value-Based-Purchasing-Demonstration-Achieves.
10. Centers for Medicare & Medicaid Services: Medicare Program; Hospital Inpatient Value-Based Purchasing Program, 76 Fed. Reg. 26490 (to be codified at 42 C.F.R. pts. 422 & 480).
11. U.S. Department of Health and Human Services. *Hospital compare*. Retrieved from http://www.hospitalcompare.hhs.gov/.
12. Centers for Medicare & Medicaid Services. *Physician compare initiative*. Retrieved from https://www.cms.gov/Medicare/Quality-Initiatives-Patient-Assessment-Instruments/physician-compare-initiative/index.html.
13. U.S. Department of Health and Human Services, Agency for Healthcare Research and Quality. (2011, February). *The patient-centered medical home: Strategies to put patients at the center of primary care*. Retrieved from http://pcmh.ahrq.gov/portal/server.pt/community/pcmh__home/1483/PCMH_Home_Papers%20Briefs%20and%20Othe%20Resources_v2 (link to downloadable PDF); and *Defining the PCMH*. Retrieved from http://pcmh.ahrq.gov/portal/server.pt/community/pcmh__home/1483/pcmh_defining_the_pcmh_v2.
14. Merrell, K., & Berenson, R. A. (2010). Structuring payment for medical homes. *Health Affairs, 29*(5), 852–858.
15. U.S. Department of Health and Human Services, Agency for Healthcare Research and Quality. (2010). *Practice-based population health: Information technology to support transformation to proactive primary care*. Retrieved

from http://pcmh.ahrq.gov/portal/server.pt/community/pcmh__home/1483/PCMH_Tools%20&%20Resources_Foundations_Health%20IT_v2.

16. Highmark's acquisition of West Penn Allegheny Health System, Insurance Department hone in. (April 20, 2012). Pittsburgh Business Times. Retrieved from http://www.bizjournals.com/pittsburgh/print-edition/2012/04/20/highmarks-acquisition-wpahs-insurance.html?page=all.
17. Foley & Lardner. (2011, November 15). *The "3-day DRG payment window."* Retrieved from http://www.foley.com/intelligence/detail.aspx?int=7769.
18. Abelson, R. (2007, May 17). In bid for better care, surgery with a warranty. *The New York Times*. Retrieved from http://www.nytimes.com/2007/05/17/business/17quality.html.
19. Mechanic, R. E., & Altman, S. H. (2009). Payment reform options: Episode payment is a good place to start. *Health Affairs, 28*(2), W262–W271.
20. Mechanic, R. E., Santos, P., Landon, B. E., & Chernew, M. E. (2011). Medical group response to global payment: Early lessons from the "alternative quality contract" in Massachusetts. *Health Affairs, 30*(9), 1734–1742.
21. Landro, L. (2010, November 21). Health care: Change the incentives. *The Wall Street Journal* CEO Council Report. Interview with healthcare cochairs Angela Braly of WellPoint Inc., William A. Hawkins of Medtronic Inc., and Klaus Kleinfeld of Alcoa. Retrieved from http://online.wsj.com/article/SB10001424052748703688704575620850148494216.html.

INDEX

Numbers

A

B

M

Q

R

T